Other monographs in the series, *Major Problems in Clinical Surgery:*

Child: *The Liver and Portal Hypertension*

Welch: *Polypoid Lesions of the Gastrointestinal Tract*

Madding and Kennedy: *Trauma to the Liver*

Spratt and Donegan: *Cancer of the Breast*

Haller: *Deep Thrombophlebitis*

Colcock and Braasch: *Surgery of the Small Intestine in the Adult*

Jackman and Beahrs: *Tumor of the Large Bowel*

Ellis and Olsen: *Achalasia of the Esophagus*

Botsford and Wilson: *The Acute Abdomen*

Colcock: *Diverticulitis*

Spratt, Butcher and Bricker: *Exenterative Surgery of the Pelvis*

Shires: *Shock*

Child: *Portal Hypertension*

PERIPHERAL ARTERIAL DISEASE

Second Edition

by

Wiley F. Barker, M.D.

Professor of Surgery,
University of California,
Los Angeles, School of Medicine

Volume IV in the Series
MAJOR PROBLEMS IN CLINICAL SURGERY

J. ENGLEBERT DUNPHY, M.D

PAUL A. EBERT, M.D.
Consulting Editors

W. B. SAUNDERS COMPANY, PHILADELPHIA, LONDON, TORONTO, 1975

W. B. Saunders Company: West Washington Square
Philadelphia, PA 19105

12 Dyott Street
London, WC1A   1DB

833 Oxford Street
Toronto, Ontario M8Z 5T9, Canada

Library of Congress Cataloging in Publication Data

Barker, Wiley F

Peripheral arterial disease.

(Major problems clinical surgery; v. 4)

Includes bibliographies and index.

1. Arteries — Surgery.   2. Arteries — Diseases.   I. Title.
  [DNLM: 1. Arteries — Surgery.   2. Vascular diseases.
  W1 MA492R v. 4 / WG510 B155p]

RD598.B35 1975   616.1'31   72–78954

ISBN 0–7216–1546–5

Peripheral Arterial Disease   ISBN   0-7216-1546-5

Last digit is the print number: 9   8   7   6   5   4   3   2   1

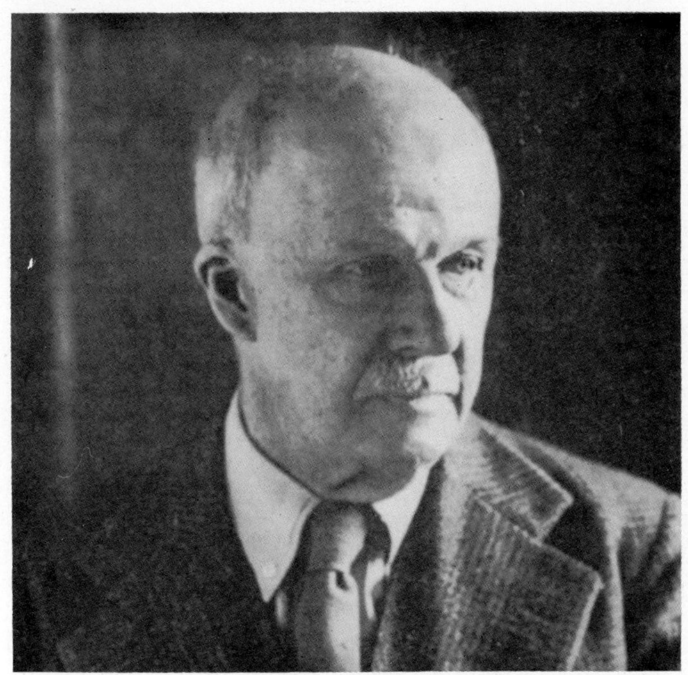

JOHN HOMANS, M.D.
*(Harvard Medical
Alumni Association)*

To the memory of
JOHN HOMANS, M.D.
1877–1954

Among the many physicians whose names have become bywords in the explosive growth of medicine and medical science John Homans stands in a special position. To those who knew him least, his is the eponymic sign of pain on dorsiflexion in the presence of deep venous thrombosis, so often misstated as Homan's sign. Osler's aphorism that a man is often known best to the world by that work which he considers his least is attested by Dr. Homans' own appraisal of this sign, expressed with typical frankness, "If you wanted to name a sign after me, why didn't you pick a good one?"

To many classes of students in Boston he was a sparkling, unpredictable, and colorful teacher and author. He was above all a clinician and a teacher of clinical surgery, and his two great textbooks *Circulatory Diseases of the Extremities* and *A Textbook of Surgery* bear clear witness to his ability to perceive basic principles and communicate them as integrated concepts to his students.

To many others he was all this as well as a tempestuous, fiery, outspoken, at times charming, at times frightening, but always stimulating mentor of clinical surgery. His barbed and keenly observant criticisms often struck with painful accuracy but their sting was always relieved by a witty and gracious dressing such that no permanent scar was left, but the goal of teaching was achieved. Such salty and irrepressible wit of course left in its wake tales galore, many apocryphal, many unrepeatable, and all told in affectionate memory. These stories share a common pattern of humor, humility, and quizzical self-appraisal. Painful honesty mixes with the quixotic support of the underdog and with thrusts at pretense and show of any kind.

It is impossible to list here all his accomplishments; many not detailed below will be met as concepts in the body of the present book. Such concepts can be recognized in the accomplishment of those in vascular surgery who worked with him. The choice of the preposition "with" is not accidental — one always had the feeling of being a partner and sharing fully in any problem with him.

The roll of names who were associated with him is a veritable honor roll in vascular surgery: Cutler, Beck, Elkin, Hufnagel, Harken, Starling, Holman, Leriche, Gross, Fontaine, Ross, Fulton, and Warren. The list goes on and on, and includes a great majority of the senior members of the Society for Vascular Surgery, who have recognized Homans' contributions by establishing a lectureship in his name.

John Homans was born in Boston. His early education at Harvard College and Harvard Medical School and his term as House Pupil in Surgery at the Massachusetts General Hospital and as Assistant to Maurice H. Richardson was an appropriate beginning for a good Bostonian. Early intimations of a pioneering and uninhibited spirit were promptly manifested by his further training in Baltimore, in London, and in New Haven before his return to Boston to participate with David Cheever under Harvey Cushing in the development of the new Peter Bent Brigham Hospital.

John Homans left an impression on the periodical literature smaller in numbers than many of his associates; almost half of his publications dealt with some form of vascular disease. His first published paper concerned the pathology and histology of the mitral and aortic valves. His later conceptual and technical contributions to the careful dissection of the region of the saphenofemoral junction, the treatment of the varicose long saphenous vein by stripping it from the thigh, and the physiologic origins of the postphlebitic syndrome in disease of the communicating veins remain as landmarks. He was the first to undertake portacaval shunt on the human in this country. His recognition of the role of the interruption of the femoral veins in the prevention of pulmonary embolism and his early espousal of lumbar sympathectomy in the treatment of peripheral occlusive disease merely add to the list of the many areas of surgery that will always bear his imprint.

Without John Homans the field of vascular surgery would undoubtedly have developed much as it has today, but it could never have been quite the same. I am certain that the many associates of John Homans, great and small alike, support my wish to dedicate this book to a remarkable scholar, a keen observer, and a beloved man — Dr. John Homans, Surgeon.

WILEY F. BARKER

Los Angeles

Contributors

WILEY F. BARKER, M.D.

Professor of Surgery, University of California, Los Angeles, School of Medicine, Los Angeles, California.
Introduction; Anatomy; Physiology (With Victor E. Hall); Pathology and Pathogenesis; Diagnostic Problems; Conservative Measures, the Role of Sympathectomy; Aortoiliac Reconstruction; Femoral-Popliteal Reconstruction; Combined Aortoiliac Femoropopliteal Lesions; Results of Arterial Reconstruction for Chronic Occlusion; Arterial Trauma; Extrinsic Arterial Compression Syndromes (With J. H. Grollman, Jr.); Arterial Aneurysms; Arterial Embolisms in the Extremities; Complications of Vascular Surgery.

WILLIAM K. EHRENFELD, M.D.

Associate Professor of Surgery, University of California School of Medicine, San Francisco; University of California Medical Center, San Francisco, California.
Surgical Techniques for Hemodialysis Access

JULIUS H. GROLLMAN, JR., M.D.

Associate Professor of Radiology, University of California, Los Angeles; Chief, Adult Cardiovascular Section, University of California, Los Angeles, Center for the Health Sciences, Department of Radiological Sciences, Los Angeles, California.
Extrinsic Arterial Compression Syndromes (With Wiley F. Barker)

VICTOR E. HALL, M.D.

Emeritus Professor of Physiology, University of California, Los Angeles, School of Medicine, Los Angeles, California.
Physiology (With Wiley F. Barker)

JOSEPH J. KAUFMAN, M.D.

Professor of Surgery/Urology, Chief, Division of Urology, University of California, Los Angeles, School of Medicine; Consultant, Mt. Sinai Hospital, St. John's Hospital, Santa Monica Hospital, Veterans Administration Hospital, Los Angeles, U.S. Naval Hospital, Long Beach; Attending Urologist, Veterans Administration Hospital, Sepulveda, California.
Diseases of the Renal Vessels

JESSE E. THOMPSON, M.D.

Clinical Professor of Surgery, University of Texas Southwestern Medical School, Dallas; Attending Surgeon, Baylor University Medical Center, and Parkland Memorial Hospital, Dallas, Texas.
Cerebrovascular Insufficiency

FRANK C. SPARKS, M.D.

Assistant Professor of Surgery, Division of Oncology, University of California, Los Angeles, Medical Center; Assistant Chief, Surgical Service, Veterans Administration Hospital, Sepulveda, California.
Mesenteric Vascular Disease

Foreword

It is nearly ten years since the First Edition of this volume of Major Problems in Clinical Surgery appeared. In that edition a comment was made in the foreword that vascular surgery had "been coming of age and falling increasingly within the range of the broadly trained general surgeon." In the interval, vascular surgery has indeed come of age, to such an extent that it can no longer be considered the province of the general surgeon unless he has had substantial and extensive training in this field. Vascular surgery has undergone such a revolution and is so dependent upon precise judgments and careful technique that it is indeed to a considerable extent a specialty in its own right. That it should become a recognized subspecialty within general surgery is now the opinion of the majority of leading vascular surgeons.

This superb monograph by Dr. Barker will not make a vascular surgeon of the untrained general surgeon, but it will be welcomed by all general surgeons who have already had experience in vascular surgery, and will do much to keep them abreast of this very rapidly moving field. It will also have appeal in specialty areas where renovascular or cerebrovascular surgery is presently being performed. Most particularly, it will become the *vade mecum* of all young surgeons who plan to acquire and maintain broad experience and competence in this field. As did the previous monograph, Dr. Barker's contribution will rank among the classic references in vascular surgery for the next decade.

J. Englebert Dunphy, M.D.

Preface

The goals of this Second Edition are the same as of the First: to bring the point of view of the author and the opinions of some of his experienced colleagues into focus on common problems in the treatment of peripheral arterial disease. Particular attention has been directed to the trouble spots that are responsible for difficulties in this sphere of surgery. The First Edition encompassed a significant proportion of the bibliography on vascular disease; however, in the few years since publication of that book the literature of vascular surgery has so expanded that only a small portion of it can be included in this edition. Undoubtedly, many important contributions have been omitted. Their exclusion can be justified only because this edition is an attempt to present a book that is convenient rather than encyclopedic.

The Second Edition has been expanded to include a wide variety of arterial problems, rather than to solely concentrate on occlusive arterial disease. Particular help in this expansion was received from the contributions of Drs. William Ehrenfeld, Julius Grollman, Victor Hall, Joseph Kaufman, Frank Sparks, and Jesse Thompson. In addition, Dr. Donald Mulder made important, though untitled, contributions regarding the management of thoracic aneurysms.

Others to whom thanks are due for their special assistance include Luciano Barajas (for his special help with the work on Pathology), Jack A. Cannon, W. A. Dale, M. E. DeBakey, Edward A. Edwards, W. Sterling Edwards, J. Harold Harrison, Robert R. Linton, T. B. Massell, D. E. Szilagyi, G. W. Taylor, Richard Warren, Irving S. Wright and E. J. Wylie.

Again I want to express my particular thanks for the assistance and tolerance of Mrs. Justine Walker, Mrs. Diane Richie, and my wife, Nancy K. Barker.

Part of the work in this book was supported by U.S. Public Health Service grants HE-0793 and HE-11946, as well as by the Blalock Foundation.

Contents

Chapter One

INTRODUCTION

Clinical recognition of the true patterns of peripheral arteriosclerosis occurred late in the history of medicine. Arteriosclerosis developing in the coronary arteries, the cerebral vessels, and the smaller
peripheral branches was readily recognized because of the dramatic
sequelae that followed upon occlusion of these vessels, but it was only
in relatively recent times that study of amputation specimens led to
the recognition of both diabetic and nondiabetic arteriosclerosis and
Buerger's disease in the peripheral arteries.

Von Winiwarter[44] and Buerger[4] were the first to report on the condition that has since become known as Buerger's disease. Frequently,
the distal arteries were found to be involved in cases of nondiabetic
arteriosclerosis to the extent that gangrene developed and amputation
became necessary. Isolated proximal lesions often did not become
gangrenous, and the frequent occurrence of obstructive lesions in vessels of a size that could be corrected surgically was not appreciated
until Leriche described surgical treatment of aortoiliac disease.[30, 31]

Impetus for this form of treatment was provided by dos Santos's
development of arteriography of peripheral vessels.[11]

Embolectomy had been the first procedure to be applied with any
great frequency to the larger arteries, but the presence of advanced arteriosclerosis long limited its successful application, and palliative
sympathectomy remained the most useful procedure for many years.

Introduced by Leriche[28, 29] as periarterial sympathectomy, the
procedure was modified as paravertebral ganglionectomy by Hunter[19]
and Royle.[38] Adson and Brown[1] were the first to make wide use of

1

sympathectomy in peripheral vascular disease, and it remained the only useful treatment until the work of J. dos Santos.[10]

Although Carrel[5] had defined the principles of arterial repair in the early 1900's, this technique was rarely employed outside the surgical laboratory. Dos Santos utilized the line of cleavage between the diseased intima and the relatively normal media in the larger arteriosclerotic arteries to dissect free the obstructing atheromatous intima and its contained thrombus; the operation was termed thromboendarterectomy. This procedure did not meet with favor in the United States until publication of the reports of Wylie[46] in 1951 and Barker and Cannon[2] in 1953. Since then the procedure has gained increasing popularity and has been used in a variety of anatomical sites for the treatment of atherosclerosis.

Arterial replacement was also first undertaken by Carrel, but his work lay dormant until the early 1940's, when Hufnagel,[20, 21] Gross,[18] and Deterling[9] revived interest in it. The first arterial homografts were used by Gross in the treatment of coarctation of the aorta.[18] In 1950 Holden was the first to succeed with replacement of the femoral artery by a venous graft, using the autologous superficial femoral vein as a reversed end-to-end graft,[19] and Julian and his associates[24] also used venous grafts during this period. Kunlin[26, 27] in France and Linton[32, 33] in the United States applied the principle of end-to-side anastomosis to bypass arterial obstructions. Venous and arterial homografts and prostheses were commonly used. The popularity of arterial homografts waxed,[9] then rapidly waned as Szilagyi[42] and others reported marked degeneration in the transplanted segment.

The introduction and subsequent popularity of fabric prostheses followed upon an observation by Voorhees that a loose thread within the lumen of the auricle became covered with endothelium.[45] Ivalon, nylon, Orlon, Dacron, and Teflon prostheses have since been introduced.[7, 13, 20, 21, 38] Knitted or woven Dacron remains the most popular and effective fabric, but its limitations indicate that there is still need for improvement in fabric prostheses.

Although the widest experience has been in the treatment of atherosclerosis of the aorta and of the iliac and femoral arteries, disease in other areas has been successfully treated by use of combinations of the techniques just described. Freeman[14] was among the first to report the successful removal of a renal arterial atheroma. The bifurcation of the carotid artery soon came to be recognized as a major and correctable cause of strokes, and Eastcott,[12] DeBakey,[8] and Cooley[6] were among the first to attempt carotid reconstruction. Klass,[25] Shaw,[39] and Mikklesen[35] had successfully treated mesenteric vascular occlusions, but such occlusions occur far less frequently than those in other sites. Longmire performed endarterectomy successfully in the coronary arteries in 1958.[34] Endarterectomy of the coronary arterial tree has been superseded, however, by bypass procedures which most commonly use the saphenous vein to reach from the root of the aorta to one or even three distal coronary arteries. This operation has become in some centers one of the most commonly performed cardiac operations.[14, 16]

The only other pathological processes causing arterial obstruction in arteries large enought to permit surgery are the lesions grouped together loosely as "fibromuscular hyperplasia," which affects the renal arteries.[36, 37] A similar process has been seen only infrequently in the internal carotid and mesenteric arteries, and possibly in the femoral arteries.[3]

In the last five years Tyson[43] and Garrett[17] have extended the distal limits of bypass procedures to the tibial vessels even at a distal level, although this type of reconstruction is not fully accepted.

The experiences of vascular surgeons in Vietnam have greatly expanded the interest in the reconstruction of the acutely injured artery.

The lesions of Buerger's disease, or thromboangiitis obliterans, develop primarily in the small peripheral vessels and are not suitable for direct surgical attack. Many misconceptions have arisen concerning Buerger's disease, and many authors doubt its existence as a pathological entity; nevertheless it is of clinical concern, regardless of its pathological "pedigree." Much of the importance of Buerger's disease derives from use of the term to describe — incorrectly — *any* occlusive disease of the arterial tree, without verification of the presence of correctable lesions.

The most severe arterial occlusions commonly associated with diabetes mellitus develop in the smaller vessels and are thus not amenable to arterial reconstruction. Operable lesions are seen in the major arteries of diabetics, but not more frequently than in the non-diabetic population, and many of these lesions are rendered inoperable because of the multiplicity and the diffuse nature of advanced associated peripheral lesions.

The techniques of reconstructive surgery for occlusive disease have, during the period of development, become applicable with high degree of success to aneurysmal disease. The treatment of aneurysms, however, includes almost of necessity the use of materials to replace the diseased artery. Familiarity with such replacement materials and the techniques of their use has increased the popularity of bypass techniques at the expense of the popularity of thromboendarterectomy.

The only major areas of importance to the vascular surgeon that will not be included in subsequent chapters are those related primarily to the coronary arteries. The scope of this volume will therefore be considerably greater than that of the initial volume on peripheral arterial surgery in this series.

REFERENCES

1. Adson, W. A., and Brown, G. E.: Treatment of Raynaud's disease by lumbar ramisection and ganglionectomy and perivascular sympathetic neurectomy of the common iliacs. J.A.M.A. *84*:1908, 1925.
2. Barker, W. F., and Cannon, J. A.: An evaluation of endarterectomy. Arch. Surg. *66*:488, 1953.
3. Barker, W. F.: Unpublished data.
4. Buerger, L.: Thromboangiitis obliterans: a study of the vascular lesions leading to presenile spontaneous gangrene. Am. J. Med. Sci. *136*:567, 1908.
5. Carrel, A.: Technique and remote results of vascular anastomoses. Surg. Gynec. Obstet. *14*:246, 1912.
6. Cooley, D. A., Al-Naaman, Y. D., and Carton, C. A.: Surgical treatment of arteriosclerotic occlusion of common carotid artery. J. Neurosurg. *13*:500, 1956.
7. DeBakey, M. E., Cooley, D. A., Crawford, E. S., and Morris, G. C., Jr.: Clinical application of a new flexible knitted Dacron arterial substitute. Arch. Surg. *77*:713, 1958.
8. DeBakey, M. E., Crawford, E. S., Cooley, D. A., and Morris, G. C., Jr.: Surgical considerations of occlusive disease of innominate, carotid, subclavian and vertebral arteries. Ann. Surg. *149*:690, 1959.
9. Deterling, R. A., Jr., Coleman, C. C., Jr., and Parshley, M. S.: Experimental studies of the frozen homologous aortic graft. Surgery *29*:419, 1951.
10. dos Santos, J.: Sur la désobstruction des thromboses artérielles anciennes. Mém. Acad. Chir. *73*:409, 1947.
11. dos Santos, R., Lamas, A., and Caldas, P.: L'artériographie des membres, de l'aorte et de ses branches abdominales. Bull. Mém. Soc. Nat. Chir. *55*:587, 1929.
12. Eastcott, H. H. G., Pickering, G. W., Rob, C. G.: Reconstruction of internal carotid artery in a patient with intermittent attacks of hemiplegia. Lancet *2*:994, 1954.
13. Edwards, W. S., and Tapp, J. S.: Chemically treated nylon tubes as arterial grafts. Surgery *38*:61, 1955.
14. Favoloro, R. G.: Saphenous vein autograft replacement of severe segmental coronary artery occlusion. Ann. Thoracic Surg. *5*:334, 1968.
15. Freeman, N. E., Leeds, F. H., Elliott, W. G., and Roland, S. I.: Thromboendarterectomy for hypertension due to renal artery occlusion. J.A.M.A. *156*:1077, 1954.
16. Garrett, H. E., Kinard, S. A., and Dennis, E.: Personal communication cited by Morris, G. C., Jr., Howell, J. F., Crawford, E. S., Reul, G. J., Chapman, D. W., Beazley, H. L., Winters, W. L., and Peterson, P. K.: The distal coronary bypass. Ann. Surg. *172*:652, 1970.
17. Garrett, H. E., Kotch, P. I., Green, M. T., Jr., Diethrich, E. B., and DeBakey, M. E.: Distal tibial artery bypass with autogenous vein grafts: An analysis of 56 cases. Surgery *63*:90, 1968.
18. Gross, R. E., Bill, A. H., Jr., and Peirce, E. C., II: Methods for preservation and transplantation of arterial grafts. Surg. Gynec. Obstet. *88*:689, 1949.
19. Holden, W.: Reconstruction of femoral artery for arteriosclerotic thrombosis. Surgery *27*:417, 1950.
20. Hufnagel, C. A.: Resection and grafting of the thoracic aorta with minimal interruption of the circulation. Presented at Forum on Fundamental Surgical Problems, American College of Surgeons, Los Angeles, 1948.
21. Hufnagel, C. A., and Rabil, P.: Replacement of arterial segments, utilizing flexible orlon prostheses. Arch. Surg. *70*:105, 1955.
22. Hunter, J. I.: The influence of the sympathetic nervous system in the genesis of ridigity of striated muscle in spastic paralysis. Surg. Gynec. Obstet. *39*:721, 1924.
23. Julian, O. C., Deterling, R. A., Jr., Su, H. H., Dye, W. S., and Belio, M. L.: Dacron tube and bifurcation arterial prostheses produced to specification. Surgery *41*:50, 1957.
24. Julian, O. C., Dye, W. S., Jr., Olwin, J. H., and Jordan, P. H.: Direct surgery of arteriosclerosis. Ann. Surg. *136*:459, 1952.

25. Klass, A. A.: Acute mesenteric arterial occlusion: restoration of blood flow by embolectomy. J. Internat. Coll. Surg. *20*:687, 1953.
26. Kunlin, J.: Le traitement de l'ischémie artéritique par la greffe veineuse longue. Rev. Chir. Paris *70*:206, 1951.
27. Kunlin, J.: El problema del injerto vascular en la arteritis de los miembros. Angiologia *10*:1, 1958.
28. Leriche, R.: De la causalgie envisagée comme une névrite du sympathetique et son staitement par la dénudation et l'escision des plexus nerveux periarterials. Presse Méd. *24*:178, 1916.
29. Leriche, R.: Surgery of the sympathetic system; indications and results. Ann. Surg. *88*:449, 1928.
30. Leriche, R.: De la résection du carrefour aorticoiliaque avec double sympathectomie lombaire pour thrombose artéritique de l'aorte; le syndrome de l'oblitération termino-aortique par artérite. Presse Méd. *48*:601, 1940.
31. Leriche, R., and Morel, A.: Syndrome of thrombotic obliteration of aortic bifurcation. Ann. Surg. *127*:193, 1948.
32. Linton, R. R.: Some practical considerations in the surgery of blood vessel grafts. Surgery *38*:817, 1955.
33. Linton, R. R., and Menendez, C. V.: Arterial homografts: a comparison of the results with end-to-end and end-to-side vascular anastomoses. Ann. Surg. *142*:568, 1955.
34. Longmire, W. P., Jr., Cannon, J. A., and Kattus, A. A.: Direct-vision coronary endarterectomy for angina pectoris. New Eng. J. Med. *259*:993, 1958.
35. Mikklesen, W. R.: Intestinal angina: its surgical significance. Am. J. Surg. *94*:262, 1957.
36. Poutasse, E. F.: Occlusion of a renal artery as a cause of hypertension. Circulation *13*:37, 1956.
37. Poutasse, E. F., and Dustan, H.: Arteriosclerosis and renal hypertension. J.A.M.A. *165*:1521, 1957.
38. Royle, N. D.: A new operative procedure in the treatment of spastic paralysis and its experimental basis. Med. J. Australia *1*:77, 1924.
39. Shaw, R. S., and Maynard, E. P., III: Acute and chronic thrombosis of mesenteric arteries associated with malabsorption: report of two cases successfully treated by thromboendarterectomy. New Eng. J. Med. *258*:874, 1958.
40. Shumacker, H. B., Jr., and King, H.: The use of pliable plastic tubes as aortic substitutes in man. Surg. Gynec. Obstet. *99*:287, 1954.
41. Szilagyi, D. E., France, L. C., Smith, R. F., and Whitcomb, J. G.: The clinical use of an elastic dacron prosthesis. Arch. Surg. *77*:538, 1958.
42. Szilagyi, D. E., McDonald, R. T., Smith, R. F., and Whitcomb, J. G.: A study of the biologic fate of human arterial homografts. Arch. Surg. *75*:506, 1957.
43. Tyson, R. R., and DeLaurentis, D.: Femorotibial bypass. Circulation *33*:183, 1966.
44. von Winiwarter, F.: Ueber eine eigenthumliche Form von Endarteriitis und Endophlebitis mit Gangrän des Fusses. Arch. Klin. Chir. *23*:202, 1879.
45. Voorhees, A. B., Jr., Jaretzki, A., III, and Blakemore, A. H.: The use of tubes constructed from vinyon "N" cloth in bridging arterial defects; preliminary report. Ann. Surg. *135*:332, 1952.
46. Wylie, E., Kerr, E., and Davies, O.: Experimental and clinical experiences with use of fascia lata applied as a graft about major arteries after thromboendarterectomy and aneurysmorrhaphy. Surg. Gynec. Obstet. *93*:257, 1951.

Chapter Two

ANATOMY

The major part of the arterial system to be considered in this book includes the major branches of the aorta and their peripheral continuations as the femoral, popliteal, tibial, subclavian, carotid, and brachial arteries. The basic structure of this arterial tree is shown in Figures 2–1 and 2–2. There are many variations in man and these will be discussed in subsequent pages.

The special anatomical problems of carotid and subclavian vertebral systems will be discussed in later chapters, and the special details of anatomical importance in these areas will be described in relation to the clinical situation.

THORACIC AORTA AND ITS BRANCHES

The transverse aortic arch gives rise to the major arterial branches to the head and neck and upper extremities. The classical pattern is shown in Figure 2–1.

Considerable variation may exist in the patterns of origin of the great vessels from the arch. All vessels may arise separately or there may be two common brachiocephalic trunks. The anomalous origin of the right subclavian artery from the distal posterior portion of the arch is a developmental anomaly related to persistence of the primitive right dorsal aorta and obliteration of the fourth right primitive aortic arch. As a rule, the right subclavian artery develops from the primitive right aortic arch.

6

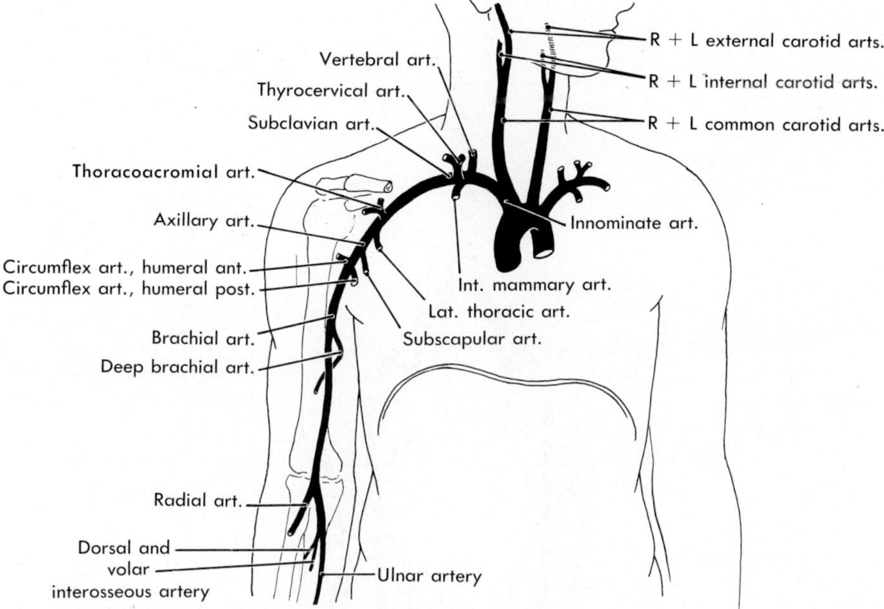

Figure 2–1.   Schema of the aortic arch, innominate subclavian and carotid vessels, and continuation of the subclavian and axillary vessels and the important branches.

The vertebral arteries are usually equal in size and join to form a single basilar artery. Marked differences in size may exist, however, on a developmental basis. Similar changes may be acquired because of atherosclerotic stenosis at the origin of the artery. Unilateral deficiency should be of little consequence to vertebral flow, however, except in those very rare circumstances in which the vertebral arteries join the circle of Willis separately and never form a true basilar artery. The details of the anatomy of the carotid bifurcation and the circle of Willis are discussed in Chapter Eleven.

Thoracic Outlet

As Edwards[3] has shown, the relative caudad movement of the shoulder girdle and heart in man causes the subclavian vessels to pass up and over the first rib. In this exposed position both the subclavian artery and vein are subjected to extrinsic pressures by the first rib (or a last cervical rib), by the anterior scalene muscle, by the clavicle, by the coracoid process or even by the head of the humerus itself, depending upon the posture of the moment. The scalenus anticus, or cervical rib, syndrome often includes neurological symptoms caused by the pressures on the lower roots of the brachial plexus. The four

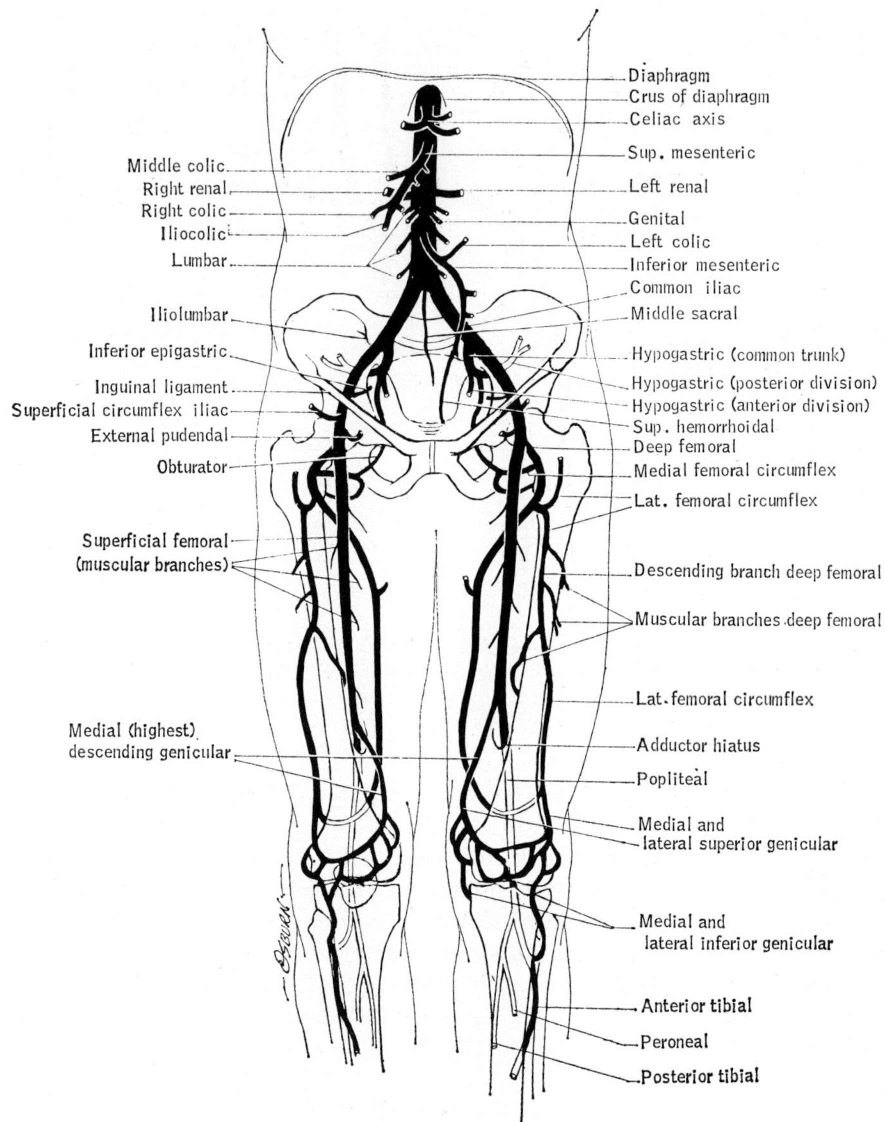

Figure 2–2.   Overall scheme of abdominal aorta, the iliac, femoral, and popliteal arteries, and the important branches of these vessels.

major points at which musculoskeletal structures can impinge on the neurovascular units are outlined in Figure 2–3.

Clagett,[2] Falconer[5] and Roos[16] have championed the concept that the first rib is the common denominator in all of the syndromes of thoracic outlet obstruction and have therefore advocated its removal for the relief of these obstructions.

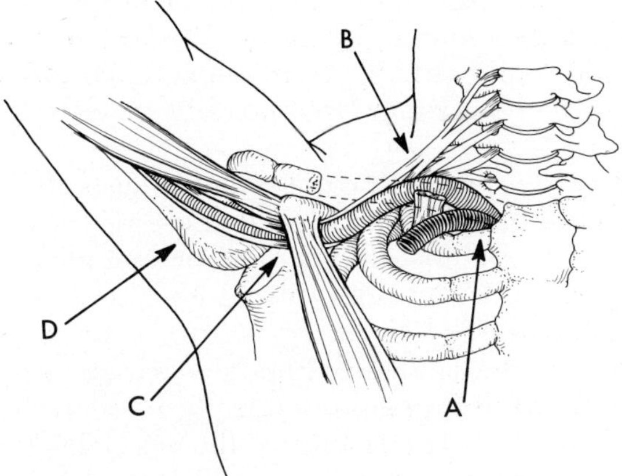

Figure 2–3. Anatomy of the structures of the right thoracic outlet showing the important points of extrinsic anatomical impression upon the subclavian and axillary artery and vein, and the brachial plexus.

The radiologic diagnosis of the thoracic outlet obstruction, as well as that of the other commonly encountered entrapment syndromes, will be discussed in greater detail along with their management in Chapter Fifteen.

ABDOMINAL AORTA

The aorta enters the abdominal cavity to the left of the midline through the diaphragm and within a distance of a few centimeters gives off its major visceral branches, the celiac axis, the superior mesenteric artery, and the paired renal arteries. The smaller inferior mesenteric artery is given off somewhat below the other visceral branches.

The abdominal aorta is reduced considerably in size by its contribution to the major visceral branches. The distal portion, or terminal aorta, is normally cylindrical; it curves forward somewhat convexly, returns almost to the midline, and terminates at the origin of the common iliac arteries over the lower third of the fourth lumbar vertebral body.

Lumbar Branches

Paired lumbar arteries are usually found in relationship to each vertebral segment. In the lower aorta, they usually arise near the midline; they may arise as a midline trunk with immediate lateral branches. The size of these lumbar branches depends on the physiological need for them; thus, in obstructions of the terminal aorta they may serve as the major sources of arterial supply refilling the internal and external iliac trunks (Fig. 2–4). In aneurysmal disease of the terminal aorta, however, they may become obliterated at the level of the aortic wall.

The spinal cord is among the important areas of the body partially supplied by arterial blood from the lumbar arteries. Detailed descriptions of the blood supply by Suh,[18] and other anatomists cited by him, indicate that the major blood supply of the cord is through the anterior longitudinal spinal artery. This artery in turn is fed by small arteries that course along the nerve roots; although each root carries an artery, only about one fourth (or a total of eight) of these arteries are of sufficient size to contribute significantly to the arterial supply. There are usually one or two lumbar branches, one lower thoracic, one mid-thoracic or none, one or two upper thoracic, one or two lower cervical, and one upper cervical. These arteries are about 0.87 mm. in diameter. The largest one, *arteria radicularis magna*, is in the lower thoracic or lumbar area. This is a single nonsymmetric branch, occurring 78 per cent of the time on the left side only. The artery may arise anywhere between T7 and L3, but its most common origin is from T2. Arterial anastomoses with other large branches within the cord are infrequent, hence injury to this somewhat unpredictable branch

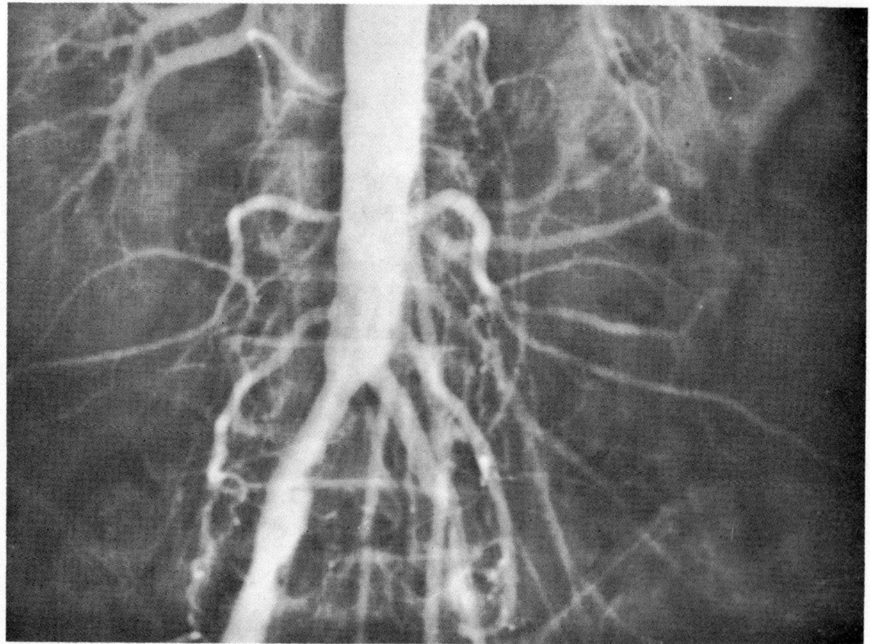

Figure 2–4. Arteriogram of extensively atherosclerotic aorta, showing large lumbar collaterals on the right.

may cause serious neurological deficit, based on injury to the cord itself. Other neurological deficits may arise from devascularization and infarction caused by injury to the much less clearly defined arterial branches supplying the nerves. In the case reported by Usabiaga, Kolodny, and Usabiaga,[20] the injury took the form of infarction of the psoas muscle and of the lumbosacral plexus and sciatic nerve.

The functional importance of this radicular branch in the vulnerability of the spinal cord to damage by aortography is also suggested by the work of Tanon,[19] who found that injection into the lumbar arteries would fill the entire arterial tree of the cord. In the thoracic cord above the level of the ninth segment, local arterial injections spread into small areas of the cord only. In the cervical segments, the area fed by each artery is slightly larger.

In studying the relationship of the ostia of the lumbar arteries, Laufman[10] found that it was safer to inject the midportion of the lumbar body than the midpoint of the intervertebral discs. In any given segment, the ostia were 3 to 12 mm. apart. In about 6 per cent of the specimens, there was a single ostium from which the paired lumbar branches arose.

Laufman concluded that from an anatomical point of view, the safest area for aorta puncture *below* the renal arteries was the level of the midportion of the second lumbar vertebra, and the safest position *above* the renal arteries was at the lower third of the twelfth thoracic vertebra.

The vessels of the dorsal root and the remaining radicular branches are insignificant.

Physiological aspects of spinal cord injury during aortography are discussed in Chapters Five and Nineteen.

There are no means available during surgery for determining the importance of any pair of lumbar arteries. In general, care must be taken to interrupt flow only to those lumbar arteries that are absolutely essential for mobilization of the aorta.

Middle Sacral Artery

The middle sacral artery is a variable midline artery arising from the posterior aspect of the aortic bifurcation. It is often absent or insignificant, but sometimes is present as a major source of collateral supply.

Terminal Aorta

The terminal aorta is the portion of the abdominal aorta between the renal arteries and the bifurcation. Normally, the length and diame-

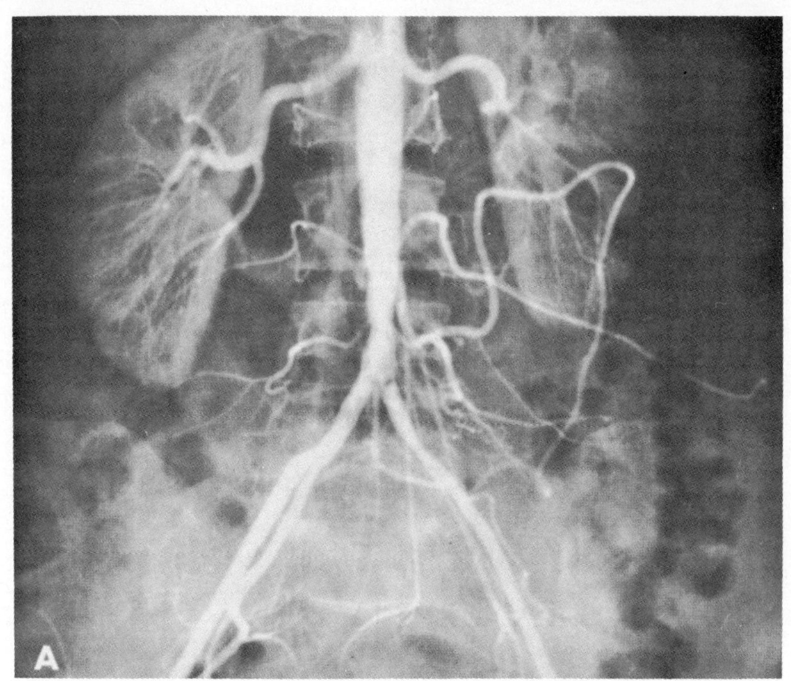

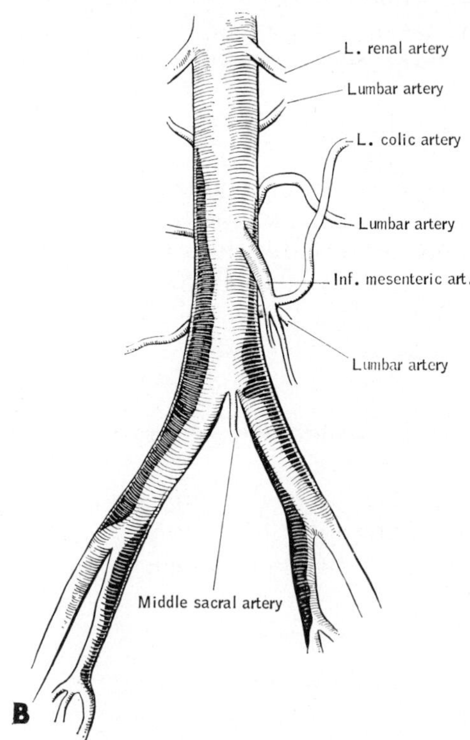

Figure 2–5.   See opposite page for legend.

ter of the segment vary considerably, and further elongation or dilatation is wrought by pathologic processes. In the adult, the diameter varies from 8 to 30 mm., although the commonest internal diameter is about 19 mm. (based on a study of 55 consecutive arteriograms). The occasional finding of a very small aorta (Fig. 2–5) suggests the presence of a diffuse hypoplastic process, and indeed there is evidence that this hypoplastic process may occur throughout the body or throughout the lower extremities. Grossman and Adams[6] have reported the occurrence of what probably are similar diminutive arteries in the coronary tree.

In three patients seen by the author, the major portion of the lower abdominal aorta was found to be absent. In the instance shown in Figure 2–6, the aorta ended at the inframesenteric level in a bulbous stump. Both renal arteries were totally occluded by a secondary atherosclerotic process; the right renal artery was well revascularized by extensive collateral supply, but the left renal artery was less well filled. The lower portion of the abdominal aorta was represented only by fragments of amorphous tissue. The pattern of a formed bifurcation could be recognized, and it appeared that the midportion of the common iliac artery had been patent at one time, but was subsequently thrombosed.

A different pathological process may produce a similar arteriogram (Fig. 2–7A). The distal aorta had become aneurysmal, and complete thrombosis had ensued. In this instance, the iliac arteries also were narrowed and took their origin from a widely spread carina (Fig. 2–7A, B, and C). Examples of this process will be found in later pages. The phenomenon is also seen in collies, which frequently are found to have arteries much smaller in relation to their body weight than dogs of other breeds.

Aortic Bifurcation

The aortic bifurcation commonly lies at the level of the lower portion of the fourth lumbar vertebra, where the two iliac arteries diverge, the branches being separated by an angle of about 80 degrees. There is much variation in this level also. In some instances the bifurcation lies as high as the second lumbar interspace, and the common iliac branches are separated by an angle of 20 or 30 degrees, or less.

Anson and McVay[1] found the level of the aortic bifurcation in 100

Figure 2–5. Arteriogram and anatomical sketch of narrow terminal aorta. Minimal atherosclerosis was present, except between L_3-L_4 intervertebral disc and common iliac bifurcation, but aorta at midportion of third lumbar body measured only 13 mm. in diameter, and the external iliac arteries (which were free of atheroma) measured only 4 and 5 mm. in diameter, respectively.

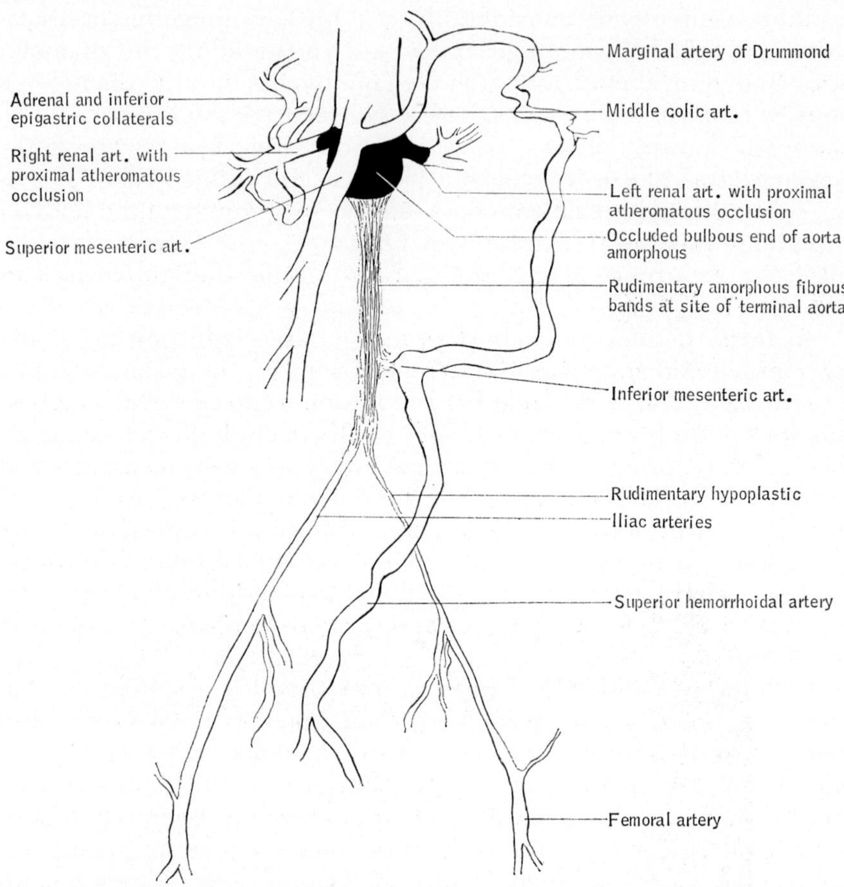

Figure 2–6. Presumed congenital absence of terminal aorta. Infrarenal aorta ended in a bulbous atheroma-filled sac which extended into the prevertebral area as amorphous fibrous strands. The middle colic artery supplied the major blood flow to this leg by way of the marginal artery of Drummond, the left colic artery, and the superior hemorrhoidal anastomoses with the hypogastric arteries.

consecutive specimens to be as listed in Table 2–1. In cases in which the bifurcation is high, the diameter of the vessel is usually abnormally small. Typically, in the Leriche syndrome,[12] the arteries are small and narrow, and form an acute angle (Fig. 2–8).

As a rule, the vena cava is close to the right lateral aspect of the aorta but is easily separable from it, a condition that is found also in most forms of occlusive disease. However, in the presence of an aneurysm of the terminal aorta, the two vessels may become adherent, so that meticulous dissection is required to separate them. Indeed, it is often simpler to develop a plane in the superficial layers of the aortic wall than to develop a plane between the two structures. No risk is involved in leaving this superficial layer of aortic wall on the caval surface.

Dissection may be made difficult by the presence of major veins in anomalous positions. Often there are major veins passing behind the aorta, to the right, from the left internal genital vein, and these veins sometimes occur as accessory retroaortic renal veins.

Occasionally a completely paired caval system is encountered.[9] The author removed one aortic aneurysm in which the two infrarenal venae cavae surrounded the aneurysm, and there were interconnecting segmental branches both in front of and behind the aorta. Fortunately, this situation is not commonly found, although a rudimentary left vena cava is often encountered and may be injured during high aortic dissection.

COMMON ILIAC ARTERIES

Normally the aorta divides into two equal common iliac arteries, each about 10 mm. in diameter and 3 to 8 cm. in length, although internal diameters varied from 6 to 13 mm. in the arteriographic studies mentioned previously (p. 13). There are no major branches from these arteries except their terminal divisions. They lie close together and adhere to the fragile underlying common iliac veins; in fact; adherence is so marked (Fig. 2–9) that the most delicate dissection is required to dissect them, and the area is properly described as the *bête noire* of the vascular surgeon.

Although the common iliac arteries are usually lacking in branches, the iliolumbar artery sometimes takes its origins from the distal common iliac artery instead of the hypogastric system.

The common iliac artery ordinarily ends opposite the level of the lumbosacral fibrocartilage. Usually, the arteries are symmetrical. They are generally equal in diameter, but the length of either may be considerably altered if the hypogastric trunk is in an anomalous high or low position.

EXTERNAL ILIAC ARTERIES

The external iliac arteries represent the continuation of the common iliac artery beyond the point of origin of the hypogastric artery. They pass laterally and anteriorly near the brim of the pelvis and terminate by entering the thigh at the inguinal ligament and becoming the common femoral artery. One or more significant branches arise

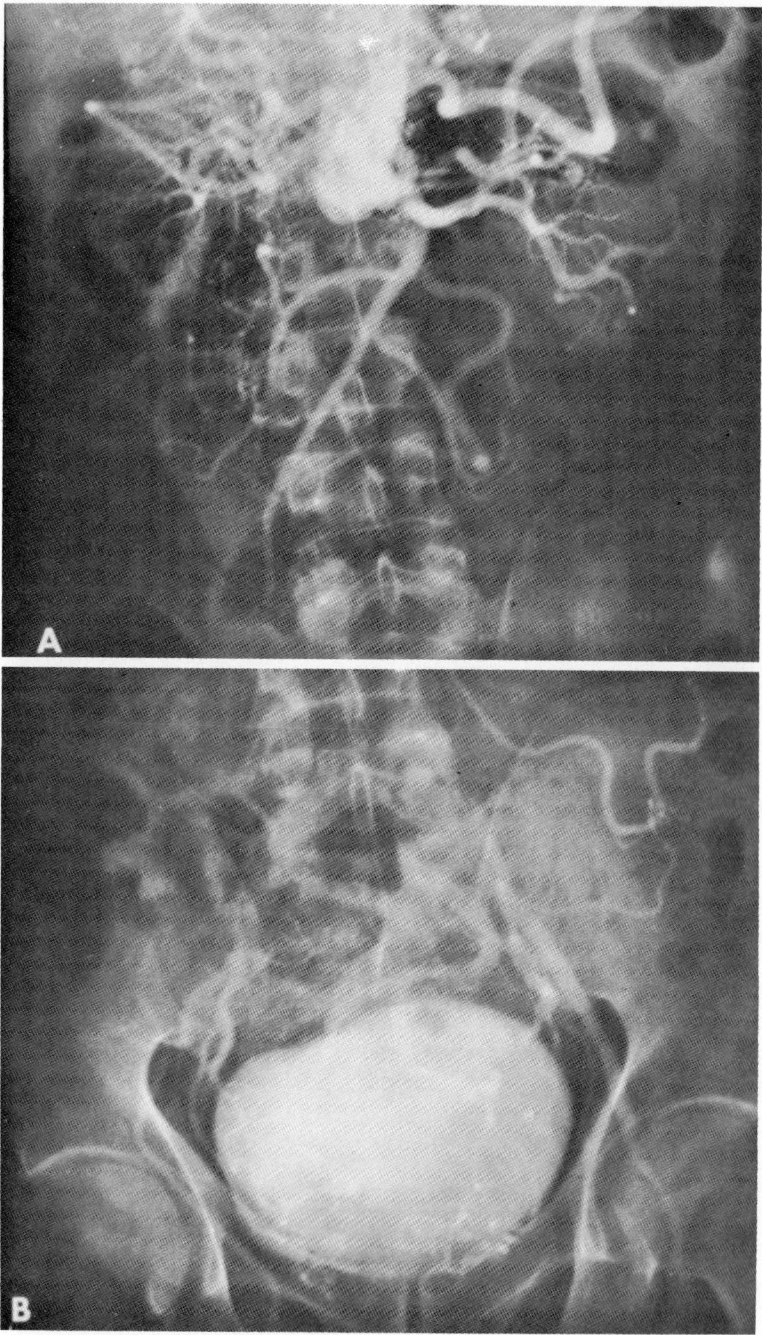

Figure 2–7.   See opposite page for legend.

(Illustration continues on opposite page.)

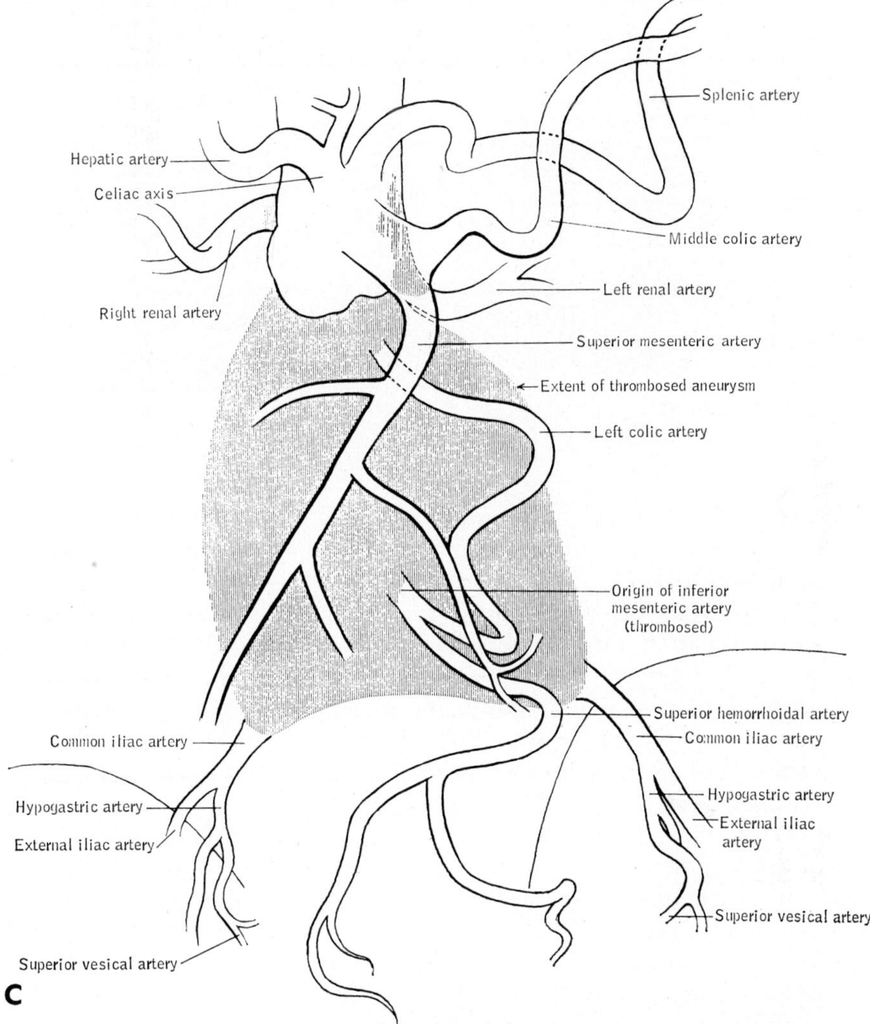

Figure 2–7. Arteriogram of patient with thrombosed aneurysm of the terminal aorta. Note collateral into the renal arteries and refilling of origin of the inferior mesenteric artery. In the pelvic portion of arteriogram, the extensive collateral between the large branches of the superior hemorrhoidal arteries and the terminal branches of the hypogastric system can be seen through the opacified bladder.

from the external iliac artery near its termination: the inferior epigastric artery, the deep iliac circumflex artery, and occasionally an anomalous obturator artery. The deep iliac circumflex artery is often an important re-entry branch of collateral supply around a proximal aortic or iliac obstruction. When serving as major sources of collateral blood supply, these vessels may measure as much as 3 to 4 mm. in diameter. These arteries are at times difficult to expose under the

Table 2–1.   Level of Aortic Bifurcation in 100 Anatomical Specimens[*]

	LEVEL	NUMBER
L_3	Upper third	0
	Middle third	0
L_3–L_4	Intervertebral disc	3
L_4	Upper third	8
L_4	Middle third	14
L_4	Lower third	32
L_4–L_5	Intervertebral disc	28
L_5	Upper third	10
L_5	Middle third	3
L_5	Lower third	1

[*]From Anson, B. J., and McVay, C. B., Anat. Rec. 67:7, 1936.[1]

shelter of the inguinal ligament, and brisk hemorrhaging may occur if they are torn. Rarely the iliolumbar artery arises from the proximal external iliac artery.

Usually, the external iliac is larger than the hypogastric artery, measuring 5 to 8 mm. When hypoplasia is found in the Leriche syndrome, however, the external iliac arteries are often not more than 2 to 3 mm. in internal diameter, as measured by calibrated rubber catheters inserted into them. This internal diameter is small even in the absence of atherosclerosis; indeed, the external iliac artery is less often affected by atherosclerotic changes than is the common iliac artery. When the external iliac artery is small, the hypogastric artery is generally larger, in a reciprocal arrangement (Fig. 2–8B). The abnormal narrowing may be present on only one side; when it is, the ipsilateral common iliac bifurcation is usually at a higher level, and the ipsilateral common iliac artery is apt to be more extensively affected by atherosclerosis than the other side.

That the anomaly does not necessarily follow the development of obstructive atherosclerosis is shown by its occasional occurrence in young people who have manifested no atherosclerosis. In time, these young people may come to show the obstructive lesions of the Leriche syndrome; this aspect of the etiology of atherosclerosis will be discussed in another section.

There are major anomalies of the aorta and the iliac system, which may explain in part some of the variations in size between the internal and external systems. Two instances have been found recently of a persistent sciatic artery (Fig. 2–10 A and B). The external iliac artery is small and continues in its normal course as the deep femoral artery. There is only a vestigial saphenous artery continuing in what might be expected to be the usual course of the superficial femoral vessel. The

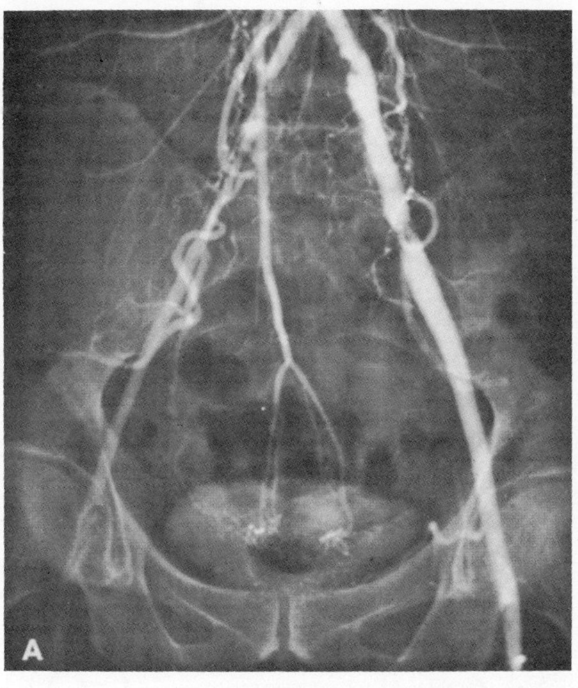

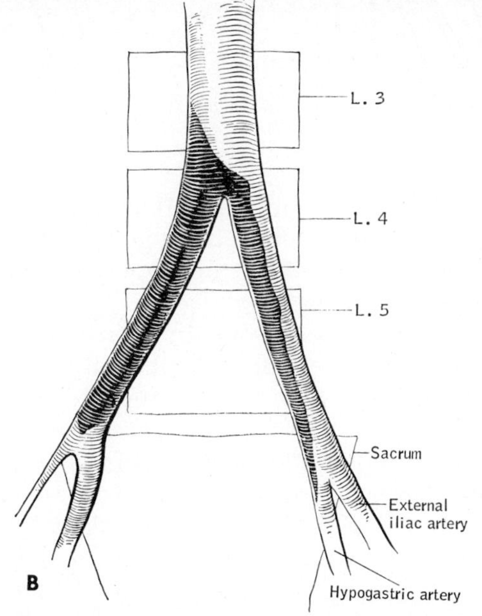

Figure 2–8. *A*, Arteriogram of patient with typical Leriche syndrome: high, narrow bifurcation with acute angle between common iliac arteries. *B*, Anatomical sketch emphasizing frequently seen reciprocal difference in size between the external and internal iliac arteries.

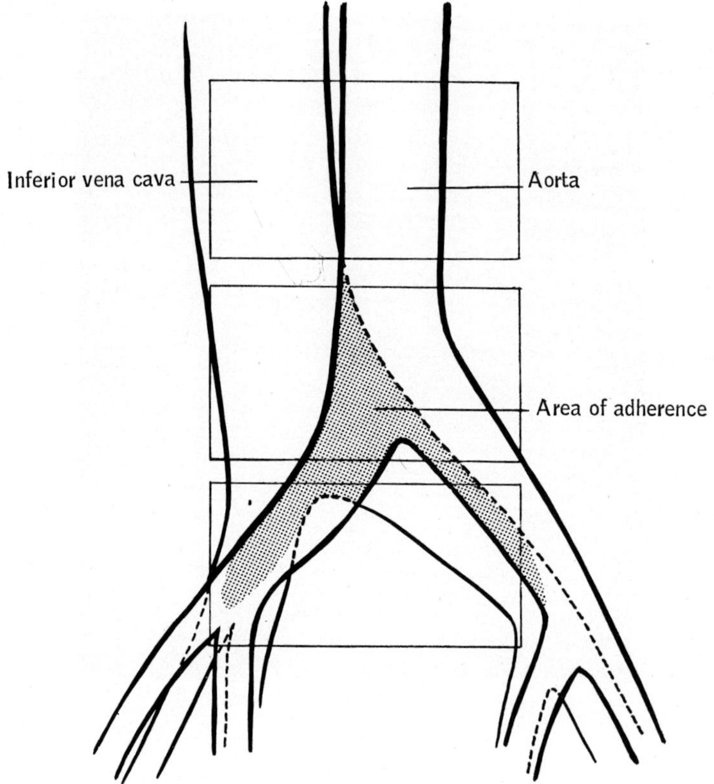

Figure 2–9.   Usual area of dense adherence between aorta and vena cava.

internal iliac artery is large and passes backward through the sciatic notch; it re-enters the thigh behind the quadratus femorus muscle and follows the sciatic nerve to reach the popliteal space, where it continues as the popliteal artery.

Another patient was seen clinically in whom the projection and the direct anterior posterior plane did not clearly demonstrate this abnormality. An oblique view, however, showed the anatomy clearly (Figs. 2–11A and B).

Another bizarre anatomic disposition of the vessels, encountered during a urological procedure on a child, is depicted in Figures 2–12A and B. An abnormally short aortic trunk gives origin to a right common iliac artery and a renomesenteric trunk. From the latter arise paired renal arteries to a solitary right kidney. The renomesenteric trunk continues in the distribution in the inferior mesenteric artery. The left lateral terminations become the posterior trunk of the left internal iliac system. The right common iliac trunk divides into internal and external arteries, and the external iliac system continues in a normal course. The major vesical branches of the right internal iliac artery continue as a large (8 to 9 mm.) artery which arches over the bladder in a subperitoneal course and re-forms a left external iliac artery through similar left vesical connections. This last, and completely unpredictable arrangement of the vessels is mentioned only to instill awe in the surgeon who finds a large anomalous vessel in this way during any dissection.

It is likely that some of the above abnormalities in size and distribution of the iliac and hypogastric system are caused by abnormal formation or premature obliteration of one of the old umbilical arteries during fetal development. Obliteration of one of these arteries may require the development of unusual and anomalous branches in order to supply sufficient amounts of blood to the developing limb.[14, 16]

There is rarely any significant adherence of the external iliac arteries to their corresponding veins. Their most important anatomical relationship is with the ureter, which drops medially into the pelvis by passing over the origin of the external iliac artery.

HYPOGASTRIC (INTERNAL ILIAC) ARTERY

The hypogastric trunk is approximately 5 mm. in diameter, but may be considerably larger. The common compensatory relationship between the size of the external and internal iliac arteries has already been mentioned.

The hypogastric trunk is usually only 3 to 4 cm. in length, passing into the depths of the pelvis in proximity to the hypogastric vein. The iliolumbar artery may arise from the proximal hypogastric trunk. The trunk usually terminates by division into an anterior and a posterior trunk.

The *anterior trunk* may exist as a true trunk or as a cluster of branches, nearly always taking origin from the posterior trunk. These branches are the superior, middle, and inferior vesical arteries; the middle hemorrhoidal; the obturator; the internal pudendal; the inferior gluteal; and the uterine and vaginal arteries in the female.

The *posterior trunk* of the hypogastric artery is, as a rule, the major channel supplying the lateral sacral and superior gluteal arteries, and often the ilolumbar artery.

The posterior trunk is the apparent direct continuation of the hypogastric artery; hence, it is possible to enter the posterior trunk through the hypogastric orifice and to remove plaques from it. Restoration of flow into the anterior branches may be accomplished because atheromata rarely extend far into the lumen of the anterior segments.

Details of the relationships within the hypogastric arterial bed are of little concern to the vascular surgeon, but the functioning of the ar-

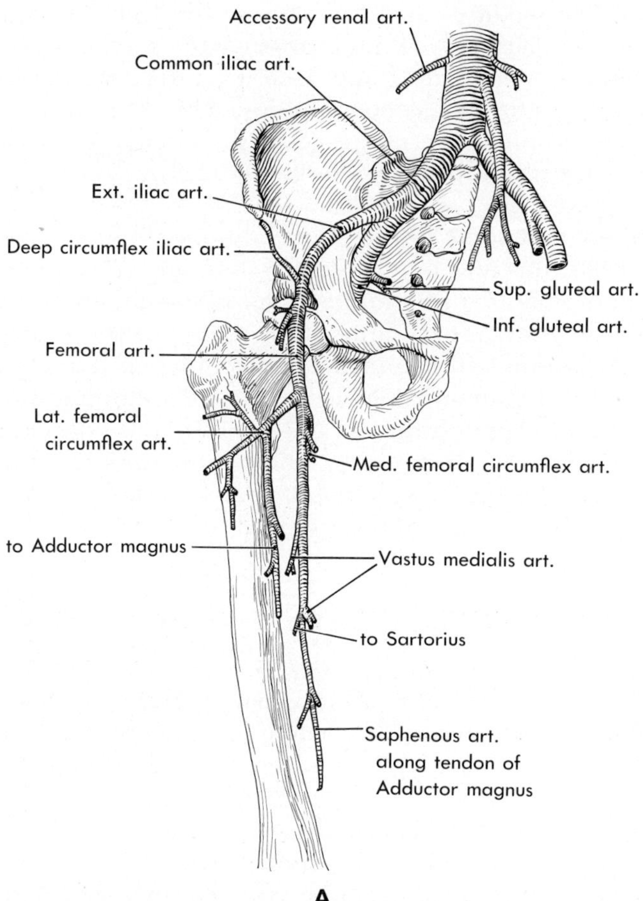

Figure 2–10. A, Anterior view of the artist's sketch of persistent sciatic artery. The external iliac artery continues down the front of the leg as the profunda femoris artery, and only the saphenous artery descends along the tendon of the adductor magnus.

(Illustration continues on opposite page.)

tery is of great importance. The hypogastric artery is one of the most frequent sites of atherosclerosis—an unfortunate circumstance, in view of its key position in the collateral network.

The anterior and posterior trunks may supply branches for collateral circulation into the hypogastric trunk from above or below; the examples of collateral circulation in the abdominal pelvis are discussed next.

COLLATERAL BRANCHES IN THE ABDOMEN AND PELVIS

The commonest pattern of collateral flow around an obstruction of the terminal aorta and both common iliac arteries is shown in Figure

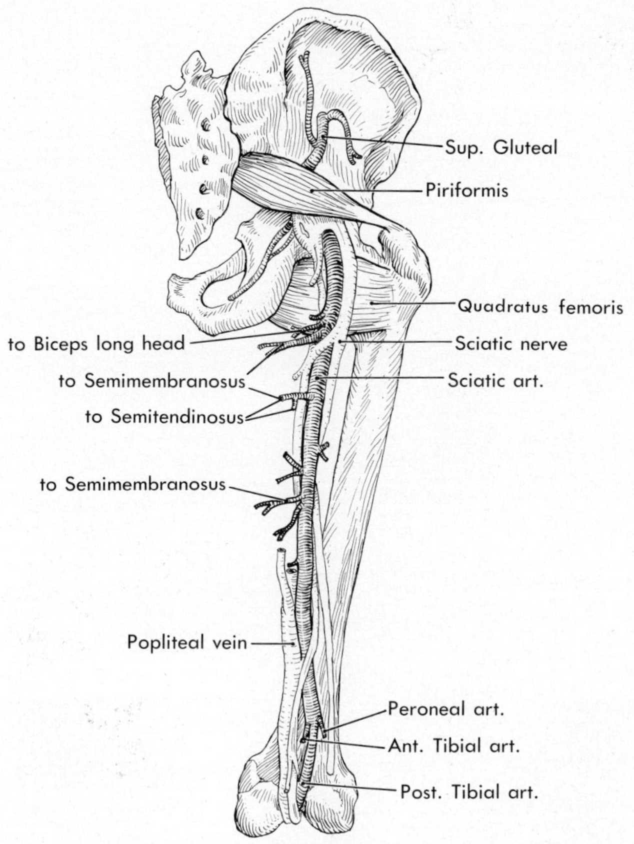

Figure 2–10 Continued. B, Posterior view of the persistent sciatic artery showing its relations to the pyriformis muscle, the sciatic nerve and its final position in the popliteal space.

2–13. Lumbar arteries supplying networks in the flank and hip muscles reenter the hypogastric bed by way of the iliolumbar and superior gluteal branches. The inferior mesenteric artery may become greatly hypertrophied in order to refill the hypogastric bed through the middle and superior hemorrhoidal anastomoses in the perirectal tissues, as shown in Figure 2–14.

In this pattern and in others relying on the inferior mesenteric arterial supply, claudication may be associated with either cramps or diarrhea attributable to presumed ischemia of the distal colon.

When only one common iliac artery is obstructed, the collateral branches that refill the affected hypogastric artery arise from the proximal lumbar arteries, as shown in Figure 2–13. The inferior mesenteric artery is rarely enlarged, but apparently there is considerable flow across the pelvis between the corresponding hypogastric

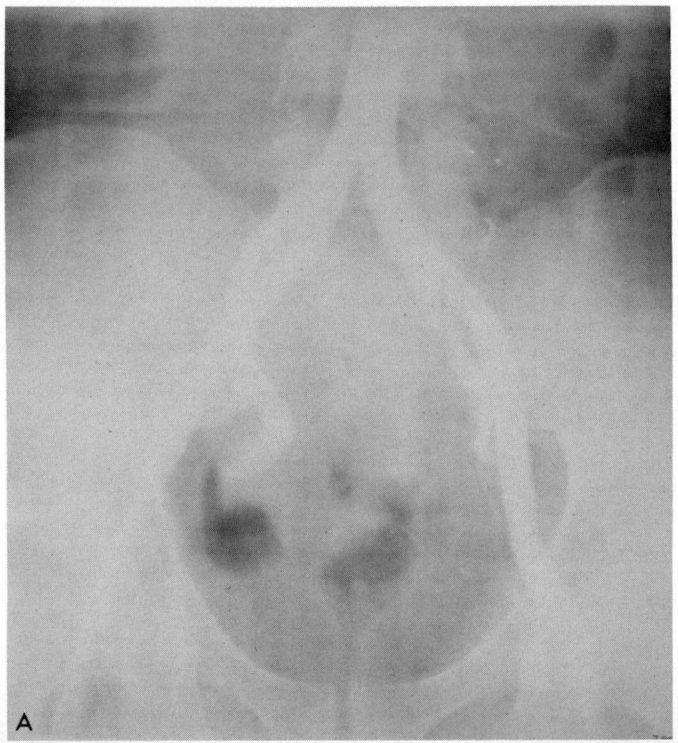

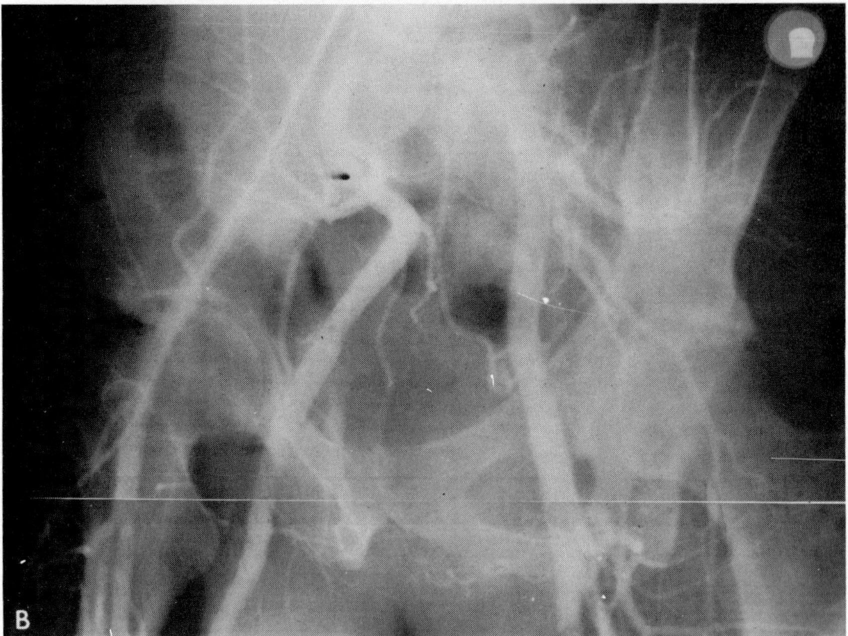

Figure 2–11. A, Anteroposterior arteriogram of a patient with a posterior sciatic artery on the right. In this projection it is hard to identify the presence of this abnormality. *B,* With the patient in the right posterior oblique position the arteriogram clearly shows the separation of the persistent sciatic artery from the anterior branches.

branches. At times, the internal pudendal artery is greatly hypertrophied and provides important collateral branches between the iliac arteries.

In more extensive involvement of the terminal aorta, the lumbar arteries contribute less and the inferior mesenteric artery, more; in this situation, the internal spermatic artery can also become greatly enlarged (to as much as 1 cm.). The re-entry site of the collateral pathway shown in Figure 2–15A was not evident, but might have been through the external spermatic and other branches of the inferior epigastric artery, perhaps communicating with the iliolumbar branches in the flank. In another case, inadvertent division of the important internal spermatic artery during ureterolithotomy led to gangrene of the leg, for which amputation had to be performed.

In extensive obstruction, when the hypogastric trunk and the common iliac trunk are occluded, the lumbar collateral branches must refill the distal hypogastric network and thence join the collateral branches from below the inguinal ligament. Some flow may return to the main line through the lumbar branches that communicate with the deep circumflex iliac artery and possibly with the inferior epigastric artery.

COMMON FEMORAL ARTERY

The common femoral artery arises at the inguinal ligament as the continuation of the external iliac artery. The deep femoral artery is given off 2.5 to 6 cm. below the inguinal ligament as a unit or a group of branches. The femoral artery as such continues down the femoral triangle and Hunter's (adductor) canal, and is usually referred to as the superficial femoral artery.

The point of origin of the deep femoral artery is quite constant in relation to the inguinal ligament. The sagging of the line of the inguinal fold of the skin sometimes causes some confusion. The inguinal fold is rarely superimposed on the inguinal ligament.

The common femoral artery gives off the three or four small branches of variable size and importance which are generally categorized as the superficial circumflex iliac, the superficial external pudic, and the deep external pudic. In some instances, the inferior epigastric, the deep circumflex iliac, and anomalous obturator arteries may arise below the ligament. Some of the other usual branches of the deep femoral artery may arise directly from the common femoral artery, and some of the usual branches of the femoral artery may arise from the deep femoral artery.

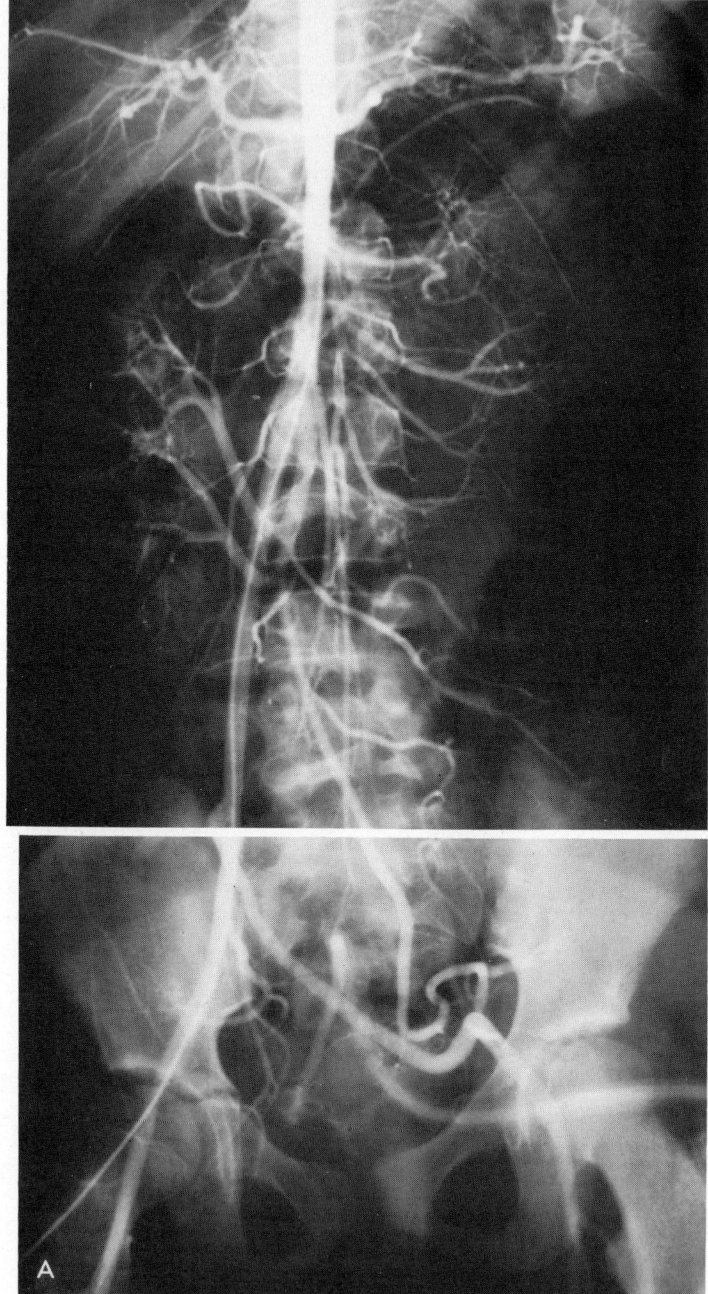

Figure 2–12. A is a composite arteriogram of a 6-year-old child who was found to have a large anomalous artery crossing the dome of the bladder.

(Illustration continues on opposite page.)

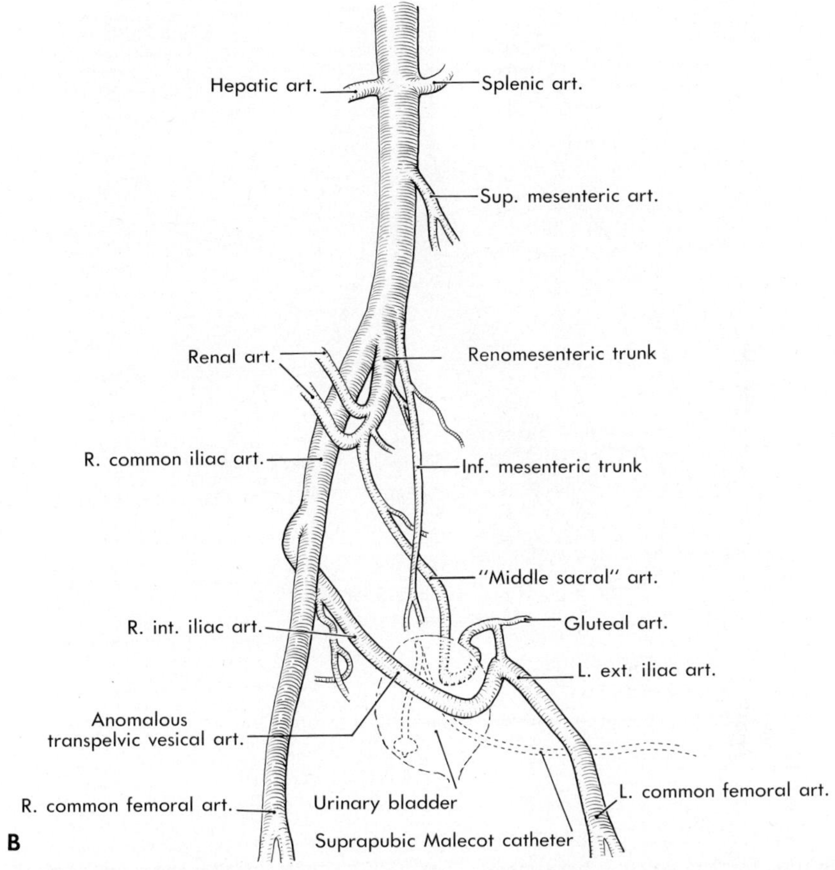

Figure 2–12 Continued. *B* is an artist's representation of the arteriogram. The aorta divides near the level of the first lumbar vertebra into a right common iliac artery and into a left nephromesenteric trunk. The right common iliac artery gives off, in a normal position, the external iliac artery and an apparently normal hypogastric artery. The vesical branches of the hypogastric artery, however, arch across the dome of the bladder and following more nearly the course of the obturator artery reassume the normal position of the left external iliac artery. At the most cephalad extent of the anomalous artery on the left side it is joined by the terminal branch of the renomesenteric trunk which lies in the retroperitoneal tissues. From the renomesenteric trunk are given off branches which apparently constitute the usual inferior mesenteric distribution as well as two large paired branches to a solitary right kidney. The superior mesenteric artery and the celiac axis are substantially within normal limits.

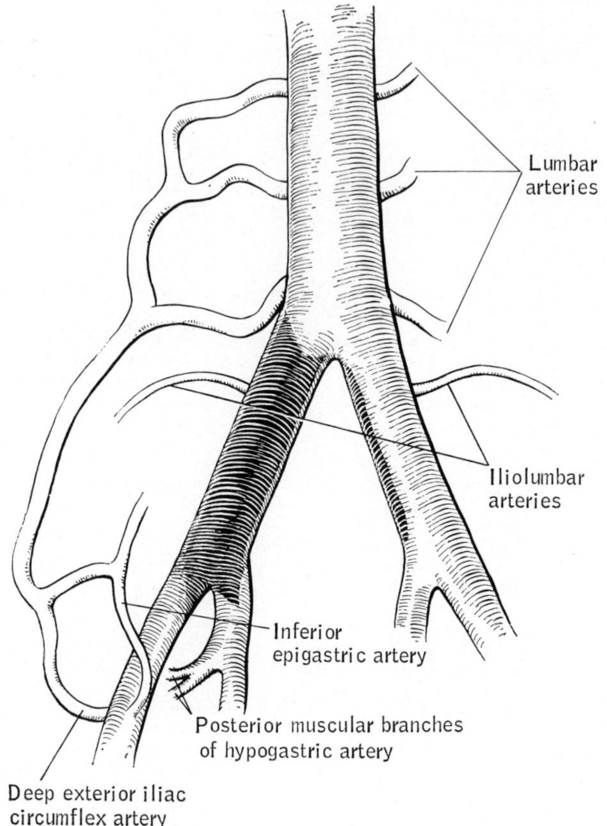

Figure 2–13.   Common collateral pathways around iliac arterial occlusion.

DEEP FEMORAL ARTERY (ARTERIA PROFUNDA FEMORIS)

The deep femoral artery is usually given off between 2.5 and 6 cm. from the inguinal ligament, and markes the end of the common femoral trunk. Rarely, it arises higher, even above the ligament. It is a short trunk and passes posterolaterally, promptly giving off a deep medial circumflex femoral artery. In its course around the femur the artery anastomoses with descending branches of the obturator artery. The main deep femoral artery continues down the leg in proximity to the medial aspect of the vastus lateralis muscle (lateral great muscle). Opposite the origin of the medial femoral circumflex artery, the deep lateral circumflex artery is given off and divides into an ascending and a descending branch. These branches anastomose with the iliac cir-

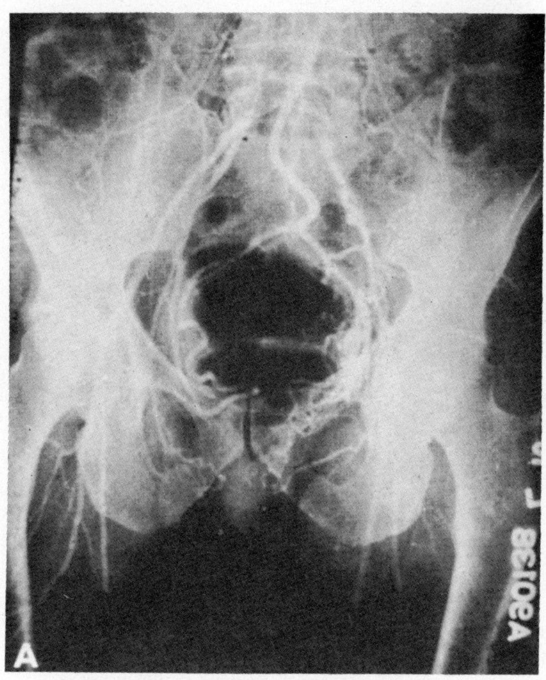

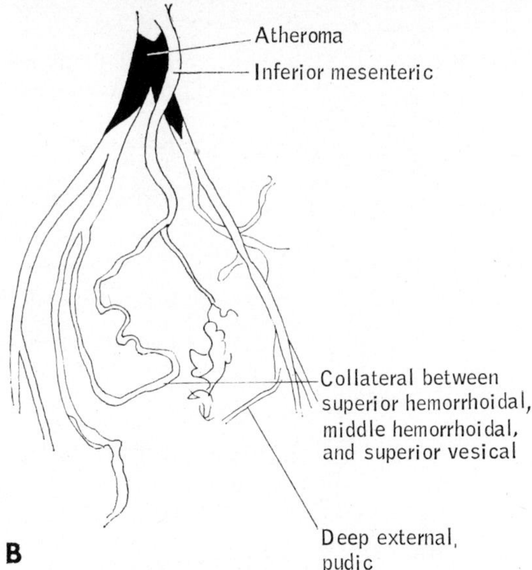

Figure 2–14. Arteriogram in case of bilateral iliac arterial occlusion. Collateral pathways through inferior mesenteric-superior hemorrhoidal anastomoses have become greatly enlarged.

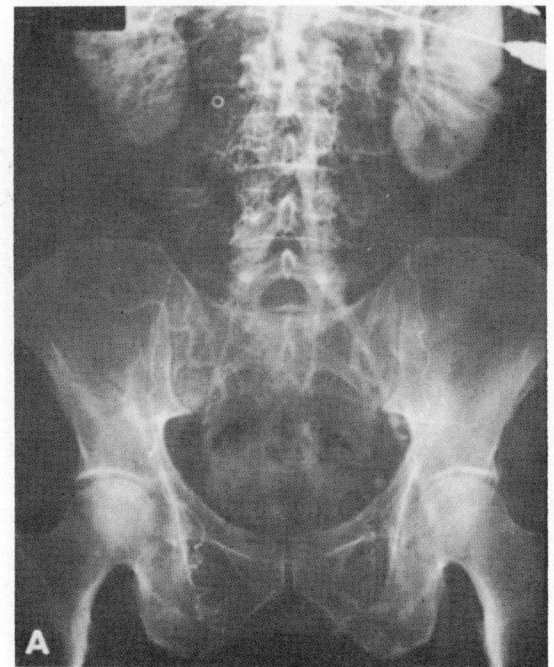

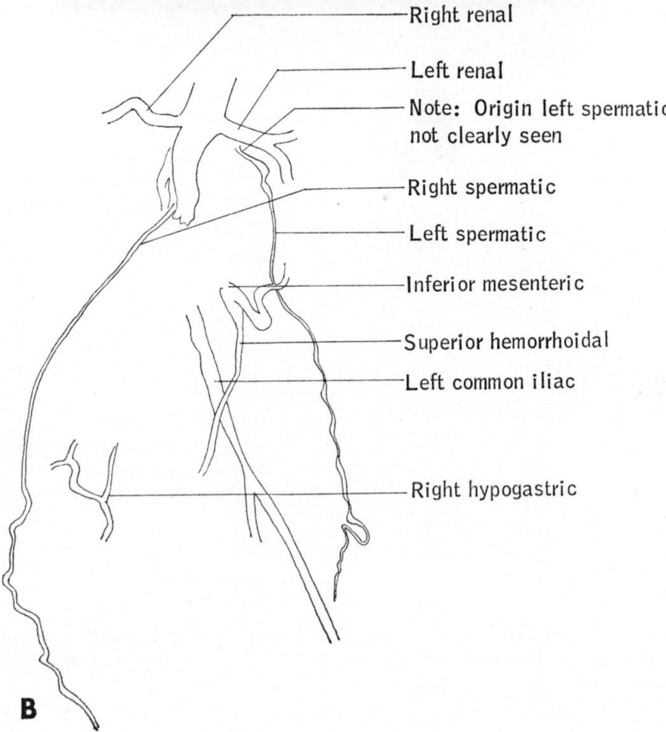

Figure 2–15. See opposite page for legend.

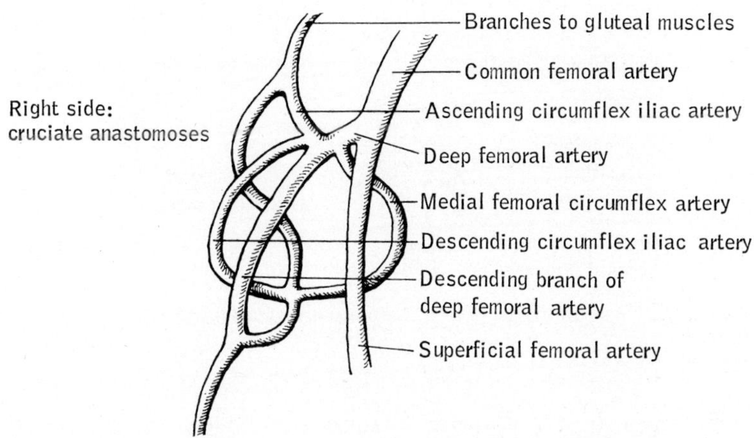

Figure 2–16. Cruciate anastomosis through which flow from gluteal area reaches the femoral artery.

cumflex artery around the femur and with the first posterior perforating branch of the main deep femoral trunk to form the cruciate anastomosis (Fig. 2–16). Either or both of the medial and lateral circumflex femoral arteries sometimes arise from the common femoral artery itself (Fig. 2–17).

SUPERFICIAL FEMORAL ARTERY

The superficial femoral artery is a continuation of the main line of the common femoral artery. Often the artery is narrowed at its origin, but beyond this area it is of normal size (Fig. 2–18). As it passes down the thigh from the femoral triangle, it comes to lie in the adductor tunnel under the sartorius muscle. The artery follows a direct course down the thigh on the anterior surface of the great adductor until it passes through the adductor hiatus in the fibrous insertion of this muscle and becomes the popliteal artery. Just at or before its passage through the adductor hiatus are given off the highest genicular arteries; usually, the larger of these is the medial branch, which often passes within the substance of the great adductor muscle for a short distance. During division of the arch of the adductor hiatus at opera-

---

Figure 2–15. *A*, Arteriogram in case of iliac arterial occlusion. Internal spermatic artery has come to participate in collateral channels. *B*, Anatomical relationships of area shown in *A*.

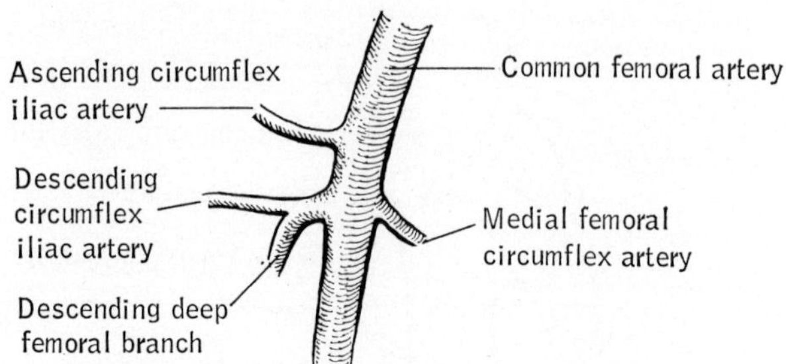

Figure 2–17.   Components of deep femoral artery arising separately from common femoral artery.

tion, this important collateral branch can easily be damaged. The lower few centimeters of the femoral artery lie close to the femoral vein; multiple anastomotic branches of the vein come to form an almost plexiform investment of this part of the artery.

POPLITEAL ARTERY

As the popliteal artery enters the popliteal space, it deviates laterally in a deep and well protected layer of fat and comes to lie in close attachment to the more superficial (that is, posterior) popliteal vein. The tibial nerve is much more superficial and is less closely attached. The several other branches listed in anatomy texts in this position of the artery are inconstant and insignificant.

Hamming[7] has described an anomalous course of the popliteal artery in a child in which the lower portion of the vessel curved posteriorly around the medial head of the gastrocnemius muscle and had become thrombosed.

There are variations of this anomalous course. The least deviation is around a simple fibrous extension of the medial head of the gastrocnemius, and the greatest involves the course of the artery around the complete substance of the medial head.

The radiographic picture seen in the presence of this pattern of entrapment is described subsequently (Chapter Fifteen).

An excellent description of the anatomy of the terminal branches of the popliteal artery is given by Morris and his associates.[13, 14]

As the artery passes superficial (posterior) to the popliteus, it gives off one of its three major branches, the anterior tibial artery.

The anterior tibial artery passes forward over the interosseous membrane and lies on the anterior surface of the interosseous membrane basically between the tibialis anterior muscle and the long extensors of the toes and of the great toe. Farther down in the leg the artery comes to lie just behind and between the tibialis tendon and the tendon to the extensor hallucis. It extends on into the foot as the dorsalis pedis artery, where it comes to lie in the subcutaneous tissue, and there it is known as the dorsal pedal artery (arteriodorsalis pedis).

The main line of the popliteal artery continues into the deep tissues of the calf beneath the soleus muscle and the two heads of the gastrocnemius muscle. Here it divides into a smaller peroneal artery and the larger posterior tibial artery, which is in substance the continuation of the popliteal artery. The peroneal artery continues down the leg on the posterior tibial muscle (musculus tibialis posterior) and medial to the short peroneal muscle (musculus peroneus brevis).

The posterior tibial artery continues down the leg on the posterior surface of the posterior muscle, lateral and posterior to the long flexor of the toes, and just deep to the soleus muscle. It is best exposed by a longitudinal incision which passes just anterior to the usual course of the saphenous vein and immediately behind the lateralmost portion of the tibia, and in the plane between the long flexor of the toes and the soleus muscle. As the artery descends further it lies medial to the continuation of the tibial nerve, with which it continues into the area behind the medial malleolus, where it is felt as the posterior tibial arterial pulsation. The surgical approach to these vessels will be described in detail in later chapters; the reader is referred to Henry's text on exposure,[8] which provides an excellent source for these and other approaches to the vessels of the extremities.

COLLATERAL BRANCHES IN THE THIGH AND THE KNEE

Obstructions of the thigh or the knee must be considered on the basis of the pathological process.

Atherosclerosis is the commonest source of obstruction. It is usually maximal at the level of the adductor hiatus, with patchy areas of obstruction extending upward. In this situation, collaterals from the descending branches of the deep femoral artery refill the network around the knee formed by the various genicular branches.

Obstructions of the popliteal artery are of several types. Occlusion of the outflow triad is apt to be associated with extensive disease in one or more of the tibial arteries. There is no suitable main line for re-entry, and the collaterals at their origin in the genicular branches must empty into relatively small channels in the calf.

In embolic occlusion at the level of the distal popliteal artery the area is better served by collateral branches than it is in chronic throm-

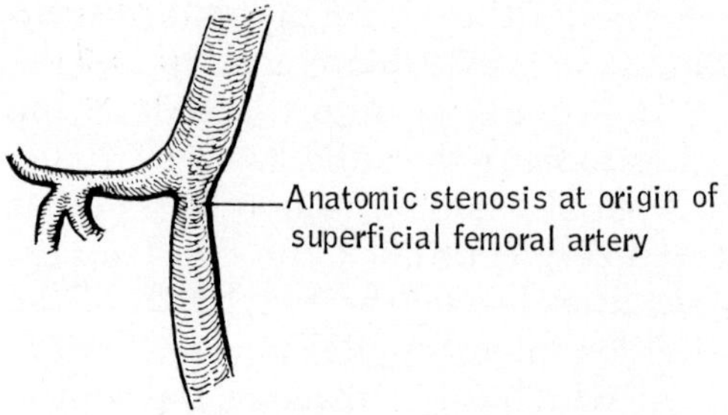

Figure 2–18. Exaggerated anatomic stenosis at origin of superficial femoral artery.

bosis, for the tibial vessels and their recurrent connections with the genicular network are usually patent.

The complications caused by thrombosis of a popliteal aneurysm depend on the level of the aneurysm and the extent to which the main line has been occluded proximally (occlusion of the proximal genicular origins) or distally (occlusion of the outflow triad and their recurrent connections with the genicular arteries).

One important anatomical sign may help define the level of an obstruction. A pulsation may sometimes be felt at the level of the patella medially if the obstruction does not extend upward to occlude the origin of the highest medial genicular artery.

SIZE OF THE FEMORAL TREE

Apparent hypoplasia of the entire femoral tree below a narrow aortic and iliac segment has been seen, most commonly in young women; in one instance, the diameters of the arteries, as measured by arteriogram, were approximately as follows:

Artery	*Diameter* (mm.)
Terminal aorta (L_3 to L_4)	10
Common iliac	5
External iliac	3
Common femoral	3
Superficial femoral	2 to 3
popliteal	2 to 3
Tibial	1 to 2

In other cases, especially when the external iliac artery is the only one of the pelvic arteries to be markedly narrowed, the common and superficial femoral trees may be of relatively normal caliber.

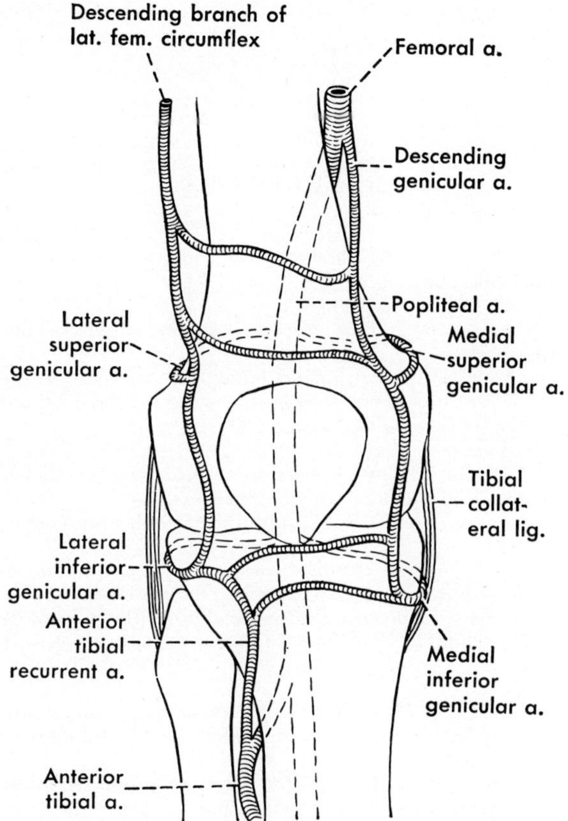

Figure 2–19. Collaterals around knee joint. (From Hollinshead, W. H.: *Anatomy for Surgeons.* New York, Hoeber Medical Div., Harper & Row, 1958, Vol. 3, p. 578.)

It often appears that there is an inverse relationship between the size of the descending branches of the deep femoral artery and that of the superficial femoral artery. When the superficial femoral artery is small, it is more apt to be occluded by a small intimal atheroma, and in these circumstances the dominant deep femoral artery may provide such excellent collateral circulation that symptoms are minimized. Part of this apparent reciprocal dominance may be the consequence of hypertrophy of the deep femoral artery in providing collateral circulation, but the two arterial patterns may be seen on arteriograms in which no occlusive disease is demonstrated.

Another aspect of anatomical variation is the size of the outflow triad from the popliteal artery. On occasion, all three major branches may be only 1 or 2 mm. in diameter; there is then considerable alteration in rates of flow and in turbulence in the distal popliteal artery.

The anterior and posterior tibial arteries also seem to share a reciprocal pattern of dominance beyond the variations imposed by atherosclerosis.

REFERENCES

1. Anson, B. J., and McVay, C. B.: The topographical positions and mutual relations of the visceral branches of the abdominal aorta: a study of 100 consecutive cadavers. Anat. Rec. 67:7, 1936.
2. Clagett, O. T.: Presidential address: Research and prosearch. J. Thor. Cardiov. Surg. 44:153, 1962.
3. Edwards, E. A.: Anatomic and clinical comments on shoulder girdle syndromes. In Barker, W. F. (ed.): Surgical Treatment of Peripheral Vascular Disease. New York, McGraw-Hill Book Company, 1962.
4. Elkin, D. C.: Exposure of blood vessels. J.A.M.A. 132:421, 1946.
5. Falconer, M. A., and Li, F. W. P.: Resection of first rib and costoclavicular compression of the brachial plexus. Lancet 1:59, 1962.
6. Grossman, L. A., and Adams, C. W.: Diminutive coronary artery syndrome. J.A.M.A. 188:1111, 1964.
7. Hamming, J. J.: Intermittent claudication at an early age, due to an anomalous course of the popliteal artery. Angiology 10:369, 1959.
8. Henry, A. K.: Extensile Exposure. Baltimore, The Williams & Wilkins Co., 1957.
9. Hirsch, D. M., and Chan, K. F.: Bilateral inferior vena cava. J.A.M.A. 185:729, 1963.
10. Hollinshead, W. H.: Anatomy for Surgeons. New York, Hoeber Medical Div., Harper & Row, Vol. 3, p. 578.
11. Laufman, H., Berggrén, R. E., Finley, T., and Anson, B. J.: Anatomical studies of the lumbar arteries with reference to the safety of translumbar aortography. Ann. Surg. 152:621, 1960.
12. Leriche, R.: De la résection du carrefour aorticoiliaque avec double sympathectomie lombaire pour thrombose artéritique de l'aorte; le syndrome de l'oblitération termino-aortique par artérite. Presse Méd. 48:601, 1940.
13. Morris, G. C., Jr., DeBakey, M. E., Cooley, D. A., and Crawford, E. S.: Arterial bypass below the knee. Surg. Gynec. Obstet. 108:321, 1959.
14. Morris, G. C., Jr., Beall, A. C., Jr., Berry, W. B., Feste, J., and DeBakey, M. E.: Anatomical studies of the distal popliteal artery and its branches. Surg. Forum 10:498, 1960.
15. Ritchie, H. D., and Douglas, D. M.: Atresia of the abdominal aorta. Brt. Med. J. 1:144, 1956.
16. Roos, D. B.: Transaxillary approach for first rib resection to relieve thoracic outlet syndrome. Ann. Surg. 163:354, 1966.
17. Senior, H. D.: An interpretation of the recorded arterial anomalies of the human pelvis and thigh. Am. J. Anat. 36:1, 1925.
18. Suh, T. H., and Alexander, L.: Vascular system of the human spinal cord. Arch. Neurol. Psychiat. 41:659, 1939.
19. Tanon, L.: Les artères de la moelle dorso-lombaire: considérations anatomiques et clinicques. Thesis, No. 98, Paris, Vigot Frères, 1908.
20. Usabiaga, J. E., Kolodny, J. E., and Usabiaga, L. E.: Neurological complications of prevertebral surgery under regional anesthesia. Surgery, 68:304, 1970.

Chapter Three

PHYSIOLOGY

VICTOR E. HALL, M.D.,
and WILEY F. BARKER, M.D.

The physiological points of importance to the vascular surgeon that will be reviewed here constitute only one aspect of vascular physiology. The reader is referred to other sources for additional details,[6, 13, 18, 20, 21, 30] and particularly to Strandness'[32] account of the pathophysiology of arterial disease. The areas to be considered include normal factors influencing flow, physiological methods controlling flow, flow through stenotic systems, and the importance of turbulence and pressure changes in a branch system such as that of the aortoiliac-femoropopliteal tree.

PHYSIOLOGICAL MECHANISMS USUALLY RESPONSIBLE FOR CONTROL OF BLOOD FLOW

Control of blood flow in the limbs is a dual process. Flow in tissues subject to sympathetic control is based primarily on one set of mechanisms; flow in tissues not so responsive to sympathetic stimuli is based on another. Preservation of an endangered extremity and protection against the hazards of minor trauma may depend on augmentation of those mechanisms increasing blood flow to the skin. On the other hand, if the sole problem is restoration of ability to do work to poorly vascularized muscle, a different means of influencing the circulation must be attempted.

Redisch[25] has estimated the relative quantities of skin and muscle as follows:

	Skin	*Muscle*
		(per cent)
Forearm and lower leg	25 to 50	50 to 77
Hands and feet	80 to 83	17 to 20

Control of Blood Flow to the Skin

The important mechanisms controlling blood flow to the skin are vasoconstriction on the one hand, and inhibition of vasoconstrictive mechanisms on the other. Active vasodilatation is almost entirely lacking, except for the bradykinin mechanism and the local effect of heat on the blood vessel itself.

Vasoconstrictive mechanisms from the sympathetic system are in a tonic state of activity. The influence of this system is primarily upon the skin of the soles and palms. Flow is reduced by restriction of the size of the terminal arteries and arterioles. Flow is increased because of the passive dilatation of the vessels which follows inhibition of the chronically active vasoconstrictor impulses. Hall[18] estimates that the usual tonic activity of the sympathetic vasoconstrictor nerves increases hindrance in the cutaneous vessels by a factor of four to six times that of the state existing in complete abolition of sympathetic tone. Total removal of sympathetic tone may arise as a reflex from heating of a distant part. Under these circumstances of *general* body heating, bradykinin, which is an active dilator agent,[14] is released.

Metabolic activity in the presence of reduced flow occasions compensatory reduction of peripheral resistance. All other things being equal, there is an increase in flow because of the accumulation of metabolic end products, because of an alteration of pCO_2, or because of hypoxia and their subsequent effects on the arteriolar and capillary beds.

Hormonal influences on blood flow due to androgens and estrogens are slight; but the adrenal medullary products, epinephrine and norepinephrine, are typically strong vasoconstrictors in the skin. However, the catecholamines secreted by the adrenal medulla have negligible effects compared with those produced by the direct sympathetic innervation.

Reflex vasoconstriction occurs as a consequence of three major stimuli. The first of these arises during hemorrhage or shock and produces its effect through the carotid sinus and the aortic nerves. The second is cooling of the body. The third is an emotional reaction. Other less important influences are deep inspiration, hypoxia, asphyxia, and hypoglycemia.

Arteriovenous Shunts in the Skin

Shunts of a caliber slightly greater than that of capillaries are known to exist in the skin. No nutritive exchange occurs through the walls of these shunts, and thus their presence potentially allows diversion of nutritive capillary flow to non-nutritive tubes. It was suggested by Atlas[2] and by Freeman, Leeds, and Gardner[15] that sympathectomy in some patients precipitated gangrene by diverting large amounts of blood through the shunts and away from nutritive vessels. This phenomenon, if it ever occurs, must be exceedingly rare. We have never known it to be the only cause of necrosis after sympathectomy. Piiper and Schoedel[24] demonstrated that following sympathectomy in animals, total flow to a limb might increase to about 45 per cent above normal. Shunt flow had been about 16 per cent of the presympathectomy flow. Whereas shunt flow was increased by 140 per cent by sympathectomy, nutritive capillary flow was increased by only 10 per cent. Clearly, sympathectomy may produce a redistribution of blood within the capillary bed. Hall suggests that under some conditions of arterial obstruction, redistribution of flow through shunts may reduce total nutritive flow.

More commonly, necrosis after sympathectomy may be precipitated by a prolonged and difficult operation, in which propagation of clot in the region of an acute or chronic arterial occlusion is facilitated by hypotension. Increased sensitivity of a previously sympathectomized extremity to ether anesthesia may contribute to some extension of the occlusive disease.[12] The rarity with which ethyl ether is currently used in anesthesia reduces the importance of this factor. Prolonged manipulation of the chain allowing a great increase of locally induced vasospastic impulses may also account for reduction of flow to a critical level.

Control of Blood Flow to Skeletal Muscle

There is more evidence of the dual role of vasoconstrictor and vasodilator mechanisms in control of flow to muscle than to skin. There are also non-nutritive shunts whose control may be under slightly different mechanisms. The primary effects on the nutritive channels are discussed in the following paragraphs.

Sympathetic nervous fibers to muscle are of two types: vasoconstrictor fibers whose activity is mediated by the release of norepinephrine, and vasodilator fibers whose activity is mediated through the release of acetylcholine.

According to Barcroft and Swan,[4] flow to the forearm may be quadrupled by blocking the brachial plexus, although such a maneuver achieves only doubling of the clearance of a deposit of radiosodium. The implication is that sympathetic tonus is present in the forearm muscles but this tonic effect is more active in restriction of flow through the arteriovenous shunts than it is in restricting flow through the nutritive channels.

There are vasodilator fibers[5, 33] in muscle, but they have little effect on radiosodium clearance when the patient is at rest and may affect primarily the arteriovenous shunts.

The *hormonal* factors that are known to be effective are primarily the catecholamines. Epinephrine—whether from the adrenal gland or from exogenous sources—normally produces a direct vasodilator effect on arterioles in muscle. Indirectly it causes an increase in blood pressure and a secondary inhibition of vasoconstrictor tone. Norepinephrine, on the other hand, has primarily a direct vasoconstrictive effect. It should be recognized that norepinephrine administered to elevate blood pressure, and so to increase flow through a reconstructed artery, may produce the reverse effect if the arterial bed beyond the area of reconstruction responds to norepinephrine by vasoconstriction. Such a means of improving flow through an internal carotid shunt may be desirable, but is not so in the peripheral arteries of the aortoiliac and femoropopliteal system.

Metabolic factors play an important role in the control of hindrance in skeletal muscle and serve as a most effective mechanism for compensatory increases in arterial flow. The accumulation of metabolic products during exercise—whether lactic acid, carbon dioxide, other metabolites, or even a change in pH or oxygen tension—produces a profound reduction in arteriolar hindrance. Hall estimates this reduction at 13 times that produced by complete sympathetic block.

Mechanical factors also can cause inhibition of flow. Barcroft and Swan[4] (p. 52) have shown that restriction of flow is evident through a muscle contracting at 25 per cent of its maximal force, and at higher levels of contraction the flow may stop completely. The effect seems to be on larger vessels, since following relaxation flow increases to a higher level than the control, which suggests arteriolar dilatation. Complete cessation of flow during exercise may occur in patients with intermittent claudication, for here the arterial lesion, if severe enough, may lower the arterial pressure distal to the obstruction so that the compression from the contracting muscle is unusually effective in arresting the blood flow into that muscle.[34]

HYDRODYNAMIC FACTORS INFLUENCING BLOOD FLOW

A great oversimplification of the classic formulation of Poiseuille is:

$$Q = K \frac{\triangle P}{R}$$

> where Q is the volume flow
> K is the constant of proportionality
> $\triangle P$ is the pressure gradient (i.e., arterial pressure minus venous pressure)
> R is a group of factors constituting "resistance"

Each of these factors can be considered separately.

Pressure

The drop in pressure across the arterial system is generally to be considered the mean arterial pressure minus the venous pressure. In later portions of this chapter, the pressures on either side of an area of stenosis in the arterial tree are considered.

It is generally true, then, that anything that elevates the arterial pressure should augment flow, provided the factor of resistance remains constant. In fact, however, many pharmacologically active substances such as the vasopressor amines increase central arterial pressure by their effect on smaller arteries and arterioles. This effect may be salutary if the elevated pressure is then directed at segments of the vascular bed in which the pharmacologic effect has not been to increase the resistance (as in the coronary bed), but it may be catastrophic in reducing flow where resistance is thereby increased (as in the renal vascular bed).

Elevation of arterial pressure does not produce a linear increase in flow, because elasticity of the vessels allows them to distend and carry more flow than the simple pressure changes would suggest. Impairment of this elasticity by such changes as arteriosclerosis reduces their capacity for allowing increases of flow, and results in characteristic systolic hypertension.

At the lower end of the pressure scale is the phenomenon of the "critical closing pressure" in vessels of arteriolar size. The forces that tend to distend such a vessel are balanced by those that tend to compress it. Laplace's law states that, at equilibrium, the tension in the vessel wall occasioned by the pressure within is proportional to the product of that pressure times the radius. Thus, at lower pressures and diameters there occurs a point at which the tensions of the muscle of the wall and the external tissue pressures cause the arterioles to collapse. The figure given for arterioles by Guyton is about 20 mm. of mercury.[17] The pressure necessary to reopen such a vessel is slightly greater. The critical closing pressure of capillaries perfused with plasma is considerably less — about 5 mm. of mercury.

Similarly, an elevation in venous pressure results in some diminution of flow. The quantitative aspects of this situation are small, but the resultant effect of increasing capillary pressure may bring about a shift in the equilibrium expressed in Starling's law so that more fluid passes through the capillary wall. This in turn may ultimately lead to increased edema and increased tissue pressure, and diminished capillary function. Clinical aspects of this phenomenon are discussed in Chapter Six.

Pulsatile flow is introduced by intermittent increases in pressure. The considerable body of information available on the aspects of pulsatile flow is made less important and the controversy concerning the merits of pulsatile or nonpulsatile flow made less meaningful by the evidence of Wesolowski.[36] Pulsatile flow in isolated perfusion systems of whole animals with intact vasomotor regulation is not more effective than nonpulsatile flow. Pulsatile flow induces more effective lymphatic circulation, and has been shown to be more effective in maintaining liver function than nonpulsatile flow, but this is a special and isolated phenomenon.[10]

Resistance

There are two major components to resistance: the viscosity of the liquid and the tube factor or hindrance, based on the size, shape, smoothness, branching, and other aspects of the vessel wall itself.

Blood is a nonhomogeneous or non-Newtonian fluid. Thus, it shows some divergence from a strict inverse relationship between flow and viscosity at constant pressure, but most of these effects and those of "plasma skimming" occur in smaller vessels in the capillary tree than will concern us. For most purposes, the viscosity of blood is dependent upon its percentage composition of red cells and plasma.[8] Whittaker and Winton[37] perfused the hind legs of dogs with blood of various hematocrit levels. If a perfusion pressure of 80 mm. of mercury and a hematocrit level of 49 per cent were used to obtain a normal flow, then increasing the hematocrit level to 65 per cent reduced the flow by 26 per cent. Decreasing the hematocrit level to 29.5 per cent resulted in an increase in flow of 22 per cent.

Red cell aggregation or sludging occurs within the smallest vessels, especially under conditions of shock, but this form of increased viscosity is a special one, again, not strictly within the purview of this discussion. Low molecular weight dextran, fibrinolysins, and heparin are all useful in controlling the tendency toward sludging.

Those factors relating to the status of the arterial wall itself—the tube factors—are of great importance to the surgeon in his understanding of clinical symptoms and ability to perform his reconstructive surgery.

Green[16] has presented figures quantitatively defining the vessel-produced resistance to flow, or hindrance, assignable to various levels of the *normal* patent vascular system:

Vessel	*Total Flow Resistance* (per cent)
Aorta to beginning of terminal arteries	2
Terminal arteries and arterioles	72
Capillaries	16
Veins	10

It may be seen from this tabulation that the normal arterial system offers little hindrance in the levels at which direct surgical intervention is feasible, and that the terminal arteries and arterioles provide most of the hindrance. Because the smaller vessels are normally subject to tonic vasoconstrictor activity by the sympathectic nerves, sympathectomy may be highly effective in increasing blood flow. (These vessels, however, spontaneously recover much of their constrictor tone within a few days after sympathectomy.)

These vessels are also, particularly in muscle, subject to vasodilatation by metabolic factors arising in exercise or in hypoxic states. These factors normally operate to adjust blood flow to the local metabolic activity by changing local resistance.

This mechanism makes possible a normal blood flow in spite of the presence of considerable arterial obstruction. It can explain how the skin of an extremity may remain warm and show a normal color even though the lumen of the feeding artery is much reduced.

However, the capacity of the arterioles to dilate in response to reduced blood flow is limited. Arterial obstruction greater than a critical value may not prevent an adequate blood flow at rest, but this may require so much vasodilatation that the additional dilatation required in exercise cannot occur. Accordingly, the blood flow increments needed to supply adequate oxygen to the muscles in exercise may not develop. Under these conditions claudication will occur.

An important consequence of these facts is that a very considerable reduction in the diameter of an artery can occur without there being much increase in total resistance. In fact, it is not until the cross-section area reaches about one-half the control that blood flow is reduced significantly.[31] If the narrowed region of the artery is one-tenth of the distance from the aortic valve to the largest arterioles, the resistance in the arteries will be raised to a level of about 5 per cent above normal. All factors being unchanged, this will reduce the flow by about 5 per cent. The fact that there is no decrease in flow results from a metabolically evoked compensatory dilatation of the arterioles sufficient to restore the flow to normal.

The single artery in which only one segment is stenotic is an ideally simplified system. In practice, such a system is modified by the collateral flow around it, and the system as a whole must be considered in terms of all resistance factors. Resistances in series in a system can be considered as additive; resistance of a system in series is determined similarly to electrical resistance.

The resistance through a series of tubes in parallel thus becomes

$$R \text{ (total)} = \cfrac{1}{\cfrac{1}{R_1} + \cfrac{1}{R_2} + \cfrac{1}{R_3} + \ldots\ldots}$$

Guyton[17] simplifies the estimation of resistance through a parallel circuit by pointing out that the resistance of a series of vessels of equal size in parallel is equal to the resistance of one such vessel divided by the number of vessels in the series.

The importance of the collateral networks will be discussed in subsequent pages, but here it may be well to emphasize that, in a system of parallel tubes arising from a single tube, the flow will be partitioned among them inversely as their individual resistances. In each case the resistance will be the sum of that in the arterioles (normally the dominant component) and that in the arteries (significant only in the presence of lesions).

Resistance to flow by a given segment of vessel, stenotic or normal, must now be considered apart from flow throughout the entire vascular tree and the compensatory mechanisms that affect it.

The most efficient type of flow is *laminar*; that is to say, all particles of the fluid are migrating in a straight line parallel to the walls of the conduit. Here, flow can be conceived of as sheets, or concentric layers, slipping over one another.

Turbulent flow is nonlaminar flow; particles move randomly in any direction, rather than parallel to the axis of the conduit. Turbulent flow is much less efficient; more energy is required to maintain a given volume with turbulent flow than with laminar flow.

Turbulent flow may arise from eddy formation, or because conditions of flow exceed the limitation of the Reynolds number.

Reynolds in 1883[26] observed flow in a smooth-walled tube and noted that usually at lower flow rates flow was smooth and axial. Disturbances of this axial pattern were soon damped out. At higher levels of flow, a critical point was reached at which turbulence ensued. The critical point was found to be dependent on the diameter of the tube, the mean velocity of the flow, and the density and viscosity of the liquid. The Reynolds number (for circular tubes) is expressed mathematically as

$$Re = \frac{V\,Dp}{\mu}$$

where V is the average velocity of flow
D is the diameter of the tube
p is the density of the liquid
μ is the viscosity

This relationship can be modified to apply to tubes of any shape.[21] The critical value usually given for the Reynolds number is about 2000, but under unusual circumstances laminar flow can be maintained at much higher figures, or turbulence may be encountered at lower figures. The latter does occur, for example, during systolic flow through the abdominal aorta of the rabbit when early turbulence appears at a Reynolds number of about 1000.[21]

The effect of introducing a curve into a straight tube is to increase the stability of the flow. One of the most critical areas of the circulatory system might be expected to be the proximal aorta; the curve of the aortic arch may provide an element of stability. The presence of major branches on the greater curvature of the arch may allow some blood at the site of maximum shear (the rate of "slippage" of one layer of fluid onto another) to be milked off into them and so to increase the stability further. Flow ordinarily follows a helical pattern around such a curve. The surgeon, therefore, need not worry if a graft or prosthesis does not pass in a perfectly straight course, for a gentle curve will not produce turbulent flow.

Flow at a bifurcation such as the aortoiliac junction is ordinarily from a region of higher to one of lower turbulence. The size of the branching vessels and the resistance—and thus the velocity of flow—play a role in these formulations. At a bifurcation into equal divisions the cross-sectional area must increase by a factor of $\sqrt{2}$ or 1.414 in order for resistance (as measured by volume flow) to remain the same. The usual figure quoted for the ratio of the areas at a bifurcation is 1.26; thus, one can ordinarily expect a higher resistance and an elevated upstream pressure.

The presence of a sharply defined projection (Fig. 3–1) would be expected to produce eddies and turbulence and to have a greater effect in critical situations, that is, in those with higher Reynolds numbers. For evaluation of the importance of a sharp-edged projection, McDonald[21] cites the following formulation

$$\frac{\epsilon}{r} < 4/(Re)^{1/2}$$

for laminar flow to be maintained. In this formulation
ϵ is the height of the sharp-edged projection

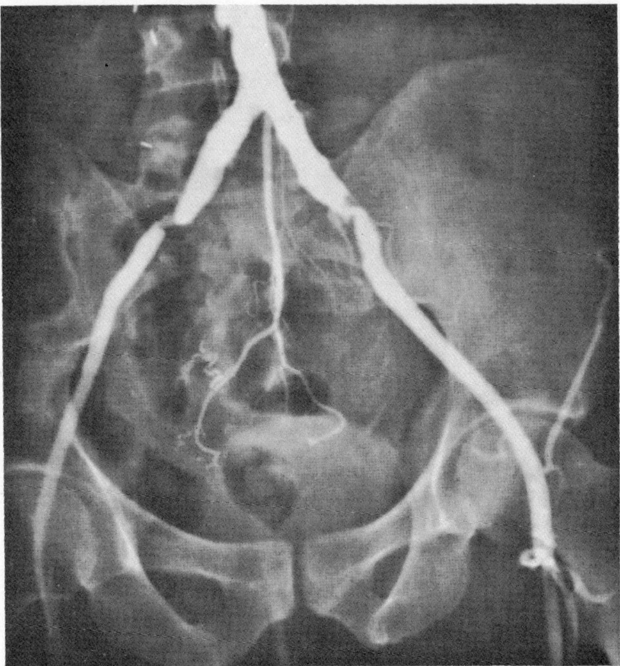

Figure 3–1.   Area of recurrent atherosclerosis suggests shape of diaphragm (believed to be at site of application of occluding clamps during aortoiliac endarterectomy that had been performed 5½ years previously) which caused a loud bruit and symptoms of severe claudication. Bypass of atherosclerotic segment brought about complete relief of symptoms.

> r is the radius of the tube and
> Re is the Reynolds number

Other types of turbulence have been described by Wesolowski.[35] They may result from local factors which cause the Reynolds number to exceed the critical level or they may simply represent the more obvious eddy formation and interference with laminar flow. The third, fourth, and fifth types of turbulence described by Wesolowski are those found at sites of anatomical expansion, those at sites of *relative* anatomical expansion (or *dynamic* expansion), and those just within the orifices of branches.

It can be seen that the introduction of stenosis is apt to introduce turbulence, and the actual reduction in flow may be greater than anticipated on the basis of calculations which do not take turbulence into consideration.

In estimating the flow of blood through a stenotic vessel, discussion usually begins with a classical relationship formulated by Poiseuille:

$$Q = \frac{K \cdot \Delta P \cdot r^4}{n\ l}$$

where Q = volume flow
   K = a constant
   ΔP = pressure drop along the tube
   r = tube radius
   n = fluid viscosity
   L = tube length

This equation holds strictly only for steady flow of a homogeneous fluid through a straight rigid tube on constant bore. Obviously, it cannot be used in quantitating flow through a stenotic area. For this Byar and associates[6] have studied fluid flow through tubes with stenoses of various degrees. In an investigation more directly applicable to flow under clinical conditions, May and others[22] have derived a mathematical model for the flow of blood through a stenotic region of a tube, based on Poiseuille's law modified to take into account the energy losses at the entrance to the stenosis ("the contraction component") and at the exit ("the expansion component"). The equation is as follows:

$$\Delta P = \Delta P_S + \Delta P_C + \Delta P_E$$

$$= \frac{8\mu L}{R_1^2} V_1 \left(\frac{A_1}{A_2}\right)^2 + \frac{4.8\mu}{R_1}\left(\frac{A_1}{A_2}\right)^{1.5} + \rho \cdot V_1^2 \left(\frac{A_1}{A_2}\right)^2$$

where ΔP = total pressure drop
   ΔP_S = pressure drop in the narrowed segment
   ΔP_C = pressure drop from the contraction
   ΔP_E = pressure drop from the expansion
   μ = fluid viscosity
   L = length of the stenosis
   R_1 = radius of the unstenosed lumen
   A_1 = area of lumen of unstenosed vessel
   A_2 = area of lumen of the stenosis
   V_1 = linear velocity of flow in prestenotic segment
   ρ = density of the fluid

The authors demonstrated the applicability of this model to segments of the aortoiliac vessels of the dog, where the pressures were measured above and below the stenoses, the flow electromagnetically, and the luminal diameters determined by latex casts of the arteries. Stenoses of varying diameters and lengths were used.

As predicted by the model, the blood through stenoses of greater narrowing showed little change until the area was reduced to 20 per cent of the original value, whereupon the flow fell precipitously with further narrowing (Fig. 3–2A). Similarly, the pressure drop across the stenosis did not exceed 5 mm. Hg until the narrowing reached an area of 20 per cent of the normal (Fig. 3–2B). As expected, the reduction of flow was an inverse linear function of the increase in pressure drop.

The length of the stenotic segment in the noncritical range of stenosis had little effect on flow, but became significant in the critical range. For example, in the presence of a stenosis reducing area to 20 per cent, a fourfold increase in stenosis length reduces flow by about 25 per cent.

In the studies of May and others,[22] the surface of the endothelium of the arteries was smooth and uninterrupted. In diseased arteries this is not the case, especially where atherosclerotic plaques deform the surface. To estimate the hemodynamic significance of this roughening, Schultz et al.[29] carried out experiments similar to those of May, except that specimens of human aorta and iliac arteries with varying degrees of narrowing, dilatation, and plaque formation from atherosclerosis were excised and perfused at various pump outputs and the pressure drop across the preparation determined. In those with minimal atherosclerotic lesions the pressure drop rose gradually with flow, but even at 50 cc. per second it remained below 5 mm. of mercury. As the lesions became more severe, especially by producing stenosis or plaques projecting irregularly into the lumen, the pressure drop increased, progressively more sharply with flow, to values as high as 30 to 50 mm. of mercury even though the stenosis never in this series reduced the patent cross-sectional area to 20 per cent of the original value (Fig. 3–3).

However, in both normal and diseased arteries the principle

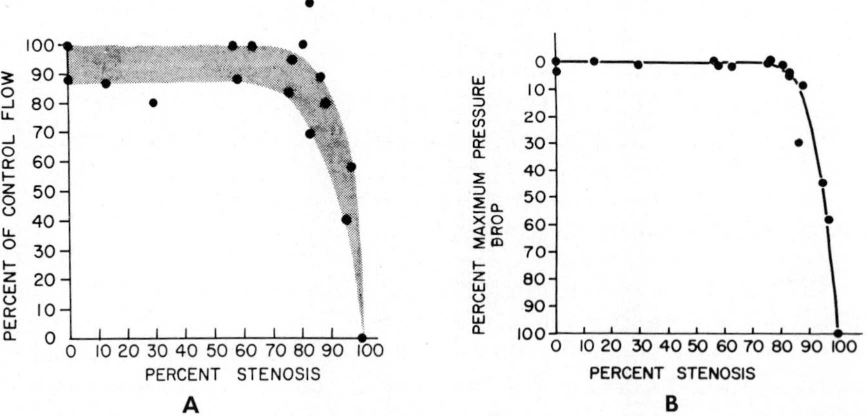

Figure 3–2. *A,* Relation of blood flow to increasing arterial stenosis. *B,* Relation of pressure drop to increase in stenosis. (From May, A. G., DeWeese, J. A., and Robb, C. G.: Surgery, 53:513, 1963.[22] Reprinted by permission of the authors and the C. V. Mosby Company.)

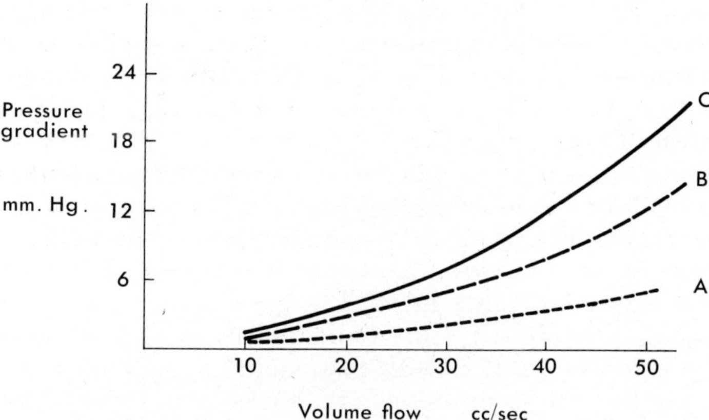

Figure 3–3. Pressure gradients generated by varying volume flow: A, normal aortoiliac specimen; B, specimen with major intimal plaques and stenosis reducing luminal area by 3 to 36 per cent; C, specimen with severe intimal disease and stenosis reducing luminal area by about 50 per cent. (Smoothed curves redrawn from Figures 3, 4 and 5 in Schultz, R. D., Hokanson, B. S., and Strandness, D. E.: Surg. Gynec. Obstet. *124*:1267, 1967.[29] Reprinted by permission of the authors and of Surgery Gynecology and Obstetrics.)

remains valid that the magnitude of the pressure drop across the stenotic segment is a function of the rate of blood flow. Accordingly, measurements of the pressure drop made immediately after exercise of the part involved provide valuable information in addition to those made in the resting state.

The role of viscosity is implied in Poiseuille's formulations. Fiddian[13] has constructed a curve of nonlinear flow rates, using both sucrose syrup and human plasma and blood, on which it can be seen that flow is greater at lower viscosities. Cranley's clinical observations[8] and Schenk's studies[28] have also shown that changes in viscosity affect rate of flow.

One further phenomenon of importance is the obliteration of palpable arterial pulsation that sometimes occurs following exercise. Ejrup[11] has studied this condition intensively, as has DeWeese,[9] who suggests that it is merely the manifestation of an increase in rate of flow through the muscle. The increase can be compared to the accentuated peak of the prestenotic pulse (proximal to an "obstruction"—this being the normal resistance of the muscle bed at rest) which is abolished when the obstruction is removed (or when the resistance falls during exercise as a consequence of the effect of the accumulation of metabolites). The weakening of the pulse is normal, but the presence of a proximal stenotic lesion accentuates the degree of weakening.

When collateral flow is satisfactory, and there may be considerable variation in peripheral resistance, measurements of pressure differentials across a stenotic lesion are apt to be confusing and not accurately indicative of the augmentation of flow that may be achieved by removal of that stenosis.

If the system is conceived of as a completely obstructed artery and its collateral branches as the "stenosis," the importance of pressure measurements in vascular surgery can be appreciated. Such measurement may not be significant in surgery of the aortoiliac-femoral systems yet it may be vital in the simpler systems of the carotid and renal arteries. Failure to demonstrate a significant gradient in pressure across a stenotic area that might for anatomical reasons be expected to be critical implies a high degree of peripheral resistance. Unless this high peripheral resistance can be reduced, correction of the stenosis will not relieve the impairment of flow. In an obstructed system of arteries in which there is an intact series of compensating mechanisms able to control (reduce) the peripheral resistance, and good collaterals, a small gradient across the major obstruction with the patient *at rest* is not necessarily ominous. Where major collateral systems do not exist, as, for instance, in the kidney, high peripheral resistance is indicated by the low gradient and suggests that restoration of arterial continuity and removal of the obstruction will not be particularly effective.

Applying Fiddian's thesis in respect to viscosity of fluid (p. 49), various investigators have found the critical reduction of the lumen to be in the range of one fourth and one fifth the cross-sectional area of the unobstructed artery. This finding should, in turn, suggest that most of the arteries we are discussing are four to five times larger than necessary. It might be said that a factor of safety of four or five exists which allows flow to continue relatively unimpeded even in face of considerable encroachment on the lumen by atherosclerotic plaques.

The smaller or hypoplastic arteries seen in the Leriche syndrome and described earlier (p. 14) thus gain added significance. Their involvement in symptomatic arterial disease may arise because their small size predisposes them to abnormalities of flow and premature localization of atheroma, or because less artheroma is required to produce encroachment of critical proportions early in the course of the disease.

Turbulent flow is important for other reasons. First, excessive turbulence gives rise to vibrations which may be recognized as murmurs or thrills. Second, if turbulence is a factor in localized deposition of atheroma, a cycle of mechanical stenotic abnormality may be initiated leading to further stenosis and atheroma.

Pulse Contours and Plethysmography

The volume changes of a digit, as determined plethysmographically, occurring during a cardiac cycle, except under extreme conditions, reflect the amplitude and time relations of the input of blood into the veins of the part, according to the study of Strandness and collaborators.[32] The amplitude normally depends, to a large measure, inversely on the degree of local vasoconstriction. The shape of the curve, normally a sharp spike with a dicrotic notch on the descending limb, reflects venous volume changes without significant arterial obstruction. With increasing arterial obstruction, the curve shape changes — first, the dicrotic notch disappears, then the peak is replaced by a rounded summit. Fourier analysis of these curves reveals that changes beyond the obstruction occur in the amplitude, not of the fundamental frequency component but of the second to sixth harmonics, which show that the arterial stenoses and irregularities result in the selective absorption of the higher frequency components of the pulse flow wave. To the extent that the lesions reduce blood flow they will also reduce the amplitude of the pulse wave.

FLOW IN COLLATERAL VESSELS

The basic patterns of collateral flow around obstructions usually follow standard anatomical pathways, i.e., lumbar and inferior mesenteric branches to hypogastric artery, lumbar and inferior mesenteric to hypogastric to deep femoral artery, or genicular artery, as seen in Figures 2–4, 2–6, 2–7, 2–13 to 2–16. Only infrequently does the surgeon encounter unexpected channels, and usually they can be recognized by adequate angiographic studies.

Widening of the internal spermatic artery, with a terminal outflow tract in the groin, predisposes the patient to distal ischemia if, because its importance is unrecognized, the vessel is injured during dissection in the region of the ureter and the spermatic artery (p. 25).

Pudendal branches communicating across the midline can also be easily damaged, with a subsequent increase in ischemia to the limb.

Congenital absence of a main trunk produces extensive collateral networks, and acquired lesions of very long standing may approximate such patterns.

It has been shown by Winblad[38] that the collateral pathways which develop when acute ligation is done were already present; that is, new branches do not arise, but the already existing pathways come into use, in many instances with a different direction of flow. With time, these channels do indeed increase in caliber, but this is a relatively slow process.

John[19] and Winblad[38] have shown that the initial stimulus to the development of collateral vessels is the rapid development of a pressure gradient across the site of sudden obstruction. The later stimulus may arise partly from a continuing small gradient with the patient at rest, but arises principally from the gradients of higher pressure brought on by diminished peripheral resistance under conditions of metabolic demand, such as exercise.

The severity of impairment to flow following acute obstruction depends first upon anatomical variation and second upon the occurrence of atherosclerosis that might require secondary arcades to be used, at the cost of considerable efficiency.

The collateral arteries themselves are usually not those of a size commonly susceptible to atherosclerosis. Their origins, however, may become affected because of continuing atherosclerosis of the main lines.

An example of the situation just described is the relatively quick recovery from an ischemic episode by a patient who happened to have a very large and dominant deep femoral artery. Occlusion of the superficial femoral artery was quickly conpensated for through the major descending branches of the deep femoral artery, and after a brief period of ischemia symptoms disappeared almost completely.

Occlusion of lower lumbar and inferior mesenteric arteries by aortic atherosclerosis is an example of the second type of difficulty in developing collaterals. In this case, occlusion of the common iliac arteries requires that collaterals descend from intercostals, from internal mammary to inferior epigastric route, or via the superior mesenteric artery, the marginal artery of Drummond and the left colic bed.

Insofar as collateral branches are almost invariably small and tortuous, and longer than the primary channel, the flow resistance is greater than that of the main artery before obstruction and, consequently, the distal pressure is reduced. Since, as stated in Poiseuille's equation, flow depends on the fourth power of the radius, vessels as small as the collaterals would each carry a very small blood flow. Consequently, many channels would be needed for effective compensation. The increased length of the channels also increases the resistance, and their tortuosity not only increases the length but makes for less efficient flow.

The comment from page 40 must be repeated here with regard to collateral flow, and this is the type of tissue through which the collateral channel passes. Retroperitoneal or subcutaneous pathways suffer only rare extrinsic encroachments. Major channels through muscle, however, may suffer considerable reduction in flow. At even the moderate contraction of 25 per cent of maximal force, restriction of flow is evident; at full contraction, flow may be completely arrested.[4, 34]

THE "STEAL" PHENOMENON

Considerable interest has been taken during recent years in such phenomena as the "subclavian steal," in which obstruction of the subclavian artery is present between the origin of the common carotid and that of the vertebral artery. Blood flow in the vertebral artery is reversed, and blood flow passes through the basilar artery into the vertebral so as to threaten brain stem ischemia and consequent functional impairment. Similar "steals" can occur in other arterial systems, for example, the "proximal steal" in patients with intermittent claudication, in whom after exercise blood flow is higher in muscles just distal to the obstruction than in those more distal.[1]

In the analysis of this phenomenon, specifically the "subclavian steal," it should first be recognized that, if all the arteries carrying blood to the circle of Willis and basilar artery were without peripheral resistance then subclavian occlusion would have no effect on either brain stem or arm blood flow. In the normal situation, in which the arterial resistance is about four per cent of the total peripheral resistance, the three afferent arteries would carry less blood to the basilar artery than would the usual four, but only slightly less, because arteriolar vasodilatation would compensate fairly effectively. Further, in the presence of abnormally high resistance in one or more of the afferent arteries, the flow and pressure will be proportionately reduced in the basilar artery.

The blood in this region will then flow into the brain stem and other head structures, and into the arm via reversed flow in the vertebral, and in inverse proportion to the resistances of the several vascular beds. Because the flow resistance in the brain is markedly less than that in the arm, it will be reduced from its relatively high normal level more than that in other tissues — with the consequent possibility of brain stem ischemia.

Thus, there are the following hemodynamic aspects of the "steal" phenomenon:

1. the presence of sufficiently high resistance in the arteries feeding the region where ischemia is significant, with consequent fall of pressure in these central arteries;
2. a decrease in central arterial pressure and consequent decrease in the total flow to the brain and involved arm; and
3. a redistribution of the decreased total blood flow between the brain and arm in inverse ratio of their local resistances.

REFERENCES

1. Alpert, I. S., Larsen, D. A., and Lassen, N. A.: Evaluation of arterial insufficiency of the legs: A comparison of arteriography and the ^{133}Xe walking test. Cardiovasc. Res. 2:161, 1968.
2. Atlas, L. N.: Lumbar sympathectomy in the treatment of peripheral arteriosclerotic disease. Am. Heart J. 23:493, 1942.
3. Berne, R. M., and Levy, M. N.: *Cardiovascular Physiology*. Saint Louis, C. V. Mosby Co., 1967, p. 123.
4. Barcroft, H., and Swan, H. J. C.: *Sympathetic Control of Human Blood Vessels*. London, Edward Arnold Ltd., 1953.
5. Burn, J. H.: Sympathetic vasodilator fibers. Physiol. Rev. 18:137, 1938.
6. Byar, D., Fiddian, R. V., Quereau, M., Hobbs, J. T., and Edwards, E. A.: The fallacy of applying the Poiseuille equation to segmental arterial stenosis. Am. Heart J. 70:216, 1965.
7. Callow, A. D., Aboulafia, E. D., and Balas, P. E.: The restrictive effect of bypass grafts upon the occluded major arterial channel and its collaterals. Surgery 49:26, 1961.
8. Cranley, J. J., Fogarty, T. J., Krause, R. J., Strasser, E. S., and Hafner, C. D.: Phlebotomy for moderate erythrocytemia. J.A.M.A. 186:206, 1963.
9. DeWeese, J. A., Van de Berg, L., May, A. G., and Rob, C. G.: Stenoses of arteries of the lower extremity. Arch. Surg. 89:806, 1964.
10. Eiseman, B.: Personal communication.
11. Ejrup, B.: Tonoscillography after exercise; new method for early diagnosis of organic arterial disease leading to intermittent claudication and for differential diagnosis of organic and functional arterial diseases with special type of apparatus adapted to this purpose. Acta Med. Scand. (Supplement 211), 130:1, 1948.
12. Felder, D. A., Linton, R. R., Todd, D. P., and Banks, C.: Changes in the sympathectomized extremity with anesthesia. Surgery 29:803, 1951.
13. Fiddian, R. V., Byar, D., and Edwards, E. A.: Factors affecting flow through a stenosed vessel. Arch. Surg. 88:83, 1964.
14. Fox, R. H., and Hilton, S. M.: Bradykinin formation in human skin as a factor in heat vasodilation. J. Physiol. 142:219, 1958.
15. Freeman, N. E., Leeds, F. H., and Gardner, R. E.: Sympathectomy for obliterative vascular disease; indications and contraindications. Ann. Surg. 126:873, 1947.
16. Green, H. D.: In Glasser, O.: *Medical Physics*. Chicago, Year Book Publishers, 1952, Vol. 2, p. 531.
17. Guyton, A. C.: *Textbook of Medical Physiology*. 3rd ed. Philadelphia, W. B. Saunders Co., 1966.
18. Hall, V. E.: In Barker, W. F. (Ed.): *The Surgical Treatment of Peripheral Vascular Disease*. New York, McGraw-Hill Book Co., 1962, Chap. 1.
19. John, H. T., and Warren, R.: The stimulus to collateral circulation. Surgery 49:14, 1961.
20. Lamport, H.: In Fulton, J. F. (Ed.): *A Textbook of Physiology*. 17th ed. Philadelphia, W. B. Saunders Co., 1955, Chap. 31.
21. McDonald, D. A.: *Blood Flow in Arteries*. London, Edward Arnold, Ltd., 1960.
22. May, A. G., DeWeese, J. A., and Rob, C. G.: Hemodynamic effects of arterial stenosis. Surgery 53:513, 1963.
23. May, A. G., Van de Berg, L., DeWeese, J. A., and Rob, C. G.: Critical arterial stenosis. Surgery 54:250, 1963.
24. Piiper, J., and Schoedel, W.: Untersuchungen über die Durchblutung der arteriovenösen Anastomosen in der hinteren Extremität des Hundes mit Hilfe von Kugeln verscheidener Grösse. Pflügers Arch. Ges. Physiol. 258:489, 1953.
25. Redisch, W., Wertheimer, L., Delisle, C., and Steele, J. M.: Comparison of various vascular beds in man; their responses to a simple vasodilator stimulus. Circulation 9:63, 1954.
26. Reynolds, O.: Phil. Trans. Roy. Soc. London A174:935, 1883.
27. Saunders, R. L.: In Redisch, W., and Tangco, F. F.: *Peripheral Circulation in Health and Disease*. New York, Grune & Stratton, 1957, Part 5.

28. Schenk, W. G., Jr., Delin, N. A., Domanig, E., Hahnloser, P., and Hoyt, R. K.: Blood viscosity as a determinant of regional blood flow. Arch. Surg. *89*:783, 1964.
29. Schultz, R. D., Hokanson, B. S., and Strandness, D. E.: Pressure flow and stress-strain measurements of normal and diseased aortoiliac segments. Surg. Gynec. Obstet. *124*:1267, 1967.
30. Shepherd, J. T.: *Physiology of the Circulation in Human Limbs in Health and Disease.* Philadelphia, W. B. Saunders Co., 1963.
31. Shipley, R. E., and Gregg, D. E.: The effect of external constriction of a blood vessel on blood flow. Am. J. Physiol. *141*:289, 1944.
32. Strandness, D. E.: *Peripheral Arterial Disease: A Physiological Approach.* Boston, Little, Brown and Co., 1969.
33. Uvnäs, B.: Sympathetic vasodilator outflow. Physiol. Rev. *34*:608, 1954.
34. Walder, D. N.: A technique for investigating the blood supply of muscle during exercise. Brit. Med. J. *1*:255, 1958.
35. Wesolowski, S. A., Fries, C. C., and Sawyer, P. N.: The production and significance of turbulence in hemic systems. Trans. Am. Soc. Artif. Int. Organs 8:11, 1962.
36. Wesolowski, S. A., Sauvage, L. R., and Pinc, R. D.: Extracorporeal circulation: the role of the pulse in maintenance of the systemic circulation during heart-lung by-pass. Surgery 37:663, 1955.
37. Whittaker, S. R. F., and Winton, F. R.: The apparent viscosity of blood flowing in the isolated hindlimb of the dog, and its variation with corpuscular concentration. J. Physiol. 78:339, 1933.
38. Winblad, J. N., Reemtsma, K., Vernhet, J. L., Laville, L. P., and Creech, O. C., Jr.: Etiologic mechanisms in the development of collateral circulation. Surgery *45*:105, 1959.

Chapter Four

PATHOLOGY AND PATHOGENESIS

The exact diagnosis, the roentgenologic and microscopical findings, and the depth of the plaque are essential details to the vascular surgeon in planning treatment for his patients; he is likely to be less concerned about cytological details, cell pedigree, and the like. The diagnosis, which will be discussed in the next chapter, depends upon clinical rather than pathologic observations. Roentgenologic observations are of great importance and will be discussed with other clinical material.

ATHEROSCLEROSIS

As far as the vascular surgeon is concerned, the commonest occlusive lesion of consequence is atherosclerosis, which he often refers to by the more descriptive clinical term, *arteriosclerosis obliterans.* The disease is distinct from arteriolar sclerosis, although the two lesions are so common that they frequently coexist.

When the vascular surgeon speaks of small vessel disease he should make it clear whether he is speaking of atherosclerosis in the smaller arteries, such as the tibial or proper digital arteries, or of arterial lesions of a much more diffuse pattern, such as arteriolosclerosis or arteriolonecrosis.

Atherosclerotic lesions are usually diffuse, but the characteristic that makes surgical intervention possible is the tendency of extensive deposits to be localized so that occlusion occurs segmentally in major arteries. Multiple diffuse lesions in many small arteries are not correctable surgically.

The earliest lesions are small yellow plaques and streaks that develop in the intima, and tend to coalesce and to enlarge (Fig. 4–1). Microscopically these deposits consist of various lipids, including cholesterol and cholesterol esters, and various triglycerides (Fig. 4–2). Lipids appear primarily in phagocytes. Fibrosis increases and portions of the plaque become amorphous and hyaline: in these areas are to be seen the cholesterol clefts so commonly described. Calcification in the areas in which lipid has been deposited is not uncommon, and is seen occasionally in roentgenograms. Loss of endothelium from the surface of the plaques results in ulceration, and mural thrombi form in the ulcerated areas (Fig. 4–3).

At times the degenerative processes of atherosclerosis cause interference with the nutrition of the blood vessel and may produce considerable softening rather than sclerosis of the vessel.

The rapidity of flow over the lesions restricts propagation of thrombi to a considerable degree. The presence of clots in various degrees of maturation suggests that they ultimately undergo incorporation as fibrous elements in the plaque. The plaque tends to become

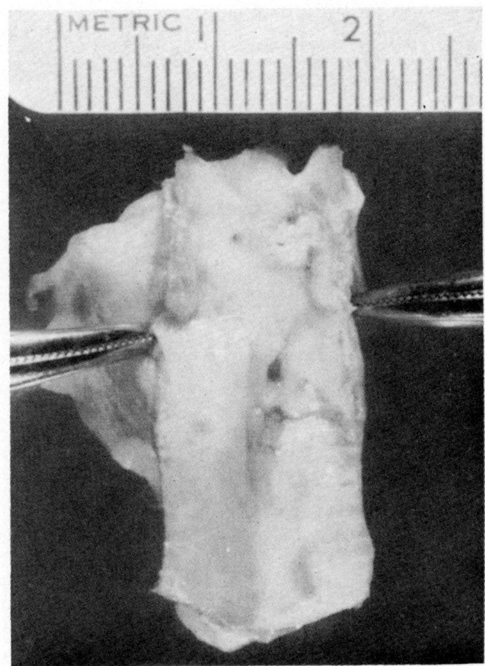

Figure 4–1. Endothelial surface of a short segment of femoral artery. Note early changes of diffuse atherosclerosis, and irregularity and thickening of intimal surface. More advanced changes are indicated by presence of small irregular well-localized opaque plaques of fatty deposits.

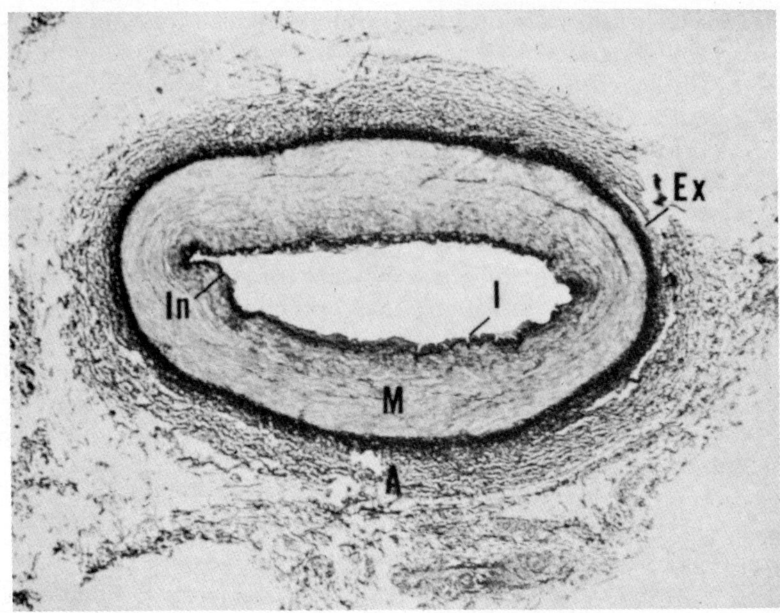

Figure 4–2. Microphotograph of cross section of small normal femoral artery. Autopsy specimen from young adult. Thin intima (I) is seen lining internal elastic membrane (In). (M) is tunica media, in which are seen a few branching elastic fibers. External elastic membrane (Ex) is densely stained. Fibrous side of tissue surrounds entire vessel. Elastic tissue stain.

self-perpetuating because of accretion of clot and also because of turbulence and pressure, which of themselves contribute to local deposition of atheroma.

Pathogenesis

That local factors as well as systemic ones contribute to the pathogenesis of atherosclerosis is suggested by the localization that occurs in the larger arteries, near bifurcations, and the infrequency with which smaller muscular arteries are involved.

Theories regarding pathogenesis are controversial and have been discussed in the literature at great length. A few of these will be mentioned briefly, and more detailed discussion will be presented regarding the surgeon's role in arterial reconstruction. Katz,[19] Windsor,[44] and Dayton[8] have written at length on these theories.

Metabolic Theory

Support for the *metabolic theory* derives from the findings of cholesterol and other lipids on the atheromatous lesions, the findings of increased atheromatous lesions in clinical conditions associated with hypercholesteremia, and the production of experimental lesions by the induction of hypercholesteremia in animals not ordinarily susceptible to atherosclerosis. Atherosclerosis does occur in the absence of what is usually recognized as hypercholesteremia; thus metabolic aspects other than absolute lipid levels must be considered.

The abnormally low proportion of cholesterol esters in atheromatous as opposed to normal aortas was described by Windaus.[42] Other abnormalities of lipid constituents have undoubted significance, including the ratio between cholesterol and phospholipids and the relationship between atherosclerosis and a high proportion of Sf 12-100 molecules.

Dietary intake is important, but its exact role is controversial. The most popular concept holds that deposition of atheroma is restricted by the ingestion of limited dietary fat, of which a high proportion is polyunsaturated. A recent observation[33] suggests that the aortic wall synthesizes some of the fat and cholesterol in the lesions. These authors believe that the factor which initiates this process stems from a deficiency of polyunsaturated fatty acids and that many local enzymic changes can be correlated with this phenomenon.

Certainly lipids other than cholesterol take part in the formation of atheromata, and excessive fat in the diet of any one kind is reflected to some degree in the composition of body fats.

The experiments of Ahrens[1] and of others[3, 5, 20, 21] indicate that plasma cholesterol levels can be reduced by low fat diets in which the limited fat content is high in polyunsaturated fats. Whether this is because of an increased output of cholesterol as bile acids or because of actual inhibition of synthesis of cholesterol is not known. It is assumed that lowered plasma cholesterol and lipid levels are favorable; it has been reported that peripheral pulses have been re-established on such a diet, but this has also happened without dietary changes.

It is difficult to obtain clear-cut evidence of the role of diet in a disease as variable as atherosclerosis when there are so many other factors. According to Rutstein's studies[31] of human aortic cells in tissue culture, each person has a characteristic level of serum triglycerides and cholesterol at which intracellular fat accumulates. Intracellular lipid deposition after ingestion of fat is directly related to the amount of fat ingested and is greater after intake of polyunsaturated fat. The increase in deposition of fat in the postprandial period is related to a rise in serum triglycerides and possibly to an increase in phospholipids, but is independent of the total cholesterol concentration, which remains constant during these short-term alimentary changes.

During fasting there is a steady rise in deposition of intracellular lipids unrelated to concentration of serum triglycerides, phospholipids, or cholesterol.

Ingestion of carbohydrate is followed by suppression in deposition of intracellular lipid, and this occurs without significant change in the concentration of any of the major serum lipids.

Rutstein has remarked on the apparent contradictions implied in these observations. He points out that there is a consistent tendency for single test meals of polyunsaturated fats to be followed by greater deposition of intracellular fat than comparable isolated meals of saturated fat. Consistent ingestion of a diet rich in polyunsaturated fat, however, tends to reduce the concentration of cholesterol in fasting serum, and lower fasting levels of cholesterol are associated in general with lower rates of intracellular deposition. He describes this difference as the "difference between the 'sea-level' effect of baseline lipid measurements in the serum and the 'fat-tide' effect of postprandial lipemia." Rutstein's important work may not be directly applicable to clinical problems.

The occurrence of atheromatous lesions on the surface of synthetic grafts[9, 10] suggests that arteriosclerosis is specifically related to the effect of serum lipids on other cellular components as well as aortic, although the pedigree of the cellular material that has grown into the fabric graft may perpetuate the metabolic pattern of the original vessel.

In the preceding paragraphs appear many statements that may seem disparate but perhaps may be drawn together in a more rational scheme by a brief discussion of the current classifications of the hyperlipoproteinemias.

These are defined by Fredrickson and others,[11, 14] and represent in plasma a sampling of the metabolic processes going on in the lipid pool. Table 4–1 shows a simple classification of the five major types.

Type I, in which hyperchylomicronemia exists, is an uncommon process encountered in childhood. It is a cause of abdominal pain but

Table 4–1.   Simple Schema of Hyperlipoproteinemias (modified after Buchwald[6])

Type	Cholesterol	Triglycerides	Electrophoresis	Carbohydrate Sensitivity	Correlation with Atherosclerosis	Diet
I	$\pm$	$\uparrow \uparrow \uparrow$	Chylomicrons $\uparrow$	No	No	Low fat
II	$\uparrow \uparrow \uparrow$	Normal or $\uparrow$	$\beta \uparrow \uparrow \uparrow$, Pre-$\beta \pm$	No	Yes	Low cholesterol Low saturated fat
III	$\uparrow \uparrow$	$\uparrow$ or $\uparrow \uparrow$	Broad β	Yes	Yes	Low CHO Low cholesterol Low saturated fat
IV	$\uparrow$	$\uparrow \uparrow \uparrow$	Pre-β, $\uparrow \uparrow \uparrow$	Yes	Yes	Low CHO Low cholesterol Low saturated fat
V	$\uparrow$	$\uparrow \uparrow$	Chylomicrons $\uparrow$ and Pre-$\beta \uparrow$	Yes	?	Low fat Low cholesterol Low CHO

is not necessarily associated with premature vascular disease.

Type V, in which hyperchylomicronemia also exists, is also associated with abdominal pains and at times with atheromatous disease. Type V may be secondary to other diseases such as pancreatitis, diabetic acidosis, alcoholism, nephrosis and hypothyroidism. The recommended therapy for these two types includes weight reduction and control of any inciting primary process.

Type III is a unique and uncommon familial recessive disorder in which normal beta-lipoproteins have an unusual affinity for triglycerides. Hypercholesterolemic levels of 400 to 600 milligrams per 100 milliliters may be found; triglycerides may be equally high. Xanthomata in the palmar creases and on the extensor surfaces may also be present. Although this is an uncommon disorder it is of importance because if it is recognized it can be treated with weight reduction, a low cholesterol diet and clofibrate, with apparent resorption of atheromata and xanthomata and relief of symptoms.[45] Heinle and his associates[14] have estimated that in coronary atherosclerosis approximately 40 per cent of patients have Type II and 40 per cent have Type IV hyperlipoproteinemias.

In Type II patients, serum drawn after an overnight fast is clear, is free of chylomicrons, and has an elevated serum cholesterol without concomitant hypertriglyceridemia. The disorder is characterized by a hyperbeta-lipoproteinemia which may be primary but may also be produced secondarily by excess dietary intake of cholesterol or by hyperthyroidism, myeloma, macroglobulinemia, liver disease, or nephrosis. Other family members should be screened for this abnormality. Treatment is not so effective as it is with Type III disorders. Diet should be low in cholesterol and saturated fats, and high in its proportion of unsaturated fat as, for instance, provided by the American Heart Association diets when one excludes egg yolks completely. Cholestyramine is the most effective drug for use in supplementing this diet. Betasitosterol, nicotinic acid, D-thyroxine, and clofibrate are much less satisfactory drugs.

Type IV hyperlipoproteinemia is a heterogenous group of disorders in which there is an excess of triglyceride in the blood, either because of excessive production from carbohydrates in the liver or because of peripheral underutilization. Overnight serum is apt to be turbid, which is indicative of the hypertriglyceridemia with a normal cholesterol level. This type of abnormality may be a secondary manifestation of diabetes mellitus, pancreatitis, alcoholism, the nephrotic syndrome, progestational hormones, weight gain, or emotional stress.

Management of Type IV hypercholesteremia is based on strict control of carbohydrate intake to maintain optimal weight. Clofibrate may be of further help if appropriate dietary management alone is not possible.

The writings of Zelis, Mason and Braunwald[45] provide a simplified and useful approach to the office understanding, diagnosis, and management of these lesions.

Other metabolic influences are clearly important. One of the commonest nondietary metabolic influences on atherosclerosis is exerted by the gonads. There is a disparity in respect to the severity of atherosclerosis and its complications in men and in women, and this situation is true particularly with regard to the younger age groups. Estrogens administered to males seem to influence atherosclerosis favorably. These clinically observed estrogenic influences have been duplicated in multiple animal experiments.[6] A large percentage of female patients who have major peripheral arterial disease have manifestations of diminished estrogen function; one fourth of the female patients in the present University of California series had had ovarian resections prior to the age of 40.

Premenopausal women have far less atherosclerotic disease than men of a comparable age, although after the menopause women become equally susceptible.

The pancreatic islets also exert an important influence on atherosclerosis in general, and the frequency with which occlusive disease involving the small arteries is seen in diabetics is a matter of common clinical knowledge. The number of diabetics who have proximal lesions in the major arteries is considerably less than might be anticipated, and it may be that the diffuse nature of the other atherosclerotic lesions removes the patients from the surgical group rather than that diabetics do not have major occlusive disease.

As a rule, the lipid level is lower in diabetics whose disease is under control than in those whose disease is not under control, but whether the former have fewer atherosclerotic complications while the disease is under good control is not clear. Certainly it is true that many patients who have serious foot infections exhibit little atherosclerosis yet have marked diabetes, and many patients who have mild diabetes manifest extensive atherosclerosis. Often these lesions are of the diffuse type affecting peripheral small vessels that is recognized clinically as the "diabetic" as opposed to the "nondiabetic."

It is not clear whether the increased incidence of atherosclerosis among diabetics is due to hyperlipemia or to other metabolic abnormalities. Certainly, any mechanism that produces hyperlipemia in dogs and other animals is associated with increased susceptibility to atherosclerosis, whether or not diabetes is present.

Some diabetic diets prescribed in the past included a relatively high proportion of fat so as to avoid a high carbohydrate intake and thus minimize the insulin requirement. It is possible that this intake of fat increased the hyperlipemic tendencies of many diabetics and contributed seriously to the development of peripheral vascular occlusions.

Thyroid deficiency also results in elevation of cholesterol levels, and conversely, thyroid has often been administered in the hope of lowering serum cholesterol level. Hyperlipemia of almost any cause in humans is associated with increased incidence of atheromatous lesions. It has been our impression, however, that elevated lipid levels were not a common finding in our patients with aortoiliac occlusive disease. Studies of total lipids have been reported so infrequently as to make confirmation of this impression difficult.

Filtration Theory

The *filtration theory* holds that there are selective ultramicroscopic gaps in the endothelium that allow filtration and accumulation of certain fat and lipoprotein elements from the serum in the wall of the artery. Hypertension has been implicated[32, 44] in the pathogenesis of atherosclerosis, and, if the filtration theory is valid, hypertension might provide a mechanism for action of a higher filtration pressure.

Lendrum[23] has presented evidence that proteins from the plasma do leak from the blood vessel lumen through the intima and into the deeper layers of the wall of the artery. Where plasma proteins can diffuse in this manner one would also expect to see lipoproteins.

Mechanical factors in the localization of atherosclerosis have long been recognized. Hypertension, as noted, has been implicated as a form of "injury" to the vessel wall, as in the development of atheroma in the pulmonary artery opposite a patent ductus arteriosus.

In a more chronic form, however, the continual tensions on the vessel can be inferentially linked to some of the common sites of atherosclerosis. Then tension on the wall of the aorta, for instance, can be calculated in terms of Laplace's law ($T = pr$) as some 170,000 dynes per cm., whereas in the capillaries the tension on the wall may be only 16 dynes per cm.[44]

Gross trauma, as in cauterization of the aortic wall, can result in formation of atheroma in the experimental animal. Figure 3–1 represents an area of atheroma resembling a diaphragm at the site of placement of occluding clamps 5½ years earlier. The endarterectomized segment was normal in appearance, and it is presumed that the reaction of the vessel to trauma took the form of deposition of atheroma at that site. If this is so, then it might be well to reduce a patient's blood lipids to the lowest possible level prior to vascular reconstruction by whatever means are available, and maintain them at this level until healing is complete. This concept is supported by Gryska,[12] who described the development of atherosclerosis in segments of the aorta in dogs after they had been made hyperlipemic.

Trauma to the arterial wall in rabbits as well as in dogs that have been made hypolipemic by dietary means results in accelerated atheroma at the site of the arterial injury.[4, 12, 28] Whether this trauma is

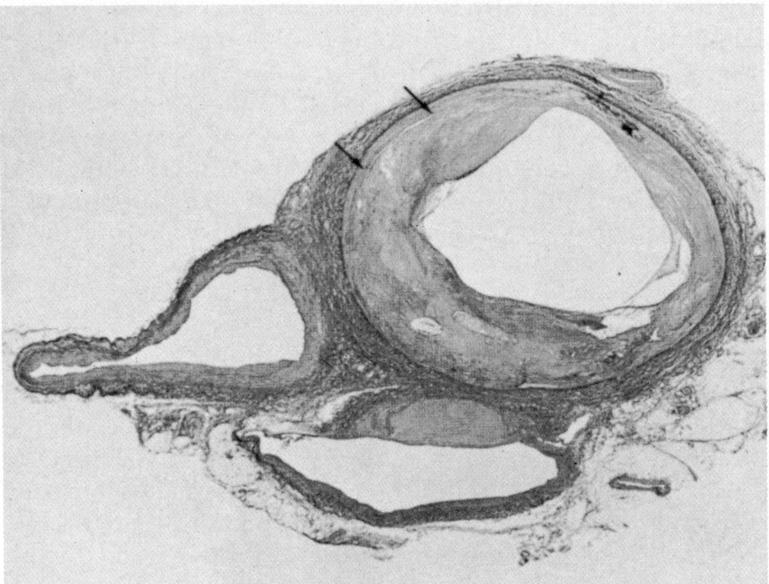

Figure 4–3. Microphotograph of cross section of femoral artery shows advanced arteriosclerotic changes in elderly male. The vessel is not completely occluded. Internal elastic membrane is inconspicuous; external elastic membrane can be seen as a thin layer beneath the adventitia. Arrows indicate clefts that separate inner severely arteriosclerotic portion of wall from less involved outer portion of muscularis and adventitia. This plane of separation is used in removal of sequestrum in endarterectomy.

caused by cauterization, damage by clamps, or actual intimectomy does not seem to be important. Whether this localization at the site of injury favors the filtration theory or whether it is simply an indication in the healing intimal tissues of a metabolic defect related to lipid abnormalities is a matter which cannot be determined at this time.

Warren's work,[38] which demonstrated the frequency with which progression of atherosclerotic lesions occurs proximal to a major obstruction, supports the thesis that proximal pressures do damage the vessel wall.

Another hemodynamic factor may be increased turbulence brought about by increased velocity of blood flow secondary to hypertension, with deposition of lipids at critical levels of the arterial tree.

Bernouilli's principle describing flow through a narrow area in a rigid tube indicates that the lateral pressure must be increased in the area above the area of narrowing so that flow of the fluid will be accelerated in the narrower channel. Such a difference in pressure, accentuated by the influence of the radius in Laplace's law ($T=pr$), is compatible with the observation of atherosclerotic localization in the common iliac artery proximal to a congenitally narrow external iliac artery that remains free of disease itself—as in the typical case of the Leriche syndrome (p. 19).

The effect of pressure changes the effect of turbulence, and the combined result of the two factors in hypercholesteremic dogs has been demonstrated by Sako.[32]

Turbulent flow may arise from several causes and must not be confused with simple mixing and eddy formation which may or may not involve turbulence of the type that is significant in atherosclerosis. All the forms of turbulence listed in the following paragraph represent flow that is less effective than laminar flow. When a considerable amount of energy is transmitted to the vessel wall, atherosclerosis is prone to develop.

The sites at which turbulence ordinarily develops have been categorized by Wesolowski[39] as follows:

1. Where flow factors exceed the Reynolds number.
2. Sites of inflow mixing (unimportant here).
3. Anatomical expansion of the arterial trunk.
4. "Dynamic" expansions at outflow sites.
5. Orifices of arteries.

The eddy currents provoked by established projections can be evaluated in terms of the following equation:[19]

$$\frac{\epsilon}{r} < 4/(\mathrm{Re})^{1/2}$$

for laminar flow to be maintained, where
ϵ = the height of sharp-edged projection in a tube
r = the radius of the tube
Re is Reynolds number

Whether the high narrow carina seen in many instances of the Leriche syndrome produces turbulence beyond that provoked by changes in size of the vessels themselves is not clear. It is not clear whether an acute angle between the two iliac arms and a straight line to the inguinal ligament is more apt to produce factors exceeding the Reynolds number, or whether a curved iliac arm may be less likely to produce turbulence and deposition of atheroma. The frequency with which the high narrow bifurcation is encountered in occlusive disease suggests that some factor is operative. It may be simply a mechanical factor; that is, it may be that the deposition of a given amount of atheroma in a small artery will more quickly produce critical stenosis than will deposition of the same amount of atheroma in a larger artery.

In any event, whether the etiologic factor is metabolic, dietary, or mechanical, many *hereditary factors* are potentially operative and little can be done about some of them, although the familial or cultural dietary pattern can be changed. When correction of an arterial occlusion is required, correction of an abnormal anatomical arrangement may be necessary for long-lasting results.

Rate of Progression

Aside from the relief of pain, one of the basic principles of reconstructive arterial surgery is that the life expectancy and the outlook for correction of the local lesion, be favorably influenced by intervention.

Because of the many anatomical and physiological variants, it is difficult to predict the course of the disease in an individual patient, and a further unknown element is the surgeon's technical skill in treating the patient's particular problem.

Warren[38] has presented a carefully followed series of 17 patients who submitted to sequential arteriograms, which made possible a graphic demonstration of the progression of the disease process. In these patients, whose initial symptom was intermittent claudication, progression of symptoms occurred in only two and symptomatic improvement occurred in five. Twenty areas of disease progression were seen in 16 legs during the period of study, only one of which was associated with worsening of the intermittent claudication, and in 18 of these instances the proximal segment of an artery was affected.

A larger retrospective study of 1850 patients has been reported by Humphries.[16] As regards the untreated patients, the conclusions were: (1) the frequency of sudden *severe* ischemia is greater, the more distal the site of the occlusion; (2) serious exacerbation is usually a sudden event and is usually of a major degree; and (3) spontaneous recovery from such an episode of sudden exacerbation is uncommon. It is of considerable interest that a higher rate of spontaneous improvement occurred in the more distal lesions also. These lesions being less stable, favorable or unfavorable change is more apt to occur in them, and an unfavorable change might be sudden and catastrophic. This group of unselected patients did not fare so well in general as the patients reported by Warren.

Humphries pointed out that his series may not reflect accurately the status of the total population afflicted with vascular disease. Some patients who experience only claudication, which can be treated adequately by their local physician, are not referred to a vascular center for arteriographic study; on the other hand, other patients, whose disease is so advanced that amputation is performed by their local physicians are also not seen in a vascular center. With allowance for these exceptions, Humphries' experience can be accepted as representative. Humphries' orginal work of 1963 has more recently been brought up to date although there are no major changes in his conclusions.[17]

The ominous prognosis in respect to patient survival and limb salvage which is associated with the diagnosis of arteriosclerosis obliterans may be seen in another report, from the Cleveland Clinic.[22] According to this report, the 5-year survival rate in nondiabetics was 59 per cent, and the amputation rate was 8.3 per cent. In diabetics, the survival rate was 52.7 per cent and the amputation rate, 20.7 per cent. DeBakey[9] has compared the survival rate of the normal population in the United States and that of patients of the same age who were undergoing treatment for aortoiliac occlusive disease. The 5-year survival rate was found to be 85 per cent for normals and 51 per cent for those treated. The amputation rate was lower in this group, but the prognosis for survival remained unfavorable.

There are other data furnished by Humphries reflecting the results of surgery in aortoiliac, femoropopliteal, and combined aortoiliac-femoropopliteal lesions. There was very little relief of claudication except in patients who were treated surgically. The over-all amputation rate was decreased, by half in the case of either isolated or combined femoropopliteal disease. Recurrence of symptoms was more common (20 per cent) in the more distal lesions. The over-all mortality rate was lower. It is not clear whether the mortality rate was lower because of the lower amputation rate, as the authors suggest, or whether the untreated groups represent truly comparable control groups or were rejected for surgical treatment because the threat to survival was too great following the development of arteriosclerosis in other sites.

THROMBOANGIITIS OBLITERANS

The other important cause of arterial obstruction is *thromboangiitis obliterans.* This condition was first described by von Winiwarter[43] but the clinical aspects were elucidated by Buerger,[7] whose name is most commonly associated with it today.

Thromboangiitis obliterans affects primarily arteries of small to medium size. It runs a progressive course, from the peripheral vessels, i.e., digital, palmar, and plantar, to the more central sites in the tibial, radial, and ulnar vessels. Clinical evidence of involvement of vessels above this level is uncommon, although the author attempted endarterectomy, which was unsuccessful, in one patient who had a characteristic lesion in the popliteal artery.

The classic description of the pathological findings is that of a segmental, sclerosing inflammatory process, in which artery, concomitant veins, and even nerves become bound in one mass (Fig. 4–5). There may be thrombosis and organization of the luminal clot, but there is only coincidental involvement by typical atherosclerosis. Microscopically, a dense inflammatory exudate composed chiefly of round cells is seen throughout all layers of the vessel wall, with proliferation of fibroblasts and endothelial cells; histiocytes, plasma cells, and even

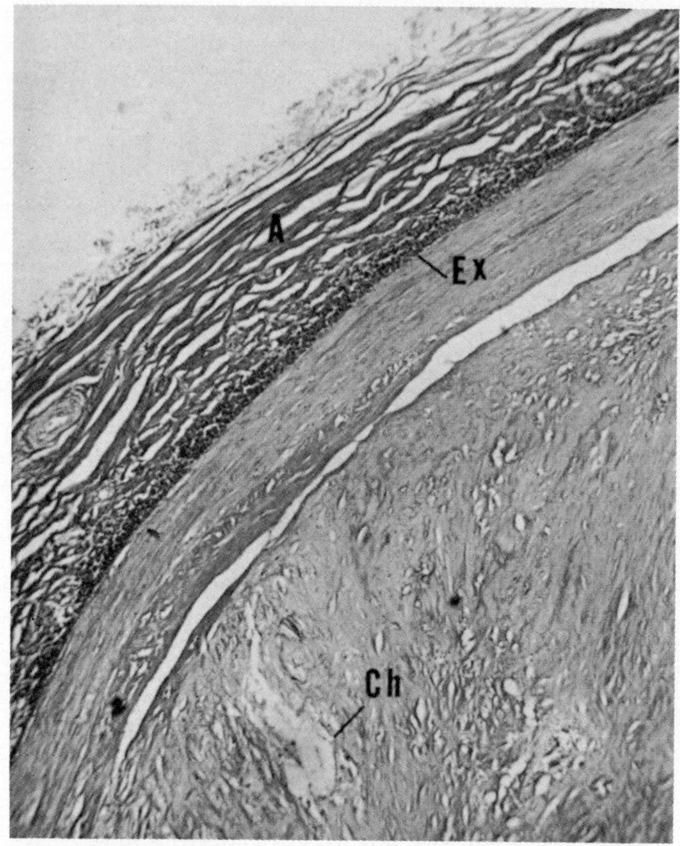

Figure 4–4.   Enlargement of area between arrows in Figure 4–3. The most involved inner part of the wall contains many cholesterol deposits (Ch), and is separated by clefts from outer parts of media. External elastic membrane (Ex) and adventitia (A) are also shown.

giant cells are found throughout all layers of the vessel. The cellular infiltration is more prominent in the intima and less so in the adventitia. In spite of the inflammatory changes, little degenerative or necrotic change is seen.[13, 18, 36]

As noted, the smaller arteries are most commonly involved, but Szilagyi has identified by arteriography "corrugation" of the superficial femoral and other arteries in some patients who exhibit the classic symptoms of the disease.

In many patients there is evidence of diffuse narrowing of the arteries. This was recognized arteriographically by Leriche,[24] who interpreted the narrowing to represent diffuse vasospasm and undertook to correct it by a combination of sympathectomy and adrenalectomy. This combined form of treatment has not been fruitful, but sympathetic ablation remains one useful palliative procedure.

There has been considerable controversy whether thromboangiitis obliterans or Buerger's disease can be regarded as a specific entity. Wessler[40] believes that the pathological process is merely an inflammatory variant of arteriosclerosis.

Some of the confusion regarding the clinical diagnosis arose because of misconceptions on the part of many pathologists concerning the clinical frequency, importance, and even the occurrence of atherosclerosis as a cause of aortic and iliac obstruction. That arterial obstruction could develop with any frequency in young men seemed unlikely to many clinicians. As a result, the clinical diagnosis of "Buerger's disease" came to be popularly applied without discrimination to all occlusive disease, especially in younger patients. When surgeons began to remove atherosclerotic plaques from the aorta and the iliac and femoral arteries in patients who were in their twenties, thirties, and forties, they found no evidence of thromboangiitis in these specimens.

Thus, it was incorrectly assumed by many surgeons that in many

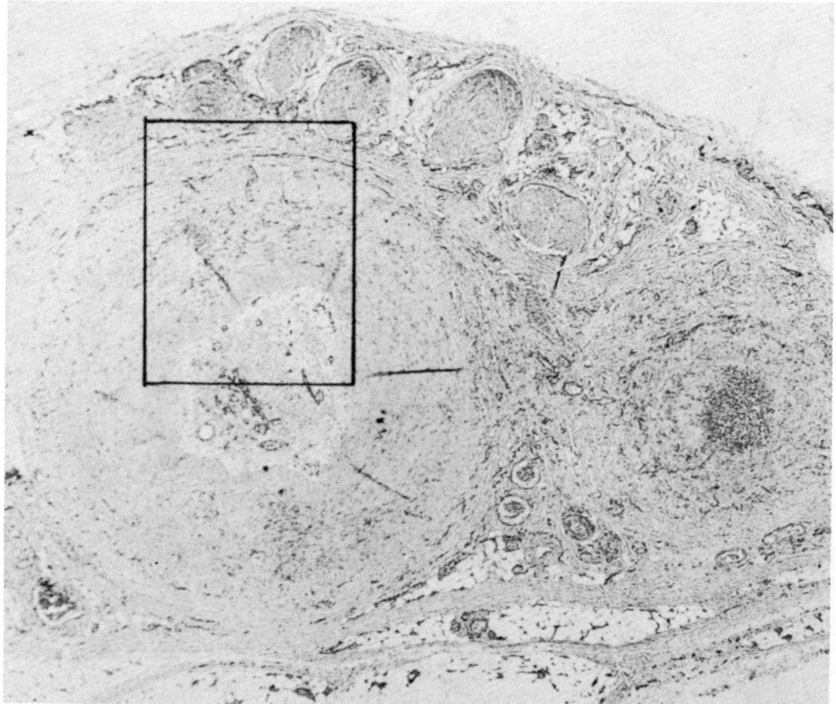

Figure 4–5. Low power view of posterior tibial artery and vein at midcalf in case of thromboangiitis obliterans. The artery, vein, and nerve trunks are involved in the process. Hematoxylin and eosin stain. (After Szilagyi, D. E., DeRusso, F. J., and Elliott, J. P., Jr.: Thromboangiitis obliterans. Arch. Surg. 88:824, 1964.)

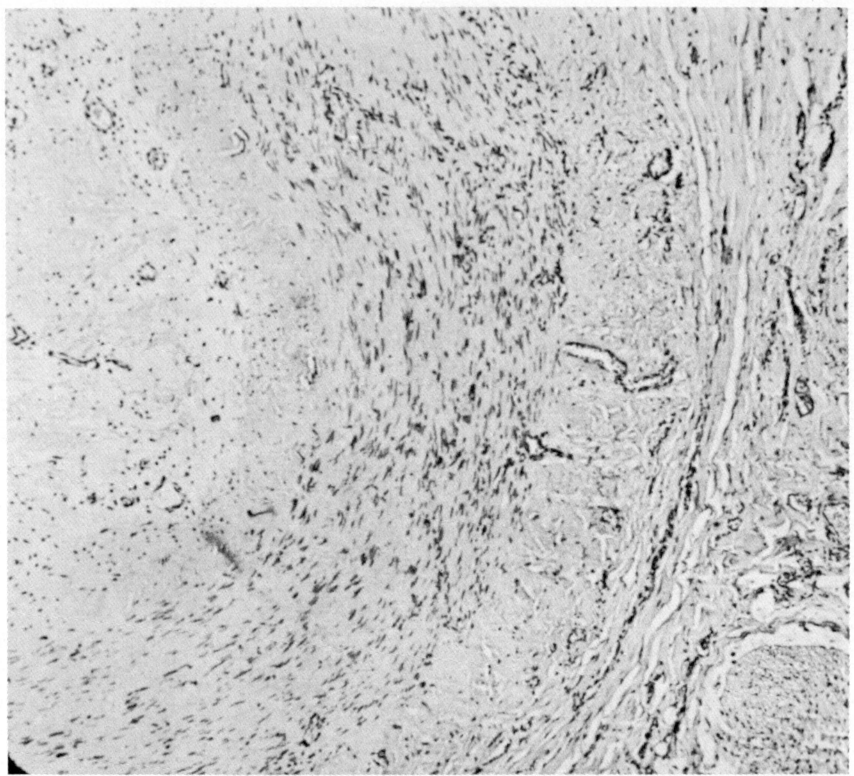

Figure 4-6. Higher power view of area defined in inset in Figure 4-5. There is a chronic inflammatory process in all coats of the arterial wall, and the intima is somewhat thickened. An intraluminal thrombus is undergoing organization. Architecture of the media is substantially preserved in spite of the fibrosis and round cell infiltration. There is little evidence of necrosis. Hematoxylin and eosin stain. (After Szilagyi, D. E., De-Russo, F. J., and Elliott, J. P., Jr.: Thromboangiitis obliterans. Arch. Surg. 88:824, 1964.)

cases peripheral occlusion had existed secondarily to unrecognized occlusion of major proximal arteries and had been misdiagnosed as thromboangiitis obliterans. Subsequent criticism of the designation of thromboangiitis as a distinct entity simply compounded confusion.

Mills and Ochsner have described myocardial scars beyond an atheromatous ulcer in a coronary artery.[25] Embolization from ulcerated atheroma in the carotid artery is recognized as a common cause of repeated episodes of localized cerebral ischemia. Major episodes of embolization in aneurysmal disease are common. Miniature emboli from proximal atheromatous ulcers may well account for patchy small vessel occlusions in atherosclerosis of the major arteries.

This phenomenon is reflected in a long-held theory that embolization of this nature is the source of the lesions of thromboangiitis obliterans. It would appear, however, that there are other clinical as well as pathological criteria to suggest that embolization alone is not sufficient to produce the syndrome of Buerger's disease.

It is the author's opinion that the argument is a futile one. There is a highly inflammatory occlusive process that does involve primarily the peripheral arteries in males. The etiology of this inflammatory process is in dispute, but there is no doubt as to the clinical diagnosis (p. 67). The pathologic features of importance include the multicentric occurrence in the small vessels which prevent the surgeon from operating successfully on an isolated segment. Because the process is an inflammatory one, the surgeon cannot perform endarterectomy locally, as he may be able to do in other areas of atherosclerosis, such as the coronary arteries.

Thus the very nature of the disease renders impossible surgical correction in the usual sense. Surgical and medical palliation so as to encourage the natural rate of formation of collaterals may be helpful in controlling the severity of the disease which, according to Allen and associates[2] "is directly proportional to the rapidity of development and extent of the arterial occlusions and is inversely proportional to the rapidity and extent to which the collateral arterial anastomoses can be developed."

The etiology of thromboangiitis is unknown. Common among Jews, it is by no means restricted to them;[26] the author has seen cases among the Chinese, Japanese (in whom it is indeed relatively common), Negroes, American Indians, contemporary Mayan Indians and all ethnic strains of the white race. It is a disease that affects males almost exclusively, although documented cases are seen rarely in women.

The relationship to tobacco is established, but the specific role of tobacco is unclear. Abstinence from tobacco during the onset of the disease is almost unheard of—evidence that the process is not thromboangiitis obliterans. Later it is almost impossible to make the patients abstain from tobacco, but if it can be managed, gradual remission usually ensues. Thus the only palliation other than good hygiene and protective measures is sympathectomy and abstinence from the tobacco.

CAUSES OF MISCELLANEOUS OBSTRUCTIONS

Ergotism is similar to thromboangiitis with respect to anatomical localization. It is different pathologically, appearing as a necrotizing thrombotic process which often involves many arteries, including those which are not amenable to surgical correction because of their small size.

Primary thrombosis may occur in certain hematologic disorders, usually secondary to another serious disorder. Cryoglobulinemic episodes, polycythemic thromboses, and similar thrombotic crises may at times involve one artery large enough to be operated on, provided the patient can tolerate surgery otherwise, in which case the general principles of surgical repair will govern the procedure.

Cystic degeneration in the wall of the popliteal artery has been seen infrequently.[15] Serious peripherally placed lesions are being encountered more and more in the several forms of *collagen disease* (including rheumatoid processes and scleroderma).

Myxomatous degeneration of the media of the carotid artery has been described by Whelan,[41] who believed that the drug Persantin, which is also implicated in retroperitoneal fibrosis, may have been responsible for this degenerative process in the form of an idiosyncratic response.

The several forms of *fibromuscular hyperplasia* with pseudoaneurysms in a beaded, accordion-like artery have been seen commonly in the renal artery in the past, but have now been more frequently encountered in the mesenteric, carotid and even femoral artery.

One of the other unusual vascular lesions which may present as either aneurysmal or occlusive disease is the *Ehlers-Danlos syndrome*. Recognition of this diagnosis is critical because the fragility of tissues including the arterial wall makes attempted surgical intervention hazardous.[41] Surgical correction depends on the status of the distal arterial tree and presents no specific problems, except in diagnosis.

ANEURYSMS

Most aneurysmal disease seen by the surgeon today is atherosclerotic, traumatic, or infectious in origin. Lues is now an uncommon cause of aneurysmal disease, but it still does occur.

The pathological processes responsible for aneurysm formation are not clearly defined, but several mechanisms may be suggested.

In an analogy to the formation of a luetic aneurysm, interference with nutrition of the arterial wall by deposition of atheroma on the intima and obstruction of vasa vasorum may result in a weakening of that wall which cannot resist internal pressures.

Elevation of lateral tensions on the wall by systemic hypertension may be a factor in the progression of aneurysmal disease, but seems an uncommon original cause. The increase in lateral mural tension associated with those vessels in which there is intrinsically a greater diameter may play an important role. It is common to see a great difference in the average diameter of vessels from one patient to another, and it is usual for the patient with an aneurysm to have vessels diffusely larger than normal at sites far distant from the aneurysm itself.

This diffuse dilatation of arteries, reaching the stage of arteriomegaly, has been commented upon by Thomas.[37]

Turbulence beyond an area of stenosis with consequent increased lateral tensions may be a factor in some circumstances, such as the infrarenal aorta, the common femoral artery and the popliteal artery, and are each associated with the common factor of a proximal arterial constriction. This is respectively an intrinsic and relative narrowing just below the renal arterial takeoff, probably related to preaortic fascial bands, the inguinal ligament, and the arch of the adductor muscle hiatus.

REFERENCES

1. Ahrens, E. H., Jr., Insull, W., Jr., Hirsch, J., Stoffel, W., Peterson, M. L., Farquhar, J. W., Miller, T., and Thomasson, H. J.: The effect on human serum-lipids of a dietary fat, highly unsaturated, but poor in essential fatty acids. Lancet *1*:115, 1959.
2. Allen, E. V., Barker, N. W., and Hines, E. A., Jr.: *Peripheral Vascular Diseases.* 3rd ed. Philadelphia, W. B. Saunders Co., 1962.
3. Anderson, J. T., Keys, A., and Grande, F.: The effects of different food fats on serum cholesterol concentration in man. J. Nutrit. *62*:421, 1957.
4. Barker, W. F., and Barakonski, A.: The use of heparin and of dextran in arterial reconstruction. Acta Chir. Scand. *387*:97, 1968.
5. Bronte-Stewart, B., Antonis, A., Eales, L., and Brock, J. T.: Effects of feeding different fats on serum-cholesterol level. Lancet *1*:521, 1956.
6. Buchwald, H.: The lipid clinic concept. Hosp. Pract. 5:119, 1970.
7. Buerger, L.: Thrombo-angiitis obliterans: a study of the vascular lesions leading to presenile spontaneous gangrene. Am. J. Med. Sci. *136*:567, 1908.
8. Dayton, S.: In Barker, W. F. (Ed.): *Surgical Treatment of Peripheral Vascular Disease.* New York, McGraw-Hill Book Co., Inc., 1962.
9. DeBakey, M. E., Crawford, E. S., Morris, G. C., Cooley, D. A., and Garrett, H. E.: Late results of vascular surgery in the treatment of arteriosclerosis. J. Cardiov. Surg. 5:473, 1964.
10. DeBakey, M. E., Jordan, G. L., Jr., Abbott, J. P., Halpert, B., and O'Neal, R. M.: The fate of dacron vascular grafts. Arch. Surg. *89*:757, 1964.
11. Frederickson, D. S., Levy, R. T., and Lees, R. S.: Fat transport in lipoproteins—an integrated approach to mechanisms and disorders. New Eng. J. Med. *276*:34, 94, 148, 215, 273, 1967.
12. Gryska, P. F.: The development of atheroma in arteries subjected to experimental thromboendarterectomy. Surgery *45*:655, 1959.
13. Hardy, J. D., Conn, J. H., and Fain, W. R.: Nonatherosclerotic occlusive lesions of small arteries. Surgery *57*:1, 1965.
14. Heinle, R. A., Levy, R. I., and Frederickson, D. S.: Lipid and carbohydrate abnormalities in angiographically documented coronary artery disease. Amer. J. Cardiol. *24*:178, 1969.
15. Holmes, J. G.: Cystic adventitial degeneration of the popliteal artery. J.A.M.A. *173*:654, 1960.
16. Humphries, A. W.: In Wesolowski, S. A., and Dennis, C.: *Fundamentals of Vascular Grafting.* New York, McGraw-Hill Book Co., Inc., 1963.
17. Humphries, A. W.: The relation of natural history of arteriosclerosis to surgical management. In Dale, A. W. (ed.): *Management of Arterial Occlusive Disease.* Chicago, Year Book Medical Publishers, Inc., 1971.
18. Kaiser, G. C., Musser, A. W., and Shumacker, H. B., Jr.: Thromboangiitis obliterans in women: report of two cases. Surgery *48*:733, 1960.

19. Katz, L. N., and Stamler, J.: *Experimental Atherosclerosis.* Springfield, Ill., Charles C Thomas, 1953.
20. Kinsell, L. W., Friskey, R. W., Michaels, G. D., and Splitter, S.: Essential fatty acids, lipid metabolism, and atherosclerosis. Lancet *1*:334, 1958.
21. Kinsell, L. W., Michaels, G. D., Walker, G., and Conklin, J.: Cholesterol synthesis in normal and abnormal human subjects. Circulation *22*:661, 1960.
22. LeFevre, F. A., Corbacioglu, C., Humphries, A. W., and de Wolfe, V. G.: Management of arteriosclerosis obliterans of the extremities. J.A.M.A. *170*:656, 1959.
23. Lendrum, A. C.: Plasmatic vasculosis, the hyaline lesion in hypertension. Presented before the Vascular Surgical Society of Great Britain and Ireland, Dundee, Scotland, November 3, 1972.
24. Leriche, R.: Causes of failure of suprarenalectomy and ganglionectomy in thromboangiitis obliterans on basis of 898 operations. Angiology *1*:432, 1950.
25. Mills, N. L., and Ochsner, J. L.: Distal thromboembolism from proximal coronary athero-sclerotic lesions. Surgery *72*:1030, 1972.
26. McDonald, D. A.: *Blood Flow in Arteries.* London, Edward Arnold, Ltd., 1960.
27. McKusick, V. A., and Harris, W. S.: Buerger syndrome in the Orient. Bull. Johns Hopkins Hosp. *109*:241, 1961.
28. Pilcher, D., and Barker, W.: Retardation of experimental atherosclerosis in endarterectomized arteries by the administration of heparin and dextran. Amer. J. Surg. *120*:270, 1970.
29. Rivin, A. U., and Dimitroff, S. P.: The incidence and severity of atherosclerosis in estrogen-treated males and in females with a hypoestrogenic or a hyperestrogenic state. Circulation *9*:533, 1954.
30. Robicsek, F., Sanger, P. W., Taylor, F. H., Magistro, R., and Foti, E.: Pathogenesis and significance of post-stenotic dilatation in great vessels. Ann. Surg. *147*:835, 1958.
31. Rutstein, D. D., Castelli, W. P., Sullivan, J. C., Newell, J. M., and Nickerson, R. J.: Effects of fats and carbohydrate ingestion in humans on serum lipids and intracellular lipid deposition in tissue culture. New Eng. J. Med. *271*:1, 1964.
32. Sako, Y.: Effects of turbulent blood flow and hypertension on experimental atherosclerosis. J.A.M.A. *179*:36, 1962.
33. Sandler, M., and Bourne, G. H.: Some new observations on human aortic atheroma. J.A.M.A. *179*:43, 1962.
34. Schlichter, J. G., Katz, L. N., and Meyer, J.: The occurrence of atheromatous lesions after cauterization of the aorta followed by cholesterol administration. Am. J. Med. Sci. *218*:603, 1949.
35. Stamler, J., Pick, R., Katz, L. N., Pick, A., Kaplan, B. M., Berkson, D. M., and Century, D.: Effectiveness of estrogens for therapy of myocardial infarction in middle-age men. J.A.M.A. *183*:632, 1963.
36. Szilagyi, D. E., DeRusso, F. J., and Elliott, J. P., Jr.: Thromboangiitis obliterans. Arch. Surg. *88*:824, 1964.
37. Thomas, M. L.: Arteriomegaly, Brit. J. Surg. *58*:690, 1971.
38. Warren, R., Gomez, R. L., Marston, J. A. P., and Cox, J. S. T.: Femoropopliteal arteriosclerosis obliterans—arteriographic patterns and rates of progression. Surgery *55*:135, 1964.
39. Wesolowski, S. A., Fries, C. C., and Sawyer, P. N.: The production and significance of turbulence in hemic systems. Trans. Am. Soc. Artif. Int. Organs *8*:11, 1962.
40. Wessler, S., Ming, S., Gurewich, V., and Frieman, D. G.: Critical evaluation of thromboangiitis obliterans. New Eng. J. Med. *262*:1149, 1960.
41. Whelan, T. J., Jr., and Baugh, J. H.: Nonatherosclerotic arterial lesions and their management. IV. Miscellaneous arterial lesions. Curr. Prob. Surg. *67*:21, 1967.
42. Windaus, A.: Über den Gehalt normaler und atheromatöser Aorten an Cholesterin und Cholesterinestern. Ztschr. Physiol. Chem. *67*:174, 1910.
43. vom Winiwarter, F.: Ueber eine egenthümliche Form von Endarteriitis und Endophlebitis mit Gangrän des Fusses. Arch. Klin. Chir. *23*:202, 1879.
44. Winsor, T.: *Peripheral Vascular Diseases: An Objective Approach.* Springfield, Ill., Charles C Thomas, 1959.
45. Zelis, R., Mason, D. T., and Braunwald, E., et al.: Peripheral vascular disease in patients with familial hypolipoproteinemia: Blood flow response following therapy. Circulation *38*(Suppl.):466, 1966.

Chapter Five

DIAGNOSTIC PROBLEMS

History, physical examination, and laboratory procedures are the essential elements in establishing the correct pathological and anatomical diagnosis.

Many aspects of a detailed history are revealing and may be of ultimate statistical importance. Among these, of course, is a family history of gangrene, coronary artery or cerebral artery disease, hypertension, diabetes, or other more specific disorders of lipid metabolism; early menopause consequent to surgery and followed by arteriosclerotic symptoms is an example.

To arrive at a diagnosis, the physician must determine the following:

1. Is there an abnormality of function in one or more of the extremities that is consistent with occlusion of the appropriate artery?

2. Is this disturbance manifested with muscular activity, or does it exist as ischemic pain when the patient is at rest?

3. Is there loss of tissue substance, which in its mildest form is atrophy and in its more advanced form is gangrene or necrosis?

4. Is there concomitant arterial disease elsewhere — e.g., in the carotid, renal or coronary arteries — that might demand prior attention because of its critical importance to survival? Or is the arterial disease that is present in another area of such a degree as to preclude, restrict, or modify surgical treatment of the presenting problem?

5. Is there nonvascular disease in another area such as neoplasia, liver disease, muscular dystrophy, mental disease, infection, or the like which would either preclude arterial reconstruction, make it futile, or necessitate deferral?

Given this framework of reference, one may then consider the basic information pertinent to diagnosis.

Until the medical profession as a whole becomes cognizant of the criteria for selection of candidates for operation, many patients will be referred to the surgeon who clearly are not suitable for any reconstructive procedure, because of the systemic involvement or by reason of the nature of local lesion. In either event, many patients must be treated medically with conservative measures. The rationale for the choice of patients is discussed in greater detail in the chapters relating to the specific arterial bed in question.

CHARACTERISTICS OF PATIENTS

Once having had experience in identifying patients with atherosclerosis, the surgeon is better able to recognize similar cases. The surgeon's outlook guides him in determining which patients are suitable candidates for surgery in his hands. In our series, the patient chosen for reconstructive surgery most frequently had symptoms of functional deficit rather than necrosis or impending gangrene and had no other major disease. The rationale for this type of patient selection is based on the high rate of success and relatively low risk of operation with such patients. On the other hand, the mortality risk is greater in patients in whom a necrotic process has begun, and there is less likelihood that the reconstruction will be successful. Hence it is exceedingly difficult to compare any two series collected by different groups.

The data to be presented concerning occlusive disease of the aorta, iliac and femoropopliteal arterial system represent two series of patients treated at the hospital of the University of California at Los Angeles. The first series were treated between 1955 and 1964 and were reported in the First Edition of this book.[3] The second were reported in part elsewhere[4] and represent a more recent group of patients. In a later chapter, two similar groups of patients with aneurysms will be compared.

Approximately 60 per cent of the series were private patients. The remainder have been treated by the resident staff. Selected patients with special problems will be described in detail. Some of the patients who do not fit within this series because of either temporal or geographic terms will be mentioned because of their specific problems.

The age and sex distribution of the patients with occlusive disease are shown in Table 5–1.

Classification of patients into two groups reflecting restriction of disease to either the aortoiliac or femoropopliteal system, and a third group reflecting combined disease is based on the clinical impression

Table 5–1. Age, Sex Distribution and Site of Disease

	MALE	AVERAGE AGE	FEMALE	AVERAGE AGE
Series I				
Aortoiliac	57	52	24	53
Femoropopliteal	33	56	10	62
Combined	43	60	17	57
Total	133	55	51	56
Series II				
Aortoiliac	32	55	15	49
Femoropopliteal	11	62	5	66
Combined	37	56	19	56
Total	80	57	39	55

that such classification accurately depicts mortality risk and risk of failure of reconstruction. The classification is based on the most accurate information available following initial careful evaluation.

The two series are very similar. The age differences between the several groups are not of significance except with regard to the fact that patients of both sexes who have femoropopliteal disease are considerably older than their counterparts who have either pure or mixed aortoiliac disease.

It is a common misconception that the majority of patients who are candidates for vascular reconstruction are diabetics. However, although it is likely that diabetes and other metabolic disorders are of contributory etiologic importance, there have been remarkably few diabetics in this group. Only 10 per cent of our patients were diabetic and most of these were only moderately afflicted. Prior to operation only a few patients had had episodes of either diabetic acidosis or coma.

Similarly, few remarkable changes in cholesterol levels were seen. The average total cholesterol was 250 milligrams per cent, which is well within the normal for our laboratory.* There have been few patients identified in this group who have the classical forms of hyperlipoproteinemia, but there were several patients who had elevated triglycerides. In those patients in whom a value for triglycerides was recorded, 60 per cent were above our upper level of normal of 135 milligrams per cent: the average was 152 milligrams per cent. This observation may mean that the importance of hyperlipemic states in man has been overemphasized; it seems more likely that we have only failed to identify the subtle and quantitative differences in lipid con-

---

*Total cholesterol levels were determined by a modification of the Babson[1] technique. Normal adult level for laboratory is between 150 and 300 mg. per cent.

stituents in patients who have peripheral vascular occlusions, and who do not have the grossly abnormal blood lipid concentrations.

The serum cholesterol levels reported by DeBakey's clinic are almost identical to ours.[19]

Selection of patients had a definite bearing on the composition of this group of patients. The surgeons were reluctant to operate on elderly patients or those who had severe diabetes. To a considerable degree this situation applied to patients with heart disease as well; many of them did not manifest extensive myocardial disease until years later (Table 5–2).

It is probable that many patients who have had myocardial infarctions later are not represented in the tabulation. That many patients with previous coronary disease were able to do well after operation seems again to reflect the selection process, in which only those who had long survived an initial coronary infarction with minimal evidence of current myocardial ischemia were selected.

The data in Table 5–2 suggest that in the second series were more patients with serious heart disease than had been accepted for operation in the first series.

Several patients in Series I subsequently died in circumstances suggesting that they had had acute myocardial infarctions, but these patients are not included in the data as certain cardiac deaths. On the basis of previously reported groups from the Veterans Administration Hospital in Los Angeles,[5] it would have been expected that more serious heart disease would occur later.

The role of early and artificial menopause must be considered in the causation of disease among the females in the group, although oophorectomy is so common in the population at large that this small

Table 5–2.   Cardiovascular Involvement in Relation to Anatomical Site and Sex

	AORTOILIAC			FEMORAL			COMBINED			
	Male	*Female*	*Both*	*Male*	*Female*	*Both*	*Male*	*Female*	*Both*	TOTAL
Hypertension only (greater than 150/90 mm. Hg)	9	5	14	12	5	17	12	0	12	43
	9	4	13	3	4	7	16	9	25	45
EKG changes, angina pectoris, or both	6	2	8	2	5	7	4	2	6	21
	4	1	5	1	4	5	8	4	12	22
Myocardial infarction prior to operation	7	0	7	7	2	9	7	5	12	28
	7	0	7	0	2	2	9	2	11	20
Later myocardial infarction or congestive heart failure	3	1	4	3	0	3	1	0	1	8
	3	0	3	1	0	1	4	0	4	8

Note: Entries in second row in each category refer to the second series of patients.

number has little significance. Seven of 24 women who had aortoiliac disease only, three of 10 who had femoral disease only, and three of 17 who had combined disease had had oophorectomies prior to the age of 40.

EVALUATION OF THE PATIENT

Symptoms and physical findings are more reliable indicators in evaluating individual problems than statistical impressions. It is assumed that in all other respects the patient is suitable for surgery before preoperative peripheral vascular studies are performed.

Symptoms

Claudication is the primary complaint that the patient notices initially. Intermittent claudication was first described by Charcot, who noted its occurrence in horses.[9] In this condition, ischemia develops in muscles which require more oxygen than the arterial system is able to provide. The resulting oxygen debt then causes claudication, as the critical point is reached. The mechanisms that allow development of maximal flow were discussed in Chapter Three.

As classically described, claudication occurs as the great calf muscles, primarily the gastrocnemius, react to the inadequate flow of blood through the femoral artery. Usually this complaint indicates femoral artery obstruction. Claudication occurring in the calf alone is a dependable sign, but when accompanied by symptoms in the hip and thigh it is not so reliable as an indicator of the anatomical site of obstruction.

The other type of claudication that occurs commonly is due to obstruction of the iliac system. The muscles of the buttocks and the thigh respond to such a deficiency either by causing pain or by causing painless paresis which is relieved by rest. At times a patient will describe his ability to force himself beyond the point of onset of iliac claudication so that deficient input to the femoral artery manifests itself as calf claudication. Under these circumstances, femoral artery disease may be suspected but may not in fact exist. If calf claudication precedes iliac claudication, or occurs coincident with it, then combined disease must be expected and sought.

With the progressive refinements in physiological evaluation brought about by more detailed arteriographic studies, the latter series of patients have seemed to demonstrate a much more diffuse involvement of both the iliac and femoropopliteal and tibial arterial systems.

Involvement of the tibial arteries alone may be manifested as pain in the foot, but the patterns of pain are too vague to be systematized. Similarly, the presence of extensive terminal aortic obstruction may cause pain in the back muscles, because of deficiency of flow into lumbar arteries. This explanation of back pain is not entirely satisfactory, and some of the pain in the lumbar area may be referred from the periaortic inflammatory process that often coexists.

Specific symptoms cannot clearly be attributed to the hypogastric arterial system. That form of sexual impotence in the male which is manifested in inability to achieve or maintain an effective erection results from inadequate flow into the hypogastric bed, or at least into one side of it. Deficient flow may be caused by common iliac disease or by hypogastric disease. If hip and thigh claudication is not present in severe degree, then primary hypogastric disease should be anticipated, as well as some degree of proximal iliac obstruction. The latter obstruction may be well compensated by lumbar or retrograde deep femoral collaterals.

An unusual syndrome which might properly be called the "pudendal steal" syndrome has recently been described by O'Hara.[36] This syndrome was seen in two patients who had aortoiliac atherosclerosis with claudication but in whom collateral circulation was sufficient to maintain sexual potency. During intercourse the patients suffered from pain and cramps in the thighs and buttocks. Treatment of the occlusive disease was followed by complete relief of these symptoms as well as by relief of the claudication.

Disease of the deep femoral system is uncommon as an isolated finding. It is of importance when there is further extensive obstructive disease in either the iliac or the femoral system.

Arteriosclerotic disease of the deep femoral system is more common than had formerly been believed. Recognition of these lesions may be accomplished more easily when oblique views of the groin are used.[6] Reconstruction of the deep femoral system when no other reconstruction has been possible is frequently advocated.[31, 32]

The ability of the patient to walk is dependent upon several factors, including his subjective responses to distress, the efficiency of his collateral tree, the efficiency of his particular gait, and the ability of his heart to maintain or increase cardiac output; hence, one cannot anticipate finding a specific lesion on the basis of the severity of symptoms.

The dependence of flow to the lower extremities on collaterals which pass through the lower gluteal area is manifested by what might be termed "claudication" which is brought about by one's sitting on a hard chair or bench, or even in a bathtub. This is not claudication, of course; it is ischemia, causing numbness, tingling, paresthesias, and other symptoms which are relieved when one stands.

Another form of claudication that may cause confusion is due to venous congestion; with walking, pain is gradually intensified, the leg feels heavy, and the patient may even have the sensation that the leg is bursting. These symptoms are relieved when he stops walking and elevates the leg, but not when he stands; whereas standing relieves the pain of arterial claudication promptly, and elevation of the leg aggravates it. This form of venous claudication can be confirmed by physical examination.

At times it is difficult to evaluate what appears to be claudication. Claudication may occur after only a few steps, but this is seen in only the most advanced stages of ischemia. When claudication occurs at such short distances, without other objective signs of advanced ischemia, one should consider the possibility of a musculoskeletal[8] or neurological abnormality.

The pseudoclaudication syndrome described by Verbiest[48] has a similar pattern of symptoms, which are probably the result of an engorgement of the vascular supply of the lumbosacral cord in the cauda equina due to an abnormal and constricting flattened, bony, spinal neural arch. Symptoms may seem to be identical with those of aortoiliac obstruction, but the prompt onset of symptoms without change of posture, that is, standing without necessarily walking, is an important clue. This is probably related to the assumption of a marked lordotic curve. When this syndrome is suspected the presence of substantially normal arterial pulsations and pressures (Fig. 5–5), especially after exercise, and a carefully performed myelogram in positions of flexion and extension may show pressures on the cord and the thecal sac consistent with this phenomenon (Fig. 5–1).

Physical Examination

The condition of the leg is a helpful guide in appraising the extent of disease. Muscular atrophy is often not recognizable unless the lesions are asymmetrical, but Leriche's original description[29] did include "global" atrophy of the lower extremities (Fig. 5–2).

The appearance of the extremity is a most helpful but somewhat subjective guide in estimating the adequacy of distal circulation and relative localization of the disease. It is usual to find no loss of hair, no atrophy of skin or loss of pulp space, and no abnormality of nail growth in the typical Leriche syndrome; it is more common to find these abnormalities in arterial obstructions restricted to the femoropopliteal artery. The changes become more pronounced, the greater the extent of the occlusion and the less efficiently the collateral circulation functions.

The simple maneuver of elevating the extremity provides some indication whether the perfusion pressure is sufficient to pump

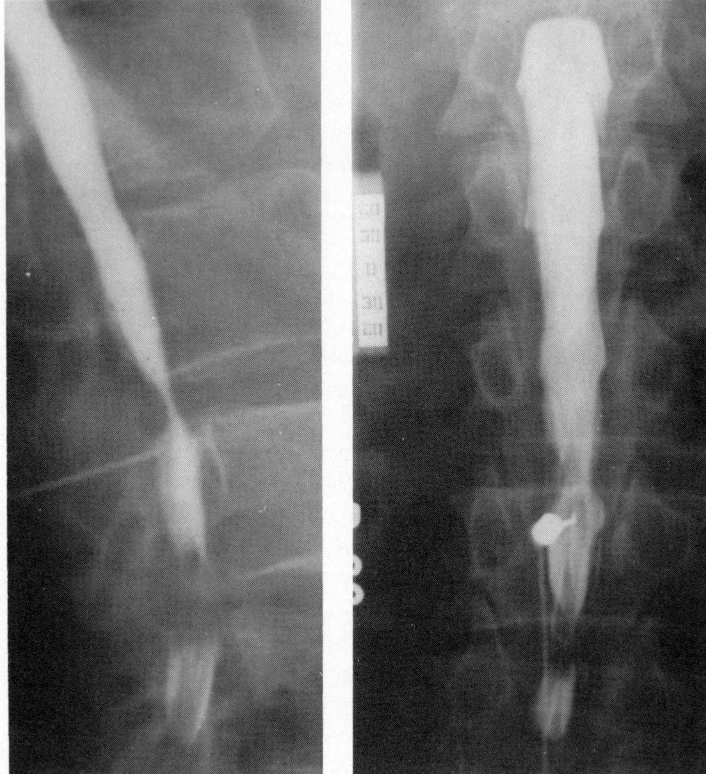

Figure 5–1. Myelogram on a patient with a neuroclaudication syndrome of Verbiest.[48]

This shows in lateral view the lumbar myelogram of a 55-year-old man. Twelve years before he had had some low back pain which disappeared. A year ago he had developed pain in the left leg which developed after walking a block or after standing for a protracted period of time. This would then progress down the back of the leg, finally appearing in the other leg, extending into the calf. The legs became heavy and weak. He could be relieved only by sitting, not simply by standing, but after five minutes of sitting he could walk on another block. He had a normal vasculature with normal peripheral pulses except for the presence of minor arterial hypertension. This radiogram shows the compression defect on the lumbar cord due to the narrowness of the neural canal. Symptoms were completely relieved by appropriate laminectomy.

blood into the foot. The normal extremity does not blanch on elevation to a 45 degree angle.

Elevation may or may not cause appreciable blanching but should cause the venous system to collapse. When the extremity is allowed to hang down two observations can be made. First is the interval required to fill the veins on the dorsum of the foot. If there is significant incompetence of the venous system, this observation is of no value, for the veins fill from the venous reflux instead of from the arterial input. In the absence of venous incompetence, the veins on the dorsum of the foot should fill in 15 to 20 seconds after the foot becomes pendent.

To the same degree that the pallor develops on elevation, abnormal rubor will follow in the same areas on pendency.

If there is rubor of any significant degree in the foot, pressure should cause it to blanch; failure to blanch indicates a very serious pregangrenous state. Prompt refilling of the blanched area is a favorable sign, whereas delayed refilling and a cyanotic hue to the rubor indicate a serious reduction of flow.

Loss of tissue substance due to cutaneous atrophy, followed by a procedure that improves the blood flow, may eventuate in warm, bright red, atrophic skin, which refills promptly after blanching. This is particularly true following sympathectomy.

Examination of pulses is the second important aspect. According to Cranley,[10] failure to feel pedal pulses indicates the occurrence of arterial disease, but failure to detect a popliteal pulse is the first indication of disease that might be corrected by operation, since it implies

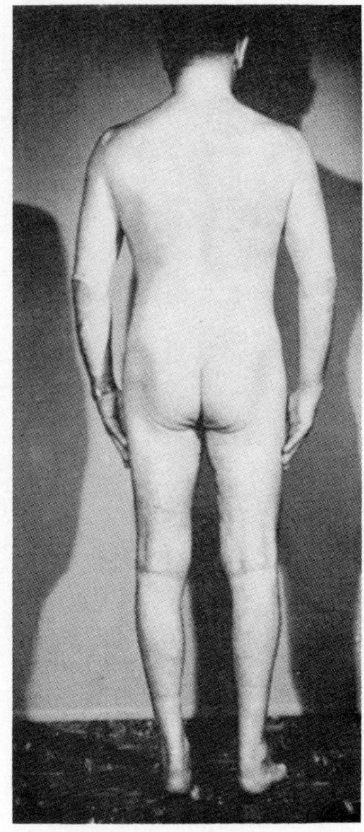

Figure 5–2. Classic Leriche syndrome in male. Note relatively well-developed upper trunk and shoulders, spindlelegs, and absence of bulk in gluteal muscles.

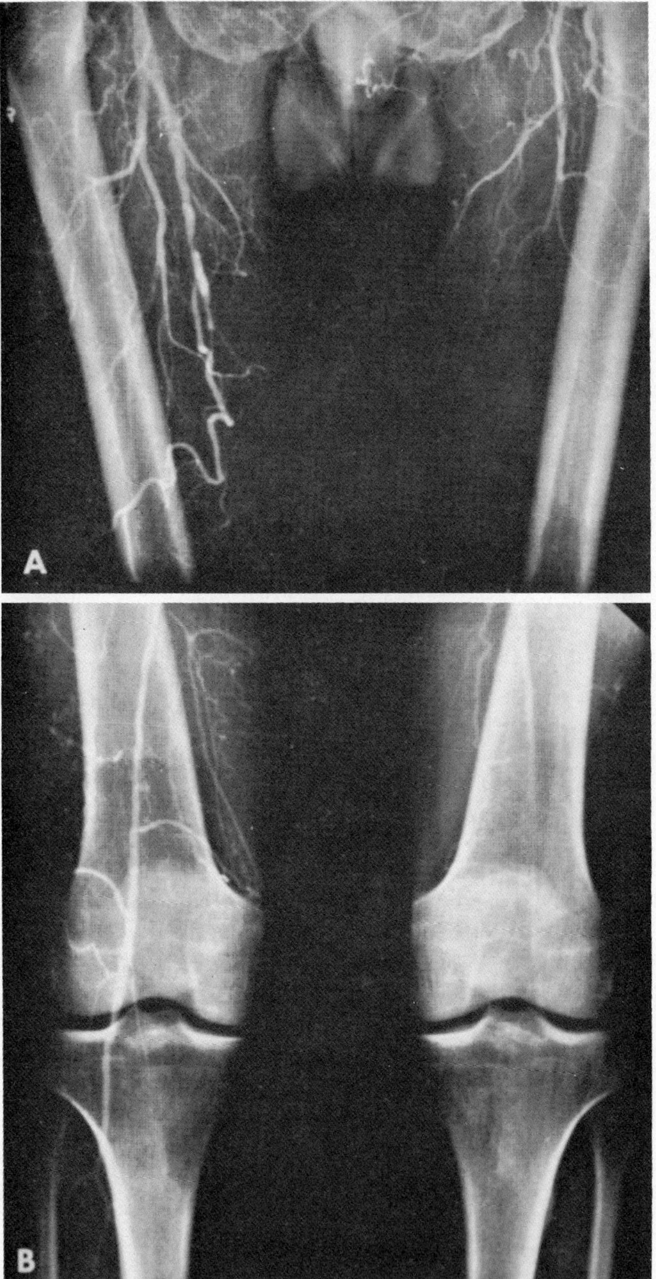

Figure 5–3.   Arteriogram in case of extensive femoral artery disease. *A*, Major collaterals can be seen, as well as very dense network of fine arterial branches. This is characteristic of collateral pathways around an obstruction. Occlusion existed in upper femoral artery, as well as in lower femoral artery. *B*, Refilling of major arterial line at level of popliteal artery. There is complete occlusion on the left and almost complete occlusion on the right.

obstruction of an artery (the femoral or iliac) that is large enough to be treated surgically.

All pulses should be examined, including the superficial temporal, internal and common carotid, subclavian, radial, aortic, common femoral, popliteal, dorsal, pedal, and posterior tibial. The examiner should estimate their volume, degree of symmetry, and the presence or absence of a bruit.

The pulses of the upper part of the body are important not only in localizing disease, but also in indicating diffuse disease. The most difficult to detect with certainty and the most important is the internal carotid pulse. Generally, when disease in the carotid or vertebral system is suspected clinically and is reinforced by arteriographic demonstration, correctable lesions should be operated upon before one undertakes other types of peripheral arterial reconstruction. Surgical correction of an internal carotid artery stenosis is considerably less apt to cause serious hypotension from acute blood loss than is major periph-

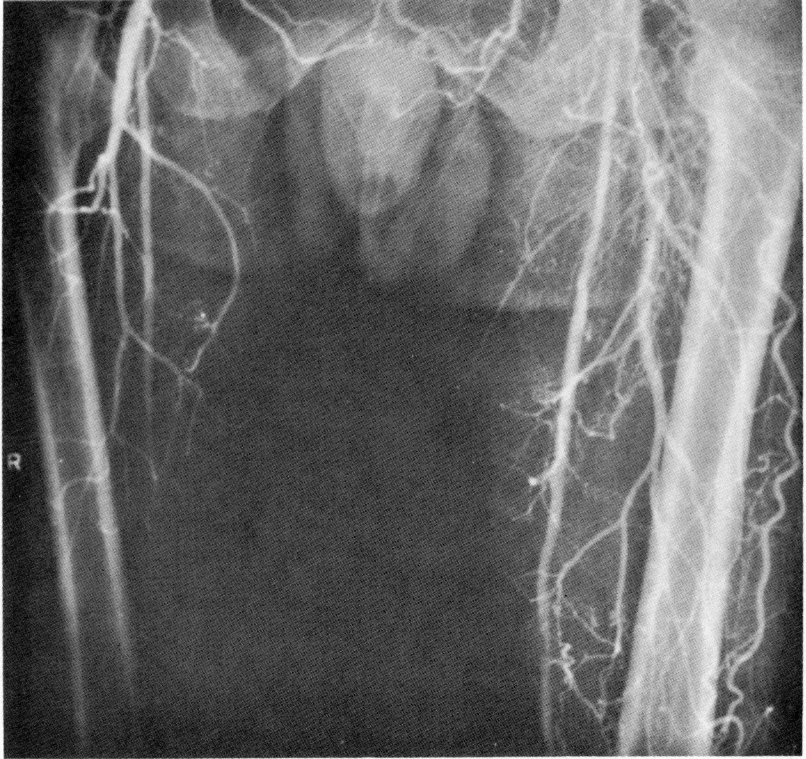

Figure 5–4.   Patient had had amputation of right thigh due to trauma some time previously. Osteoporosis and atrophy of right femur also developed. On the left are seen major collaterals, indicating major obstruction at level of orifice of superficial femoral artery. Co-existing iliac obstruction is not revealed in these arteriograms.

eral arterial reconstruction. The serious consequences of carotid thrombosis give it surgical priority. This combination of carotid artery disease and arterial disease in the lower leg is seen much more frequently with aortic aneurysms than with peripheral occlusive disease; one of the reasons for this situation is that a patient who has had a history of serious cerebrovascular symptoms is often considered unsuitable for surgery of *minor* symptomatic peripheral lesions.

The presence of carotid artery disease may on rare occasions cause some confusion in the diagnosis of peripheral arterial occlusion. A representative case is presented.

J.B., a 55-year-old man, was operated upon for an aortoiliac occlusion in 1958. He was well for only 6 months when he again experienced symptoms; these were clearly demonstrated to be due to closure of the endarterectomized segments.

A Dacron bifurcation bypass prosthesis was used to relieve the occlusion and the patient was well until 1963. He then developed indubitable right carotid stenosis, manifested by weakness of the entire left side and by intermittent aphasia. The unusually high level of carotid bifurcation made correction difficult. Milder symptoms recurred within a few months, chiefly aphasia and weakness of the left leg which developed when he walked only 50 feet—symptoms very much like the original ones. Oscillometric excursions were almost identical in the thighs, and the only other manifestation of disease was a bruit near the anastomosis of the left iliac limb of the graft. Arteriography indicated extensive stenosis of the carotid bifurcation and less marked narrowing at the anastomotic site on the left side. It was believed that the carotid stenosis was only minimally symptomatic, whereas the stenosis at the anastomotic site was the primary source of symptoms.

Correction of the carotid stenosis was done first, in June, 1964. The immediate postoperative result was excellent: not only was the patient's aphasia corrected but his claudication disappeared. No further surgical correction of the graft placement has been undertaken, and the patient was free of symptoms when last seen in 1968.

Evaluation of pulse volume in the lower extremities remains a subjective skill that depends considerably on experience. Attempts should be made to grade the pulse volume by digital examination, but even more objective and reproducible methods should be used and recorded: these methods will be discussed in later pages.

A slight pulse beyond a stenotic lesion can be distinguished from a slight pulse beyond a complete occlusion by its murmur, as described by Edwards[15] and by Wylie.[50] This observation is applicable particularly in diagnosing stenosis in the neck and the groin.

Ejrup[16] and DeWeese[12] have studied in detail the phenomenon of the disappearance of pulses on exercise, especially in patients with limited arterial input. The demonstration of pulsation at a particular site means only that the examiner's finger can *detect* a pulse wave, and that there is transient distention of the vessel by a wave generated by the heart. It carries no implications concerning flow, although these are commonly ascribed to it. As a simple analogy, the normal contour of a pulse wave might be compared with the steep-sloped, sharp upswing of the wave in the typical prestenotic contour. If the peripheral resistance in the extremity after exercise is compared with the peripheral resistance after recovery and at rest, the similarity between the "normal" and "prestenotic" contours will be recognized. Ordinarily, cardiac output can increase sufficiently so that in the normal subject this change will be minimized, but if there is a proximal arterial obstruction of critical degree, the pulse felt after exercise will be of the exaggerated poststenotic shape and may even become "impalpable," although flow is actually increased. This discussion has not taken into account the obvious difficulties of detecting major pulses in the extremities while the subject is exercising vigorously.

As indicated previously, oscillometric measurements and segmental blood pressures provide a convenient office or bedside maneuver through which one may easily identify asymmetry or gross abnormalities which are useful in evaluating the patient's symptoms, in deciding whether or not arteriography is indicated and, indeed, in interpreting more exactly the anatomical findings identified by arteriography. Sumner and Strandness[42] have been most helpful in introducing the technique of pressure measurement using the Doppler velocity sensor. They have correlated the pressures which they have measured with calf flow which was measured by plethysmography (see Table 5–3). In Figure 5–5 are outlined several of the possible variations in oscillometric excursions and segmental pressures in relationship to some of the more commonly identified arterial lesions.

The method of obtaining readings such as those shown in Figure 5–5 is simple. With the patient recumbent, bilateral brachial artery pressures are measured in the standard manner, using the cuff from the oscillometer to be sure that there is no discrepancy between the visual scale readings. It is helpful to record both systolic and diastolic pressures, as recorded by the usual auscultation of Korotkov's sounds, as well as to record systolic pressure as determined by the Doppler sensor placed over the radial artery. A suitable peripheral artery is selected as the sensor in the foot. It is helpful to see if one can hear the dorsal pedal artery in its usual position, the peroneal artery slightly lateral to this, or the posterior tibial artery. These often can be heard with the Doppler sensor equipment even when they cannot be felt. Edema, cutaneous thickening, or weakness of the pulse may all be reasons for not being able to feel the pulse digitally. The best pulse is selected for the further studies. The cuff is then placed at several levels on the leg. If a large enough cuff is available (and it may be wrapped with gauze bandage to maintain it in position) a measurement can be obtained high in the thigh of both the oscillometric excur-

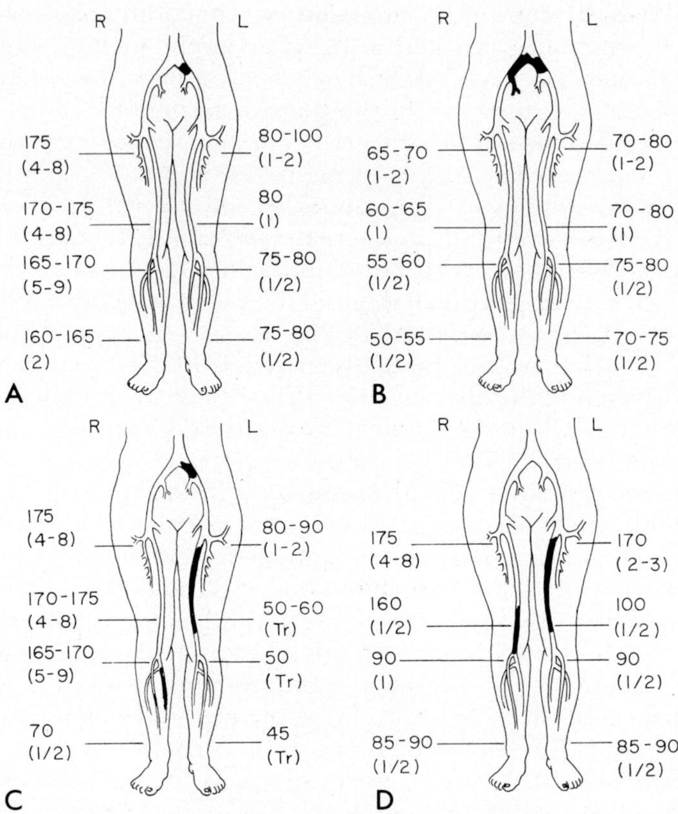

Figure 5–5.   Sketches of the arterial tree showing typical pressures as obtained by the Doppler sensor and blood pressure cuff at four levels; in parentheses typical oscillometric excursions.

A, The right side of the system is normal. The left side has a restricted aortic iliac obstruction. *B,* Bilateral aortic iliac obstruction (the classical Leriche syndrome). *C.* Shows on the right side an aortic iliac obstruction combined with a separate femoral obstruction, and in the left arterial tree a normal tree down to the level of the tibial, and in the tibial system two discrete obstructions. *D.* On the right side an isolated femoral artery obstruction and on the left side an isolated femoral popliteal obstruction. On both sides in this last example the popliteal and tibial systems have no further disease. These are meant to be representative figures, and a wide range of normal may be observed differing from these characteristic figures.

sion and the systolic pressure. The cuff is then moved to the area just above the knee, then to the upper calf, and then to the ankle.

The prolonged and marked drop in ankle blood pressure that follows exercise in the patient who has occlusive disease can be measured as follows. The site of the audible tone is marked, and a deflated cuff is placed at the ankle. The patient exercises until symptoms of claudication develop: the cuff is inflated and the pressure measured as quickly as possible. Significant delay in the return to normal occurs in proportion to the severity of the occlusive disease.

Moore and Hall[35] have used simultaneous femoral puncture to record pressures directly while the patient exercises on a treadle, in order to bring out physiological evidence of iliac artery obstruction when the aortogram does not seem to show significant encroachment. Unrecognized stenoses may be overlooked on the x-rays if the narrowing is crescentic and the ribbon of contrast material is viewed with its greatest diameter perpendicular instead of in profile.

It is difficult to establish a normal range for oscillometric readings. Individual instruments vary, and, of course, measurements may be modified depending upon the security of the cuff, kinks in the tubing, the size of the extremity, and the pressure at which measurements are made.

The expected range for calf oscillations is 3 to 10 units at a pressure midway between diastolic and systolic. Thigh readings are usually slightly lower, depending on the bulk of the thigh.

The magnitude of the oscillometric swing is related to blood flow to some degree. It is affected, however, in a positive way by the ratio of the cross section of the major artery to the cross section of the soft tissue at the level of the cuff. It is also affected positively by the size of the pulse pressure. In addition, the rapidity of the swing of the needle is indicative of the presence of an unobstructed arterial tree proximal to the cuff and, on the contrary, a slow dampened swing suggests a proximally situated obstruction. Troedsson[46] has described in detail the use of several indices relating oscillometric excursions to one another in various parts of the body.

The temperature of the extremity depends upon the environment, the availability of adequate input, and the vasomotor activity as governed by the sympathetic system.

The temperature of the surface of the extremity reflects the balance between the heat loss to the environment and the volume of centrally warmed blood being carried to the skin. Total flow to the limb

Table 5–3. Resting Blood Pressure Correlated with Calf Blood Flow Measured by Plethysmography[*]

Site of Lesion	Resting Ankle Pressure (mm. hg.)	Pressure After Exercise[**] (mm. hg.)	Resting Calf Flow (ml./100 ml./min.)	Flow After Exercise[**] (ml./100 ml./min.)
Superficial femoral artery	83	20	4	19
Iliac artery	81	10	4	15
Combined femoral and iliac lesions	61	7	4	8

[*]After Sumner and Strandness.[42]
[**]Exercise on a treadmill, usually of 5 minutes duration.

may be normal and the internal temperature of the limb normal, but diversion of blood from the skin by increased sympathetic activity may be able to alter the temperature of the skin by as much as 10 degrees C. By the same token, even with maximal vasodilatation of the skin, inadequate arterial inflow may be responsible for the inability of normal regulatory mechanisms of the skin to prevent the temperature of the surface from reflecting closely the temperature of the environment. This situation may occur in diabetic vascular disease. Increased sympathetic tone is usually easily recognized by cyanosis and increased moisture or perspiration on the skin. Significant vascular stasis because of insufficient flow may also occur without markedly increased vasomotor tone when small acral vessels such as those at the digital levels are occluded. This type of cyanosis often does not blanch on pressure. The vessels are filled with a cellular sludge containing reduced hemoglobin.

Changes in room temperature and the subsequent alterations in skin temperature are useful in evaluating the activity and effectiveness of the sympathetic nervous system. Reduction of environmental temperature serves as a challenge of the ability of the sympathetic nervous system to react. The degree to which reaction can occur may be estimated by the degree to which sympathetic blockade or paralysis reduces this capacity to react.

Tissue Necrosis

Actual necrosis of the limb takes many forms, but all have an ominous prognosis. Spontaneous gangrene or necrosis following minor trauma can be interpreted as reflecting serious restriction of blood flow. The more serious the impairment of flow, the less likely are the results of repair to be favorable and the less likely are the favorable initial results to last.

Spontaneous gangrene generally begins in the acral parts of the toes and the heel. The initial deep unblanching rubor proceeds to desiccation and darkening and thence to gangrene, with the typical black "mummified" appearance. A red flare at the margin marks the hyperemia at the level of demarcation.

Melanoma of the digit has been misinterpreted as gangrene; adequate evaluation of the arterial circulation should eliminate this error.

In some cases infection around a nail bed or under a callus or a corn leads to local necrosis. The inflammatory destructive component is more prominent. As will be noted in the section on conservative management (p. 110), infection in or between the toes may drain refluxly along the lumbrical tunnel or other peritendinous pathways to the depths of the plantar fascial compartments and present there as abscesses.

Minimal trauma to the shin, the dorsum of the foot, or the heel or toes can result in the formation of irregular necrotic ulcers. Those on the foot rarely cause diagnostic difficulty, but their implications are no less ominous. In the leg, however, the ischemic ulcer must be distinguished from the ulcer of venous stasis and the hypertensive ulcer of Martorell.[32]

The varicose ulcer is usually much less painful than either of those mentioned. At the base there is shaggy cyanotic granulation tissue, and obvious necrosis and peripheral inflammatory reaction are minimal. Edema and bronze pigmentation are often present; the edema can usually be relieved by protracted elevation of the extremity; whereas elevation of the ischemic extremity usually produces distress. Demonstration of venous dilatation and incompetence helps confirm the diagnosis, but the combination of arterial insufficiency and venous insufficiency may obscure the diagnosis. Arterial insufficiency may be suspected because of inability to detect pulses, but this may be apparent rather than actual, due to edema and thickening of the skin caused, in turn, by chronic venous stasis. Varicose ulcers almost never occur below the level of the malleoli. Oscillometry will often indicate normal levels when brawny induration prevents the digital determination of pulses.

The symmetrical shallow ulcers of Martorell[32] probably arise from local cutaneous infarcts secondary to arteriolar necrosis. The patient usually manifests little peripheral arterial insufficiency otherwise but is severely hypertensive. These ulcers are also apt to be painful. The treatment of choice is lumbar sympathectomy followed by application of split thickness skin grafts, provided the patient is a suitable candidate.

Acute occlusion of the major arteries of the femoropopliteal tree may be due to arteriosclerotic thrombosis, failure of operative intervention, embolism, or trauma. Thrombosis is apt to produce diffuse ischemia, especially if prior sympathectomy has been done, but rarely extensive acute necrosis. The other situations, arising in the absence of collaterals, may provoke acute and extensive gangrene, with severe pain. The level of demarcation and suitability for amputation depend upon the local arterial anatomy and the extent of arteriosclerosis, more specifically upon the number of collaterals obliterated.

Spotty areas of peripheral gangrene, for instance, involving one or two separated digits although separated by relatively healthy tissue, may indicate local distal thromboses. Under such circumstances, however, one should always look for a proximal site from which small emboli may have arisen, either popliteal, femoral or aortic, or proximal ulcerated atherosclerotic lesions. The phenomenon of multiple small emboli to critical areas of the brain has long been recognized in the presence of carotid stenoses; it has recently been demonstrated with regard to coronary artery stenoses.[34] This phenomenon has not been given full consideration with regard to peripheral arterial lesions, however.

The prognosis following acute ligation is indicated in Table 5–4. This table does not take into account the length of the segment obliterated nor the importance of that segment to collateral circulation, and should serve only as a rough guide.

The distinction between acute thrombosis imposed upon a *stenotic* system and acute obstruction of previously normal arterial tree without well developed collaterals depends on subtle factors.

The general status of the patient may be helpful in reaching a diagnosis. The teenager who has had atrial fibrillation and experiences the sudden onset of symptoms of acute occlusion is easily recognized as having experienced an embolism; on the other hand, the older patient who develops an acute occlusion is more apt to have coronary arteriosclerosis, in which there is mural thrombosis attributable to an infarct, embolism attributable to atrial fibrillation, or thrombosis consequent to hypotension and decreased cardiac output due to acute coronary occlusion.

Unrecognized myocardial infarction must be kept in mind in every case of acute femoral occlusion. Failure to be alert to the possibility of infarction may result in catastrophe if major surgery is undertaken. A representative case is detailed in which the outcome fortunately was successful.

B.R., a 56-year-old man who had a history of minimal diabetes, was admitted because of pain and swelling in the left calf. He also noticed red streaks along the calf. Past history included minimal claudication of several months' duration, which had suddenly become more severe a week before admission. Physical examination showed slight edema, acute superficial thrombophlebitis in the calf, prompt pallor on elevation, and absence of popliteal and pedal pulses on the left side.

Table 5–4. Development of Gangrene Following Arterial Ligation at Various Levels. All Figures Given as Percentage.[*]

Site of Ligation	Series		
	Wolff	Hendrich	Makins
Subclavian	4.8	9.7	
Axillary	15.0	9.8	
Brachial	4.0	3.1	
Aortic	—	100.0	
Common iliac	50.0	100.0	
External iliac	11.2	13.4	16.6
Common femoral	25.0	21.8	25.9
Superficial femoral	12.7	10.4	14.1
Popliteal	14.9	37.2	37.5

[*]After Key.[25]

Administration of heparin was begun. Lumbar sympathectomy and arteriography were recommended to the patient but he refused these. His symptoms responded to heparin therapy and conservative management, but successive electrocardiograms showed progression of ischemic changes in the heart.

Following recovery, the patient returned to his normal activity, and experienced angina for the first time. Had he not refused sympathectomy and arteriography, he might have been subjected to operation in the face of an unrecognized myocardial infarction.

Pain at rest is a sign of advanced arterial obstruction and often connotes either a distal level of obstruction or an extensive degree of obstruction. Such pain is often relieved by the combination of pendency and muscular inactivity; however, the resulting edema causes a further decrease in capillary perfusion, and thus increases the pain.

Another type of pain at rest has recently been described by Shaw;[41] this is pathologic malingering on the part of the patient in whom there is a true need for secondary gain from the disability of a cold, painful, edematous extremity. This situation requires careful psychiatric management as well as physical rehabilitation.

In other circumstances causalgia develops in a leg or arm which is protected from all use. In this situation the prognosis is poor, but it can be improved if the patient is properly supported psychologically and persuaded to redevelop use of the extremity.

Biophysical Methods of Diagnosis

There are various biophysical methods of evaluating blood flow through a limb, most of which are classifiable into two categories. Some were introduced at a time when the only available procedure was sympathectomy; they involve estimation of the degree of function of the sympathetic nervous system in controlling and, possibly, restricting flow. In this category are various tests of skin temperature, skin resistance, and plethysmography. Those in the second category are of greatest interest to the physiologist; many are of great significance in demonstrating the importance of clinical signs in evaluating peripheral vascular disease. Here are included digital and segmental plethysmography, as well as pulse registration,[11] impedance plethysmography,[47] and radioisotope dilution, appearance, and mobilization blood volume flow. (A detailed account of the technique and patterns of results of these tests is found in Winsor.[49]) Part of the merit of these tests is their reproducibility during various stages in the course of the patient's care.

The use of the oscillometer and the measurement of segmental blood pressures should be reemphasized here, although these methods have been discussed as an integral part of the routine examination in previous pages. The segmental pressures are a more reliable guide than is strain gauge plethysmography, according to Yao.[51]

Arteriographic Diagnosis

One can recognize clinically the patient whose condition demands treatment, and the most profitable evaluation is provided by the local and general physical examinations already discussed and by radiologic studies which indicate whether or not reconstruction is feasible.

Translumbar arteriography was first popularized by R. Dos Santos et al.[13] Local puncture of the femoral artery and arteriographic demonstration of the distal tree[2] were additional techniques subsequently introduced for evaluation.

At first the roentgenologists grudgingly tolerated the efforts of the vascular surgeons; in recent years, however, the roentgenologists have developed techniques that are of great assistance to the surgeon, and their participation has become invaluable.

Two small exceptions must be taken regarding the role of the roentgenologist in this field. First, in spite of the improvements in roentgenologic technique, the adequqncy of the *distal* tree is not always accurately represented by *proximal* arteriography. It then becomes necessary to utilize direct exposure of the arterial tree as well as injection of a contrast medium to determine the degree of adequacy of outflow system.[2]

Second is the circumstance—fortunately rare—in which an inappropriate examination is ordered by a physician who is not trained to evaluate the clinical aspects of peripheral vascular disease. The following *hypothetical* case illustrates the devastating consequences of this occurrence.

A 65-year-old diabetic who had serious coronary disease and extensive peripheral vascular disease was referred to a roentgenologist for coronary arteriography. Inadvertently, the roentgenologist was not informed that the patient was receiving warfarin sodium. The patient was entirely unsuitable for surgical treatment of either his coronary or peripheral arteries, but the examination was carried out to satisfy the apparent need for a complete and objective diagnosis beyond that already obtained by simple and orthodox means. At examination, the arterial catheter was introduced into a prominent left femoral artery, because the axillary arteries were believed to be too sclerotic and tortuous. During attempts to place the catheter in the ascending aorta the patient went into circulatory collapse and suffered a cardiac arrest. Although cardiac function was promptly restored, it soon became apparent that the catheter was no longer in the lumen of the aorta, but had entered the subatheromatous plane at the aortic bifurcation, and the opposite iliac artery had become occluded. Gangrene of the right leg promptly ensued, and amputation was performed because of the patient's poor general condition. A hematoma at the site of the puncture—actually an aneurysm of the femoral artery—became infected. Secondary hemorrhage from the artery required ligation of that femoral artery, with subsequent amputation of the second limb.

It is incumbent upon the radiologist to question the reason for requests for arteriography. He must be assured that the surgeon has already made a careful and critical evaluation of the entire vascular tree, and he must assure himself that the projected study is necessary not only in establishing a diagnosis, but to the care of the patient as well.

The surgeon is fortunate who is associated with radiologists who combine the safeguards just described with technical skill and professional interest.

The details of the arteriographic procedure have been outlined by Riley et al.,[38] by Hanafee,[21] and by Seldinger,[40] and will simply be summarized here.

A modification of the Seldinger tecnhique is frequently used. An appropriate artery is chosen and a needle is introduced. A flexible wire is then introduced through the needle and guided under control by an image intensifier that minimizes the fluoroscopic dose of irradiation. When the guidewire is clearly in the descending thoracic aorta, the needle is withdrawn and the double catheter system is threaded over it. By maneuvering the wire and a curved tip on one of the catheters, catheterization can be done of any of the major visceral branches. For opacification of the distal arterial tree, a preliminary test injection is made at the level of the infrarenal aorta and observed with an image-intensifying device as it passes into the lower leg. A second full injection outlines the bifurcation and three automatic moves of the table in 10 inch increments allow the rapid cassette changer to record films of the contrast material as it fills the vessels of the leg. On the basis of the fluoroscopic examinations and by estimating the changes in flow secondary to the anticipated extent of the disease, the sliding table can be programed to follow the progress of the radiopaque material down the legs.

Because of a large number of local complications at the site of arterial puncture, there has been some trend back to translumbar aortography. The catheter is placed in the aortic lumen through a modification of the Seldinger method, using, however, the posterior approach. It is not possible to utilize this route for wide manipulation of the catheter, but repeated injections can be made for proper visualization of the lower abdominal aorta and all of its distal branches. It is probably hazardous to use this method in the presence of coagulation defects or hypertension, for there is no way to apply local pressure to control bleeding at the site of the aortic puncture.

There are undoubted risks in aortography. Local injury can occur, or a false aneurysm may develop at the site of arterial puncture. With

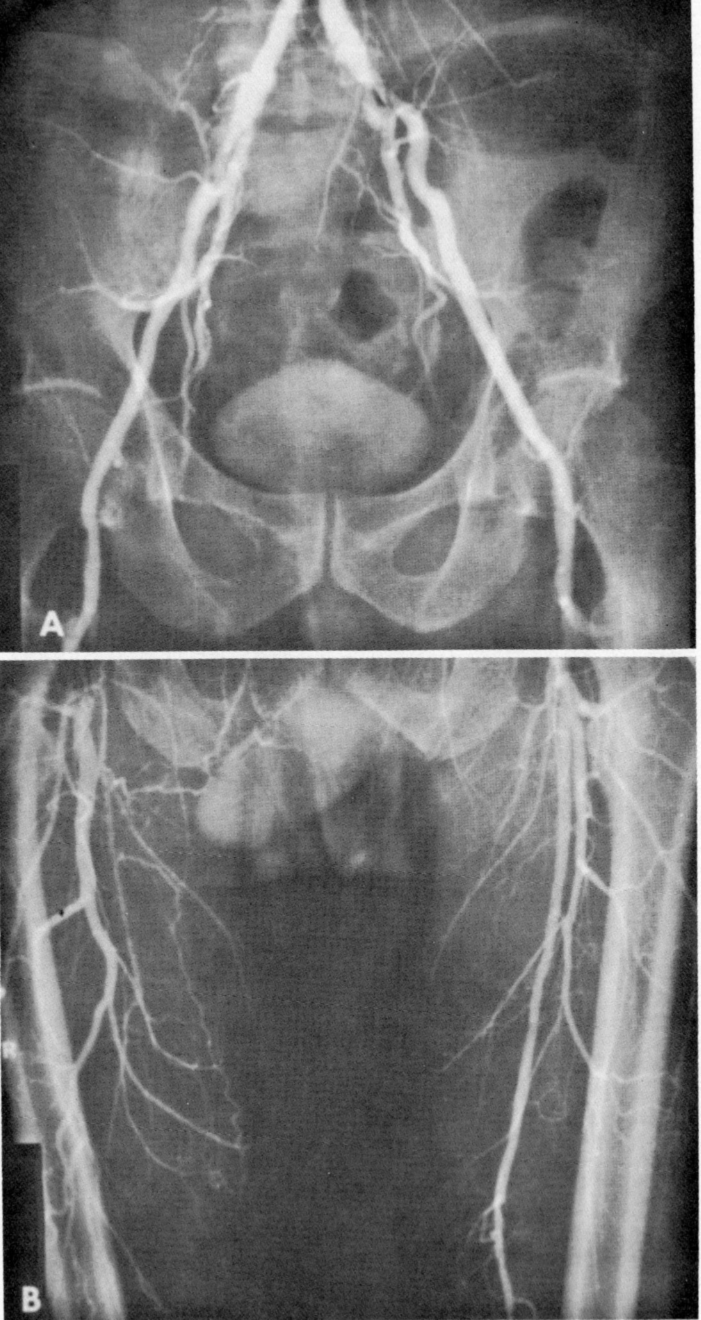

Figure 5–6.   See opposite page for legend.

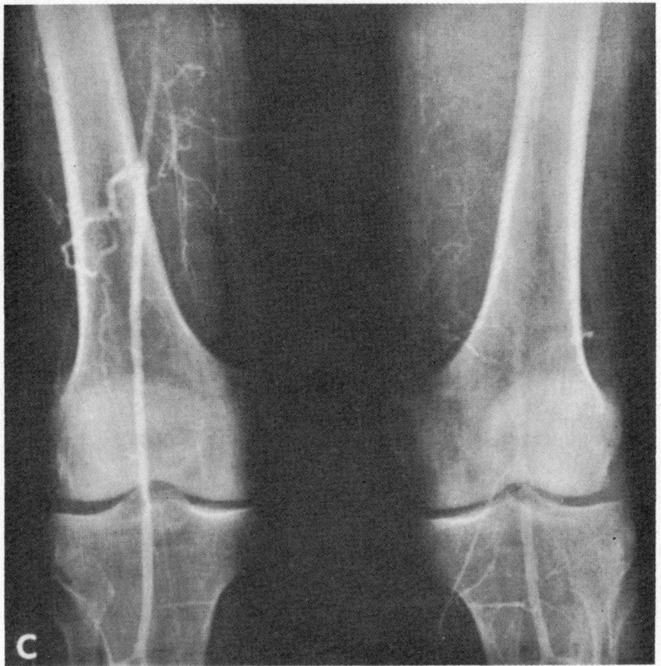

Figure 5–6. Arteriogram in case of extensive disease. *A,* Stenosis with patchy incipient aneurysmal disease at iliac vessels. *B,* Collaterals are seen with hypertrophic deep femoral artery and complete obstruction of upper superficial femoral artery. *C,* Left popliteal artery is seen to be completely refilled. Note large collaterals in region of lateral superior genicular artery. Radiopaque material has passed almost entirely through left superficial femoral artery. Left superficial femoral artery is slightly stenotic, as demonstrated in *B,* but passage of dye through femoral artery in *C* makes it appear that there is an occlusion of lower femoral artery.

care at the time of puncture, the two-catheter technique, and maintenance of local pressure after the procedure, false aneurysms should be rare. Idiosyncratic responses to the contrast medium are always possible, but preliminary test injections and use of a relatively innocuous contrast medium should minimize these.

Machleder has summarized his experience with false aneurysms in brachial arterial catheterizations.[30] His findings indicate that repeated punctures and prolonged catheterization are more likely to result in arterial injury. Arterial injury may manifest itself by hemorrhage. Hemorrhage may result in a false aneurysm which identifies itself so clearly that repair becomes necessary. Arterial thrombosis secondary to intimal injury or arterial spasm is the other complication which is often undertreated with dismal results. The use of the Doppler Velocity Sensor to measure pressures peripheral to the site of arterial puncture and to compare them with the opposite side has been very useful in identifying the severity of the arterial puncture injury. With increasing experience in the management of patients with such arterial puncture injuries it has become our practice to proceed promptly with arterial exploration if the pulse is lost or if the Doppler Sensor shows a pressure drop of more than 15 or 20 millimeters of mercury, which persists after a brief period of observation. Furthermore, under some circumstances a cuff of platelet and fibrin debris may form on the catheter. Mechanical dislodgment of this cuff may cause its embolization into the arterial tree either beyond the site of arterial puncture or elsewhere. Heparinization during the procedure or the use of truly thrombosis-resistant catheters should reduce this hazard to a minimum.[45]

Toxic reactions to high local concentrations of the medium occur, primarily in the spinal cord and kidneys. Injury secondary to aortography has been discussed in considerable detail in the literature.[17, 18, 26, 27, 37]

Critical dosage levels are recognized for each concentration of each drug, but there is considerable variation in individual sensitivity to the drugs. The position of the catheter tip must not be opposite the orifice of the major lumbar branch feeding the anterior spinal artery (see p. 11); for distal opacification the tip of the catheter is best placed about 3 cm. above the bifurcation of the aorta.

Multiple injections into renal and other branches should be avoided because the initial injection seems to provoke changes in capillary permeability that make subsequent injections more hazardous.[37] For peripheral arteriography, it has proved to be safe[38] to give an initial injection of 10 ml. of contrast material and to follow the rate of filling of the distal vessels in order to plan the movement of the table to follow the course of the initial injection of 25 ml.* If disease is more extensive on one side, and if flow is greatly delayed down that side, a second injection and series of films may be necessary, with a slower movement of the table to follow the contrast material down the more diseased side. Videotape recordings may be made from the input to the monitor of the image intensifier and may be shown repeatedly to provide a clear understanding of the actual rate of flow in the system being studied.

The amount of material injected can be handled satisfactorily by the kidneys under most circumstances, but care should be taken to have the patient well hydrated. The common practice of having the patient abstain from breakfast should be avoided. If it is necessary that the patient have no food, then he should be given adequate amounts of intravenous fluid to assure adequate renal output.

Some additional protection to the central nervous system during cerebral arteriography may be afforded by antecedent injection of

---

*Angio-Conray or 76 per cent Renografin.

procaine, 20 per cent glucose, or low molecular weight dextran; however, the mechanism of this protection is not clear.[11]

The use of the prone position as suggested by Killen and Foster[26] has not seemed important when the catheter technique just described is used. Almost all arteriography done with the catheter is carried out under local anesthesia in order to achieve the cooperation of the patient and to avoid use of barbiturates.

The therapeutic technique developed by Dotter,[14] which is an outgrowth of transbrachial arteriography, has provoked great interest. This percutaneous dilatation of stenotic vessels will be described in a subsequent chapter.

Szilagyi[44] and Blaisdell[7] have advocated the use of angiography performed on the operating table or in the early postoperative period in order to ascertain that the arterial reconstruction has been adequate. We have not in the past used it as a routine measure but it is becoming more and more popular. Operative angiography used in this way has been one of the means of assuring a successful reconstruction. The electromagnetic flowmeter has also been of great value at the operating table in assessing the success of the reconstruction. An interesting sidelight of the use of the flowmeter at the operating table at UCLA has been the use of intra-arterial vasodilators such as Papaverine to estimate the degree to which flow will increase after recovery from the early postoperative period.[20] Most helpful in following the patient after he leaves the table, however, has been the continued reassessment using the oscillometer or segmental pressure measurements, as outlined previously, or both together.

REFERENCES

1. Babson, A. L., Shapiro, P. O., and Phillips, G. E.: A new assay for cholesterol and cholesterol esters in serum which is not affected by bilirubin. Clin. Chim. Acta 7:800, 1962.
2. Barker, W. F.: Distal operative angiography as an aid in endarterectomy. Surgery 36:233, 1954.
3. Barker, W. F.: *Peripheral Arterial Disease*, Philadelphia, W. B. Saunders Company, 1966.
4. Barker, W. F., In Dale, W. A.: *Management of Arterial Occlusive Disease*. Chicago, Year Book Medical Publishers, Inc., pp. 383–398, 1971.
5. Barker, W. F., and Hart, J.: Arterial reconstruction by endarterectomy. Four-year follow-up study. Am. J. Surg. *100*:165, 1960.
6. Beales, J. S. M., Adcock, F. A., Frawley, J. S., Nathan, B. E., McLachlan, M. S. F., Martin, P., and Steiner, R. E.: The radiologic assessment of disease of the profunda femoris artery. Brit. J. Radiol. *44*:854, 1971.
7. Blaisdell, F. W., Lim, R. Jr., and Hall, A. D.: Technical result of carotid endarterectomy. Arteriographic Assessment. Am. J. Surg. 114, pg. 239, 1967.
8. Cannon, J. A.: Intermittent claudication—what it is and isn't. Calif. Med. *102*:301, 1965.
9. Charcot, J. M.: Sur la claudication intermittente observée dans un cas d'oblitération complète de l'une des artères iliaques primitives. Mém. Soc. Biol. *1*, 225, 1858.

10. Cranley, J. J., Krause, R. J., and Strasser, E. S.: Limb survival with and without definitive surgical treatment in obliterative arterial disease. Surgery *45*:32, 1959.
11. Darling, C. R., Raines, J. K., Brenner, B. J., and Austen, W. G.: Quantitative segmental pulse volume recorder. Surgery *72*:873, 1972.
12. DeWeese, J. A.: Pedal pulses disappearing with exercise. New Eng. J. Med. *262*:1214, 1960.
13. dos Santos, R., Lamas, A. C., and Caldas, J. P.: *Artériographie des Membres et de l'Aorte Abdominale.* Paris, Masson et Cie; 1931.
14. Dotter, C. A.: Cardiovascular catheterization and angiographic technics of future promise. Presented at Pan-Pacific Surgical Association, 1963.
15. Edwards, E. A., and Levine, H. D.: Peripheral vascular murmurs; mechanism of production and diagnostic significance. Arch. Int. Med. *90*:284, 1952.
16. Ejrup, B.: Tonoscillography after exercise: new method for early diagnosis of organic arterial disease leading to intermittent claudication and for differential diagnosis of organic and functional arterial diseases with special type of apparatus adapted to this purpose. Acta Med. Scand. (Suppl. 211) *130*:1, 1948.
17. Foster, J. H., Killen, D. A., Sessions, R. T., Rhea, G. W., Winfrey, E. W., III., and Collins, H. A.: The relative toxicity of angiographic contrast media. Vascular Dis. *1*:8, 1964.
18. Foster, J. H., Sessions, R. T., and Killen, D. A.: Studies in the prevention of toxic reactions incident to contrast angiography. Bull. Soc. Int. Chir. *21*:122, 1962.
19. Garret, H. E., Horning, E. C., Creech, B. G., and DeBakey, M. E.: Serum cholesterol values in patients treated surgically for atherosclerosis. J.A.M.A. *189*:655, 1964.
20. Golding, A. L., and Cannon, J. A.: Application of electromagnetic blood flow meter during arterial reconstruction. Results in conjunction with Papaverine in 47 cases. Ann. Surg. *164*:662, 1966.
21. Hanafee, W.: Axillary artery approach to carotid, vertebral, abdominal aorta, and coronary angiography. Radiology *81*:559, 1963.
22. Humphries, A. W., Young, J. R., DeWolfe, V. G., LeFevre, F. A., and Beven, E. G.: Severe ischemia of the lower extremity due to arteriosclerosis obliterans. Arch. Surg. *87*:175, 1963.
23. Humphries, A. W., In Dale, W. A. (Ed.): *Management of Arterial Occlusive Disease.* Chicago, Year Book Medical Publishers, Inc., 1971, pp. 67–78.
24. Keitzer, W. F., Fry, W. J., Kraft, R. O., and DeWeese, M. S.: Hemodynamic mechanism for pulse changes seen in occlusive vascular disease. Surgery *57*:163, 1965.
25. Key, E.: Embolectomy on vessels of the extremities. Brit. J. Surg. *24*:350, 1936.
26. Killen, D. A., and Foster, J. H.: Spinal cord injury as a complication of aortography. Ann. Surg. *152*:211, 1960.
27. Killen, D. A., Foster, J. H., and Scott, H. W., Jr.: Toxic reaction incident to Urokon aortography as related to the volume of contrast medium injected. Ann. Surg. *155*:472, 1962.
28. Lassen, N. A., Lindbjerg, I. F., and Dahn, I.: Validity of the Xenon[133] method for measurement of muscle blood flow evaluated by simultaneous venous occlusion plethysmography. Circ. Research *16*:287, 1965.
29. Leriche, R.: De la résection du carrefour aorticoiliaque avec double sympathectomie lombaire pour thromboise artéritique; le syndrome de l'oblitération termino-aortique par artérite. Presse Méd. *48*:601, 1940.
30. Machleder, H. I., Sweeney, J. P., and Barker, W. F.: Pulseless arm after brachial-artery catheterization. Lancet, Pg. 407–409, Feb. 19, 1972.
31. Martin, P., Frawley, J. F., Barabas, A. P., and Rosengarten, D. S.: On the surgery of the profunda femoris artery. Surgery *71*:182, 1972.
32. Martorell, F.: Las úlcers supra maleolares por arteriolitis de las grandes hipertensas. Actas Cuerpo Fac. Inst. Policlín. Barc. *1*:6, 1945.
33. Miller, T., Niazmand, R., and Barker, W. F.: Femoral artery reconstruction under local anesthesia, maximal results from minimal risk. Am. J. Surg. *122*:513, 1971.
34. Mills, N., and Ochsner, J. L.: Distal thromboembolism in proximal coronary arteriosclerotic lesions. Surgery *72*:1030, 1972.

35. Moore, W. S., and Hall, A. D.: Unrecognized aortoiliac stenosis: a physiologic approach to the diagnosis.

36. O'Hara, V.: Personal communication.

37. Rhea, W. G., Jr., O'Neill, J. A., Killen, D. A., and Foster, J. H.: Toxic reactions incident to aortography. The hazard of repeat injection. Circulation 29:Suppl.: 161, 1964.

38. Riley, J. M., Hanafee, W., and Weidner, W.: Left axillary approach to the abdominal aorta. Radiology 84:96, 1965.

39. Sawyer, R. B., and Moncrief, J. A.: Dextran specificity in thrombus inhibition. Arch. Surg. 90:562, 1965.

40. Seldinger, S.: Catheter replacement of needle in percutaneous arteriography; new technique. Acta Radiol. 39:368, 1953.

41. Shaw, R. S.: Pathologic malingering. The painful disabled extremity. New Eng. J. Med. 271:22, 1964.

42. Sumner, D. S., and Strandness, D. E. Jr.: Relationship between calf blood flow and ankle blood pressure in patients with intermittent claudication. Surgery 65:763, 1969.

43. Szilagyi, D. E., Rodriguez, F. J., Smith, R. F., and Elliott, J. P.: Late fate of arterial allografts. Observations 6 to 15 years after implantation. Arch. Surg. 101:721, 1970.

44. Szilagyi, D. E., Smith, R. F., and Whitney, D. G.: The durability of aorto-iliac endarterectomy. Arch. Surg. 89:827, 1964.

45. Takaro, T., Pifarre, R., Wuerflein, R. D., Hall, A. D., Gage, A. A., Scott, S. M., Dart, C. H. Jr., and Price, H. P.: Acute coronary occlusion following coronary arteriography: mechanisms and surgical relief. Surgery 72:1018, 1972.

46. Troedsson, B. S.: Oscillometric arterial circulatory norms. J.A.M.A. 172:141, 1960.

47. Van de Water, J. M., Dmochowski, J. R., Dove, G. B., and Couch, N. P.: Evaluation of an impedence flowmeter in arterial surgery. Surgery 70:954, 1971.

48. Verbiest, H.: A radicular syndrome from the development narrowing of the lumbar vertebral canal. J. Bone Joint Surg. 36B:230, 1954.

49. Winsor, T.: *Peripheral Vascular Disease.* Springfield, Ill., Charles C Thomas, 1959.

50. Wylie, E. J., and McGuinness, J. S.: The recognition and treatment of arteriosclerotic stenosis of major arteries. Surg. Gynec. Obstet. 97:425, 1953.

51. Yao, S. T., Weedham, T. N., Gourmos, C., and Irvine, W. T.: A comparative study of strain gauge plethysmography and Doppler ultrasound in the assessment of occlusive arterial disease of the extremities. Surgery 71:4, 1972.

Chapter Six

CONSERVATIVE MEASURES. THE ROLE OF SYMPATHECTOMY

Conservative measures are an important part of treatment in peripheral vascular disease. The patient about to undergo surgery may need a period of conservative management preoperatively or postoperatively just as much as the patient being managed medically.

The surgeon employs these conservative measures according to personal opinion, for objective proof of their value is biased by the patient's responses, which are apt to be unpredictable by either objective or subjective criteria. An example of the variation in results that can be effected by the patient's wish that the medicine help him is the case of a patient who was observed in a double blind study; he insisted that his claudication was greatly improved—and was found later to be receiving the placebo!

Conservative management includes systemic measures and local measures.

SYSTEMIC MEASURES

Medication for relief of symptoms of peripheral arterial insufficiency has been largely ineffectual.

Of course, other diseases that may be present require drug therapy, as heart disease with digitalis, diabetes with insulin, and so forth.

At times methods of therapy may appear to be contradictory. The patient who must have some relief of hypertension discovers that with the use of antihypertensive medication his legs are not well perfused, even though his blood pressure is near the normal level, and that the distance he can walk before claudication develops has decreased.

Vasodilators

Vasodilators may be divided into centrally acting drugs, those acting peripherally on autonomic ganglia, as adrenergic blocking agents, and those acting directly on the vessel.

The centrally acting drugs include primarily the dihydrogenated ergot alkaloids (dihydroergocornine, dihydroergocristine, and dihydroergokryptine [Hydergine]) and ethyl alcohol.

The primary effect of the dihydrogenated ergot alkaloids is central but they also have an adrenergic effect on the neuroeffector organ in blood vessels. Clinically, they are of greatest value in vasospastic conditions of the upper extremities.

Ethyl alcohol, although not practical in all situations as a chronic medication, remains one of the best drugs in view of its central vasodilating effect, its mild sedative effect, and its direct local effect—although minor—on the blood vessel. It is an excellent drug for use in the hospitalized patient.

The ganglionic blocking agents, such as mecamylamine (Inversine) and chlorisondamine (Ecolid), are not generally useful in the management of the ambulatory patient.

Adrenergic blocking agents include phenoxybenzamine (Dibenzyline) which is of value in combination with tolazoline (Priscoline); phentolamine (Regitine) which is more useful in the diagnosis of pheochromocytoma than it is in arterial disease; and azapetine (Ilidar). Azapetine is sympatholytic and adrenergic and also has a direct effect on the blood vessels; it can cause serious postural hypotension and must be used with care.

The direct acting drugs include, in addition to ethyl alcohol, Priscoline, betapyridil carbinol (Roniacol), and nitroglycerin.

Priscoline is perhaps one of the most widely used drugs in peripheral vascular occlusions. In spite of its side reactions of palpitation, formication and other cutaneous symptoms, and gastric secretory stimulation, it is usually well tolerated. Not only does it act directly on the vessel, but it also has an adrenergic blocking and sympatholytic effect.

Roniacol, the alcohol corresponding to nicotinic acid, is a relatively innocuous agent of special merit in treatment of the upper limbs.

Nitroglycerin has a very transient effect on the peripheral circulation but may be of use in the treatment of the restless legs syndrome, which may be completely unrelated to arterial occlusive disease.

Papaverine, one of the first vasodilating drugs, has been almost forgotten in clinical practice. It is not suitable for chronic use, and other drugs have replaced it; however, because of its direct effect on the blood vessel, it may be useful when blood flow seems to be unduly restricted after arterial reconstruction, even when combined with sympathectomy. Although this effect may be transient, it may be of prognostic value, as is indicated in the following case.

A 46-year-old man had extensive atherosclerosis of a very narrow aorta, and of the common femoral and iliac artery system bilaterally. A bypass graft was placed from the aorta into the common femoral arteries bilaterally after bilateral lumbar sympathectomy. Initial flow measurements in the graft were apparently adequate at 300 ml. per minute on the right and at 145 ml. per minute on the left. After 15 mg. of papaverine had been injected into the artery, flow rose to 900 ml. per minute, and 500 ml. per minute, respectively. These increases were transient but were believed to indicate that the distal tree would accept a high rate of flow. The clinical outcome of the reconstruction was highly satisfactory and much more compatible with the higher flow rates measured with use of papaverine than the lower flows initially obtained. Other drugs may serve as well as papaverine, but the drug should not be overlooked.

One other agent deserves particular mention. This is phenyl-2-butyl norsuprifen (Arlidin). Arlidin has a direct effect on the blood flow to skeletal muscles and an inotropic effect that increases cardiac output and coronary artery flow, and mean arterial pressure. It should therefore be valuable in relieving claudication, but it must be used cautiously in patients with angina, significant myocardial disease, paroxysmal tachycardia, or hyperthyroidism.

A more detailed description of these drugs may be found in standard pharmacological references or textbooks.[2, 54]

The improvement effected by the use of any of these drugs is slight and unpredictable. Theoretically, their generalized effect on peripheral resistance could cause blood to be shunted *away from* the area affected by stenosis, rather than augment flow where needed.[4] That a favorable response to these drugs sometimes occurs suggests that such shunting does not always occur. This situation might be brought about by diffuse and symmetrical involvement of the arterial tree, by a highly subjective response on the part of the patient, or by increased sensitivity to the drugs in the distal tree beyond an obstruction. In any case, a trial of these drugs is certainly warranted but their benefits are subject to question and they do not represent a good alternative to appropriate surgical intervention.

The local use by arterial injection has greater rationale. Priscoline has commonly been used by this route, but the frequency with which

injections are required limits its use. More recently, intra-arterial injection of reserpine in doses up to 1 milligram for injection will at
times have an effect lasting a month or more on the more classical
vasospastic syndromes involving the hand.[36] The addition of guane-
thidine in doses of 10 to 30 milligrams per day orally supplements the
intra-arterial reserpine.

Anticoagulants

The evaluation of anticoagulants is equally difficult. In the cerebral and coronary arteries, for example, dramatic episodes constitute
clear-cut evidence of further arterial occlusion, yet in spite of such objective end points the use of anticoagulant drugs is still the subject of
much controversy: the effectiveness of heparin and of prothrombin antagonists such as warfarin in preventing further occlusions must be
balanced against the increased hazard of hemorrhage. The end points
in peripheral vascular disease are less clearly recognized and the most
severe manifestations may be tempered by the presence of a potentially much more efficient collateral vascular flow. Therefore it becomes even more difficult to assess accurately the value of anticoagulant therapy in conservative management.

In acute occlusions the use of heparin followed by a later protracted course of sodium warfarin offers some protection against further propagation of an intravascular thrombus and further deterioration of collateral efficiency. Statistical proof of this statement is
lacking, and in fact would be difficult to obtain because of general
unpredictability regarding the outcome of acute occlusions. Furthermore, general reliance on anticoagulants as an effective aid also makes
it difficult to withhold such therapy. It would also be difficult to match
control cases against treated cases, because of the great variability
among patients with regard to general physical status, local anatomic
variability, potential collaterals, and acquired pathologic disorders.

Equally difficult to evaluate is the effect of long-term sodium warfarin therapy after the acute phase has passed. There are some specific
situations in which objective observations support the use of the drug;
for example, sodium warfarin apparently produces a thinner and presumably more adherent lining within a fabric graft.[19] More common is
the use of sodium warfarin in the type of patient now described.

A 72-year-old male had been seen initially in 1955 by a vascular surgeon,
who believed that the patient's bilateral femoral artery obstruction could be
treated by arterial reconstruction. The patient refused operation and was
placed on sodium warfarin therapy. When treatment was begun he had a
claudication distance of only 50 feet, and oscillometric excursions of 2 units
on the left and 1/4 unit on the right, just below the knee.

By 1960 he had improved to the point that he could walk 5 miles without
stopping, and oscillometrics were measured at 2 units bilaterally in the calf.

It may be that the natural history of many cases of arterial obstruction is just as has been described, and that the prolonged period of study and the repeated contacts required to maintain control of the prothrombin content have merely served to reveal the course. Characteristically, however, one would expect deterioration of the peripheral circulation to occur during this period. Carefully controlled studies of this mode of treatment should be made. Wright[55] has had favorable experience in the pharmacologic management of occlusive disease.

This use of sodium warfarin is to be distinguished from the role of sodium heparin as an agent for clearing the serum of lipids. Even the efficacy of the use of heparin as an antilipemic agent in this situation has been questioned by Wright.[56]

The importance of agents that reduce the adhesiveness of platelets, as opposed to drugs that affect other parts of the clotting "waterfall" mechanism, has recently come into prominence.[12] It is of particular importance in some arterial operations and diseases to prevent the aggregation of platelets on damaged arterial intima, intimectomized arteries, suture lines and venous grafts.

Dextran, especially of the higher molecular weights,[45] is very effective in preventing platelets from "seeing"[41] one another or other sticky surfaces. Dextran, however, has its limitations because of the requirements that it be given by the intravenous route every 24 hours. Oral medications which are available which are also effective in reducing the stickiness of the platelets include aspirin, sulfinpyrazone, cyproheptadine hydrochloride (Periactin, Dipyridamole, Persantine). Table 6–1 shows the commonly recommended dosages.

Each drug has its own disadvantages. Aspirin is probably the simplest and best known of all the agents, and is a relatively effective platelet antagonist. Anturane is very effective. It is, however, a uricosuric drug and must be observed carefully in the patient during therapy. It is contraindicated in the presence of an active ulcer or in the

Table 6–1.   Commonly Used Antiplatelet Agents

Listing of the Agents	Daily dosage	Comments
Aspirin	600–1200 mg.	Hazardous in the presence of ulcer disease
Anturane*	400–800 mg.	Uricosuric; contraindicated in ulcer and kidney disease
Periactin*	12–16 mg.	Should not be used in elderly or debilitated patients. Contraindicated in presence of monamine oxidase inhibitors
Persantin*	100–150 mg.	

*Not released by the Federal Drug Administration for active use of antiplatelet agent.

presence of kidney disease. Periactin is also an effective agent but is not specifically cleared by the Federal Drug Administration for use as a platelet antagonist. Its use is associated with drowsiness. It should not be used in elderly or debilitated patients or in the presence of monamine oxidase inhibitors. Persantine is another potent agent, originally recommended as a coronary vasodilator. It has been used in the treatment of headache. It has also been thought to be implicated in the development of retroperitoneal fibrosis.

Fibrinolytic agents offer some advantages in the treatment of established thrombosis,[28] but share a paradoxical hazard. If the agent is potent enough to accomplish dissolution of an established thrombus it is likely to cause hemorrhage at the site of venous or arterial puncture or at the site of a recent surgical wound and bleeding through the interstices of a plastic graft. The efficiency of the agent, therefore, limits its very use.

The use of platelet antagonists and the evaluation of the effectiveness of antithrombic agents cannot be guided by simple laboratory tests as can therapy with heparin or therapy with the prothrombin antagonists. For this reason the dosage levels are empiric and control is uncertain.

Metabolic Control

Dietary measures directed at the basic metabolic error that leads to atherosclerosis are desirable. Certainly, inborn errors in the metabolism of fat, mechanical factors resulting from the configuration of vessels, and secondary acquired defects such as diabetes, hypothyroidism, and premature oophorectomy are of great importance, but dietary intake is one factor that is subject to control. Caloric intake should be restricted, with few fats, and a high proportion of these fats should be polyunsaturated. Some individuals may have greater benefit from dietary control than others. Details of classification and management of the hyperlipoproteinemias are discussed in Table 4–1.

Careful dietary management may be necessary even in the nondiabetic with relation to the proportion of carbohydrate in the diet. Diabetics must not be allowed to increase their fat intake at the expense of their insulin requirements. If Rutstein's findings[39] are applied to the economy of the whole organism, rather than tissue culture only, it can be seen that even in normal subjects there may be less deposition of lipids in the aortic cells if intake of carbohydrate is high.

The actual restriction of weight is of symportance not only because it reduces the likelihood of atheroma formation, but also because with less weight less effort is required on the part of the legs and heart.

How the amount of work imposed on the legs may be reduced by weight loss so as to achieve maximal flow into the legs is exemplified by a 60-year-old patient who had had a lumbar sympathectomy after an acute femoral thrombosis. Although his condition is favorable for a reconstructive procedure, he has declined further operation. Because he has reduced his weight by more than 20 pounds, he experiences no claudication within his normal range of activities, which include walking two blocks at a brisk pace; however, if he carries a 10 pound briefcase, he can walk only 50 to 75 feet without experiencing claudication.

Although maintenance of hemoglobin levels near normal is generally desirable, Cranley has demonstrated the damaging effect of polycythemia on peripheral blood flow.[8, 9] Schenk's study[42] indicates the marked effect of changes in the viscosity of the blood on regional blood flow. The long-term use of low molecular weight dextran to reduce viscosity is questionable, although it may be useful in acute episodes.

LOCAL MEASURES

Prominent among local measures are those that are designed to improve local collateral circulation or to assist a failing circulation. For example, in the first category there may be an exercise, such as walking to the point of claudication. Not only is walking beyond this point unnecessarily painful, but it might actually be harmful, whereas walking to the point of distress is one means of increasing collateral flow by an intermittent increase in demand.

When circulation is very severely endangered, the use of Buerger's exercises is of slight but definite benefit. The patient elevates his legs so that all venous blood is emptied from them. The capillary bed becomes even more hypoxic, and maximal stimulus to vasodilatation is produced, so that when the patient lowers his leg, arterial blood, assisted by gravity, fills the capillary tree beyond the obstruction. Mild exercise performed with the legs dependent helps maintain peripheral arterial resistance at a low level and helps pump some venous blood out of the legs. The legs are then returned to the horizontal position for a period of rest.

The useful cycle of exercise (which may be modified by individual needs) is as follows:

1. Legs elevated (on a chair turned so that the seat faces the floor) for 1 minute.

2. Legs lowered; patient exercises for 2 or 3 minutes.

3. Legs at rest horizontally for 5 to 7 minutes (Fig. 6–1).

This cycle should be repeated at least three times a day. A hospitalized patient may be able to spend much of his time doing such exercises.

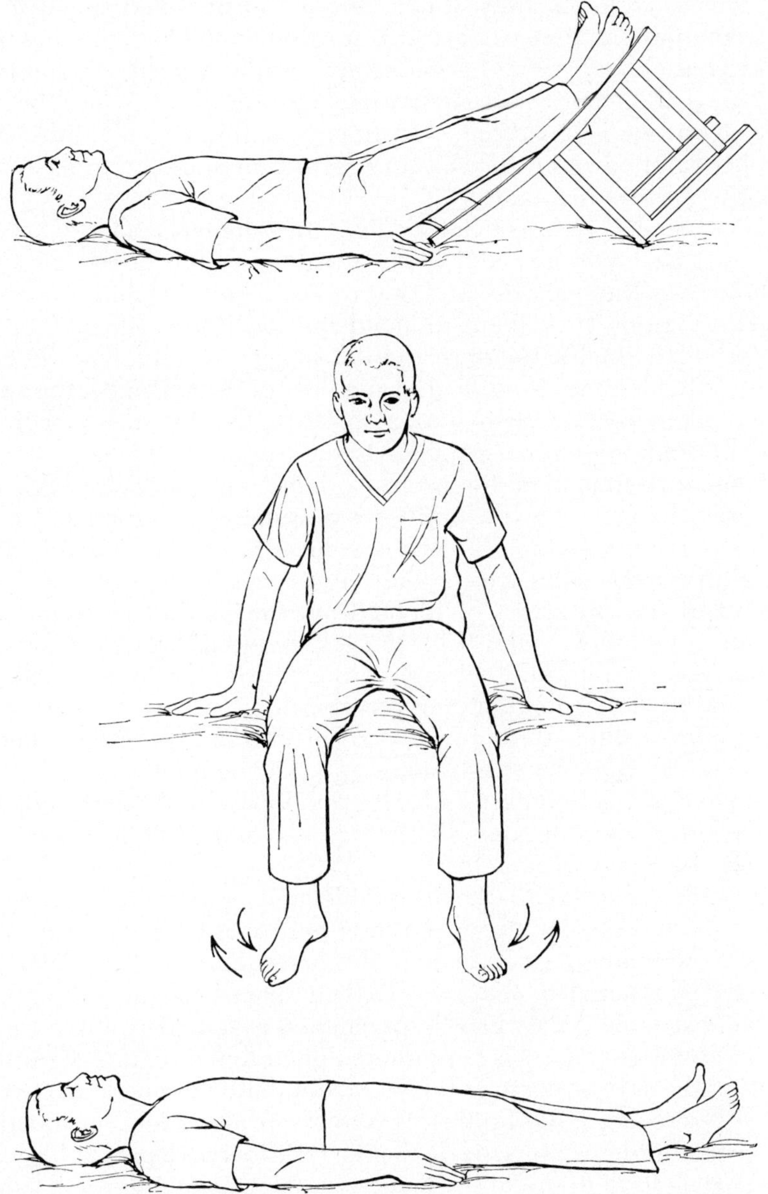

Figure 6–1. Top, patient elevates feet; middle, patient gently exercises his dependent feet; bottom, patient rests in horizontal position.

In more critical situations the patient is unable to do the work of Buerger's exercises. Continuous filling and emptying of blood in the peripheral vasculature may be provided by an oscillating bed.

Local protection is of utmost importance. Avoidance of excessive heat or cold, trauma, tight shoes, minor injuries, and the like may make amputation unnecessary; Arthur Allen is said to have shown that 80 per cent of cases of gangrene began with a *preventable* injury.

The patient must give meticulous attention to his feet, keeping them clean, well lubricated, and free from fungus infections. Nails must be trimmed carefully so as to prevent incidental trauma and the formation of ingrown nails.

In acute disease, especially among hospitalized patients, special care must be taken to avoid pressure sores on the heels, decubitus erosions over the malleoli, and other clearly preventable injuries.

The patient must learn to avoid the local use of heat. The skin metabolism is unable to adjust to the external warmth, and the blood supply is inadequate for diffusing the flow of heat. Hence, the skin is burned more readily than normal tissues. By the same token, the ischemic limb is more susceptible to cold injury.

The appearance of hypostatic edema may signal irreversible ischemic changes. As the patient experiences freedom from pain when the leg is pendent, he learns to let it hang over the side of the bed. Further, he soon learns that any use of his muscles demands blood, and the diversion of blood from the painful ischemic areas produces even more pain. With the leg pendent the pain is relieved but the venous pumping system of the leg is thus put at rest. The combination of rest and pendent position shortly causes an accumulation of edema fluid. With edema, greater arterial pressure is needed for effective capillary perfusion—and an ominous cycle is thus established. Early in the course of its development the use of intermittent elevation, as in Buerger's exercises, may help, but later the condition may be irreversible.

The toes are particularly vulnerable, and a minor infection here or in the fissures between the toes often progresses to major septic crises with development of deep plantar abscesses. Patients in whom an infection is restricted to the toes may be spared the development of plantar abscesses if they can be persuaded to spend as much time as possible lying prone, so as to promote dependent drainage of purulent material; the supine position favors accumulation of purulent material, with seepage along the lumbrical tunnels or along tendon sheaths.

Just as mild muscle activity that is described as a part of Buerger's exercises is done in the hope of increasing collateral flow, so can the patient utilize walking, provided there is no associated necrosis. The patient should walk only to the point that discomfort develops. He should not force himself to the point that he has severe pain, but should rest until the discomfort passes, and then continue his walking.

It has been suggested[6] that division of the Achilles tendon would relieve *calf* claudication due to femoral artery obstruction. As the gastrocnemius muscle is rendered powerless, the patient now must learn to use a new gait: he uses femoral and gluteal muscles supplied from above the site of obstruction to initiate each step. Dividing the Achilles tendon seems a poor procedure at best, and is of no value in the treatment of iliac artery occlusion. A much less drastic measure, based on the same principle, is the prescription of lifts on the heels of shoes to reduce the work of the gastrocnemius muscle.

Walking is of greater value than bicycling because walking places the demand on the calf muscles where collateral supply is most needed.

Amputation

A vascular occlusion may progress to the point that amputation becomes the only therapy possible. In general, amputation for peripheral vascular disease must be performed with greater caution than for trauma and neoplastic disease. The primary goal of amputation is the creation of an intact integument with freedom from pain; simultaneous restoration of function is desirable, but must be secondary.

Technique must be as simple as possible. The utmost attention must be paid to Halsted's principles of gentleness, minimal trauma during hemostasis, closure with fine suture, but without tension or dead space, and delayed primary closure when necessary. Only the simplest flaps should be created, and a tourniquet must never be used. Tight wrapping for early molding of a stump immediately following amputation is exceedingly hazardous; it has at times provoked further tissue loss and has even been the critical factor in causing death.

The introduction of immediate plaster dressing and immediate weight bearing has been a boon for many patients whose protracted inactivity might interfere with their rehabilitation. Burgess[7] describes the use of the immediate weight bearing prosthesis. The greatest care and skill must be exercised in applying the plaster so that the dressing is not too tight.

In the face of wet gangrene and other forms of virulent sepsis, a guillotine amputation is necessary; however, the skin of the debilitated arteriosclerotic patient may not tolerate skin traction, and this may preclude its use. One useful procedure is a planned reamputation; i.e., initial local open amputation of a distal process to provide control of the virulent sepsis, followed by definitive amputation at a later date, at which time complete closure may be accomplished.

Piecemeal amputation of a limb beginning with amputation of the toes and progressing to amputation of the thigh is to be avoided. Nevertheless, since arteriosclerotic vascular disease is not predictably a progressive disease, conservatism is a virtue, when practiced wisely. Local amputation is acceptable if the stump is likely to heal or if it is part of a staged amputation. Thus, amputation of one or more dry gangrenous toes is fruitless in a patient in whom occlusion has developed from the aorta to the ankle. Unless reconstruction of the artery is feasible, one of two courses is desirable: The patient can be treated very conservatively in the hope that autoamputation and subsequent healing will take place;[40] or, early in the course, an adequate midthigh amputation can be performed — as high as necessary to assure healing. The additional procedure of superficial femoral vein interruption is desirable if the patient does not have a fresh groin wound. Vein interruption[49] reduces pulmonary complications without promoting edema in the stump, when performed at this level.

The selection of an appropriate site for amputation is critical. If the arterial supply is normal or has been restored to normal, digital amputation may be expected to heal provided necrosis has not spread into the forefoot.

If blood supply to the foot is inadequate, or in the event three or more toes must be removed, amputation at the transmetatarsal area is often favorable for healing.[50] A transmetatarsal amputation usually heals even in the absence of popliteal pulsation, but a popliteal pulse makes healing much more likely.

The most vulnerable area in the transmetatarsal amputation is the dorsal skin over the distal third and fourth metatarsals. Necrosis may develop that is totally resistant to local treatment, and further amputation may become necessary. In some cases part of the plantar flap is lost at the site of trophic ulcers or calluses. Under these last two circumstances the Syme amputation may be useful. If the other leg is unaffected, the patient can ambulate when necessary and need not wear a prosthesis, as, for example, when he wakens at night to use the bathroom. If the other leg had previously been removed, the use of the Syme amputation preserves extra leg length and makes walking easier than does a second thigh amputation. If the transmetatarsal amputation fails, however, and no local sites of failure are responsible and if the blood supply is tenuous, then the Syme amputation is apt to fail also.

Amputation below the knee is not desirable in peripheral vascular disease except in the case of thromboangiitis obliterans and diabetic vascular disease, in which local tissue destruction has made amputation necessary even in the presence of adequate blood supply to the calf. Under most other circumstances, the patient with generalized arteriosclerosis has such scant muscle bulk and such thin skin that the end of the stump repeatedly breaks down (even though the stump is not weight bearing). Although others[11, 25, 33, 47, 48] have advocated wider use of this type of amputation, the author has rarely seen a completely satisfactory below the knee stump that allowed full use of the prosthesis, when performed for nondiabetic arteriosclerosis.

The low thigh and midthigh amputations remain the most satisfactory levels and are the most nearly certain to heal. The prostheses available for thigh amputations are of such excellent design that an extensive range of activity is possible even for the bilateral amputee. There are many patients, however, who will never be able to use a prosthesis. Under these circumstances amputation should be carried out without hesitation at a high enough level to assure healing.

Conservative and unorthodox methods of amputation which consist of little more than debridement and closure with placement of local flaps or grafts may well be done at the same time as a tenuous reconstructive procedure performed for salvage.[46] Even transitory success of the reconstruction will allow this type of amputation to heal. Once the amputation has healed, failure of the process may not necessarily lead to further necrosis.

Major upper extremity amputations should be as conservative as possible, for modern prosthetic techniques allow fitting of almost any length of stump. Reconstruction at the hand becomes a problem of specific importance to the hand surgeon if there is loss of the thumb. Lesser digital amputations fall into two categories. When the strength and breadth of the hand must be preserved simple flaps and amputation through the midportion of the phalanx are satisfactory. Amputation through a joint must include excision of the cartilaginous surfaces. In the presence of the most distal and localized forms of the disease, one may at times carry out digital amputation in the form of amputation of the entire digital ray, removing all or most of the metacarpal. Such extensive reconstruction may be precluded by the presence of extensive disease proximal to the palmar arch.

SYMPATHECTOMY

In 1916, René Leriche first undertook to accomplish ablation of tonic sympathetic nervous activity in the peripheral blood vessels of the extremities by means of periarterial sympathectomy.[26, 27] Lumbar sympathectomy was introduced in an attempt to reduce the muscular rigidity that occurred in certain neurological conditions.[21, 38] The incidental observation that the extremities were rendered warm and cutaneous blood flow was increased led to the utilization of lumbar sympathectomy in Raynaud's disease by Adson and Brown.[1]

For many years lumbar sympathectomy remained the only operative procedure of any avail in the treatment of occlusive or vasospastic arterial disease. Its value was deprecated when arterial reconstruction was introduced, but it has again come to be recognized as a critical and useful procedure.[2, 4, 15, 17, 20, 22, 29, 32, 35, 51]

As described in Chapter Three, ablation of the sympathetic nerves results in denervation of the small vessels of the skin, and to some degree denervation of the blood vessels of the muscles, with subsequent increase in blood flow. These vessels are ordinarily under chronic tonic contraction in response to sympathetic motor activity, and ablation of the sympathetic nerves not only renders the blood vessels unable to respond by marked vasoconstriction to hemorrhage, shock, cold, emotion, and so forth, but also allows them to be distended maximally by intravascular pressures. Arteriolar and capillary pressures are more frequently maintained above the critical closing pressures and flow presumably remains at a greater level.

Although some of the vasoconstrictor fibers do supply muscle, the greater effect is on the skin of the distal portions of the extremities. Sympathetic ablation does increase flow through the arteriovenous shunts. Despite the dilatation of these shunts, the nutritive capillaries usually receive a larger absolute quantity of blood, although this represents a smaller proportion of the total flow to the skin.

The admonition made by Atlas[4, 5] and by Freeman[17] that sympathectomy might cause paradoxical gangrene has not been borne out in clinical observations.

Sympathectomy cannot be relied upon to augment blood flow to muscles to any important degree in either an upper or lower extremity. Its major effect is on the skin. Figure 6–2 illustrates the area of the leg denervated by lumbar sympathectomy when L1, L2 and L3 are removed, and compares it with removal of L2 and L3. In order to denervate the hand the cervical chain from T1 down through T3 or T4 should be removed if possible.

The effect of sympathectomy becomes maximal almost immediately, but in the course of the following 7 to 10 days sensitization to circulating adrenergic hormones causes temporary return of a considerable degree of sympathetic activity. This temporary reversal is followed by gradual stabilization with augmentation of flow that is less marked than that which occurred immediately after the procedure.

In some patients vasoconstrictor activity returns to such a degree that the effect appears to have been dissipated. According to Malan and Puglionisi,[30] patients in whom this occurs probably did not have complete extirpation of sympathetic channels, and the alternative pathways have become more easily utilized as time has passed.

Two of the most carefully studied series of sympathectomies are those of Edwards[15] and of Palumbo.[32]

In Edwards' series of 100 patients there was an initial loss of 10 limbs in the first year; there were no further amputations until the sixth year, and only five more over the rest of the 10 year period. To be sure, only 42 of the 100 patients survived the full 10 years. Amputation was performed in 29 per cent of those who died in the first 5 years, as

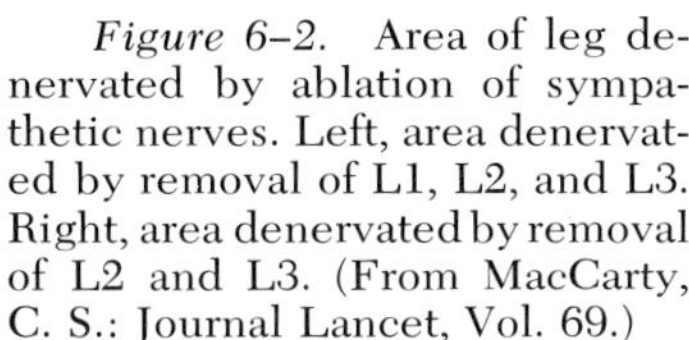

Figure 6–2. Area of leg denervated by ablation of sympathetic nerves. Left, area denervated by removal of L1, L2, and L3. Right, area denervated by removal of L2 and L3. (From MacCarty, C. S.: Journal Lancet, Vol. 69.)

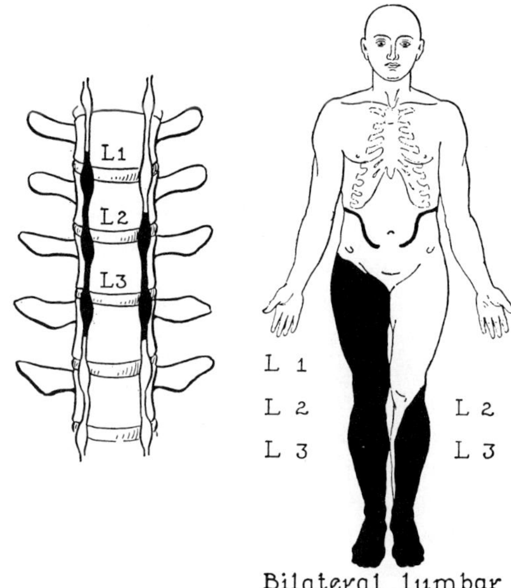

opposed to only 8 per cent of the survivors. The patient who has arterial disease of the limbs so serious as to require amputation is apt to have other cardiovascular disease endangering his life.

Another observation by Edwards is that no limb became more critical without major extension of the arterial occlusion, and that even in the event of a major occlusion significant protection to the limb was afforded by the prior sympathectomy. This phenomenon is illustrated in the following case.

A 59-year-old woman had had a right lumbar sympathectomy in 1955 for diffuse arteriosclerosis; the outstanding symptoms were attributable to occlusion of the femoropopliteal tibial system. Sympathectomy had been done on the left side in 1958 for similar symptoms. Her limbs remained relatively warm and well nourished, in spite of continued claudication, until December 1964, when she complained that her right leg felt heavy. The right femoral pulse could no longer be detected, and oscillometric readings on the left were barely detectable. Nevertheless, the foot remained warm, pink, and viable and was preserved with simple conservative supporting measures.

It has been demonstrated by Robertson and Smithwick[35] that a considerable vasomotor activity returned after sympathectomy. A successful sympathectomy was equated with inability to respond to a cold environment by a decrease in skin temparature and a decrease in blood flow to the skin; return of the ability to respond to environmental changes signaled return of vasomotor activity. In spite of this demonstrated loss of sympathectomy effect, which was more pronounced in the arm than in the leg, the clinical results in the patients remained satisfactory.

We have relied heavily on the protracted protection afforded by sympathectomy in patients who were not suitable for reconstructive procedures as well as in those who were, and in whom sympathectomy was done as an adjunct to reconstruction. It was hoped that sympathectomy would prevent the development of an ischemic crisis in the event of late failure of the reconstructive procedure, and we believe this has held true, although we lack data to prove it statistically. We have seen, however, that sympathectomy appears to protect individuals against later major occlusion.

In our earlier experience with arterial reconstruction we utilized sympathectomy in aortoiliac reconstruction only when one or both femoral arteries were severely sclerosed. In some cases sympathectomy was done only in the affected side; in a small series, however, the ratio of the number of late femoral occlusions in the *untreated* side to the number of occlusions in the sympathectomized side was 8 to 1. Although some occlusions may not have been recognized, we are convinced that the protection offered by sympathectomy is valid.

As the protection described in the previous paragraph became recognized, we began to use lumbar sympathectomy in almost every patient who underwent an arterial reconstruction.[40] Usually these procedures were performed at the same operation.

It is difficult to determine how much of this success results from increasing skill in selecting suitable surgical candidates and how much from improvements in technique. Certainly the addition of lumbar sympathectomy to arterial reconstruction has been associated with an increasing initial success rate; what effect it may have had in that improvement is not clear.

The maximal effect of sympathectomy is promptly reached; it reduces peripheral resistance when maintenance of a high flow rate through the reconstructed segment is critical. This initial enhancement of flow may be a critical factor responsible for an increased rate of early success.

The sequence in most flow measurements that we have made at the operating table has been the following: before sympathectomy, after sympathectomy, and after reconstruction. This sequence is followed because we prefer to perform sympathectomy prior to reconstruction. The case described is illustrative of the effect when sympathectomy is performed *after* reconstruction.

A 68-year-old male was operated upon for a resection of a large aortic aneurysm associated with occlusion of the right iliac artery and stenosis of the left. The condition of the distal collateral run-off tree was not known; at operation, however, an adequate bilateral femoral tree was seen below the stenotic areas. Following resection of the aneurysm, plethysmographic studies revealed poor digital flow, principally on the left. Bilateral lumbar sympathectomy was done, and it brought about a prompt increase in flow on both sides; in fact, flow became equalized (see Figure 7–2).

The experiments of Kountz[24] in the dog illustrate the phenomenon of restriction of flow after temporary interruption, followed by amelioration with sympathectomy; the case just cited appears to be an example of this phenomenon occurring in the human. Such findings confirm our impression of the merit of sympathectomy performed at the time of reconstruction.

On the other hand, reports questioning the merit of sympathectomy must be considered.[18]

Indications for Sympathectomy

One cannot rely on prior testing to foretell the ultimate beneficial results of sympathectomy. If the goal of sympathectomy were simply immediate ablation of increased sympathetic tone, then diagnostic paravertebral nerve block would be fairly accurate in defining the presence of increased tonus. Equally convincing might be plethysmographic evidence of strong vasomotor control by the sympathetic nervous system. However, the long-term result of lumbar sympathectomy is not necessarily reflected by the increased skin warmth and decreased skin conductivity which are used as the criteria of successful lumbar block.

If the patient is not a suitable candidate for arterial reconstruction, but can tolerate sympathectomy, we recommend this only. There is no absolute upper age limit, but few patients have been operated upon who were past the age of 70. Diabetes in itself does not constitute a contraindication to operation.

Ozeran[31] has studied the vasomotor tone in a series of diabetic patients and confirms the clinical observation that many diabetics have lost their sympathetic activity. This is presumably due to a neuritis involving the sympathetic nerves. In a few diabetic patients the irritative phenomena associated with the neuritis have led to a transient hyperactivity of the sympathetic system. This is then followed by progression to normal tone and, finally, to an autosympathectomized state. If serious symptoms occur during this period of hyperactivity, however, sympathectomy may be justified.

We shall mention briefly a few other indications for sympathectomy.

Raynaud's disease, when uncontrollable by other conservative treatment, should be considered for sympathetic ablation when loss of tissue impends.

Thromboangiitis obliterans is commonly treated by sympathectomy; this may not correct the basic pathological process but it may reduce the severity of symptoms. Many miscellaneous forms of distal arterial occlusions that occur in the hands, frequently in women, are nearly indistinguishable from thromboangiitis obliterans. These include the arteritis associated with rheumatoid arthritis and the collagen diseases, and in particular scleroderma.

Sympathectomy in scleroderma will not effect softening of sclerotic lesions and contractures of the skin, but it may augment cutaneous flow just enough to allow healing skin of defects, such as gangrenous spots and amputation sites.

One must keep in mind that in diffuse disease processes, it may become necessary to perform sympathectomy on more than one limb—perhaps all the limbs, because hematometakinesia may develop, and aggravate symptoms in the untreated limbs.[4, 13] Furthermore, the more sympathetic activity of the limbs is destroyed, the greater will be the possibility of truncal hyperhidrosis, which occurs primarily in response to the body's need to dispel excess heat, rather than as a response to emotion.[44]

Technique of Lumbar Sympathectomy

The surgeon's aim in performing sympathectomy is to remove the ganglionated chain between the top of the second lumbar vertebra and the bottom of the third lumbar disc. On the basis of dissections he had done, Edwards demonstrated that this technique assured removal of the second and third lumbar rami in substantially all cases.[14] Removal of the fourth ganglion is unnecessary, for no gray rami arise below the third segment. Removal of the first ramus is necessary only in sympathectomy of the upper and medial thigh. The merit of removing higher ganglia, including the twelfth thoracic and first lumbar ganglia, at least, and the second and third lumbar rami, as advocated by Lilly[29] and by Hohf[20] has not been clearly demonstrated.

When we perform sympathectomy only, our approach is through an oblique abdominal incision that extends nearly from the tip of the twelfth rib to the margin of the rectus sheath at the level of the umbilicus. Minor improvement in exposure can be obtained by placing pillows or folded sheets about 2 inches thick under the lower ribs and hips, by slight flexion and adduction to the ipsilateral hip, and by breaking the table at not more than 10 to 15 degrees of flexion.

The type of anesthesia and its administration are important. Ether anesthesia is contraindicated, especially when both sides are involved, because of the extreme sensitivity of the sympathectomized arteries to this anesthetic.[16]

Conduction anesthesia is excellent if a sufficiently high level is obtained, and inhalational anesthesia is equally satisfactory if it affords comparable relaxation. Whatever the type of anesthesia, two things are required; maintenance of blood pressure at a safe level, and exposure sufficient to allow expeditious removal of the chain.

The lower medial and upper lateral portion of the subcutaneous incision is undermined so as to allow the longest possible incision in the external oblique fascia and muscle. Next, this muscle is undermined. In most cases the underlying internal oblique and transverse muscles are similarly split parallel to their fibers and undermined, but if it appears that the gridiron incision will not allow adequate exposure, then the internal oblique muscle may be divided parallel to the incision in the external oblique muscle. The lowest intercostal nerves should be retracted and spared, if possible.

The peritoneum is retracted and mobilized forward. There is little need for mobilization of the peritoneum from the undersurface of the anterior portion of the wound. Mobilization of the peritoneum in the flank is accomplished easily with a sponge stick, and with it the ureter should also be mobilized forward and protected. Tears in the peritoneum should be repaired promptly with interrupted sutures. Peritoneal tears are infrequent if dissection in the anterior portion of the wound is avoided. Initial retraction of the edge of the muscles is accomplished by means of retractors; long Deaver retractors replace the Richardson retractors as the deepest part of the wound is reached and the peritoneum must be retracted.

The level of the vertebral interspaces in relation to the iliac crest may be identified preoperatively by a roentgenogram. Edwards' anatomic study relates the levels of the several lumbar ganglionic segments and the lumbar vertebrae.[14] The chain is identified by palpation in the groove between the aorta (or vena cava) and the medial margin of the psoas major, resting on the lateral portion of the vertebral column. The chain has the consistency of a firm cord. Excessive palpation should be avoided in order to reduce the number of noxious distal impulses. If the chain cannot be identified promptly, the region should be infiltrated with a local anesthesic, and dissection can then proceed safely.

The chain is identified at the distal level and divided there. A metal clip is placed at the point of division for hemostasis and for roentgenologic identification. The chain is grasped with a long clamp and retracted upward; individual rami are dissected and divided as far from the ganglia as possible to include as much as possible of ganglionated tissue. The chain is dissected upward from the bottom of the third lumbar disc to the level of the top of the second lumbar vertebra, where it is clipped or ligated and then divided.[14] All vascular branches are controlled with clips or ligatures, or cautery if need be. Excessive bleeding from lumbar veins can cause additional difficulty, and preliminary control of this factor is desirable.

If it is desired to remove the first lumbar ganglion, the chain can be dissected further, being followed into the substance of the crus of the diaphragm. All branches of the chain are clipped or ligated, primarily to control bleeding. We have seen no reduction in postsympathectomy neuralgia by ligation of the rami and chain. In some cases the right lumbar chain is so situated that the vena cava overlies it, and careful dissection and mobilization are necessary to expose the chain.

The surgeon must carefully avoid causing trauma to the genitofemoral nerve complex as it crosses the psoas muscle.

After meticulous hemostasis, closure of the wound is performed with interrupted fine sutures to the individual muscle layers and subcutaneous tissue, and routine closure of the skin. Drainage is not done.

Transabdominal sympathectomy is usually performed at the same time as exposure of the aorta and great vessels. This approach may be used in bilateral sympathectomy without a concomitant vascular procedure or in sympathectomy when reoperation is to be done. Exposure is obtained through a midline or paramedian midabdominal and upper abdominal incision. A bilateral extraperitoneal approach can be done, but is often difficult to achieve and unnecessary. Bilateral exposure through a transverse incision across the rectus muscles is also possible, but this incision is generally undesirable because of the necessity of dividing the big collateral channels of the inferior epigastric arterial trunks.

After the peritoneal cavity is opened, the vessels at the root of the small bowel mesentery may be approached in the same manner as the aorta and vena cava. As a rule, the lumbar sympathetic chains are more accessible if the left and right colon are mobilized in turn, thereby achieving essentially the same kind of exposure as in the usual flank approach.

Technique of Cervicodorsal Sympathectomy

The removal of the paravertebral ganglia T1 through T3 or T4 can be accomplished by any one of several routes. General anesthesia is required as a rule but local anesthesia can be used by a gentle operator using the supraclavicular approach. This exposure is also the one which does allow bilateral operation at the same sitting, although a stage procedure is usually to be preferred. Resection of the ganglia is more effective than the formerly practiced preganglionic ramisection.[23]

SUPRACLAVICULAR APPROACH

With the patient supine the neck is extended and the head turned slightly to the opposite side. A collar incision is made one to two centimeters above the clavicle and extending laterally from the posterior margin of the sternomastoid muscle. The platysma and the clavicular head of the sternomastoid are divided. The omohyoid fascia and muscle are divided (the muscle may later be approximated). The prescalene fat pad is mobilized laterally to expose the anterior scalene muscle, with the phrenic nerve crossing it obliquely from medial to lateral. The nerve should be carefully mobilized and protected. The anterior scalene muscle is divided carefully to avoid injury to the brachial plexus laterally and posteriorly and to the subclavian post-inferiorly. It is often necessary to divide the thyrocervical trunk. The superior margin of the first rib can now be palpated.

If a cervical rib is present it may be removed at this point, although its encroachment on the brachial nerve routes and subclavian artery is well relieved by complete division of the anterior scalene muscle and all of its accessory slips. Careful retraction of the brachial plexus laterally and of the subclavian anteriorly now enables one to divide the slips of Sibson's fascia and to mobilize the apical pleura from the neck and the posterior portion of the upper three or four ribs. By palpation one should be able to identify the stellate ganglion lying on the neck of the first rib. With the aid of a mobile light source or a lighted retractor one can now divide the stellate ganglion, and dissect downward along the chain. Tantalum clips should be used to achieve perfect hemostasis. Under most circumstances one can easily reach and remove T3, and sometimes as far as T5.

Closure of the wound after removal of the chain is accomplished by simple closure of the platysma and the skin, but the ends of the omohyoid muscle and the clavicular portion of the sternocleidomastoid may be reapproximated if desired. Details in the classical points of this technique are well described by Ross.[37]

If the pleura has been torn the lung should be expanded and a tube used to drain the pleural space through the wound for several days. If not, a suction catheter drain can be used for 24 hours in the retropleural space.

The supraclavicular approach has the merit of minimal morbidity, but the exposure can be difficult. It is most useful when one expects encroachment by the scalene muscle on the neurovascular structures. It may be undesirable to use this approach if the operation is performed for causalgia.

TRANSAXILLARY APPROACH

With the patient in the true lateral decubitus position, a transverse incision is made at the inferior margin of the axillary hair. It is carried forward short of the position of the anterior thoracic nerve and posteriorly to the level of the thoracodorsal nerve. This incision is ordinarily no more than three inches in length. The incision is carried down to the rib itself and then dissection carried upward on the surface of the thoracic cage to the second interspace. An intercostal incision is made here, entering the pleural space. A lighted malleable retractor depresses the dome of the lung after a small rib spreader has been introduced and the space opened as much as possible. The stellate ganglion and upper thoracic chain can then be identified through the pleura, which will be incised with a bistoury. The stellate ganglion is divided as before in its midportion and dissected downward as far as necessary, using care to maintain hemostasis with tantalum clips. No closure of the pleura over the site of the removed chain is attempted.

The pleural space is drained with an anteriorly placed chest tube. Closure of the wound requires only two paracostal sutures and a running suture in the muscle, followed by closure of the subcutaneous tissue and skin.

At times the intercostal approach results in considerable pain, but its advantage is that almost no structures are cut except the skin and intercostal muscles. It may be exceedingly difficult in the face of old pleural adhesions from tuberculosis; it is possible, however, if such adhesions are encountered to proceed with an extra-pleural approach. Good chest films should ordinarily eliminate this as an unexpected finding. This approach was described by Atkins, and details can be found in his work.[3]

POSTERIOR APPROACH

This approach was well described by White and Smithwick.[52] The patient is in the prone position and a vertical incision, 7 centimeters in length, is made in the paraspinous position opposite the second and third spinous processes. The trapezius and rhomboid muscles are divided and the longissimus cervicis muscle is split. Through this split the third rib is resected over a distance of about 5 centimeters. The pleura is then mobilized and the third intercostal nerve divided. The nerve is dissected medially, dividing the gray and white rami in the dorsal branch of the nerve. The second intercostal nerve is similarly dissected. White and Smithwick resected the ganglionated chain by mobilizing the chain from below upward from the third ganglion and dividing the midportion of the stellate ganglion. The wound was then closed in layers.

Although this approach is favored by some neurosurgeons, its relatively poor exposure, the face down position, and the frequency of postoperative pain make it a less popular approach in the hands of peripheral vascular surgeons.

TRANSTHORACIC ROUTE

A classical high anterolateral thoracotomy incision can also be used to expose the apex of the pleura. There is better exposure of the proximal left subclavian artery available through this approach if concomitant direct surgical attack on this vessel is contemplated. The right subclavian artery can be managed through a strictly supraclavicular approach as long as the innominate artery is not involved.

Complications

The most common complication is femoral neuralgia, which occurs unpredictably regardless of the method of ligation or other variables. It is distinct from the neuritis that is due to trauma to the genitofemoral complex. The neuralgia is felt in the tissues of the thigh, usually on the inner aspect, and is often associated with exquisite hyperesthesia of the skin of the thigh. It usually comes on by the tenth postoperative day and lasts for a few weeks; in rare instances it has remained severe for 9 months. It may be so severe as to require narcotics, or may be so slight that it may be controlled by use of salicylates and reassurance. It is most important to reassure the patient that the onset of the pain does not indicate aggravation of the disease. A similar phenomenon occasionally occurs following cervicodorsal sympathectomy. Treatment with Dilantin and Tegretol is described in Chapter Nineteen.

Hemorrhage into the retroperitoneal or retropleural tissues is common when anticoagulant therapy is employed, unless hemostasis is done meticulously. Paradoxical gangrene as described by Atlas[4] and by Freeman[17] has not been recognized. In one case, seen in another hospital, progression of an extensive femoral thrombosis followed sympathectomy. In this instance, however, the anesthetic was unsuitable, the procedure was exceedingly difficult and prolonged, and several serious and prolonged episodes of hypotension occurred. Sympathectomy was accomplished, but the foot remained cold and painful, ultimately it became gangrenous and required amputation. There was no evidence of any increased flow through cutaneous shunts.

Protracted ileus occasionally follows lumbar operation, presumably as a reflex resulting from retroperitoneal dissection and hemorrhage, rather than as a direct neurological effect.

The effect of lumbar sympathetic denervation on sexual activity is often misunderstood and misrepresented to the patient. Bilateral excision of the first lumbar ganglion renders a considerable number of patients unable to ejaculate externally; the internal vesical sphincter is unable to close at the moment of ejaculation, and the discharge is directed into the bladder instead of out through the urethra. Sensation and actual potency remain unchanged.[53]

The specific complication of Horner's syndrome following cervicodorsal sympathectomy deserves special mention. This syndrome consists of miosis, palpebrotosis, enophthalmos and unilateral loss of fascial sweating. It does not represent any significant deformity under most circumstances. When it follows bilateral sympathectomy its symmetry makes it almost impossible to recognize. The occurrence unilaterally is usually an acceptable compromise if the indications for the operation were sound in the first place. Furthermore, in a dark eyed person the pupillary changes are difficult to distinguish. The ptosis is rarely troublesome after the first few days, except when the patient is excessively fatigued. The enophthalmos and diminished fascial sweating do not represent a problem.

REFERENCES

1. Adson, A. W., and Brown, G. E.: Treatment of Raynaud's disease by lumbar ramisection and ganglionectomy and perivascular sympathetic neurectomy of the common iliacs. J.A.M.A. *84*:1908, 1925.
2. Allen, E. V., Barker, N. W., and Hines, E. A., Jr.: *Peripheral Vascular Diseases.* Ed. 3. Philadelphia, W. B. Saunders Co., 1962.
3. Atkins, H. J. B.: Sympathectomy by axillary approach. Lancet *1*:538, 1954.
4. Atlas, L. N.: Lumbar sympathectomy in the treatment of peripheral arteriosclerotic disease. Am. Heart J. *23*:43, 1942.
5. Atlas, L. N.: Application of the physiologic principle of hemometakinesia to the technique of lumbar sympathectomy. Surgery *37*:130, 1955.
6. Boyd, A. M., Ratcliffe, A. H., Jepson, R. P., and James, G. W. H.: Intermittent claudication; a clinical study. J. Bone Joint Surg. *31-B*:325, 1949.
7. Burgess, E. M.: Below knee amputations with immediate-fit prostheses. In Dale, W.: *Management of Arterial Occlusive Disease.* Chicago, Year Book Medical Publishers, Inc., 1971, p. 449.
8. Cranley, J. J.: In Discussion of Schenk, W. G., Jr., Delin, N. A., Domanig, E., Hahnloser, P., and Hoyt, R. K.: Blood viscosity as a determinant of regional blood flow. Arch. Surg. *89*:783, 1964.
9. Cranley, J. J., Fogarty, T. J., Krause, R. J., Strasser, E. S., and Hafner, C. D.: Phlebotomy for moderate erthrocythemia. J.A.M.A. *186*:206, 1963.
10. Crawford, E. S., Creech, O., Jr., Cooley, D. A., and DeBakey, M. E.: Treatment of arteriosclerotic occlusive disease of the lower extremities by excision and graft replacement or bypass. Surgery *38*:981, 1955.
11. Dale, W. A., and Jacobs, J. K.: Lower extremity amputation. Ann. Surg. *155*:1011, 1962.
12. Danese, C. A., and Haimov, M.: Inhibition of experimental arterial thrombosis in dogs with platelet deaggregating agents. Surgery *70*:927, 1971.
13. DeBakey, M. E., Burch, G., Roy, T., and Ochsner, A.: The "borrowing-lending" hemodynamic phenomenon (hemometakinesia) and its therapeutic application in peripheral vascular disturbances. Ann. Surg. *126*:850, 1947.
14. Edwards, E. A.: Operative anatomy of the lumbar sympathetic chain. Angiology *2*:184, 1951.
15. Edwards, E. A., and Crane, C.: Ten-year status after sympathectomy for arteriosclerosis. J.A.M.A. *175*:677, 1961.

16. Felder, D. A., Simeone, F. A., Linton, R. R., and Welch, C. E.: Evaluation of sympathectomy neurectomy in Raynaud's disease. Surgery 26:1014, 1949.
17. Freeman, N. E., Leeds, F. H., and Gardner, R. E.: Sympathectomy for obliterative vascular disease: indications and contraindications. Ann. Surg. 126:873, 1947.
18. Fulton, R. L., and Blakeley, W. R.: Lumbar sympathectomy: a procedure of questionable value in the treatment of arteriosclerosis obliterans of the legs. Am. J. Surg. 116:735, 1968.
19. Hamming, J. J.: Vascular prostheses and anticoagulant therapy. J. Cardiov. Surg. 4:681, 1963.
20. Hohf, R. P., Dye, W. S., Olwin, J. H., and Julian, O. C.: Low thoracic-high lumbar sympathectomy for vascular diseases of the legs. J.A.M.A. 156:1238, 1954.
21. Hunter, J. I.: The influence of the sympathetic nervous system in the genesis of rigidity of striated muscle in spastic paralysis. Surg. Gynec. Obstet. 39:721, 1924.
22. King, R. D., Kaiser, G. C., Lempke, R. E., and Shumacker, H. B., Jr.: Evaluation of lumbar sympathetic denervation. Arch. Surg. 88:36, 1964.
23. Kirgis, H. D., Reed, A. F., and Pearce, J. Y.: The relative effectiveness of sympathectomy, ganglionectomy and section of preganglionic fibers in activation of smooth muscle. Surgery 28:941, 1950.
24. Kountz, S. L., Eschelman, L. T., and Cohn, R.: The effect of aorto-iliac occlusion and sympathectomy on aorto-iliac blood flow. An experimental study. Am. J. Surg. 104:316, 1962.
25. Lempke, R. E., King, R. D., Kaiser, G. C., Judd, D., and Nahrwold, D.: Amputation for arteriosclerosis obliterans. Arch. Surg. 86:406, 1963.
26. Leriche, R.: De la causalgie envisagée comme une névrite du sympathetique et de son traitement par le dénudation et l'excision des plexus nerveux périartériels. Presse Méd. 24:178, 1916.
27. Leriche, R.: Surgery of the sympathetic system; indications and results. Ann. Surg. 88:449, 1928.
28. Leveen, H. H., and Diaz, C. A.: Venous and arterial occlusive disease treated by enzymatic clot lysis. Arch. Surg. 105:927, 1972.
29. Lilly, G. D., Smith, D. W., Biggane, C. F., Jr., and Jana, J. T., Jr.: An evaluation of "high" lumbar sympathectomy in arteriosclerotic circulatory insufficiency of the lower extremities. Surgery 35:1, 1954.
30. Malan, E., and Puglionisi, A.: Effects de la ganglionectomie lombaire sur la fonction vasculaire. Acta Neuroveg. 14:190, 1956.
31. Ozeran, R. S., Wagner, G. R., Reimer, T. R., and Hill, R. A.: Neuropathy of the sympathetic nervous system associated with diabetes mellitus. Surgery 68:953, 1970.
32. Palumbo, L. T., Gray, G. W., and Claman, M. A.: Lumbar sympathectomy in the treatment of peripheral vascular diseases. Arch. Surg. 74:596, 1957.
33. Perry, T., Jr.: Below-knee amputation. Arch. Surg. 86:199, 1963.
34. Poole, J. C. F., Sabiston, D. C., Jr., Florey, H. W., and Allison, P. R.: Growth of endothelium in arterial prosthetic grafts and following endarterectomy. Surg. Forum, 13:225, 1962.
35. Robertson, C. W., and Smithwick, R. H.: The recurrence of vasoconstrictor activity after limb sympathectomy in Raynaud's disease and allied vasomotor states. New Eng. J. Med. 245:317, 1951.
36. Romeo, S. G., Whalen, R. E., and Tindall, J. P.: Intra-arterial administration of reserpine. Its use in patients with Raynaud's disease or Raynaud's phenomenon. Arch. Intern. Med. 128:825, 1970.
37. Ross, J. P.: *Surgery of the Sympathetic Nervous System.* London, Bailliere, 1956.
38. Royle, N. D.: A new operative procedure in the treatment of spastic paralysis and its experimental basis. Med. J. Australia 1:77, 1924.
39. Rutstein, D. D., Castrelli, W. P., Sullivan, J. C., Newell, J. M., and Nickerson, R. J.: Effects of fat and carbohydrate ingestion in human beings on serum lipids and intracellular lipid deposition in tissue culture. New Eng. J. Med. 271:1, 1964.
40. Samuels, S. S.: *Management of Peripheral Arterial Diseases.* New York, Oxford University Press, 1950.

41. Sawyer, P. N., Stanczewski, B., Pomerance, A., Cohen, M., Lucas, T., and Srinivasan, S.: Utility of anticoagulant drugs in vascular thrombosis, an electron microscopic and biophysical study. Surgery 74:263, 1973.

42. Schenk, W. G., Jr., Delin, N. A., Domanig, E., Hahnloser, P., and Hoyt, R. K.: Blood viscosity as a determinant of regional blood flow. Arch. Surg. 89:783, 1964.

43. Schwartz, D. I., Pennock, L. L., Pessolano, C. J., and Littman, D. S.: A clinical evaluation of subcutaneous Achilles tenotomy as an aid in the treatment of intermittent claudication. J. Bone Joint Surg. 34-A:619, 1952.

44. Shelley, W. B., and Florence, R.: Compensatory hyperhidrosis after sympathectomy. New Eng. J. Med. 263:1056, 1960.

45. Silver, D.: An evaluation of dextran in the prevention and treatment of thrombosis. Acta Chir. Scand. (Suppl.)387:69, 1968.

46. Taylor, G. A.: Personal communication.

47. Thompson, R. C., Jr., Delblanco, T. L., and McAllister, F. F.: Complication following lower extremity amputation. Surg. Gynec. Obstet. 120:301, 1965.

48. Tolstedt, G. E., and Bell, J. W.: Failure of below-knee amputation in peripheral arterial disease. Arch. Surg. 83:934, 1961.

49. Veal, J. R.: Prevention of pulmonary complications following thigh amputations by high ligation of the femoral vein. J.A.M.A. 121:240, 1943.

50. Warren, R., Crawford, E. S., Hardy, I. B., Jr., and McKittrick, J. B.: The transmetatarsal amputation in arterial deficiency of the lower extremity. Surgery 31:132, 1952.

51. Weisman, R. E., and Upson, J. F.: The use of lumbar sympathectomy as an adjunct to reconstructive arterial surgery. Ann. Surg. 154:788, 1961.

52. White, J. C., and Smithwick, R.: *The Autonomic Nervous System.* New York, The Macmillan Co., 1947.

53. Whitelaw, G. P., and Smithwick, R. H.: Some secondary effects of sympathectomy with particular reference to disturbance of sexual function. New Eng. J. Med. 245:121, 1951.

54. Winsor, T.: *Peripheral Vascular Diseases; An Objective Approach.* Springfield, Ill., Charles C Thomas, 1959.

55. Wright, I. S.: The treatment of occlusive arterial disease. J.A.M.A. 183:186, 1963.

56. Wright, I. S. Personal communication.

Chapter Seven

AORTOILIAC RECONSTRUCTION

GENERAL CONSIDERATIONS IN ARTERIAL RECONSTRUCTION

The prime indication for operation in peripheral vascular disease is the need for restoration of function, which may be defined as the ability to perform needed muscular work, or to heal the integument or maintain its integrity. Function may also refer to maintenance of a vascular supply sufficient to keep the limb free of ischemic pain while at rest. In some cases pain on walking may be severe enough to require surgical treatment, but in others a less drastic procedure may be sufficient if it assures preservation of a viable limb.

Surgical treatment represents a series of compromises: at best the disease is a temporarily localized process which is likely to become generalized; at worst it presents so diffusely as to make operation of any kind unfeasible. A few examples may clarify this statement.

A 67-year-old man had been unable to walk more than 200 feet because of dypsnea due to extensive pulmonary fibrosis secondary to tuberculosis in childhood. He had experienced mild symptoms of fatigue in one thigh just before his dyspnea made him stop. On examination he was found to have unilateral iliac atherosclerosis with complete occlusion of the iliac artery, but no obvious disease process on the other side. The foot was well nourished and there was no evidence of cutaneous change. Full arterial reconstruction was thought to be ill advised, and lumbar sympathectomy was done on the affected side.

Four years later, the patient was free of peripheral vascular symptoms, but he returned to the hospital with the symptoms of transient confusion, aphasia, weakness of the left side, and a loud bruit over the right carotid artery. Stenosis of the carotid bifurcation due to atherosclerosis was diagnosed and was corrected by endarterectomy. The patient made an uneventful recovery and has been well for a follow-up period of 3 years.

A 34-year-old janitor had developed progressive hip and thigh claudication that severely affected his ability to work. Examination revealed no abnormality except a typical aortoiliac occlusion of the Leriche type. Following aortoiliac endarterectomy and bilateral sympathectomy he experienced complete relief of symptoms.

A 65-year-old retired carpenter entered the hospital with a a gangrenous abscess on the sole of his right foot; the abscess was secondary to gangrene in two toes. He had had diabetes for 20 years, and several episodes of coronary occlusion with subsequent angina. Examination demonstrated evidence of a long area of femoral arterial obstruction on the affected side. Lumbar sympathectomy was performed, but during and after the operation there was great difficulty in maintaining the patient's blood pressure. No arterial reconstruction was considered, and only local amputation and debridement were performed. Almost a year was required for the foot to heal, but thereafter the patient was able to walk short distances without pain. His foot is deformed but functioning, and the patient remains well 2 years later.

Several principles guide the surgeon in his choice of operation, but these may be disregarded in certain circumstances:

1. The lesion should produce symptoms.

2. Lesions that cause restriction of activity only must be considered in respect to inconvenience, interference with the patient's livelihood, or endangerment to life or limb.

3. The mortality risk of the operation must be evaluated in relation not only to the immediate relief to be anticipated but also to the patient's longevity and the other atherosclerotic complications that may arise.

4. Some visceral lesions, such as renal or carotid artery stenosis, may be so critically life-threatening that reconstruction may be undertaken with less regard to general conditions that might otherwise contraindicate operation.

The presence of certain complications of atherosclerosis, and related conditions such as diabetes, may make the risk too great in lesions that are not actually life-endangering.

There is no wisdom in offering a procedure of even moderate risk to a patient who cannot benefit from it because of other incapacities; on the other hand, there is no reason to withhold even hazardous procedures if they are likely to improve a life-threatening situation. Since the situation is critical, the greater risks may indeed be acceptable. A poor prognosis may lead one to choose between two similar procedures, selecting the quicker, simpler, or safer operation even if it appears to offer less immediate or long-term benefit.

AORTOILIAC ENDARTERECTOMY

Wide exposure is required in any abdominal approach to the aorta and iliac arteries. Preparation and draping of the skin should include not only the *entire* abdomen but the lower left chest and the anterior aspect of both legs to midthigh. Seldom will it be necessary to expose the femoral arteries, and even more seldom to enter the thorax (or divide the costal margin and diaphragm) to expose the high abdominal aorta. However, the hazards of venturing these maneuvers without asepsis are too great to risk, and preliminary precautions are readily accomplished.

The general condition of the patient is pertinent. Anemia (hemoglobin below 10 grams per cent) should be corrected. Phlebotomy should be considered for patients with polycythemia. Blood may be drawn preoperatively in a quantity sufficient to lower the hematocrit to less than 48 per cent and the platelets to less than 400,000 per cubic milliliter. This same blood may then be used for the patient during his operation without subjecting him to the usual hazards of banked blood. With lesser degrees of polycythemia it may be a simple practice to replace lost blood during the operation with dextran or other plasma expanders instead of whole blood in order to bring the hemoglobin (and viscosity) to a safer level.[19, 20]

There are no special preoperative studies, and it is presumed that specific diagnostic studies have already been done. Cholesterol, triglycerides and blood sugar levels should be known. Renal function usually is estimated adequately by a serum creatinine determination. The presence of two functioning kidneys should be known. Determination of cryoglobulin levels before institution of heparin therapy may also be advisable in specific instances (see Chapter Nineteen).

Preparation of a patient with known myocardial disease should at times include prophylactic digitalization even when there is no apparent evidence of cardiac failure. Willman[81] has revived this procedure in the management of heart operations, but it applies equally to major arterial reconstructions.

Any localized areas of sepsis should preclude elective surgery and may modify emergency procedures. The presence of an infection in one area of the body has been implicated in an increased incidence of infection in other operative wounds, and this hazard should be avoided whenever possible.[39]

A liquid diet for 2 days and intestinal intubation are helpful; additionally, the colon should be emptied by enemas and the bladder decompressed by temporary catheterization.

The use of preoperative antibiotics is controversial. If used they must be started early enough to have a level well established before the operation begins. The blind administration of a routine antibiotic is decried. The agent must be given in bactericidal doses and, if possible, should be effective against any known pathogenic bacteria that can be cultured from the patient's nose and throat or urinary tract. Even under these conditions there is hazard of superinfection which must be acknowledged. If a plastic prosthesis is not used the course of antibiotics should be brief unless it is redirected at specific postoperative complications.

It has been the author's practice to use intestinal antibiotic or chemotherapeutic prophylaxis in those instances in which manipulation and dissection of the colon and poor colonic blood supply—which may be reduced further by the need to sacrifice inferior mesenteric artery—may combine to produce ischemic symptoms in the colon. Elective resection of an abdominal aneurysm is an example; however, this need to protect the colon against ischemia is not very frequently encountered in operations for pure occlusive disease.

A steady level of anesthesia must be maintained. Adequate relaxation at all times is desirable, but complete control is *essential* during the critical moments of dissection and repair. Exposure of the deep retroperitoneal areas is difficult and should not be complicated by inadequate anesthetization.

The anesthesiologist should also serve as a monitor for the surgeon by recording blood loss, heart rate and rhythm, and occasionally the contour of the electrocardiographic and electroencephalographic tracings. The percutaneous placement of an arterial line from which continuous monitoring of the arterial blood pressure may be read is of great value to both surgeon and anesthesiologist. Furthermore, assessment of either the central venous pressure or pressure in the pulmonary artery is also of great importance in defining the receptivity of the cardiovascular system to further fluid load. When a subclavian central venous line or a pulmonary artery line must be placed, it should be done prior to the operation so that an x-ray can be obtained to confirm the position of the line and the absence of a pneumothorax or pleural effusion. The competent anesthesiologist accepts and understands this role completely; indeed, major arterial surgery must not be undertaken without the help of a competent and cooperative anesthesiology staff. They should determine the choice of anesthetic; either general or conduction anesthesia is appropriate when properly managed.

The skin may be prepared by any of the standard methods. The author prefers several days of skin preparation with a soap or detergent containing hexachlorophene, an immediately preoperative shave, the use of aqueous iodine or iodophore as skin germicide, and the application of one of the imprevious plastic adherent sheets to exclude as much skin surface as possible.

Incision and Exposure

A long midline or left paramedian incision is most commonly used. It may be carried into the costoxyphoid angle if necessary so that the intestines can be lifted up and out of the field. Very rarely is it necessary to modify this incision for exposure of the upper abdominal aorta, left renal artery, celiac axis, or superior mesenteric artery, but, if it is, the incision may be extended across the left costal margin at the level of the fifth to the seventh interspace. The diaphragm may be incised and the pleura entered if necessary, but division of the costal margin and only partial splitting of the diaphragm may give adequate exposure without the pleural cavity being entered. The splenic flexure may be mobilized medially, or the spleen, tail of the pancreas, and splenic flexure may all be mobilized as one unit.

Very high abdominal exposure is not so commonly necessary in the treatment of occlusive disease as it is in aneurysmectomy or renal arterial operations. If the intestines are to be fully mobilized and placed outside the abdomen during the operation, a high extension to the incision is very helpful.

Imparato[41] tilts the patient sharply to the right so that gravity assists in holding the intestines out of the field.

Rob[56] has advocated a long oblique incision for exposure of the abdominal aorta. This incision has the merit of being extraperitoneal and of giving good exposure at a high level, although the right paravertebral sympathetic ganglia are not easily reached by this route, nor is the right external iliac artery. It has the disadvantage of cutting across many small collateral channels and some important ones that may not have been anticipated. It should be used only after the surgeon has had considerable experience with vascular repair. One disadvantage of the extraperitoneal approach is that it does not allow exposure and exploration of the intraperitoneal structures.

If the transperitoneal route is chosen the initial step should include careful exploration. The most common incidental lesions of importance are cholelithiasis and duodenal ulcer. Unsuspected carcinomas of the kidney, stomach, and pancreas have also been encountered. Cholelithiasis usually warrants cholecystectomy at the same operation, as acute cholecystitis has been known to follow major arterial operations with considerable frequency. Few other lesions warrant concomitant operation, but the finding of a carcinoma for which the prognosis was poor might well cancel an extensive arterial procedure. The management of any carcinoma would usually have priority over the arterial operation.

There are circumstances, however, in which the arterial operation should precede the treatment of a carcinoma, but these usually entail the combination of a superior mesenteric artery obstruction, collateralization by means of the inferior mesenteric artery, and a carcinoma of the left colon that would demand resection of that major collateral. Under such circumstances restoration of superior mesenteric flow should precede treatment of the neoplasm. Although potentially contaminating procedures are often done at the same time as arterial reconstructions, it is generally safer to stage them wherever possible.

Initial evaluation of the aorta and its bifurcation and the common and external iliac arteries can be obtained at this time by palpation. The presence of aneurysmal dilatation or of very small external iliac vessels (see Chapter Two, p. 18), especially when they are involved in the thrombo-occlusive process, may make a bypass procedure preferable to endarterectomy. The critical size of the external iliacs below which endarterectomy should not be undertaken is somewhat arbitrary. The author usually proceeds with endarterectomy if the vessels are uninvolved by atherosclerosis and will accept a No. 10 or No. 12 French catheter. Involvement by a tail of atheroma may be disregarded; if the degree of narrowing endangers adequate flow a lateral patch may be used. If the external iliacs are so diseased as to require extensive endarterectomy, it should be possible to insert intraluminally a No. 14 French catheter, at least. Aneurysmal dilatation is equally an indication for the use of a graft instead of endarterectomy. If complete occlusion of an aneurysmal segment is present it may be bypassed; if significant flow is present, the segment should be excised and replaced by a graft.

At this stage, it is important to decide which procedure to use. It is poor judgment to spend several hours trying to achieve an endarterectomy, only to have to sacrifice the dissected vessels and fall back on a grafting procedure. The bypass grafts in the abdomen are so effective that they should be used without hesitation if endarterectomy is not feasible. The less experienced surgeon should probably elect the bypass operation more frequently than the experienced surgeon.

Direct exposure of the involved vessels is obtained by an incision at the root of the small bowel mesentery (Fig. 7–1). This incision may be extended as high as necessary, running medially to (that is, to the right of) the inferior mesenteric vein as far as the angle formed by the duodenum and the dextrad deviation of the vein, near its termination in the splenoportal system. The incision may be extended down along the course of the right iliac artery, avoiding the ureter and sparing the spermatic vessels. Full mobilization of the structures in the ileocecal region usually is not required, but if it is, a peritoneal incision may be carried up laterally to the cecum and the entire superior mesenteric pedicle may be lifted upward and to the right. The intestinal contents may be placed in a plastic Lahey bag. For very high exposure, the left renal vein, which has excellent collaterals, may be divided as far to the right as possible.[70] Mobilization of the splenic flexure, spleen and pancreas allows the surgeon an even higher approach to the left lateral aspect of the highest abdominal aorta. The inferior mesenteric vein may also be divided if necessary.

If such extensive mobilization is not necessary, excellent expo-

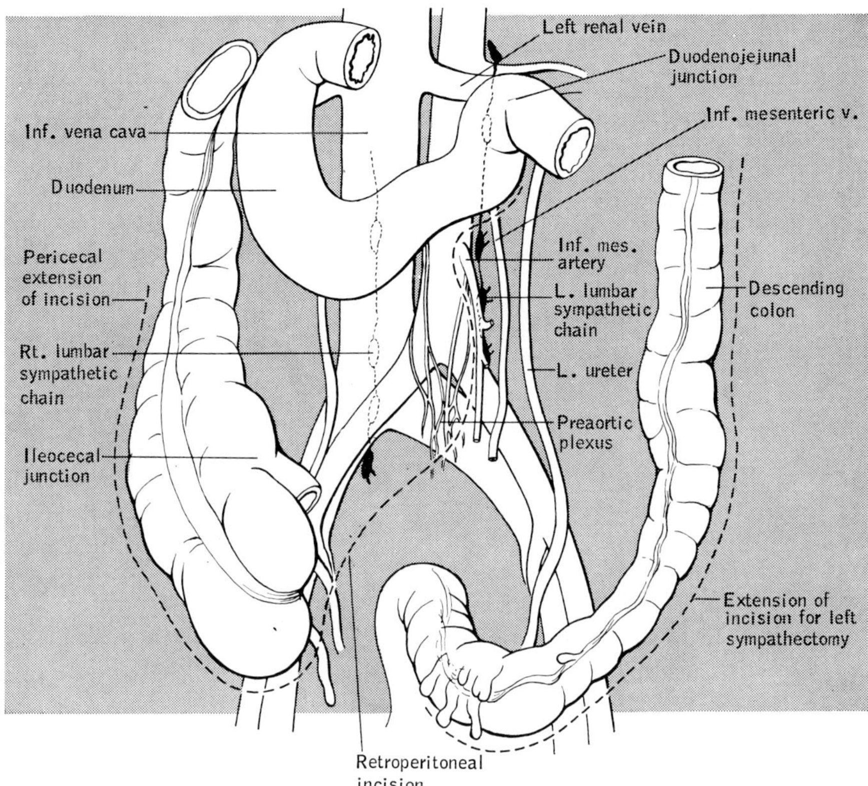

Figure 7–1. Anatomical exposure of aortic bifurcation, showing structures of major importance. Retroperitoneal tissues are incised along the dotted line as indicated over aortoiliac area. Intestinal tract is reflected to the right. Incision may be extended around tip of cecum so as to achieve greater mobility. Incision indicated by dotted line lateral to left colon may be used in full or in part to expose distal left iliac artery or left lumbar chain.

sure may be obtained by the following routine: After exploration, gauze pads are placed over the wound edges and either a large deep Balfour or medium Finochetto, or a similar self-retaining retractor, is put in place. The posterior peritoneal incision is made as shown in Figure 7–1. A moist towel is laid on the right side of the incision, the small intestine is lifted out and onto it, and the towel is folded over the displaced intestine. The towel is less irritating to the serosal surfaces than gauze and has sufficient body to hold the intestines in place. A sheet of plastic offers even more protection.

Sympathectomy

If sympathectomy has not been done previously, it should be done before arterial reconstruction or heparinization.

The left lumbar chain may be exposed by dissection at the left lateral margin of the aorta near its bifurcation. It is difficult to extend this dissection as high as is desired because of the presence of the inferior mesenteric artery. An easy procedure, although one that requires more extensive retroperitoneal dissection, is to mobilize the descending colon, ureter, and spermatic vessels and mesenteric vessels, to the right. This dissection, although extensive, should be practically bloodless, and allows good exposure of the portion of the chain to be divided, namely, from the top of the second lumbar vertebra to the bottom of the third lumbar disc.

The right sympathetic chain is usually easily reached by the direct route along the right side of the vena cava, but the right colon may be mobilized if necessary.

Many surgeons[32] disagree with the use of sympathectomy as a routine concomitant of arterial reconstruction, believing that it is not necessary. The author has no reason to believe concomitant sympathectomy has done any harm and continues to use it in hopes that it may provide some protection against the progression of the disease in years to come. The argument for its use to achieve an immediate effect is based on the augmentation of flow which has been mentioned in Chapters Three and Six. Inasmuch as flow to the skin and the muscles is under sympathetic control, release of the sympathetic tonus should augment flow during the early period, when the reconstruction is most subject to failure. Augmentation of flow rates decreases the possibility of failure.

The effect on flow of sympathectomy following arterial reconstruction[1] is illustrated by the case of a 65-year-old man who was admitted to the hospital with the complaints of arterial insufficiency and hypertension.

An abdominal aneurysm was detected, and the femoral and pedal pulses were reduced but symmetrical. The aneurysm was resected and replaced by a bifurcation prosthesis of Dacron. The obstructive symptoms had apparently been brought about by elongation of the aorta which had caused kinking of the common iliac arteries.

Continuous monitoring of the peripheral circulation by plethysmography revealed an expected marked diminution of flow when the aorta was cross-clamped. As soon as flow was restored along the right arm of the graft, flow returned to the right toes; similar prompt return occurred on the left. Within the next 20 minutes there was a gradual diminution of pulsations in the toes bilaterally, presumably due to spasm. There was no obstruction at the site of attachment of the graft. Bilateral lumbar sympathectomy was followed by prompt reversal of the spasm and return to the previous level of flow (Fig. 7–2).

Arterial Mobilization

Blunt dissection with a large right angle clamp such as a Moynihan is used to secure a tape around the lower abdominal aorta above the area of occlusion. This is where the occluding clamp will be

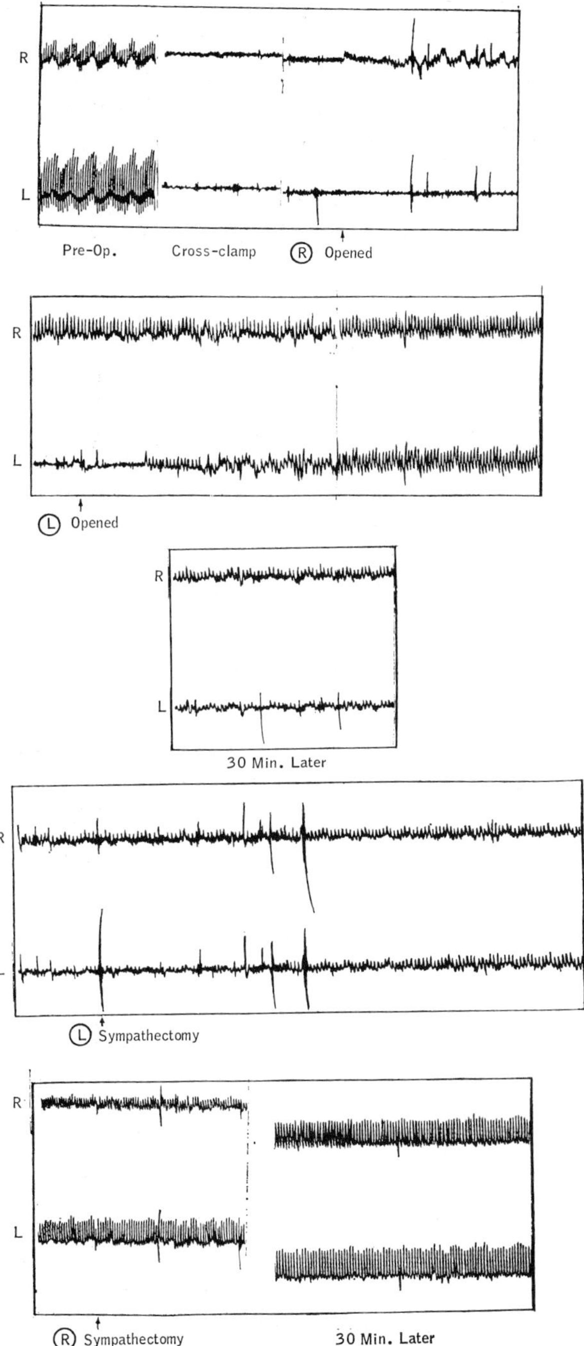

Figure 7–2. Digital pulse registration during resection of aortic aneurysm: tracings taken during preoperative period; during cross-clamping; after right and left sides restored; 30 minutes later; after left and right lumbar sympathectomy; and 30 minutes later.

placed, hence there should be no extensive calcified plaques at the level chosen. The clamp should be placed below as many lumbar arteries as possible to allow maximal collateral flow to the spinal cord and to minimize trauma to those lumbar arteries that must be controlled. The lumbar arteries below the encircling tape may be isolated and controlled with tapes, heavy temporary ties, small bulldog clamps or lightly placed tantalum clips which may be removed at the conclusion of the operation. The middle sacral artery may require similar treatment.

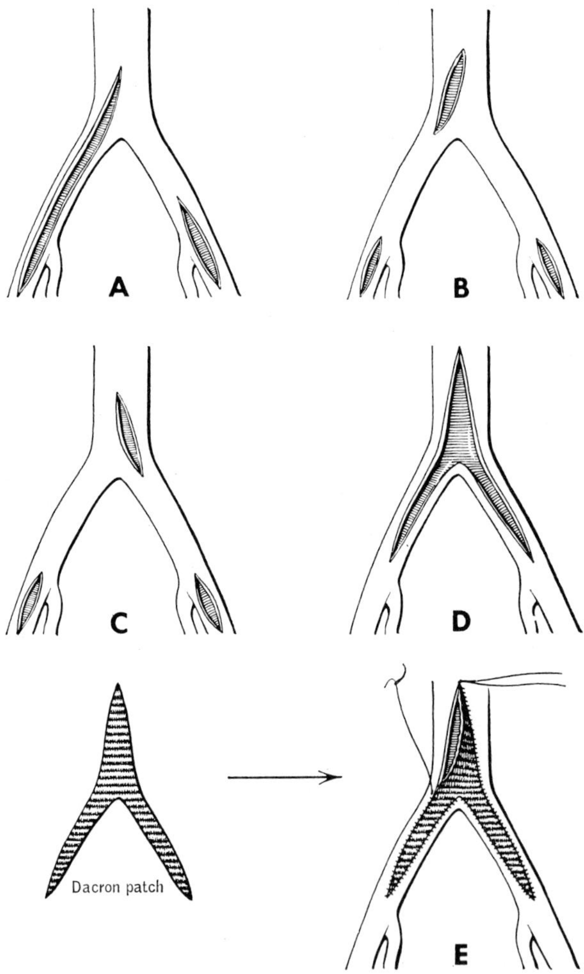

Figure 7–3.   Aortic and iliac arteriotomies. *A,* Continuous right aortoiliac and separate left iliac arteriotomy. *B,* Bilateral iliac arteriotomies and separate aortic incision directed down the right side for initial right-sided restoration; *C,* Same as *B,* but left-sided restoration. *D,* Y-shaped incision. *E,* Closure of Y-shaped incision by Y-shaped patch, made of Dacron in this case.

Although circumferential control by tapes provides a certain factor of safety and moral support for the surgeon it may not always be necessary. The direct clamping without dissection behind the aorta saves time and sometimes troublesome bleeding. A reliable clamp must be used and must be well protected against dislodgment while it is in place.

The common iliac arteries near their origin from the aorta should now be dissected and encircled with tapes. The posterior attachment of the iliac artery to the underlying iliac veins is a critical point, for a tear in the vein may cause potentially disastrous hemorrhage (Fig. 2–9, p. 20). Tapes are similarly placed around the hypogastric artery and the external iliac artery beyond the area of occlusion.

Incisions to be used in the vessel wall and the operating sequence need to be decided upon early.

Ordinarily, the side with less degree of occlusion should be chosen first for operation on the assumption that collateral circulation will be more efficient on the more seriously affected side. Endarterectomy and closure of the arteriotomy can be completed and flow restored along the first side; then the other side can be treated, with the operating team under less pressure.

If both iliac arteries are occluded, i.e., if the aorta is occluded, there may be little choice of one side over the other. In this case, it is more practical to restore flow to the right external iliac artery; then, without interrupting the right iliac arterial flow, the left iliac artery may be operated upon both above and below the sigmoid mesocolon.

The pattern of incisions may vary, as shown in Figure 7–3 A, B, C. The aorta and one iliac artery may be opened in one continuous incision. This may be difficult on the left side, as the incision must be made under the mesocolon. It does, however, assure a perfectly clean endarterectomized segment. The time required for closure of the longer arteriotomy may be a factor, but the time may be decreased by the use of a straight arterial needle (Fig. 7–11).

Intimal Dissection

It is usually desirable to perform the endarterectomy through two or more discrete incisions in the artery (Fig. 7–3B, 3C). At the site of one or both of these incisions, a plane of dissection can be developed between the diseased sequestrum of atheromatous material and the healthy wall that remains. A tunnel can be dissected in this plane to join the two arteriotomies with a blunt Freer dissector or a loop dissector. We have commonly used a loop similar to Cannon's[14] but made of a heavier gauge metal and with a blunter leading edge. This modification makes the instrument serve as a blunt dissector rather than as a sharp one, with less likelihood of being deformed by a plaque of calcium, or of tearing the media (Fig. 7–4A).

Another type of dissector has been described by LeVeen,[47] it is in the form of an open blunt tipped helix (Fig. 7–4B). It is said to be inserted more easily, and to be less apt to tear the remaining medial wall, for the dissection is done as the instrument is withdrawn.

If endarterectomy is performed through two separate arteriotomies, it is essential that a smooth surface be left on the media. Repeated passes with a loop dissector, or with a gauze swab held in a bayonet or alligator forceps and pulled through, will serve to clean the surface. A compromise must be made between undue trauma to the vessel wall and inadequate dissection.

Sawyer[60, 64] introduced a technique of gas endarterectomy in which part of the initial dissection of the thickened intima is performed in the same way as outlined in previous pages. A cannulated needle or spatula is used, however, to continue the dissection the length of the obstructed segment. With experience this technique allows extensive endarterectomy and removal of even fine extensions into small branches. The dissection ordinarily proceeds rapidly and with minimal trauma to the arterial wall. It may be difficult to be sure that the remaining arterial wall is truly free from adherent remnants of intima and may require further intraluminal passages of pledgets of gauze.

The Y-shaped incision shown in Figure 7–3D should be avoided if possible; the junction of the two iliac arms represents a weak point in the suture line. If such an incision is required in order to remove the plaques in the carina of the aortic bifurcation, or if it is made inadvertently, a satisfactory repair can be accomplished by means of a patch of suitable material. This patch, shaped like an inverted V or Y, avoids the need for T-shaped suture lines (Fig. 7–3E). Either autologous saphenous vein or a portion of Dacron prosthesis serves adequately. The use of this V-shaped patch will be discussed elsewhere (p. 136). Dissection of the autonomic plexus over the bifurcation of the aorta should be as limited as possible in the male to reduce the possibility of impotence occurring. The incision in the aorta may be carried to either side of the midline of the vessel to protect this plexus, but extensive dissection of the vessels beyond that needed for control is unnecessary.

Preservation of the inferior mesenteric artery and its surrounding neural plexus is highly desirable.

Heparinization in the distal arterial tree is desirable during the period of occlusion. Heparin may be given systemically by the anesthetist, or by the surgeon who may inject it directly into the aorta. We prefer to place catheters in the arteries at the distal limit of the diseased segment as soon as flow is interrupted and the arteriotomies

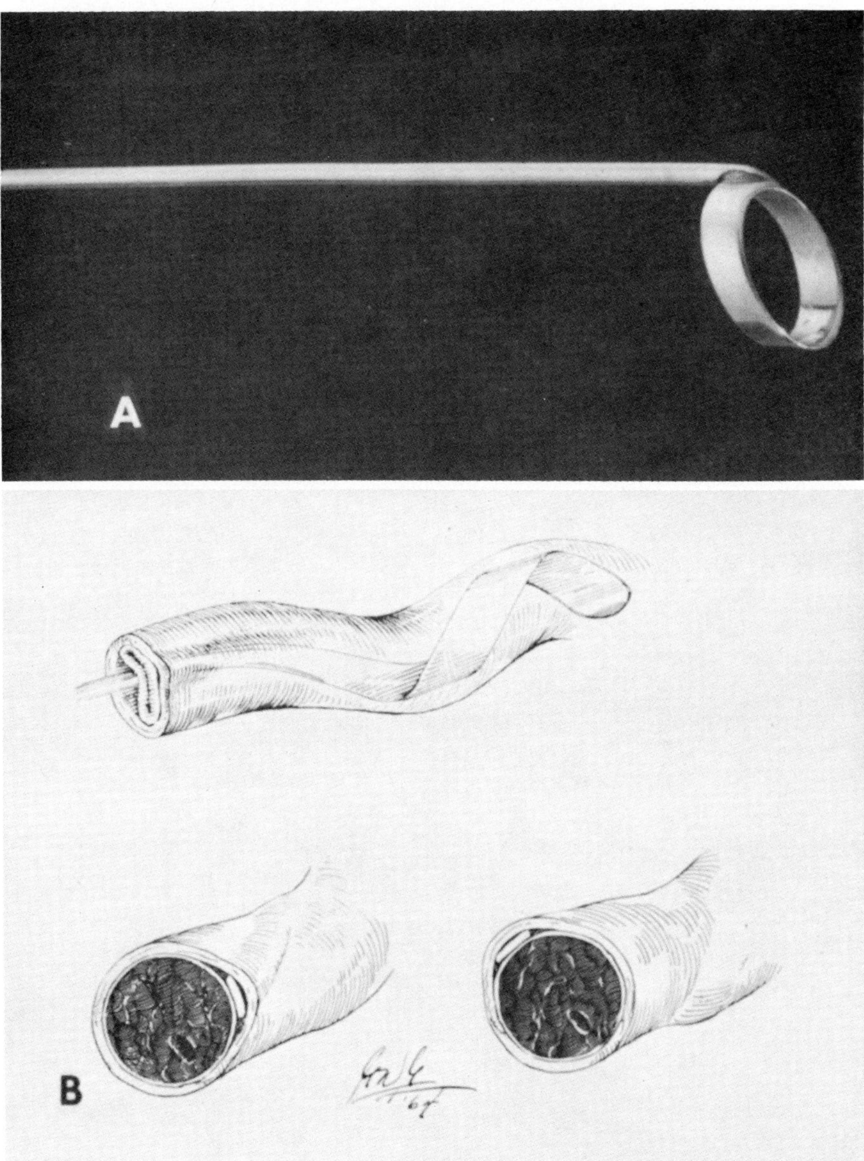

Figure 7–4. A, Author's modification of Cannon's intraluminal loop-dissector; it is made of heavier gauge steel and has a blunter leading edge. B, LeVeen's helical loop dissector. The instrument is advanced by its corkscrew motion, but dissection is carried out by *withdrawing* it; dissection must not be accomplished by pushing. (From LeVeen, H. H.: Technical features in endarterectomy. Surgery 57:22, 1965. Reprinted with permission of publisher.)

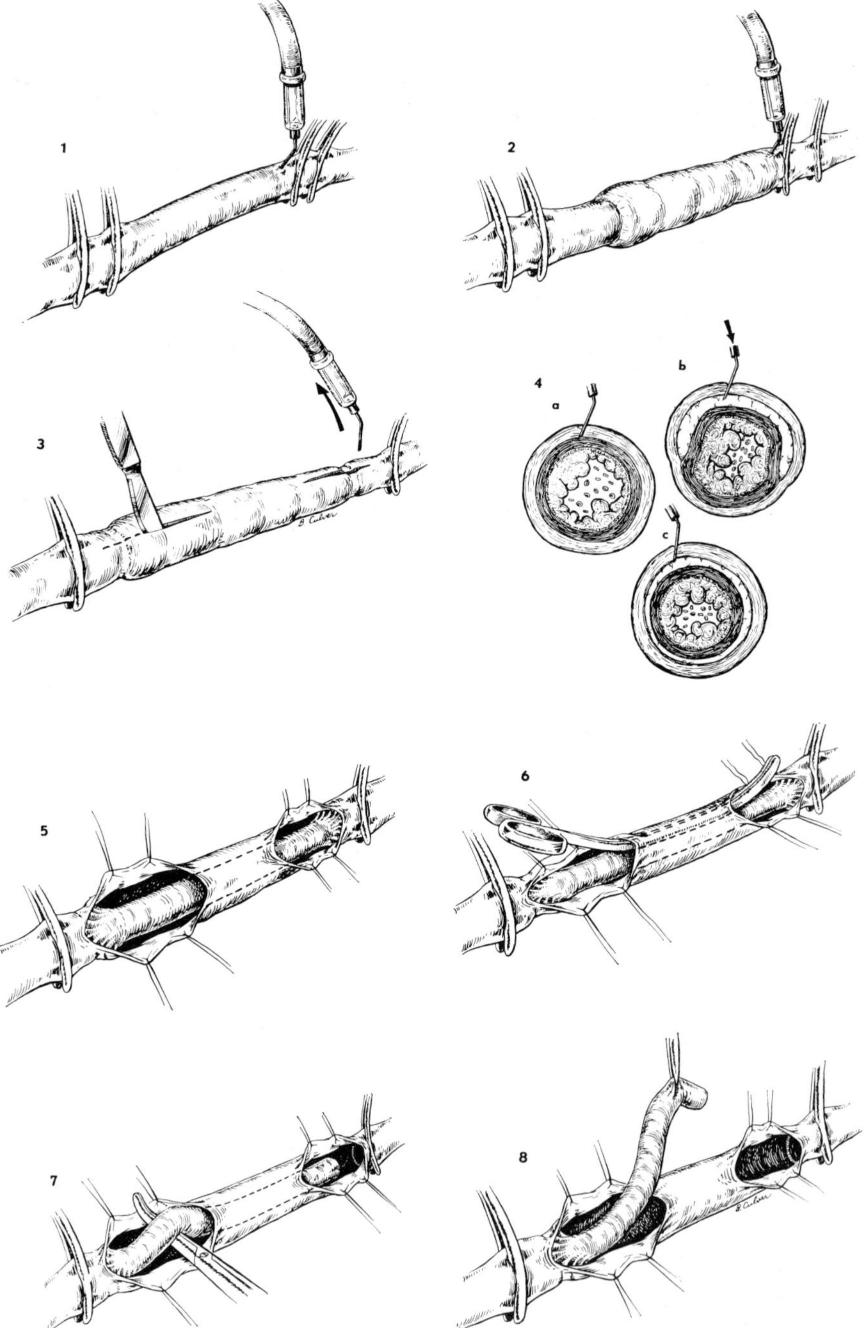

Figure 7–5. Several stages in the performance of gas endarterectomy. *1*, Isolated vessel is doubly clamped on either end and the needle which is the source of the gas is inserted between the arterial media and the inner intima "sequestrum." *2*, The gas dis-

(Legend continued on opposite page.)

made. These catheters then can serve as a gauge of the size of the artery, as a means of occluding the vessel (by drawing down the encircling tapes), as a means of direct investigation, mechanically or by injection of radiopaque contrast material, and to provide continuous administration of dilute heparin into the distal tree until flow is restored. Generous volumes of a dilute heparin solution (containing 10 units per ml.) may be injected by this route, but the total dose should be considered if one chooses to use other systemic anticoagulants or antiplatelet drugs.

Ten milliliters may be injected every 10 minutes during the arterial repair. Since the entire reconstruction of the bifurcation of the aorta should rarely require more than 2 hours, not more than 2500 to 3000 units of heparin is given by this route. Intravenous heparin, in the amount of 2500 to 5000 units, may be given at this time, either as an alternative or as a supplement. Reversal with protamine sulfate may be done if desired at the termination of the procedure.

Cross-clamping of the aorta can be done with any vascular clamp of standard design. Each surgeon develops a personal preference. Modern vascular clamps are relatively nontraumatic but must inevitably cause some distortion of the intima and some trauma to it. This distortion, if extreme, may lead to subintimal hemorrhage and even to dislodgment of the intima. Even when not extreme, the injury may result in the development of atheroma at the site of cross-clamping, as is described on page 46. Gaspar[34] has used the crushing clamp as a means of sealing the intima to the media, although this method has not been consistently reliable when employed by others. A Satinsky clamp, or a Potts ductus clamp, or an angled DeBakey clamp will serve well as an occluding clamp. The clamp is placed at the site of dissection marked by the tape, and the tape is left in place to facilitate later replacement of the clamp if necessary. Distal control can also be obtained by the use of doubly encircling tapes pulled tight, standard vascular clamps, or bulldog clamps. Once the distal artery has been opened, rubber catheters fitting snugly into the lumen of the vessel allow for easy occlusion by tightening the encircling tapes, and also grant access to the distal arterial tree.

We prefer to make a longitudinal incision in the vessel, although advocates of the transverse incision believe the latter is less likely to

---

sects along the artery to the more proximal of the two clamps at the other extremity of the vessel. 3, Arteriotomies are made to enable removal of the atheromatous "sequestrum." 4, *a*, *b*, and *c*. Stages of the circumferential dissection of gas in cross section. 5, 6, and 7, Removal of the "sequestrum" from the endarterectomized tube of media. Distal intimal flaps should be treated as shown in Figures 7–6 and 7–7. (From Sobel, S., Kaplitt, M. J., Reingold, M., and Sawyer, P. N.: Gas endarterectomy. Surgery, 59:517, 1966.)

narrow.[21, 24] Our reasons for favoring the longitudinal incision are the following:

1. Its level of placement is not so critical and it may be extended up or down as needed.

2. In our experience the dehiscence of suture lines in endarterectomized vessels has occurred almost exclusively in transverse incisions.

3. The risk of narrowing the vessel during closure of the arteriotomy seems not to be great, provided meticulous care is given to placement of sutures. Even if such narrowing threatens, the use of a patch graft will obviate the hazard.

The initial intimal dissection is begun distally. If it is possible to reach below the "tail" of the common iliac atheroma, often the tip can be lifted and mobilized in a proximal direction. A finger placed under the vessel[83] helps to flatten it so that a dissector can reach the tip of the plaque. Careful incision of the intima with a knife may be necessary (Fig. 7–6).

A procedure in which the external iliac artery or, indeed, the entire aortic bifurcation with the iliac system attached is removed, everted and endarterectomized has been described.[17, 43] Such extensive mobilization is not necessary if one uses appropriate long arteriotomies, and this mobilization may increase the development of recurrent atherosclerosis.

One must not yield to the temptation to continue an easy plane of dissection distally beyond the level at which one has sufficient control and exposure of the artery to discontinue the dissection safely lest subintimal dissection by the flow of blood obstruct the distal lumen.

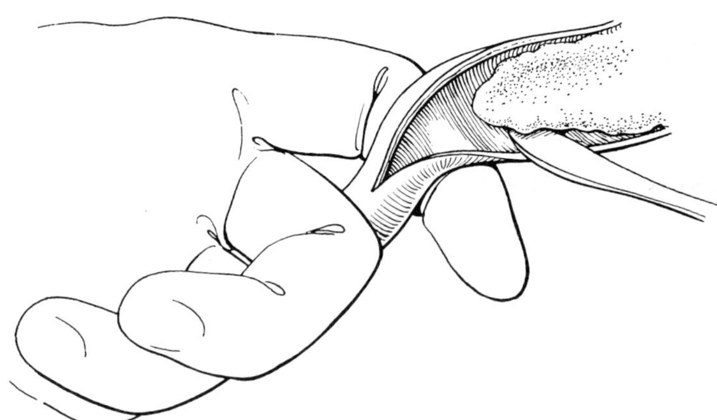

Figure 7–6. Arteriotomy opened, with finger behind longitudinal arteriotomy. Tip of dissector lifts pointed extremity of atheromatous plaque from wall of artery. (From Wylie, E. J., Binkley, F. M., and Albo, R. J.: Femoropopliteal endarterectomy. Am. J. Surg. *108*:215, 1964.)

If no clear-cut line of demarcation exists between atheroma and healthy intima at this level, consideration must be given to extending the arterial dissection further distally, or suturing down the thickened flap of intima at the orginal level chosen for arteriotomy (Fig. 7–7).

The decision to carry the operation distally may be governed by several criteria. If there is extensive plaque formation in the external iliac artery, and especially if the external iliac artery is relatively narrow, the advisability of using a bypass graft instead of an endarterectomy should be considered. This question is best resolved before the artery is opened, as arteriotomy for attachment of the distal limb of the graft would of necessity be done in the distal external iliac or common femoral artery.

A second criterion concerns the size of the blood vessel involved. Extensive endarterectomy in an external iliac artery 3.5 ml. (No. 10 French) or less in internal diameter is ill advised. Either a bypass graft or a long on-lay patch[21, 23, 24, 27] may be desirable under these circumstances.

Blodgett[7] has suggested use of an angioplastic technique (Fig. 7–8) which allows the intima to be sutured down in the narrow iliac arteries close to the division of common into external and hypogastric vessels, and the longitudinal arteriotomies in the two iliac arteries to be closed by the "reverse Finney" technique that leaves a patent lumen

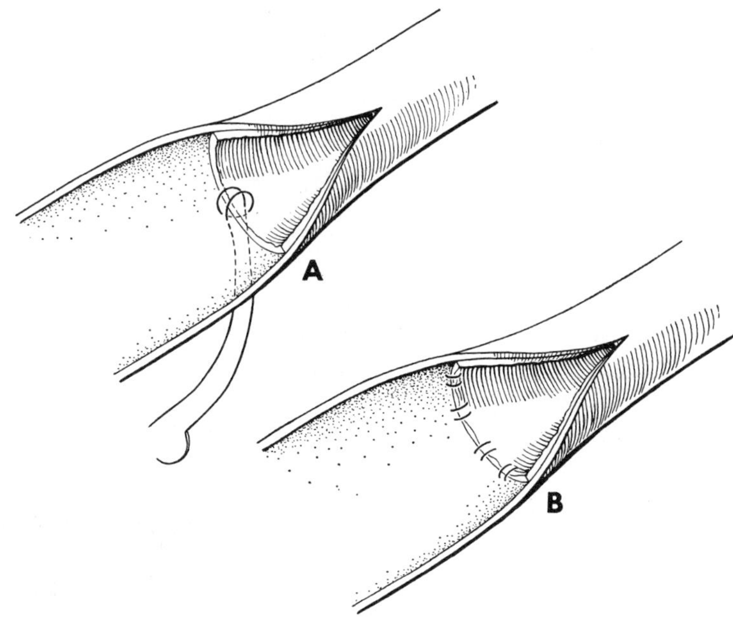

Figure 7–7. Mattress sutures placed to hold loose intima against media. Knots are *outside*: suture passes in through endarterectomized vessel and out through intima and media to avoid lifting intima away from media.

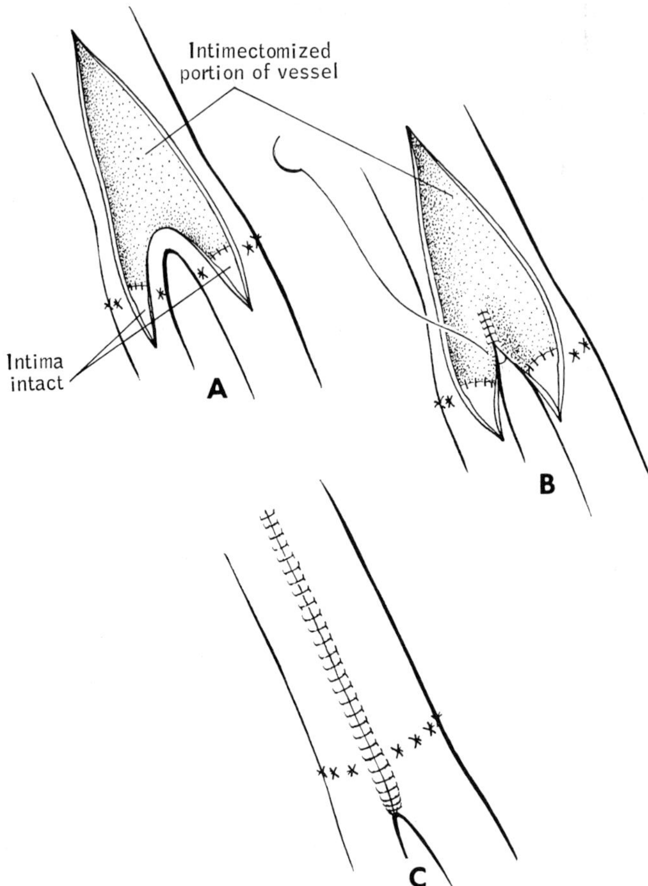

Figure 7–8.   Angioplasty converting proximal endarterectomy which extends below bifurcation into endarterectomy which is extended into larger vessel. (After Blodgett, J. B., and Viguri, J. J.: Bifurcation angioplasty to extend the usefulness of endarterectomy. Surg. Forum 6:266, 1955.)

in the endarterectomized vessel with no raw media in either narrow
iliac. This technique can be employed only when the area of disease
ends near the bifurcation of the common iliac artery or the common
femoral artery. Before this site is left, however, a check should be
made to be certain that no intimal flap or projection remains to hinder
flow; it may be excised or may be sutured in place with mattress sutures. The mattress sutures are placed from outside the vessel, passing
in through endarterectomized media, over the edge of intima, and
back out through intima and media (Fig. 7–7). The knots are tied
loosely to avoid cutting and distortion or puckering. This basic principle remains a critical point that must not be neglected.

When the subintimal plane is entered, the distal intimal flap is controlled, and the distal catheters are placed, the proximal dissection may be carried out. With gentle traction on the mobilized intima and atheroma, the sequestrum may be freed further by blunt dissection with a dull dissector. If it is desirable to leave an intact medial tube between arteriotomies, one selects a blunt stripper the size of the arterial segment and insinuates it under the media (Fig. 7–6). By palpating and applying countertraction digitally on the vessel, the surgeon usually can dissect the core cleanly from the medial wall.

The chief reasons for failure of the loop dissector are the use of too small a dissector to pass around the hard parts of the sequestrum, choice of too large a dissector to pass through even the elastic medial tunnel, impingement on a plaque of calcium or in the wrong layer of the wall, or impingement at a point of angulation or at the origin of a major vessel. If there is doubt whether the loop has passed safely, then the artery *must* be exposed at the point where the loop is caught to be certain of clean dissection without trauma to the wall.

The distal arteriotomy should usually extend beyond the bifurcation of the common iliac artery and should thus expose on the posterior wall of the open artery the orifice of the hypogastric artery.

Usually a segment of atheromatous material extends for several centimeters down this vessel, and this core can be freed by gentle ma-

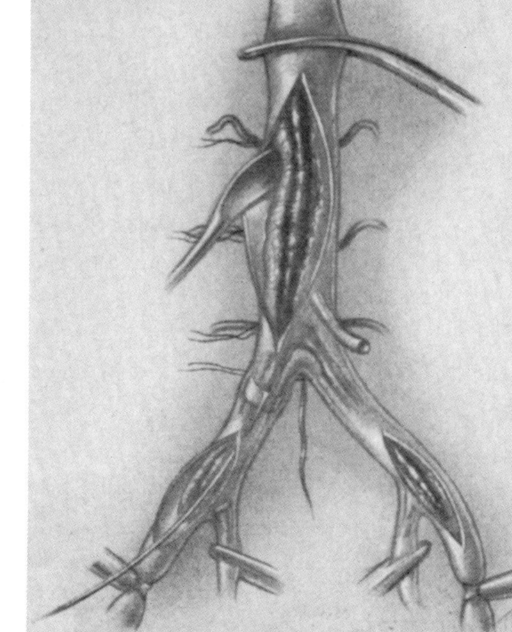

Figure 7–9. Loop dissector, Cannon type, being used in iliac region. (Redrawn from Figure 5 in Cannon, J. A., Kawakami, I. G., and Barker, W. F.: Arch. Surg. 82:813, 1961. Redrawn with permission of publisher.)

nipulation with a Freer dissector or a loop and with cautious traction applied to the atheroma. Often a pointed tip comes free, leaving an unobstructed distal channel. At other times the core extends down one of the major branches, usually anterior, and the orifice of the main posterior (muscular) trunk is freed so that flow can be restored into it even if flow into the anterior visceral trunk is less satisfactory.

Having dissected up to the level of the aortoiliac junction, the surgeon should open the aorta to a point no closer than 5 mm. from the occluding clamp.

Dissection is performed through the aortotomy until the major aortic and iliac segments are free of atheroma and clot as far as the level of the cross-clamp on the aorta. The carina is easily torn and must be dissected with care.[84]

The cross-clamp on the *opposite* iliac artery should be 1 cm. or more distant from the bifurcation, so that dissection into the proximal part of that iliac artery may be done. When the atheromatous plug is freed, the iliac occluding clamp (or tape) should be moved as near the bifurcation as possible. This will allow removal of the iliac atheroma on the second side from below without further handling of the aorta (Fig. 7–10).

There is often a loose plug of atheromatous material, old clot, and fresh clot above the aortic clamp that measures several centimeters in length. It is almost invariably present when both iliacs are occluded, but may form even when only one is completely obstructed. Removal of this loose plug is vital, for if it is not removed it will be carried into the reconstructed arterial tree and promptly precipitate thrombosis. Its consistency may be such that it is not easily felt through the wall and its existence not recognized. In order to be sure that he has removed it, the surgeon should place the fingers of one hand at the level of the renal arteries, and the aorta should be occluded manually. The aortic clamp is released but not displaced with the other hand, and the fingers are used to milk the plug from the aortotomy. If necessary, the infrarenal aorta below the fingers may be explored digitally, or with a pair of grasping forceps or a large curved hemostat. Fragments of the plug may be washed out with saline, and final irrigation performed by releasing the fingers for one or two pulse beats, flushing the channel from above with blood.

One must be careful not to displace debris and fragments of intima into the lumina of the renal arteries. Full exposure of the renal vessels and direct removal of atheroma at the level of the renal orifice through the open aorta is much less hazardous than inadvertent and unrecognized renal obstruction.

A small dose of heparin (2500 units) should now be given intravenously unless a heparinizing level has been achieved by the distal irrigation with heparin.

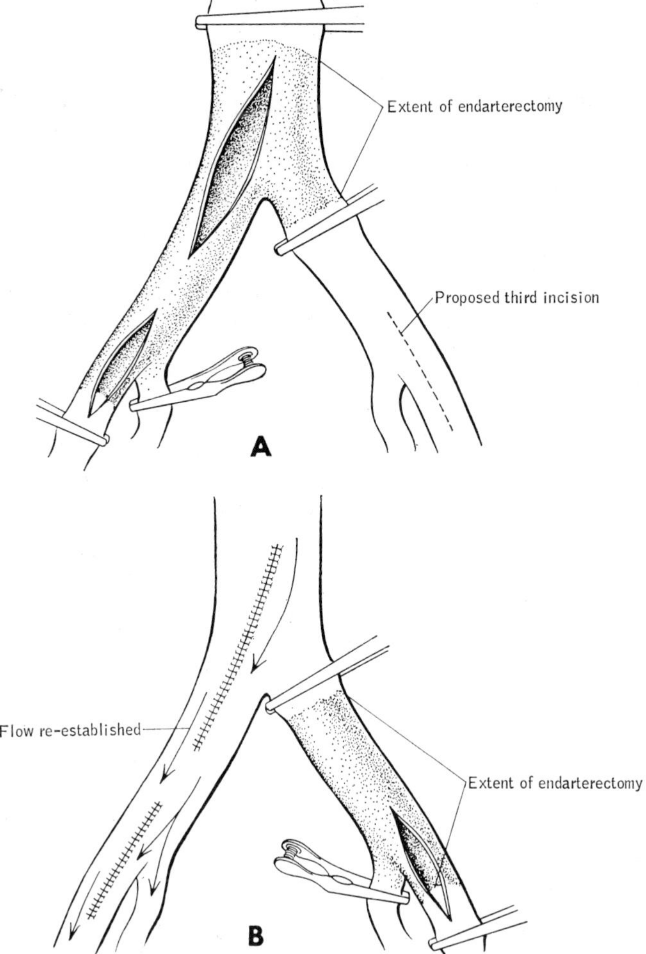

Figure 7–10. Replacement of iliac cross-clamps to allow restoration of flow along one side while endarterectomy of opposite side is done through single arteriotomy.

Arterial Repair

Arterial repair is usually best begun distally, or where the artery is narrowest. It is performed over a catheter which is used as a stent; the size should be as large as placed for the reconstructed lumen. The last few millimeters of the repair must of course be performed without the stent after the catheter is removed. In this situation, as whenever repair of a longitudinal incision is attempted without the use of a stent, special care must be taken to avoid encroaching unduly on the circumference of the vessel so as to create an isthmus. The last sutures may be placed as interrupted sutures before the stent is removed. These may be displaced for the removal of the stent and tied later.

Fine arterial suture material carried on a straight needle is most useful for rapid closure of an arteriotomy, provided there is sufficient exposure for lengthwise movement of the needle. A short straight hemostat with transverse serrations in its jaws makes a convenient needle holder. The surgeon may follow his own suture, holding it with one hand to assure proper tension (Fig. 7–11).

With the needle held near its eye, the point is advanced through both arterial walls. The grasp of the hemostat is loosely repositioned near the tip of the needle, pulled forward far enough to regrasp and hold the needle where it will be ready for the next bite. The transverse serrations automatically replace the needle perpendicularly to the axis of the needle holder. No other manipulation of the needle is required as is usually the case with a curved needle. There is also less risk of inadvertently causing contamination by puncturing the surgeon's glove, since the needle is handled less. With experience in this technique, the surgeon can sew three or four times as fast as with the curved needle. The curved needle is useful, nevertheless, in su-

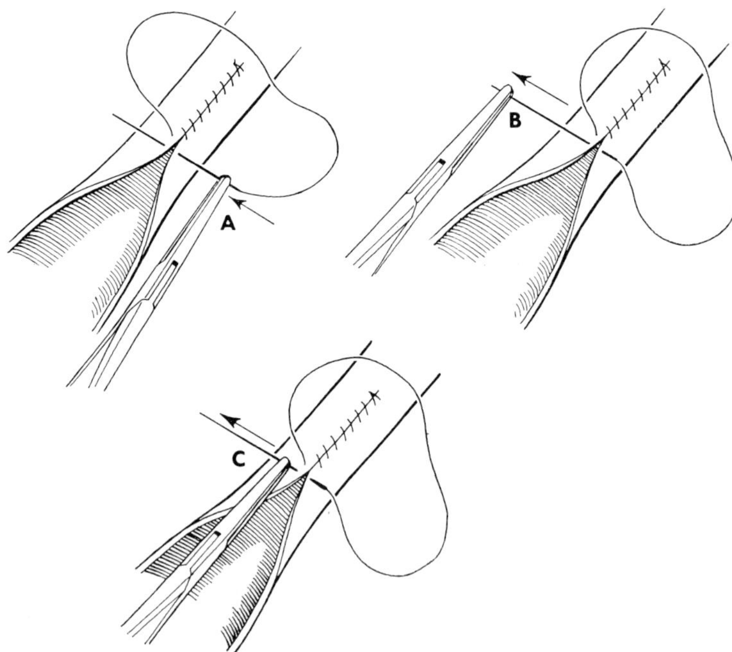

Figure 7–11.   Use of straight needle to close arterial incision.

turing deep recesses of the wound and suturing at the angles of the arteriotomy, especially the final few millimeters.

The suture material depends upon the surgeon's preference; the author uses 5–0 silk Mersilene, coated with Dacron, or polypropylene sutures. Monofilamentous sutures may damage the arterial wall less because of their smoother surface and so may cause less suture bleeding. They are better able to resist infection and, although late brittleness and loss of strength may be a problem they may offer many advantages.

When all but the last few millimiters of the suture line are complete, the catheter stent is withdrawn and the raw medial wall is irrigated with a few milliliters of dilute heparin. Reflux from the distal tree should be prevented by maintaining snug control with the occluding tapes or by reclamping the vessel so that blood will not lie stagnant in the reconstructed segment during the remaining minutes of closure. Before the final sutures are placed it is important to reopen the aortic clamp and flush *freely* for one or two pulse beats to remove all proximal clots. It is well to be sure that there is a moderate level of systemic heparin effect at this moment to inhibit clotting just above the clamp for the time that occlusion must be continued.

The distal clamp should be removed first, not only because this occasions less stress on the suture line, but also because such a test may reveal any major leaks from the reconstructed segment and result in less loss of blood. If any *major* leaks are found, the vessel should be milked free of blood, the distal clamp applied, and the defect carefully closed with a mattress suture. Care must be taken not to impinge on the lumen. The distal clamps may be removed, and if no serious leaks remain, the proximal clamps removed. As full proximal pressure is introduced into the reconstructed area, there will often be leakage at a few points. Intra-arterial pressure will soon adjust tension along the continuous suture line, and most leaks will stop. Even bleeders of considerable size may be controlled by local pressure and application of one of the absorbable sponges, such as Surgicel.

The absorbable sponge may either be removed before the end of the operation or left in place; in a series of experimental procedures conducted by the author,[78] Surgicel could not be identified as a noxious residue on grafts or endarterectomies in canines after 2 weeks.

Gallagher and Geschickter[33] have advocated the use of electrostatically charged gold leaf surgery. Eastman polymeric adhesive is very effective in controlling hemorrhage from lacy suture lines in experimental animals, but the polymers currently available are not suitable for routine use in humans because of the fibrotic response they produce. Powdered dry collagen has been used as an experimental agent for the control of lacerations of the spleen and liver and may be of value here.

Unilateral Iliac Arterial Occlusion

A compromise procedure consisting of anastomosis between the two sides of the arterial tree is often useful. This operation was originally introduced as a means of providing a simpler way of devascularizing an ischemic extremity in a very poor risk patient whose primary disease was occlusion of one iliac system. It can be performed as either a femoral-femoral bypass, which can be done under local anesthesia, or an ilioiliac or iliofemoral bypass, which may require more than local anesthesia but which can with care in thinner patients be done quite expeditiously. It was also introduced as an extra-anatomic bypass to avoid areas of infection within the abdomen. More recently, however,[8, 25, 76] it has been noted that this operation may indeed be the primary choice for revascularization of unilateral iliac disease if there is no significant disease on the donor side above or below the graft. This leaves the abdomen untouched in case later procedures should become necessary. It is a procedure which certainly leaves less in the way of adhesions and fibrosis for a later surgeon than does even a unilateral extraperitoneal endarterectomy.

The length of the graft required is usually a little less than a unilateral aorto-femoral graft. The graft can often be placed so it crosses no groin crease, but it does place a graft in a hazardous area as far as the risk of infection is concerned. Vetto[76] orginally believed that placement of such a graft reduced the risk of progression of the disease in the donor iliac artery above the graft, and this appears to be borne out by the opinions of recent authors.

One of the limitations of this excellent procedure is the failure to recognize a much greater extent of atherosclerosis existing in the aortoiliac segment than had been indicated by x-ray.

The surgical technique is simple. Either oblique femoral incisions are used to expose the femoral artery or a suprainguinal extraperitoneal approach, similar to the classical hernia incision, is used to expose the distal iliac artery. The best choice of material for the graft is probably Dacron of one of the more porous recent introductions. The saphenous vein is usually too small. A bovine carotid heterograft can also be used. The anastomosis is made side-to-end on the donor side and may be made either end-to-side if the recipient iliac artery is open, or end-to-end if the recipient internal iliac artery is thrombosed. A graft may be led across the abdomen in a properitoneal position. The subcutaneous position is much more easily used; however, it is theoretically more easily encroached upon by external pressure and there are apocryphal stories of occlusion of the subcutaneous graft during intercourse.

One should be sure in performing this crossover graft that a differential pressure exists in order to maintain flow through the prosthesis. If one attempts to improve the arterial tree itself on the affected side, and for even a brief period succeeds in restoring flow by removing some of the most recent clot from an atheromatous iliac artery, this may eliminate the gradient between the two sides. Under these circumstances the prosthesis will promptly become obliterated, and in short order the original thrombosis of the iliac system will recur and the patient will be exactly where he was before the operation began. It may even be desirable to obliterate the external iliac artery above the attachment of the graft unless one desires to achieve bidirectional flow, that is, flow both distally into the femoral artery and proximally into the external iliac and internal iliac system.

Axillary femoral bypasses are almost never indicated as primary procedures for pure aortoiliac lesions and will be discussed later in Chapter Ten.

Declamping Hypotension

Sudden removal of the clamps and full restoration of flow into the distal tree is often followed by severe hypotension.[29, 31, 38, 50, 51, 55, 68] Three mechanisms may cause this hypotension.

First and most obvious is the occasional hemorrhage from a leaky suture line (or graft). Correction may require reocclusion, in which case care must be taken to empty the reconstructed segment (or just the graft, if a bypass has been used) to preclude the occurrence of thrombosis that would mean failure of the graft. Minor leaks can be controlled by application of local pressure without reocclusion, but blood loss must be replaced. Accuracy in suturing increases with experience, so that serious blood loss from such a defect occurs less frequently.

The other two mechanisms probably coexist always, but are not so important if complete occlusion has developed before operation, or a stenotic system has been bypassed and flow has been intermittently maintained during placement of the bypass. With this latter maneuver, one avoids a low perfusion pressure and hypoxia of the distal tree during repair.

One source of hypotension is that attributed to "bleeding" into the distal tree. The presumption is that during periods of occlusion, the tone of the vascular bed is reduced as the local intravascular volume is reduced, so that when flow is re-established there is a transient disparity between blood volume and potential capacity of the blood vessels.

To counteract this situation, it has been suggested that sympathectomy not be performed before reconstruction, so as to avoid further reduction in vascular tone. Others have advocated the use of vasopressors, either intra-arterially or locally.[31, 38, 68] These agents are effective in ameliorating hypotension but may transiently decrease total flow. Rader[55] indicates the acidosis in the stagnant area is a significant factor.

The third mechanism was suggested by Malette,[50, 51] who was able to demonstrate the effect of vasodepressor substances by cross-circulation techniques. The production of vasoactive substances is dependent upon a period of hypoxia lasting more than 90 minutes. According to Malette,[50] there is a similarity between these vasoactive substances and bradykinin. Their effect can be counteracted by salicylates, at least experimentally.

No other specific means of counteracting hypotension caused by these substances is available at present. Insofar as the return of these substances to the circulation is brought about by perfusion of the distal tree and flushing of the stagnant capillary blood into the venous system, the same techniques are used that are effective against bleeding into the distal tree: use of a shunt during occlusion;[29] gradual restoration of flow; titration of flow against arterial hypotension; use of vasopressors;[38, 55, 68] and augmentation of systemic blood volume. With the last, overtransfusion can occur and polycythemia may develop along with hypervolemia in patients whose ability to handle hypervolemia may be restricted.

Hypotensive episodes are of greater frequency in aortic and iliac arterial reconstruction than in femoral, but similar problems arise when the site of operation is the leg. The severity of hypoxia (due to less satisfactory collateral circulation)[29] and its duration during prolonged femoral reconstruction may require greater use of vasoactive substances.

If care is taken to prevent hypotensive episodes and overtransfusion, acute renal failure should occur infrequently; as a matter of fact, only one instance of anuria was encountered in our series. Adequate hydration is probably one of the effective means of preventing acute renal failure.[62, 63] Mannitol[54] has been used extensively but its role is probably no more than an obligatory osmotic diuretic that forces urine flow as long as tubular function continues; as such it may have prognostic if not therapeutic value. Ethacrynic acid or furosemide may be of more specific value in protection of the kidneys.[28, 66]

The use of a large amount of banked blood in which citrate has been used as an added coagulant and in which calcium is therefore deficient may result in catastrophic diminution in ventricular function, as Cooper and his associates[18] have demonstrated. Recalcification and heparinization of the blood may prevent this kind of collapse associated with declamping hypotension or any other circumstance requiring massive transfusion; equally effective is the administration of one ml. of 10 per cent calcium chloride for every 100 to 150 ml. of

banked ACD blood administered per minute, given through any venous line except the central venous pressure monitor.

Sometimes when the proximal aortic suture line is completed a
narrow area is created proximal to a dilated area (Fig. 7–12). In this
event, a patch may be inserted to widen the narrow area.

If the vessel at this level appears to be too thin to withstand continued aortic pressure, a sleeve of Dacron may be sutured around the
area, thereby providing not only immediate tamponade for any persistent leaks, but also later structural support.[26]

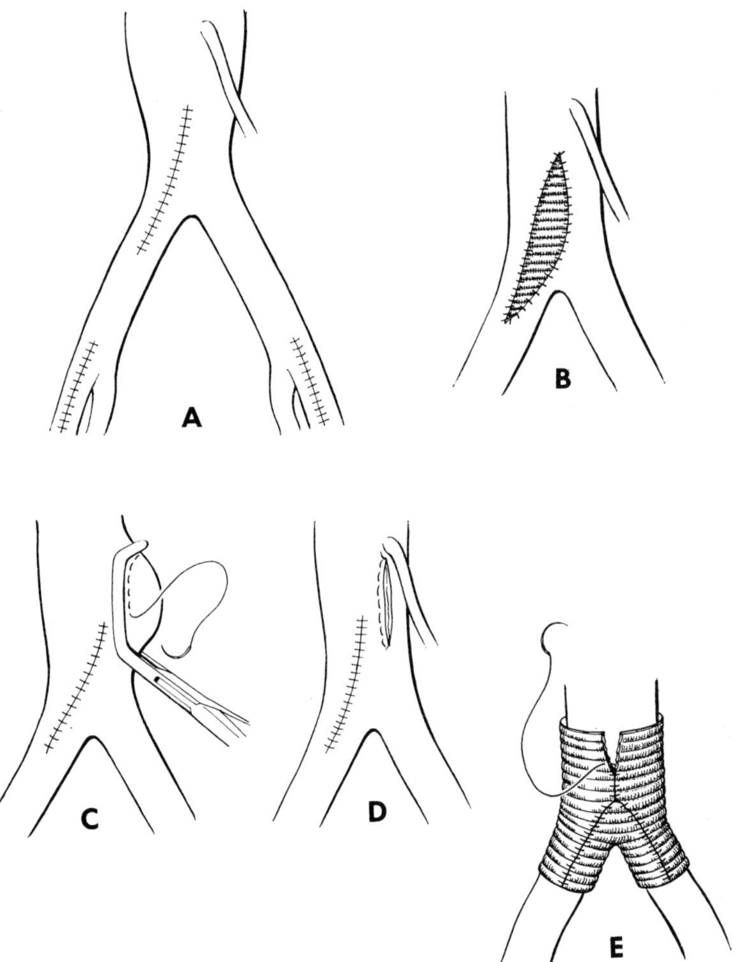

Figure 7–12. Aortotomy with stenotic isthmus after repair. *B,* Repair with patch.
C and *D,* Narrowing of proximal bulge. *E,* Bolster of Dacron sleeve for thin-walled residual vessel. *C* and *D* represent least preferred techniques.

It is highly desirable to be able to make arteriographic studies while the wound is still open in order to be certain that there is no correctable operative error. Arteriography at the time of operation as advocated by Plecha[53] allows one to correct the error immediately. The provision of adequate operative equipment for this procedure is becoming more important for the peripheral vascular surgeon.

When adequacy of flow, propriety of anatomical reconstruction, and hemostasis are assurred, the posterior peritoneum must be carefully closed over the suture lines in the vessels. Aortoenteric fistulas are much more infrequent with endarterectomy than with fabric prostheses[61, 65] but they are a potential hazard even with endarterectomy. Interposition of as much of a peritoneal layer as possible is desirable. Closure of the peritoneum lateral to the sigmoid mesocolon is desirable but not mandatory. It is debatable whether hematoma should be confined to a retroperitoneal site or allowed to drain freely into the peritoneal cavity. Drains to the surface should rarely be used, but suction catheters are preferred to simple drains if drainage is deemed necessary.

Postoperative Management

The prophylactic use of antibiotics is controversial (see page 129). Should sepsis, gangrene, or a break in surgical technique occur, antibiotics should be used during the operation or, if appropriate, preoperatively.[9, 39] The agent should be chosen in terms of the specific bacteriologic risk; when fabric prostheses are used, a broad spectrum antibiotic and one of the synthetic penicillins may be used according to criteria outlined on page 129.

Routine postoperative measures must be employed to treat ileus, which frequently is resistant, to observe for continued bleeding, and to assure proper tracheal toilet.

The use of anticoagulants presents a special problem. The most favorable endarterectomies are performed in a situation of high flow and on a large vessel, but some must be done under less favorable circumstances. If the vessels are small and flow is restricted, an appropriate agent should be used to inhibit the development of red clot on the vessel wall.

It has been demonstrated in canine endarterectomies that the presence of heparin allows prompt endothelization over a thin layer of fibrin and platelets.[5] If red clot develops on this layer, endothelization does not follow until final organization by granulation tissue occurs. During this interval, clotting can occur on such sites of granulation tissue. Later, with maturation of such areas, there may be strictures, webs, and other defects, which have been described by Warren[77] as a cause of late failure in endarterectomy. It seems appropriate, therefore, to prevent accretion of platelet thrombi and later whole red clot.

We have used heparin for this purpose; there have been, however, *few* instances of hemorrhage from the wound in our experience. Others[58] have had greater difficulty than we have, and this difficulty has led to a reassessment of the use of heparin. An analysis of our most recent series of patients has indicated that wound hematomas are just as common without heparin as with it.

There is significant hazard from venous thrombosis that must also be considered, particularly in lengthy operations, in those for correction of stenosis rather than complete occlusion, and in those in which femoral arterial dissection is necessary. In the last instance, the proximity of the femoral vein and the femoral artery as well as the plexus of venous branches around the distal femoral artery plays an important role.

Salzman[58] has suggested that the most important use of heparin is to protect the organism against fibrin formation in areas of stagnant flow. When flow is more rapid and protection is needed against mural accretion of fibrin and platelets, macromolecular dextran has been advocated. Our experience with dextran in humans is limited but has been favorable. We have used approximately 1 unit of dextran per day in the postoperative period which has been given at the time of operation in place of blood replacement. The dual function of volume replacement and platelet inhibition is thus served. There is a potential hazard of hypervolemia developing but in the dose of 1 unit per day for 5 days this does not seem to be likely.

Other antiplatelet drugs such as aspirin, Periactin, Persantin, and Anturane may be effective in controlling the deposition of platelets but they show no significant antilipemic effect.

A potential source of late complication is the atheromatous cicatrix that forms, as well as the formation of atheroma at the point of minor intimal injury where the vessels are cross-clamped. It is conceivable — although it has not been proved — that the lipid clearing effect of heparin may be useful during this postoperative healing period to reduce the amount of atheroma deposited in the scar in the vessel wall. This lipid clearing effect of heparin is quite separate from the anticoagulant effect, and can be achieved by much smaller daily doses. The beneficial role of heparin in protecting against later atherosclerosis is suggested by a study of 12 patients who experienced a late occlusion. Most patients subjected to endarterectomy at the University of California at Los Angeles have received heparin for a week or more. As a rule, only those patients whose reconstruction was most dramatically successful in restoring peripheral flow received small doses of heparin or none at all. There were four patients in whom the clear progression of atherosclerosis in a site not operated upon indicated a continuing susceptibility. The endarterectomized segment remained open in these four patients; three of these patients received full doses of heparin, and one received only limited heparin post-operatively.

There were eight patients whose operated site showed serious reaccumulation of atheroma. Five of these patients had had such a good response initially that *no* heparin had been used, and in three heparin was limited to only a few days' use. Heparinization has not been perfect protection against re-formation of atheroma, but our continuing observations are in close agreement with the course of these 12 patients.

Physical activity is not restricted as long as the reconstructive procedure is limited to the abdomen, but if a suture line or graft crosses the groin or affects the femoral artery, the patient is kept at bed rest for 6 or 7 days.

Patch Graft Closures

Under most circumstances there is little reason to use a patch for simple closure of a longitudinal arteriotomy.[23] With precise technique and utilization of optical magnification, fine closely placed sutures, and an intraluminal stent, closure should not be difficult. Indeed, the use of a patch has been criticized because it is either a biological graft of autologous material and has limited structural strength or, being a plastic fabric, constitutes a foreign body. In any case, only a small patch should be used because of the tendency to form an area of localized dilation that may even progress to become a true aneurysm and become the site of local thrombosis and the source of distal embolization. One may use Laplace's law, which states that tension on the wall is proportional to the product of pressure and the diameter, to explain formation of an aneurysm in this situation. The small fabric patch is well tolerated,[23] being quickly matured by endothelial growth from the edges of the vessel; however, it is unwise to use the patch in areas of flexion. More frequent use of the patch, as opposed to direct closure, probably is merited when other methods of closure are unsatisfactory, and under other specific conditions. Furthermore, the use of a plastic patch carries with it greater hazards if infection occurs than does endarterectomy.

The narrow external iliac artery seen in the Leriche syndrome has been described (Fig. 2–8, p. 18). In a young patient, two goals are important in treatment: restoration of flow, and the correction of any anatomical abnormalities that may have contributed to the premature deposition of atheroma and might therefore predispose the patient to an early recurrence of atheromatous occlusion.

A long patch might be used to widen the external iliac artery as one part of the reconstruction, as a means of reducing the difference in mural tension that exists between the larger common iliac and narrower external iliac artery (Fig. 7–13).

One (hypothetical) way to widen the angle between the two iliac arteries is to insert the prosthesis so that it lowers and widens the angle of the bifurcation (Fig. 7–14A, B). Removal of a segment of common iliac artery might be necessary. Two or four circular suture lines would be needed, and the method seems unwarranted under most circumstances.

In a minor restorative procedure (Fig. 7–3E) an inverted V-shaped patch widens the common iliac arms and lowers the bifurcation somewhat.

The most reasonable reconstruction is probably the one in which a Dacron fabric bifurcation prosthesis is placed to restore anatomy to the most favorable condition possible (Fig. 7–14C). It is unfortunate that technical reasons currently preclude the manufacture of a Dacron graft with proper hemodynamic characteristics, although Buxton has recently introduced a graft which has an improved aortoiliac relationship.[10, 11]

BYPASS PROCEDURES

Choice of Operation

Under certain circumstances placement of an arterial prosthesis (usually as a bypass) may be desirable. The indications for this procedure are as follows:

1. When the patient's *general* condition demands a shorter opera-

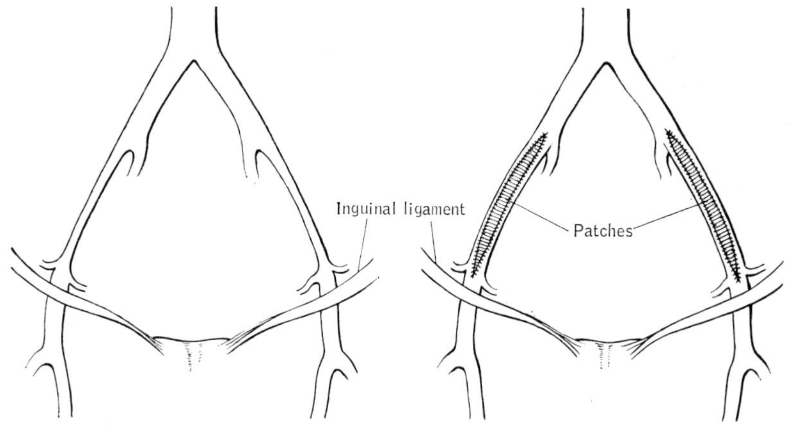

Figure 7–13.   Patch closure to widen narrow external iliac artery.

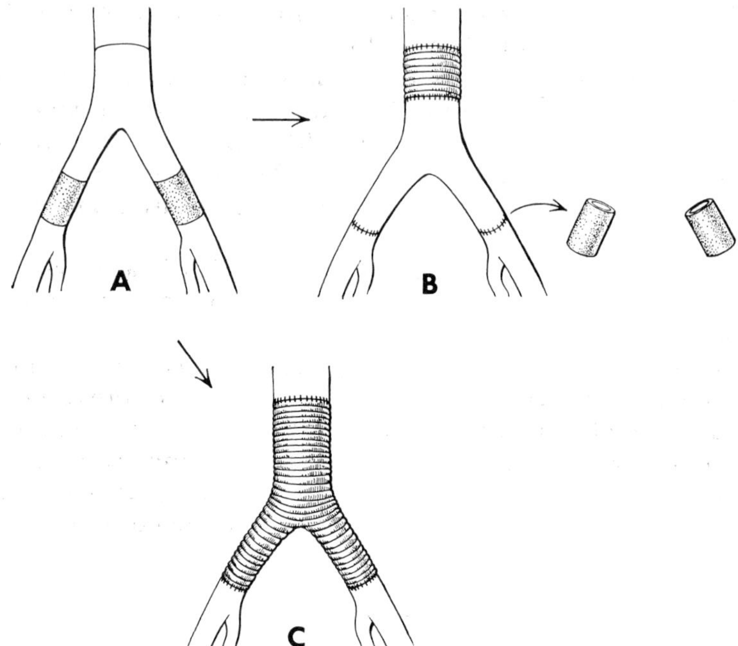

Figure 7–14. A and B, Modification of aortic bifurcation by interposition of proximal tube C, by replacement with Dacron bifurcation.

tive procedure than endarterectomy. The surgeon's experience may govern this choice.

2. When *local* conditions make endarterectomy impractical, such as the presence of an aneurysm in the terminal aorta or the iliac arteries, fragility of the wall following endarterectomy, inadvertent trauma such as to destroy the integrity of the wall, or the extreme narrowing described on pages 18 and 157.

3. When reconstruction is necessary to form a more favorable anatomical and mechanical situation.

The ease with which many well-trained surgeons can learn to place a graft has increased the popularity of this procedure at the expense of endarterectomy. Where conditions are favorable for endarterectomy, and if the surgeon is trained to do this operation, it remains the procedure of choice.

Exposure

It may be possible to make the decision to do the bypass procedure instead of endarterectomy before the retroperitoneal area is fully exposed. In this case, dissection may be limited to an incision at the root of the mesentery that exposes the terminal aorta only. From this site a tunnel can be developed retroperitoneally to the site of distal attachment of the prosthesis, whether it is in the external iliac or in the femoral artery distal to the inguinal ligament. The prosthesis should usually pass under the ureter, and a sufficient length of ureter must be mobilized to allow it to cross the prosthesis without tension, so as to avoid both obstruction and necrosis of the ureter. This situation must be individualized, for in some circumstances the anatomical relationships dictate placement of the graft *over* the ureter, just so long as in this position the ureter is not compressed. Such a circumstance occurs when the common iliac bifurcation dips into the pelvis and the three iliac arteries form a "Y" through which the ureter passes.

Technique

If sympathectomy has not been done, it should be performed as described on page 134.

The aorta may be completely or partially occluded during the anastomosis. Although complete occlusion makes anastomosis easier, more dissection is required, including that necessary to control the lumbar vessels. Partial occlusion with a curved clamp not only obviates such dissection but also interferes less with distal perfusion during the brief period of placement of the prosthesis (Fig. 7–15), if either

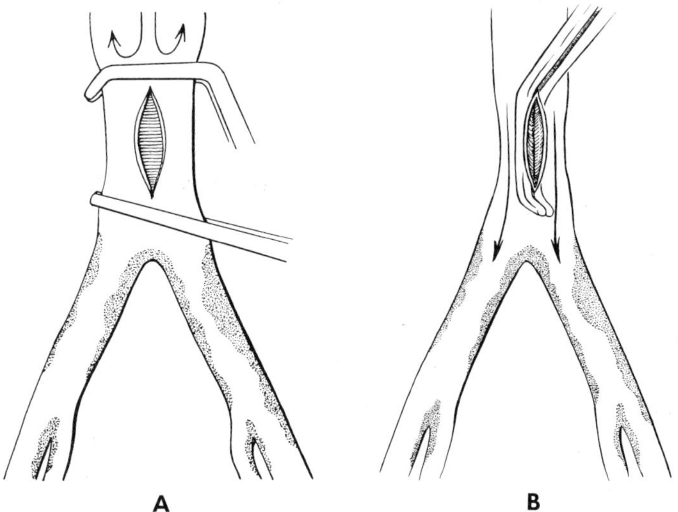

A   **B**

Figure 7–15. A, Cross-clamping of aorta interrupts iliac flow completely. B, Partial occlusion clamp makes arterial repair more difficult but allows flow to continue down iliac arteries. The arteriotomy should be placed anteriorly as in A.

iliac artery is not completely occluded. Such occlusion may be of little consequence in regard to viability of the limb; however, when a partially occluded vessel is cross-clamped temporarily, the distal vascular bed becomes hypoxic and hypovolemic, and a hypotensive crisis may follow removal of the cross-clamps and restoration of circulation. In brittle diabetics, in whom the hazard from such hypotension is greatest, bypass grafting is the safest procedure. Partial occlusion techniques should reduce the hazard of distal ischemia and hypotension following declamping.[29]

Because of better flow characteristics and a lesser risk of aortoduodenal fistulization, it may be desirable in the presence of complete aortic occlusion to resect a portion of the infrarenal aorta and to perform an end-to-end anastomosis between the aorta and the prosthesis. If one follows this procedure it may become necessary to perform an endarterectomy on the aorta between the renal arteries and the level of the anastomosis.

Choice of Material for the Prosthesis

Although the choice of prosthesis is governed by personal preference, certain factors must always be considered.

Porosity. Wesolowski[79, 80] has demonstrated that ultimate healing of the prosthesis, with provision of the most secure lining, depends on maximal porosity during final healing. Initial porosity, however, may occasion undue bleeding at operation. Composite prostheses having an initial low porosity and a later high biological porosity have been proposed but have not yet proved themselves.

TYPES. Teflon has the advantage of great strength which is unaffected by passage of time, absorption of water, or dissipation of plasticizers. It has been difficult to extrude Teflon in fibers sufficiently fine to make a knitted fabric. When woven tightly in order to prevent undue bleeding at operation it lacks necessary biological porosity.[22] The knitted fabric prostheses made of teflon may have the advantages of strength and durability, which make up for less satisfactory incorporation in the body.

Dacron prostheses are either woven or knitted.[13, 15, 48, 55, 56] The chief advantages of knitted ones are their resistance to fraying and their high degree of biological porosity; some, however, are difficult to handle because of their bulk.

Sauvage has advocated a Dacron graft coated externally with velour, and reports a better rate and degree of endothelialization because of presumed better ingrowth of fibroblasts.[59] Buxton has used a Dacron graft lined with velour, and reports similar good results.[11] A combination of internal and external velour may be the most satisfactory graft, but technological problems have delayed its introduction.

A certain amount of elasticity is desirable in a graft. Szilagyi[69] has used Helanca and certain other yarns which are easy to handle and are not bulky. Raveling can be avoided by sealing the cut edge with a hot cautery or treating the edge *after* preclotting with an electrocautery unit of the Bovie type. When a prosthesis of this material is placed so that the ends are cut perpendicularly to its long axis, the ends may be turned back like cuffs to further reduce the possibility of fraying.

Other woven prostheses are crimped to produce elasticity and prevent kinking during placement, but none maintains this elasticity after healing and infiltration with granulation. One cause of late failure of prostheses has been kinking and dislodgment of the lining when flexion of the tube occurs (Figs. 8–5 and 8–6). This is most marked at the knee but also occurs at the groin. Only biological grafts such as vein grafts can resist the kinking. Endarterectomized segments also have this attribute of flexibility.

Wesolowski,[79, 80] Krippaehne,[44] and Cannon,[12] among others, have advocated the use of a compound prosthesis composed of a basic plastic fiber and a filler of collagen fiber which is ultimately absorbed and replaced by endogenous scar.

According to Szilagyi,[73] the appropriate size of a tube graft should usually be 1.0 to 1.3 times the diameter of the vessels.

As indicated in Chapter Three, the ideal bifurcation should have a ratio of 1.414 to 1 between the cross sectional area of the two iliac limbs of the graft and the aorta. Most grafts in current use have a ratio of 1 to 2, although Buxton has advocated a graft with a ratio of 1 to 1.5.[10, 11]

Clamps used to occlude vascular grafts should be padded or shod with rubber; toothed or ridged clamps may injure the fabric and cause bleeding.

Suture Material

Any nonabsorbable suture material will suffice, but the primary requisites are bulk to reduce the risk of cutting through the host vessel and a needle that will easily penetrate plaques at the operative site which are often dense. Silk, Mersilene (Dacron), Mersilene coated with Teflon, linear polyethylene or polypropylene are all satisfactory. Stoney and Wylie[67] report that broken silk sutures have been instrumental in the development of false aneurysms at the anastomotic site. The use of monofilamentous sutures may be associated with less bleeding through the suture holes.

Although very fine suture material has wide application in vascular surgery, aortic anastomosis is often best accomplished with 3-0 or 4-0 suture, which has less tendency to cut through the wall. Larger bites than are generally used not only help to maintain union of the fabric and the vessel until healing has occurred, but also are likely to reduce bleeding from the suture line. Most vascular surgeons early in their experience have encountered false aneurysms developing from the vessel-graft suture line.[67] Generally, they may be attributed to local leakage, with formation of a pulsating hematoma and false aneurysm, or to inadequate suturing (see p. 168).

Placement

Resection of the infrarenal aorta and the bifurcation, followed by end-to-end replacement (Fig. 7–14) is usually unnecessary although it may be desirable if there is aneurysmal dilatation of the distal vessel, and incomplete occlusion. The procedure is comparable to the placement of the prosthesis for an aortic aneurysm. The use of the bypass principle as originally advocated by Kunlin[45] and popularized by Linton,[24, 48, 49] by Crawford and DeBakey,[21] and by others is a simpler procedure. It should be noted that there is a small but definite risk in resecting the infrarenal aorta if there is any flow through it, because of the risk of possible encroachment on the anterior spinal arteries.[36] The risk must be accepted in removal of the aortic aneurysm but when performed for partial occlusive disease of the aorta it may be hazardous.

Szilagyi[73] has shown that if the graft is placed at an angle of about 30 degrees to the distal limb of the vessel, flow is virtually unimpeded through the stoma. This angle of placement protrudes less and consequently there may be less possibility of an aortoenteric fistula developing. The ascending limb of the duodenum overlies the prosthesis and becomes adherent to it. In order to reduce the risk of aortoenteric fistula, one should attach the prosthesis at a narrow angle and should interpose flaps of retroperitoneal tissue between fabric and duodenum.[65] A segment of omentum may be mobilized and sutured in place over the fabric graft if retroperitoneal tissue is unavailable. One should take care to be sure no aperture exists through which small bowel may prolapse and become obstructed. Graft exposed in the peritoneal cavity *may* heal, but it may also mature slowly, and graft adherence and fistula formation may supervene.

Incision into the aortic wall is done with a knife, then extended with Satinsky scissors. It is best to excise a window from the anterior wall of the vessel. Local endarterectomy may be necessary to remove thickened plaques, especially when such calcified plaques interfere with the placement of sutures. If redundant intima is present, it should be trimmed back. It is often desirable to suture the loosened intima to the media[3] to assure a smooth suture line (Fig. 7–16).

The suture line is usually begun proximally; double armed suture with a curved needle is convenient. Figure-of-eight matress sutures

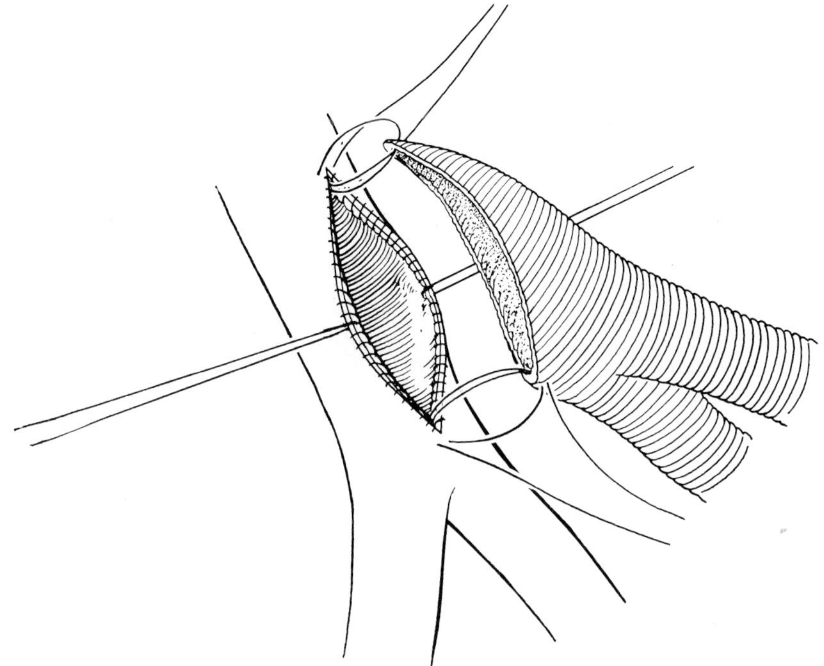

Figure 7–16. Bypass graft secured with four stay sutures, and with running suture securing ragged intima to media for more satisfactory suture line.

secure the opposed ends of the stoma of graft to the appropriate site in the aorta. Other stay sutures centered so as to convert the suture lines into quadrants facilitate matching the segment of prosthesis and host vessel and avoid inadvertently catching the opposite side of the anastomosis with a suture. This procedure is an extension of the Carrel technique.

As a rule, the attachment of the prosthesis can be satisfactorily performed as described above. At other times, when thick but friable plaques are present in the wall, or when the vessel wall has been rendered fragile by local endarterectomy into deeper layers than usual, it is possible to encircle the aorta with a sling of the prosthetic fabric.[26] The edges of the vessel are sutured to the folded edge of the prosthesis (Fig. 7–17) and the sling is passed behind the aorta and sutured to the sling from the opposite side. The folded edge can be sutured in this way as is done with a cuffed prosthesis. The sling not only helps keep the attachment secure, but also acts as a tamponade on the suture line. If a lumbar vessel interferes with placement of the sling, a slit may be made in the sling to accommodate the vessel. These additions should rarely be necessary, but may be vital at times.

As soon as the aortic suture line is completed, the clamps should be removed so as to restore flow through the stenotic aorta and iliac ar-

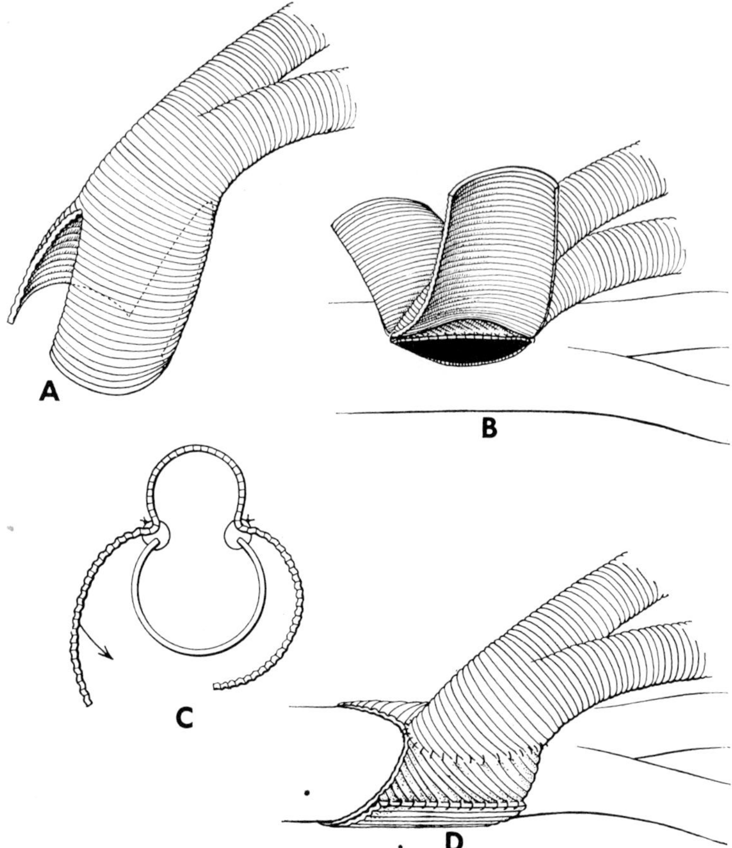

Figure 7–17.   Oblique bypass graft is secured with extra flaps of Dacron that allow graft to hold aorta as a "sling." A, Cutting of graft. B, Attachment. C, Cross section of anastomosis. D, Sling wrapped around aorta at completion of anastomosis.

teries (Fig. 7–18). The clamps are immediately reapplied to the prosthesis after one or two pulse beats to flush any clots from behind the clamps out through the open graft. Bleeding from the suture line can be controlled by temporary tamponade, by additional suturing, or by use of one of the absorbable sponges.

Selection of the site for implantation of the iliac limb of the prosthesis depends on several factors. First, the distal implantation must be beyond any area of major obstruction in the iliac or femoral system. It may be necessary to carry the prosthesis under the inguinal ligament and implant it in the common femoral artery. Second, the shorter the bypass the better, so long as the qualification just mentioned is met. Third, it is preferable to keep the prosthesis entirely within the abdomen.[24, 67] A prosthesis that extends past the fold of the groin is

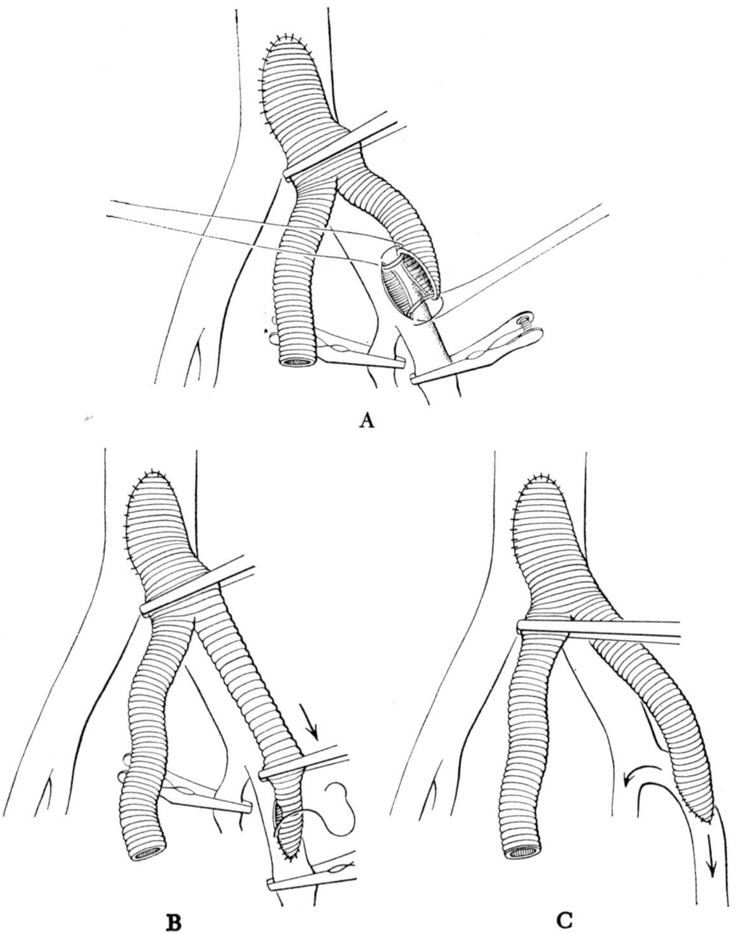

Figure 7–18.   A, Restoration of flow down arms of graft. Clamps are first placed as shown in A, and flow continues down right iliac system if there is any channel remaining. When first iliac suture line is complete (left, in figure), distal bulldog clamps are released and backflow from distal (left) iliofemoral system is assured. These lower clamps should be replaced and left iliac arm cleared of all blood. Right arm should be cross-clamped and proximal cross-clamp moved to the most proximal position on left arm; right arm is then flushed by removing distal occluding clamp temporarily. to blow any clots in region of upper anastomosis out of right arm. Right arm is then reclamped, distal clamps are removed from the iliac vessels, and the proximal clamp is removed from the left arm of the graft to restore flow as quickly as possible into the left limb. The clamp on the aortic portion of the graft must be as near the aortic suture line as possible, preferably higher than is shown here.

B, Graft being placed into external iliac artery under tension. When clamps are removed and flow is restored C, anastomosis pulls the external iliac artery up so that flow is directed both ways, into internal iliac system as well as femoral system. B and C show the attachment of the graft to a slightly more distal site than does A.

subject to flexion, with its attendant hazards, and as pointed out by Darling and Linton[24] this has greatly reduced late success in patency.

To provide a more flexible graft across the bend of the groin, Wylie[67, 82] has advocated the use of an autologous artery. The source of the artery may be the external or common iliac artery which has been resected and endarterectomized, or an occluded superficial femoral artery which has been treated similarly. Autologous saphenous vein (Fig. 7–19) can also be used for this purpose.

Stoney's figures[67] indicate that false aneurysms following femoral end-to-end anastomosis develop far less frequently, but, of course, ligation of the proximal end of the femoral artery and end-to-end anastomosis of the prosthesis with the distal femoral artery removes the source of reflux into the external and internal iliac arteries.

Gaspar[35] has advocated temporarily placing the graft under extreme tension, dividing the external iliac artery carrying the graft under the inguinal ligament, and thus performing the anastomosis easily under adequate exposure in the groin. When the anastomosis is completed the elastic prosthesis will withdraw to the peritoneal area above the inguinal ligament. End-to-end anastomosis was suggested for this procedure, but it can be performed end to side after dividing the external iliac proximally in order to allow it to reach below the ligament. After the graft to host anastomosis has been completed, the cut ends of the proximal external iliac artery can be reanastomosed to assure reflux into the hypogastric bed (Fig. 19–3). Connolly has advocated removing entire arterial segments from the body in order to perform "bench" endarterectomy.[17]

These measures have been described as alternate maneuvers to avoid attaching the prosthesis in the common femoral artery, because of the reported increase in rate of failure, when such a prosthesis crosses the groin. In spite of these factors, other circumstances may at times make it necessary to attach the prosthesis directly to the femoral artery. Further explanations for the dissatisfaction with the anastomosis to the femoral artery should be considered. Three local factors function to make this anastomosis an unsatisfactory one. First, the pointed toe of the fabric graft tends to fray and must be handled with care. Second, there is continued tension on the suture line because of the movement of the hip. Stoney and Wylie[67] consider this factor most important in the genesis of aneurysms at this site. Third, to secure the toe of the prosthesis, the surgeon may unwittingly place sutures that reduce the circumference of the artery (Fig. 7–20A). Taylor[74] and Lazzarini-Robertson[46] suggest the use of a square-toed graft in a T-shaped incision (Fig. 7–20B). This shape approximates the shape of the venous graft as Kunlin[45] and Linton[48, 49] originally described cutting it. This configuration allows the surgeon to place several sutures in the toe of the graft which provide a mechanical advantage because they

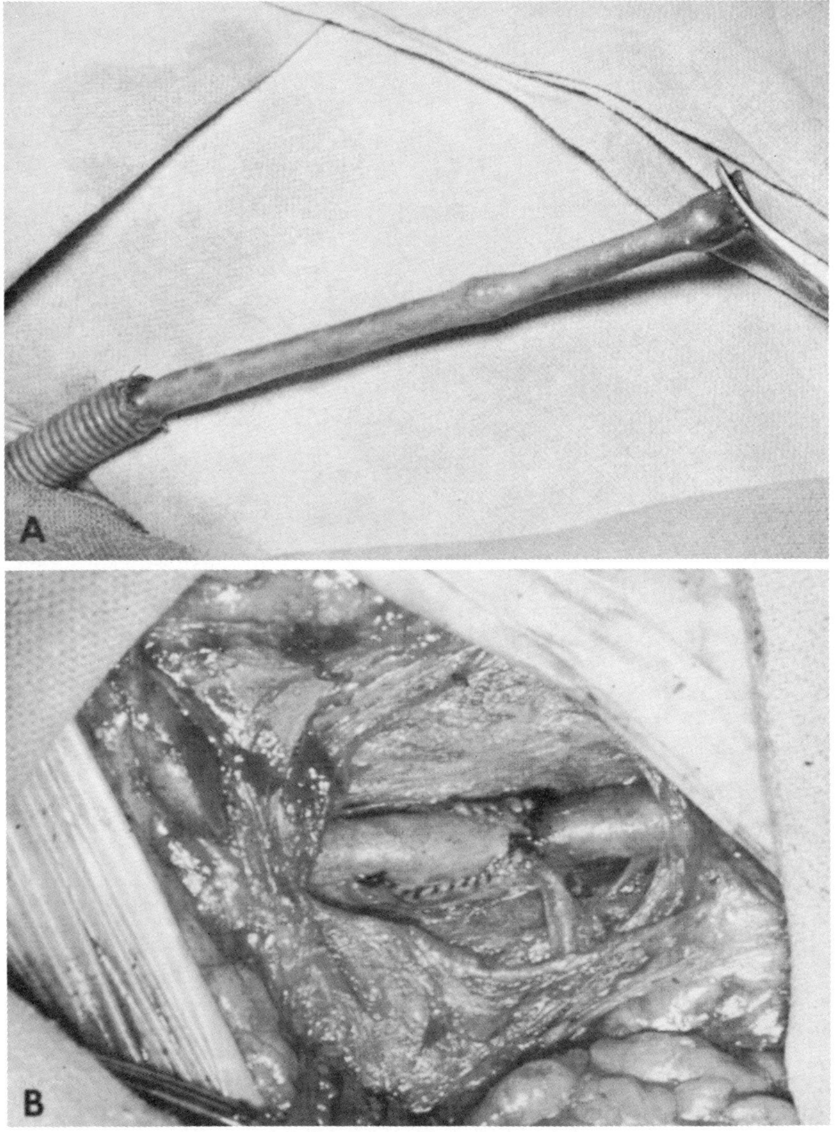

Figure 7–19. *A*, Saphenous vein graft has been attached end-to-end to a segment of Dacron in order to cross the groin. The vein is not yet distended to match the diameter of the fabric prosthesis. *B*, Attachment of the bell-shaped vein graft into a T-shaped arteriotomy.

are parallel to the axis of the artery and along the line of tension. For added security a flap of graft can be left beyond the tip of the toe and secured to the artery (Fig. 19–4). This procedure is rarely necessary, but is useful if the artery is dangerously thin walled.

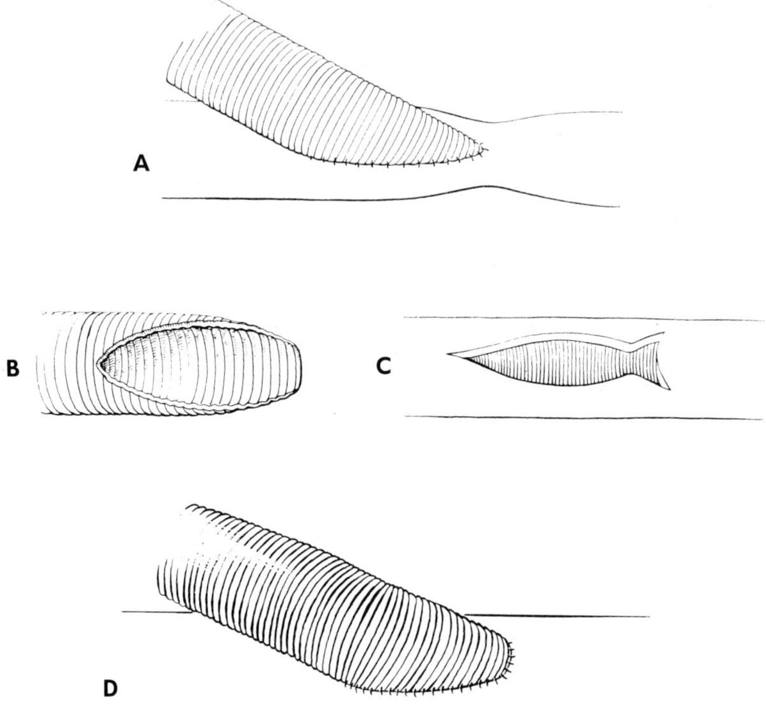

Figure 7–20.   *A*, Stenosis in the host artery at the tip of the plastic prosthesis because of unnecessarily wide bites at the tip of the prosthesis. *B*, Square-cut prosthesis or graft. *C*, T-shaped arteriotomy. *D*, Proper prosthesis–host relationship without stenosis.

Another complication that may develop with a prosthesis placed in the groin is infection. The anastomotic site lies under skin which is particularly hard to disinfect. The groin is rich in lymphatics which, even when not infected, encourage the collection of fluid, and consequently the development of secondary infection. Furthermore, the anastomotic site is superficial and only skin is present as a protective covering. The sartorius muscle may be mobilized to cover the graft as is commonly done in a radical groin dissection. Szilagyi[71] has described the groin as the commonest site from which dangerous wound infections develop, and suggests prophylactic antibiotics against the organism Staphylococcus aureus.

The most proximal site in which one can place the iliac limb of the graft is the distal portion of the common iliac artery. Anastomosis is done just as in proximal anastomosis, although it is best to cross-clamp all three vessels. Insertion of the toe of the graft widens the orifice of the external iliac artery thereby assuring direct flow into the hypogastric bed (Fig. 7–18A). More commonly, the graft is placed in the external iliac artery. In this position the end-to-side (T) anastomosis resembles an inverted Y (Fig. 7–18C). The proximal arm of the Y allows for hypogastric perfusion and the distal arm allows for femoral perfusion. Flexion of the hip joint does not cause any significant movement of the graft.

The external iliac artery is usually less affected by arteriosclerosis than other arteries. If extensive plaques are present, local endarterectomy may be done, provided the usual safeguards are observed and no intimal flap remains that may turn up into the bloodstream.

If plaques occur in only one part of the circumference, an unaffected portion may often be chosen, the vessel being rotated so that anastomosis may be done in the healthy portion of the vessel.

When the iliac limb must be placed in the femoral artery, the tunnel is made by blunt dissection from the abdominal side along the medial and superior aspect of the course of the external iliac artery. It is easy to let the tunnel remain too tight at the level of the ligament—actually from the ilopectineal line past the lacunar ligament. The finger may be forced through this relatively rigid portion of the tunnel without establishing enough space to ensure that there will be no encroachment on the prosthesis. Enlargement of the tunnel beyond that obtainable by blunt dissection is necessary, and this can be done by incising the edge of the lacunar ligament or the undersurface of the inguinal ligament. It should be done under direct vision in order to avoid damaging major collaterals, such as the inferior epigastric artery, or an aberrant obturator artery arising from the femoral artery.

A word should be said regarding restoration of flow through the graft and correct sequence in flushing. On page 164, we mentioned that cross-clamps should be removed from the aorta and placed on the proximal portion of the prosthesis as close to the aorta as possible. Immediately after cross-clamping the prosthesis, all blood should be sucked out of the distal portion, using saline irrigation if necessary. Clot left in the prosthesis for even a few moments may increase the hazard of occlusion of the reconstruction.

Restoration of flow should be to the side having less involvement, for that side has less satisfactory collaterals and can tolerate occlusion for a shorter period than the more seriously affected side.

When only 5 to 7 mm. of the first distal suture line remain to be closed, the clamps should be removed distally to be sure that there is backflow. Pressure is exerted on the thigh to milk back any clots and assure flow from the femoral system. If there is any possibility that fresh clot remains in the major vascular tree, a Fogarty catheter should be passed down the vessel as far as possible, the balloon inflated and withdrawn.[30] Arteriography may be used as further diagnostic evaluation if prior arteriography had not adequately shown the extent of atheroma in the distal tree, and if the possibility of atheromatous as well as thrombotic occlusion in the distal tree must be considered. Distal irrigation with dilute solution of heparin (10 units per ml.) may diminish the chance of further deposition of clot at this time.

If there is retrograde flow, the clamp should be applied to the distal vessel and the suture line completed. The proximal limb of the graft on the side already anastomosed should now be occluded and free flow developed from the untreated limb so as to force out clots that have developed in the short cul de sac between aorta and clamp. The aorta may then be reoccluded and the distal clamps on the anastomotic side removed in order to fill the prosthesis with blood. As soon as the graft is filled, the clamp on the aortic end of the prosthesis is opened and flow established, while the opposite unanastomosed arm is occluded at the most proximal level possible. As indicated in the legend of Figure 7–18, graded restoration of flow down first, the internal iliac and then the external iliac systems not only may reduce the severity of declamping hypotension but also may divert any loose bits of clot or atheromatous debris into the internal iliac system, where they will be less likely to cause harm than they would in the external iliac system.[42] The blood is then sucked out of this arm, and the second side is now sutured in place. Immediately prior to final closure, distal flow is checked as described, then distal clamps are reapplied so as to prevent additional blood from flowing back into the graft. Closure is completed, the distal clamps are removed, and the graft is filled with blood. Only then should the proximal clamp on the iliac limb be released.

To recapitulate:

1. Use no vascular clamps on the Dacron prosthesis; simple Satinsky clamps or rubber-shod vascular clamps will occlude it without damaging it.

2. Stagnant blood should not be allowed to remain in the graft any longer than absolutely necessary, and this should be only seconds.

3. Distal clamps should be removed first to force air out of the prosthesis without putting undue pressure on either suture line.

Postoperative Management

As a rule, anticoagulants are unnecessary postoperatively. Rarely will they maintain patency in a graft which would have failed otherwise. It has been suggested, however,[37] that protracted use of antiprothrombin agents might assist in the formation of a thin, firmly attached, and well matured lining in fabric prosthesis. This protection is afforded by preventing the late deposition of fibrin clot. As mentioned, however, there may be less likelihood of atheroma formation in the cicatrix if the patient continues to receive heparin in doses large enough to clear the serum of lipids.

In contrast to our usual practice with endarterectomy, when fabric prostheses are used, prophylactic antibiotics are usually prescribed for a week or more. If contamination of the prosthesis has occurred, antibiotics should be administered locally through catheters placed down to the prosthesis.[16, 75]

Any area of reconstruction, whether done with a prosthesis or by endarterectomy, that crosses a joint is subject to abnormal stress; movement should be prevented until a measure of fibroplasia has occurred. Whereas early ambulation is desirable in purely aortoiliac reconstructive operation, any reconstructive procedure that extends into the femoral artery should be followed by 5 or 6 days of inactivity, with proscription of ambulation.

In general, reconstruction of the aortic and iliac arteries, although fraught with hazards in the absence of necessary precautions, has become an accepted operation. In the hands of an experienced surgeon the mortality and morbidity rates are very low, and there is a high rate of successful restoration of flow.

REFERENCES

1. Barcroft, H., and Swan, H. J. C.: *Sympathetic Control of Human Blood Vessels.* London, E. Arnold, 1953.
2. Barker, W. F. (Ed.): *Surgical Treatment of Peripheral Vascular Disease.* New York, McGraw-Hill Book Co., Inc., 1962.
3. Barker, W. F.: Lateral arterial anastomosis: a point of technique. Angiology *10*:90, 1959.
4. Barker, W. F., and Cannon, J. A.: Technique of endarterectomy. Am. Surgeon *25*:912, 1959.
5. Barker, W. F., Cannon, J. A., Zeldis, L. J., and Ah'Tye, P.: Anatomical results of endarterectomy. Surg. Forum *6*:266, 1955.
6. Berger, K., Sauvage, L. R., Rao, A. M., and Wood, S. J.: Healing of arterial prostheses in man. Its incompleteness. Ann. Surg. *175*:118, 1972.
7. Blodgett, J. B., and Viguri, J. J.: Bifurcation angioplasty to extend the usefulness of endarterectomy. Surgery *56*:361, 1964.
8. Brief, D. K., Alpert, J., and Parsonnet, V.: Crossover femoral-femoral grafts: Compromise or preference: a reappraisal. Arch. Surg. *105*:880–919, 1972.
9. Burke, J. F.: The effective period of preventive antibiotic action in experimental incisions and dermal lesions. Surgery *50*:161, 1961.
10. Buxton, B. F., Wukasch, D. C., and Cooley, D. A.: The dimensions of the aortoiliofemoral arterial segment. Austral. New Zeal. J. Surg. *42*:204, 1972.
11. Buxton, B. F., Wukasch, D. C., Martin, C., Liebig, W. J., Hallman, G. L., and Cooley, D. A.: Practical considerations in fabric vascular grafts. Introduction of a new bifurcated graft. Am. J. Surg. *125*:288, 1973.
12. Cannon, J. A.: Discussion of paper by Krippaehne, W. W., Deshpande, P. J., Jackson, D. S., and Dunphy, J. E.: Reaction of connective tissue to collagen-dacron prostheses: an experimental study. Am. J. Surg. *110*:186, 1965.
13. Cannon, J. A.: *A Current Technique of Aortoiliac and Femoropopliteal Endarterectomy for Obliterative Atherosclerosis.* Springfield, Ill., Charles C Thomas, 1965.

14. Cannon, J. A., and Barker, W. F.: Successful management of obstructive femoral arteriosclerosis by endarterectomy. Surgery 38:48, 1955.
15. Cannon, J. A., Kawakami, I. G., and Barker, W. F.: Present status of aortoiliac endarterectomy for obliterative atherosclerosis. Arch. Surg. 82:813, 1961.
16. Carter, S. C., Cohen, A., and Whelan, T. J.: Clinical experience with management of the infected dacron graft. Ann. Surg. 158:249, 1963.
17. Connolly, J. E., and Stemmer, E. A.: Simplified technique of eversion endarterectomy for aorto-ilio-femoral occlusive disease. Arch. Surg. 105:520, 1972.
18. Cooper, N., Brazier, J., Hottenrott, C., Mulder, D. G., Maloney, J. V., and Buckberg, G. D.: Myocardial depression following citrated blood transfusion — an avoidable complication. Arch. Surg. 107:756, 1973.
19. Cranley, J. J.: Discussion of paper by Schenk, W. G., Jr., Delin, N. A., Domanig, E., Hahnloser, P., and Hoyt, R. K.: Blood viscosity as a determinant of regional blood flow. Arch. Surg. 89:783, 1964.
20. Cranley, J. J., Fogarty, T. J., Krause, R. J., Strasser, E. S., and Hafner, C. D.: Phlebotomy for moderate erythrocythemia. J.A.M.A. 186:206, 1963.
21. Crawford, E. S., and DeBakey, M. E.: The by-pass operation in the treatment of arteriosclerotic occlusive disease of the lower extremities. Surg. Gynec. Obstet. 101:529, 1955.
22. Creech, O.: In Barker, W. F. (Ed.): *Surgical Treatment of Peripheral Vascular Disease.* New York, McGraw-Hill Book Co., Inc., 1962.
23. Dale, W. A., and Lewis, M. R.: Lateral vascular patch grafts. Surgery 57:36, 1965.
24. Darling, R. C., and Linton, R. R.: Management of the late failure of arterial reconstruction of the lower extremities. New Eng. J. Med. 270:609, 1964.
25. Davis, R. C., O'Hara, E. T., Mannick, J. A., Vollman, R. W., and Nabseth, D. C.: Broadened indications for femoral-femoral grafts. Surgery 72:990, 1972.
26. Derrick, J. R.: A technique of attaching a synthetic graft to the side of a severely arteriosclerotic aorta. Surgery 50:782, 1961.
27. Edwards, W. S.: Composite reconstruction of small leg arteries after endarterectomy. Surgery 51:58, 1962.
28. Eng, K., and Stahl, W. M.: Correction of the renal hemodynamic changes produced by surgical trauma. Ann. Surg. 174:19–23, 1971.
29. Engler, H. S., Ellison, L. T., Moretz, W. H., Simpson, J. G., Gleaton, H. E., and Freeman, R. A.: Shock following release of aortic cross-clamping. Arch. Surg. 86:791, 1963.
30. Fogarty, T. J., Cranley, J. J., Krause, R. J., Strasser, E. S., and Hafner, C. D.: A method for extraction of arterial emboli and thrombi. Surg. Gynec. Obstet. 116:241, 1963.
31. Fry, W. J., Keitzer, W. F., Kraft, R. O., and DeWeese, M. S.: Prevention of hypotension due to aortic release. Surg. Gynec. Obstet. 116:301, 1963.
32. Fulton, R. L., and Blakeley, W. R.: Lumbar sympathectomy: A procedure of questionable value in the treatment of arteriosclerosis obliterans of the legs. Am. J. Surg. 116:735, 1968.
33. Gallagher, J. P., and Geschickter, F.: The use of charged gold leaf in surgery. J.A.M.A. 189:928, 1964.
34. Gaspar, M., Discussion of paper by Wylie, E. J., Binkley, F. M., and Albo, R. J.: Femoropopliteal endarterectomy. Am. J. Surg. 108:215, 1964.
35. Gaspar, M., Discussion of paper by Stoney, R. J., and Wylie, E. J.: False aneurysm after arterial grafting. Am. J. Surg. 110:153, 1965.
36. Golden, G. T., Sears, H. F., Wellons, H. A., Jr., and Muller, W. H., Jr.: Paraplegia complicating resection of aneurysms of the infrarenal abdominal aorta. Surgery 73:91, 1973.
37. Hamming, J. J.: Vascular prostheses and anticoagulant therapy. J. Cardiov. Surg. 4:681, 1963.
38. Hohf, R. P., and Sutton, G. C.: The experimental use of a vasopressor at the end of temporary aortic occlusion. Surg. Gynec. Obstet. 110:693, 1960.
39. Howard, J. M.: Postoperative wound infections. The influence of ultraviolet irradiation of the operating room and of various other factors. Ann. Surg. (Supplement) 160:1, 1964.
40. Humpert, E. L., Quinn, E. L., Dienst, S. G., and Szilagyi, D. E.: Infection of the

well-incorporated Dacron graft caused by septicemia. Surg. Forum 23:234, 1972.

41. Imparato, A.: Personal communication.

42. Imparato, A. M., Berman, I. R., Bracco, A., Kim, G. E., and Beaudet, R.: Avoidance of shock and peripheral embolism during surgery of the abdominal aorta. Surgery 73:68, 1973.

43. Inahara, T.: Endarterectomy for occlusive disease at the aorto, iliac and common femoral arteries. Evaluation of results of the eversion technique endarterectomy. Am. J. Surg. 124:235, 1972.

44. Krippaehne, W. W., Deshpande, P. J., Jackson, D. S., and Dunphy, J. E.: Collagen-dacron prostheses: an experimental study. Am. J. Surg. 110:186, 1965.

45. Kunlin, J.: Le traitement de l'ischémie artéritique par la greffe veineuse longue. Rev. chir. Paris 70:206, 1951.

46. Lazarrini-Robertson, A. A., Jr.: Hemodynamic principles and end-to-side vascular anastomoses. Arch. Surg. 82:384, 1961.

47. LeVeen, H. H.: Technical features in endarterectomy. Surgery 57:22, 1965.

48. Linton, R. R.: Some practical considerations in the surgery of blood vessel grafts. Surgery 38:817, 1955.

49. Linton, R. R., and Darling, R. C.: Autogenous saphenous vein bypass grafts in femoropopliteal obliterative arterial disease. Surgery 51:62, 1962.

50. Malette, W. G.: Mechanisms in declamping hypotension. Presented before The Society of Clinical Surgery, Lexington, Ky., April, 1965.

51. Malette, W. G., Armstrong, R. G., and Criscuolo, D.: A second mechanism in hypotension following release of abdominal aortic clamps. Surg. Forum 14:292, 1963.

52. Moore, W. S., Rossan, C. T., Hall, A. D., and Thomas, A. N.: Transient bacteremia. A cause of infection in prosthetic vascular grafts. Am. J. Surg. 117:342, 1969.

53. Plecha, F. R., and Porries, W. J.: Intraoperative angiography in the immediate assessment of arterial reconstruction. Arch. Surg. 105:902, 1972.

54. Powers, S. R., Jr., Boba, A., Hostnik, W., and Stein, A.: Prevention of postoperative acute renal failure with mannitol in 100 cases. Surgery 55:15, 1964.

55. Rader, L. E., Jr., Keith, H. B., and Campbell, G. S.: Mechanism of hypotension following release of abdominal aortic clamps. Surg. Forum 12:265, 1961.

56. Rob, C.: Extraperitoneal approach to the abdominal aorta. Surgery 53:87, 1963.

57. Rosenberg, D. M. L., Glass, B. A., Rosenberg, N., Lewis, M. R., and Dale, W. A.: Experiences with modified bovine carotid arteries in arterial surgery. J. Surg. 68:1064, 1970.

58. Salzman, E. W.: The limitations of heparin therapy after arterial reconstruction. Surgery 57:131, 1965.

59. Sauvage, L. R., Berger, K., Wood, S. J., Nakagawa, Y., and Mansfield, P. B.: An external velour surface for porous arterial prostheses. Surgery 70:940, 1971.

60. Sawyer, P. N., Pasupathy, C. E., Fitzgerald, J., Kaplitt, M. J., Costello, M., Keates, J. R. W., O'Malley, G., and Lapousky, A.: Six year follow-up study in the use of gas endarterectomy. Surgery 72:837, 1972.

61. Shaw, R. S., and Baue, A. E.: Management of sepsis complicating arterial reconstructive surgery. Surgery 53:75, 1963.

62. Shumacker, H. B., Jr., Hawtof, D., Herendeen, T., Judd, D., Webb, M. L.: Osmotic diuresis and experimental renal ischemia. Surgery 55:687, 1964.

63. Smith, L. L., Saito, S., and Hinshaw, D. B.: The prevention and treatment of acute renal failure in surgical patients. Am. J. Surg. 110:192, 1965.

64. Sobel, S., Kaplitt, M. J., and Sawyer, P. N.: Gas endarterectomy. Surgery 59:517, 1966.

65. Sproul, G.: Rupture of an infected aortic graft into jejunum: resection and survival. J.A.M.A. 182:1118, 1962.

66. Stone, A. M., and Stahl, W. M.: Effect of ethacrynic acid and furosemide on renal function in hypovolemia. Ann. Surg. 174:1, 1971.

67. Stoney, R. J., and Wylie, E. J.: False aneurysms after arterial grafting. Am. J. Surg. 110:153, 1965.

68. Strandness, D. E., Jr., Parrish, D. G., and Bell, J. W.: Mechanism of declamping shock in operations on the abdominal aorta. Surgery 50:488, 1961.

69. Szilagyi, D. E., France, L. C., Smith, R. F., and Whitcomb, J. G.: The clinical use of an elastic dacron prosthesis. Arch. Surg. 77:538, 1958.

70. Szilagyi, D. E., Smith, R. F., and Elliott, J. P.: Temporary transection of the left renal vein: a technical aid in aortic surgery. Surgery 65:32, 1969.

71. Szilagyi, D. E., Smith, R. F., Elliott, J. P., and Vrandecic, M. T.: Infection in arterial reconstruction with synthetic grafts. Ann. Surgery 176:321, 1972.

72. Szilagyi, D. E., Smith, R. F., Elmquist, J. G., Gonzalez, A., and Elliott, J. P.: Angioplasty in the treatment of peripheral occlusive arteriopathy. Arch. Surg. 90:617, 1965.

73. Szilagyi, D. E., Whitcomb, J. G., Schenker, W., and Waibel, P.: The laws of fluid flow and arterial grafting. Surgery 47:55, 1960.

74. Taylor, G. W.: personal communication.

75. Van de Water, J. M., and Gaal, P. G.: Management of patients with infected vascular prostheses. Am. Surgeon. 31:651, 1965.

76. Vetto, R. M.: The femoral-femoral shunt: An appraisal. Am. J. Surg. 112:162, 1966.

77. Warren, R., and Villavicencio, J. L.: Iliofemoral arterial reconstructions for arteriosclerosis obliterans. New Eng. J. Med. 260:255, 1959.

78. Webb, R. W., and Barker, W. F.: Unpublished observations.

79. Wesolowski, S. A., Fries, C. C., Domingo, R. T., Liebig, W. J., and Sawyer, P. N.: The compound prosthetic vascular graft: a pathologic survey. Surgery 53:19, 1963.

80. Wesolowski, S. A., Fries, C. C., Karlson, K. E., DeBakey, M. E., and Sawyer, P. N.: Porosity: primary determinant of ultimate fate of synthetic vascular grafts. Surgery 50:91, 1961.

81. Willman, V. L., Cooper, T., and Hanlon, C. R.: Prophylactic and therapeutic use of digitalis in open-heart operations. Arch. Surg. 80:860, 1960.

82. Wylie, E. J.: Vascular replacement with arterial autografts. Surgery 57:14, 1965.

83. Wylie, E. J., Binkley, F. M., and Albo, R. J.: Femoropopliteal endarterectomy. Am. J. Surg. 108:215, 1964.

84. Wylie, E. J., and McGuiness, J. S.: The recognition and treatment of arteriosclerotic stenoses of major arteries. Surg. Gynec. Obstet. 97:425, 1953.

Chapter Eight

FEMORAL-POPLITEAL RECONSTRUCTION

INTRODUCTION

In the five years between 1965 and 1969 we have seen dramatic changes in the surgical approach to occlusive disease of the femoral artery and its distal branches. Thromboendarterectomy has been almost entirely replaced except in the management of very short femoral artery occlusions, and the various shunting procedures have taken its place. The technique of endarterectomy was difficult to learn and difficult to perform well without special training. Semi-closed methods by means of the intraluminal dissecting loops were often disappointing if incomplete endarterectomy or trauma to the wall occurred.[87] The full-length patch on an open endarterectomy was too long an operation for most surgeons and most patients. Gas endarterectomy obviates some of these problems but has found limited acceptance.

Furthermore, the distal limit of dissection has often been so far down the tibial system that endarterectomy of such a long and narrow segment is virtually impossible. The success and popularity of the long grafts have led to continued problems regarding the type of material to be used for the bypass when a good autologous saphenous vein is not available. At the same time that the technical feasibility of the long graft has been proven the merit of such procedures in the care of the overall patient has been seriously questioned by Stoney[77] and by Cannon,[13] except under unusual circumstances with operation for limb salvage. This chapter will present the classical details of endarterectomy technique because of its importance as a method that still can be of value in some patients, and because of its important historical role, but emphasis should be placed on the use of the bypass procedures and the several methods and materials that are available.

GENERAL CONSIDERATIONS

Everything that pertains to the general preparation of the patient for aortoiliac surgery pertains also to the patient with femoral artery occlusion. The general status of patients with femoral artery disease is often not as favorable as that of patients with purely aortoiliac disease, as the former tend to be older (see Chapter Five, p. 77), and often have more advanced arteriosclerosis. LeFevre[51] and Hines[39] have described the serious mortality risk in arteriosclerosis obliterans of the femoral artery. Also, diabetes is more frequently a complicating factor.

Generally, the obstructed segment is longer and the vessel is narrower. The outflow tract may be restricted, by either anatomic or pathologic processes. The collateral vessels around the obstructed segment may be injured during dissection. The intimate anatomic association of the femoral vein may be responsible for the development of venous thrombosis after operation.

Szilagyi has noted the frequency with which infections in arterial reconstructions arise in wounds placed in the groin.[80] Lymphatic drainage from infected or ischemic changes in the foot may make groin wounds particularly hazardous.

The use of the autologous saphenous vein is safest in the presence of infection, but at times other substances must be used, with the recognized associated hazard of foreign bodies in the presence of infection.

In some instances necrosis of the limb will occur in a patient who has a curable arterial lesion. Areas of sepsis must be drained and treated. Mechanically, the reconstruction is longer and narrower, and will support less flow; it is also more apt to be subjected to movement, especially flexion, as well as to external compression, compared to aortoiliac reconstruction.

For all these reasons, reconstruction of the femoropopliteal segment is a much more exacting procedure, and is likely to be less successful. Compromises in treatment must often be accepted, rather than risk the patient's life.

It is often true that the more extensive the disease in the femoral-popliteal-tibial system, the more grave is the vascular disease of the coronary system. This relationship places serious responsibility on the surgeon, who must balance the chance for a technically successful result in the peripheral vessels against the quality of survival of the rest of the patient. At times these patients become candidates for multiple procedures on the coronary,[83] carotid and other peripheral vessels, and the ethical responsibility for embarking on such a series of procedures in the face of the unlikelihood of surgically induced immortality must always be in the mind of the peripheral vascular surgeon.

As with aortoiliac procedures the author continues to believe firmly in the immediate and late value of lumbar sympathectomy as a preliminary procedure important in arterial reconstruction in the leg. Not only does it exert specific effects which are beneficial in themselves, but by reducing peripheral resistance and augmenting cutaneous flow, and albeit to a lesser extent, flow through muscle,[2] it increases the likelihood of a successful reconstruction.

Insofar as the flow augmented by sympathectomy soon returns toward normal,[71] there is reason to perform sympathectomy at the same time or a few days before the major arterial procedure. However, the frequency with which anticoagulants must be used during the arterial reconstruction is hazardous in terms of the retroperitoneal sympathectomy wound; hence it is often desirable to perform the operations at least 48 hours apart.

As a rule the obstruction will have been defined accurately by preoperative arteriography. It is of prime inportance to ascertain the patency of the distal arterial tree; if patency has not been proved by preoperative radiologic study, it may be necessary to perform direct exploration and distal angiography.[3]

Distal angiography may be performed as follows: The popliteal artery is exposed as described on page 179. Blind exploration of the tibial vessels in order to obtain an arteriogram is more difficult to accomplish than that of the main popliteal trunk. Fortunately, modern techniques with delayed multiple exposures of the x-ray can usually show which of the tibial vessels should be sought as a site for distal bypass, hence direct blind exploration may be infrequently needed. The popliteal artery in its distal branches may be exposed as described on page 181, and Figure 8–1. Exposure of the anterior tibial artery in the upper calf is almost impossible from this medial approach. A lateral approach to the anterior tibial artery is also described on page 182. If a soft and collapsible vessel is found, suggesting that arterial repair is feasible, a small catheter (No. 8 to No. 12F) can be placed in the artery through a longitudinal arteriotomy. If retrograde bleeding occurs, an umbilical tape is doubly looped about the artery and carefully tightened. Dilute heparin may be injected cautiously, and contrast material injected to assure accurate delineation of the distal tree at the site of dissection as well as in the calf below the area of direct visualization. As soon as x-ray films have been taken, the vessel is flushed with dilute heparin (10 units per ml.) and papaverine or priscoline. Spasm induced by injection of the contrast material may

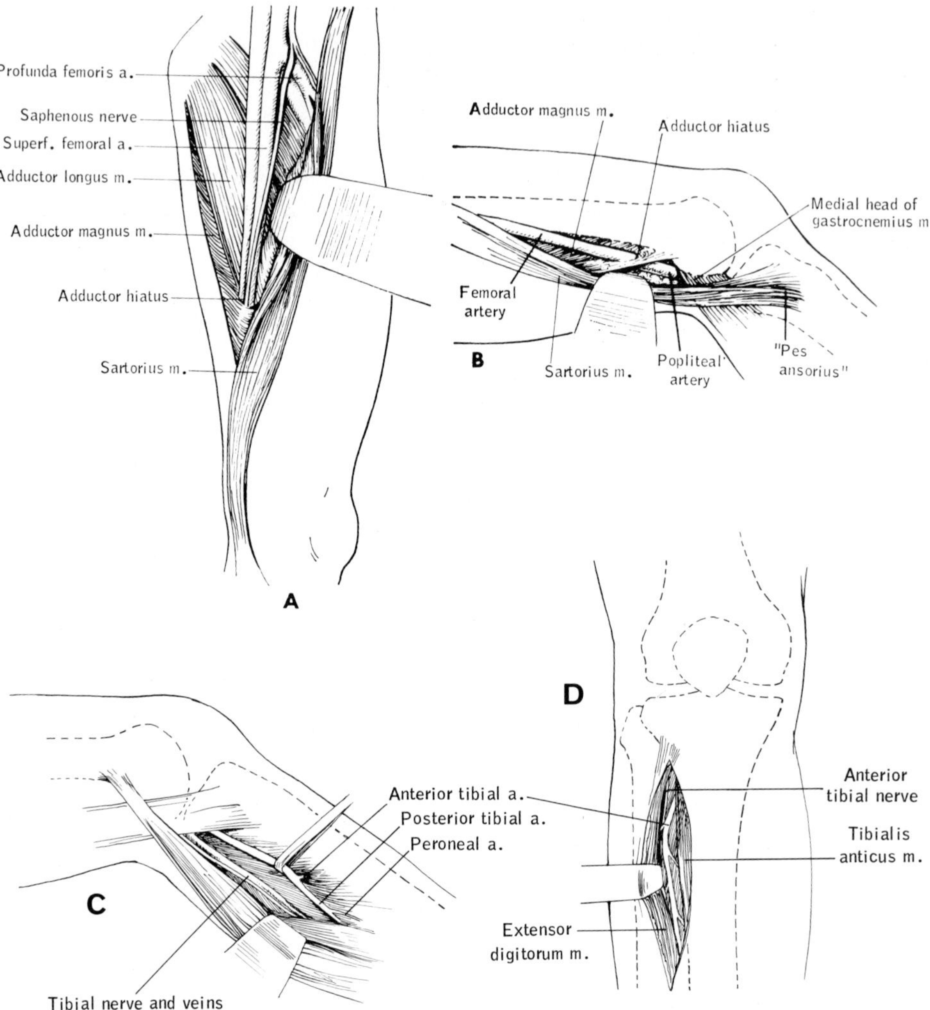

Figure 8–1.   Surgical relationships in the femoral popliteal artery and vein and the major muscles and nerves.

provoke propagation of arterial thrombus or may reduce perfusion of the calf to the extent that the contrast material remains in the veins and provokes venous thrombosis. Either of these complications is serious.

The radiologic procedure is dependent upon the equipment available. Superior films are obtained if a grid is used. Some operating tables are equipped with a Bucky grid, but satisfactory films can sometimes be obtained with a film placed in a cassette holder with a portable grid under the operating table mattress. If this arrangement has not been made, the cassette may simply be wrapped in sterile sheets or pillowcases and placed directly under the leg. It is possible to obtain films of better quality if the operating room is provided with a 220 volt power supply.

INCISION AND EXPOSURE

A longitudinal cutaneous incision is more versatile than a transverse one and is less apt to damage major collaterals. Its upper portion lies almost vertically over the femoral artery. The incision at the knee and extending down into the leg should be midlateral on the medial aspect. This incision does not handicap flexion. The upper portion easily exposes the upper popliteal artery, the lower femoral artery, and the adductor hiatus. Posterior reflection of the sartorius muscle grants access to the popliteal space from the medial aspect. The distal limb allows exposure of the lower portion of the popliteal artery and the origin and upper portion of the posterior tibial artery. As described, the lower portion of this incision is made at the origin of the medial head of the gastrocnemius and the pes anserinus, the fibrous attachments of the semimembranous, semitendinous, and the sartorius muscles, and one must dissect around these muscular structures (Fig. 8–1).

The skin of the thigh may be left intact between the incisions in the groin and the knee. If the full length of the thigh must be incised, placement of the incision is important. If there is *no* reason to anticipate using the saphenous vein, the incision should follow the course of the femoral artery and should be carried down to deep fascia without undermining the skin in the subcutaneous layer. If, however, there is *any* reason to believe that the saphenous vein will be needed either as a patch or as a tubular bypass, then the course of the vein should be followed (Fig. 8–2) to the level of deep fascia. Skin necrosis because of excessive undermining may lead to deeper sepsis in which the arterial reconstruction itself is involved—a potential catastrophe.

Dissection of the popliteal artery from the medial incision must be done at a considerable depth, because the popliteal artery shortly passes from the adductor hiatus to lie in a lateral position in the popliteal space. The artery is adherent along much of its length to the popliteal vein, and separation of the two vessels must be performed most cautiously. Once the artery is freed, it may be mobilized by lifting it with a cloth or rubber tape. Either material may cause trauma to the vessel unless used with caution.

Dissection in the region of the adductor hiatus must be performed with greatest caution. It is desirable to divide the fibrous arch of the

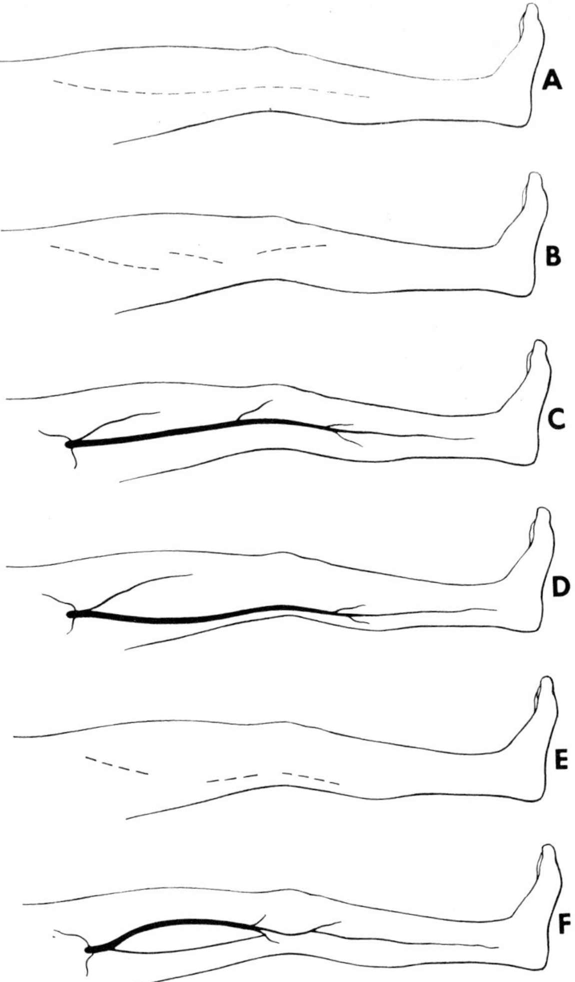

Figure 8–2.   *A*, General course of most common incision is to expose the entire length of the femoral popliteal vessels. An incision can be made along any part or all of the dotted line shown. With extensive subcutaneous dissection the posterior part of the flap in the thigh is prone to develop necrosis. *B*, Separate incisions that can be used to expose the same vessels. *C*, The usual course of the saphenous vein, which is well exposed by the incisions in *A* and *B*. *D*, The commonly encountered posterior course of the saphenous vein is shown. If incisions of *A* or *B* are used to dissect this vein free, the hazard of necrosis is increased. *E*, The incisions in the thigh which are more appropriate to the course of the vein shown in *D*. *F*, Course of the vein which makes *A*, or an incision placed even more anteriorly, more feasible.

great adductor muscle, but in so doing care must be taken not to injure the genicular arteries which arise here and which are essential to the collateral network around the knee.

Further exposure of the superficial femoral artery in the thigh may be necessary for open endarterectomy, but is unnecessary for the bypass procedures. If this exposure is necessary it is obtained by mobilization of the sartorius muscle. The lower portion of the artery lies anterior to and deep to the sartorius, the central portion of the artery lies under the midportion of the sartorius, and the upper portion of the artery lies posterior and deep to the muscle (Fig. 8–1 A, B). Extensive mobilization of sartorius muscle is necessary for full visualization of the femoral artery, but mobilization of the muscle must be done cautiously with respect to two points: First, the incision in the deep fascia must often be placed in line with the saphenous vein. The point at which the line of dissection crosses the sartorius muscle lies in the region of the junction of the middle and lower thirds of the thigh. Furthermore, care must be taken to protect the blood supply to the sartorius which is normally derived almost entirely from the superficial femoral artery. Collateral branches from the deep femoral branches must be protected.

Exposure of the terminal part of the popliteal artery and the origins of the anterior and posterior tibial arteries is obtained by incising the loose attachments of the medial belly of the gastrocnemius to the posterior edge of the tibia. The posterior tibial vein lies between the operator and the posterior tibial artery and must be mobilized with care. It is so fragile that it is often injured. When so injured it should be specifically interrupted just below the next more proximal branch and below the site of injury in order to avoid postoperative hemorrhage or uncontrolled postoperative venous thrombosis (Fig. 8–1C).[11, 58]

The anterior tibial artery can best be exposed using an anterior approach. The skin incision is made vertically, halfway between the tibia and fibula. The fascia is incised between the bellies of the tibialis anterior and the extensor digitorum muscles. When these muscles are separated, the anterior tibial artery, vein and nerve are found in the depths of the groove, and may be dissected easily. The choice of a course for a bypass graft from this area may be difficult. It can be led out the lateral side of the wound and up the lateral side of the knee, but this is an area where it is subject to serious extrinsic encroachment. It may be led directly anteriorly between the two muscle bellies and then subcutaneously and up the medial aspect of the thigh. It is possible to do the anastomosis on the posteromedial or medial aspect of the artery and to dissect a tunnel blindly into the popliteal space. A third approach is through a generous tunnel made by incising some of the deeper fibers and the fascia over the tibialis muscle, crossing subcutaneously well below the tibial tubercle and thence up the medial aspect of the thigh, either subcutaneously or under the muscle fascia.

Farther down in the leg, the anterior tibial artery is exposed by a vertical incision made one finger's breadth lateral to the fibular side of the tibial crest. The fascia is opened in this same line, just lateral to the tendon that lies next to the tibial, that is, the tibialis muscle tendon, and medial to the second tendon, which is the tendon of the extensor hallucis. Dissection between these two tendons exposes the neurovascular bundle composed of artery and veins and the deep branch of the peroneal nerve.

An approach to the anterior tibial artery popularized by Elkin[32, 33] can be made by removing the head of the fibula. A longitudinal incision is made over the head of the fibula and extended downward. The common peroneal nerve must be defined carefully as it passes down behind the head of the fibula and as it comes out from behind the attachment of the biceps femoris tendon to the head of the fibula. This nerve is mobilized with great care and retracted forward. It lies in a groove between the peroneus longus muscles and the soleus muscles, and this groove is incised. A strip of the peroneus muscle reaches laterally over this nerve and must be divided for accurate exposure. When this is done the peroneus muscle can then be turned forward, with the nerve attached to it.

The proximal portion of the fibula is then resected subperiosteally. The muscles can be detached from it by dissecting *upward* with a periosteal elevator, working from forward to backward. The interosseus membrane is the last attachment to be removed, and when this has been done the dissection must then be carried downward. The biceps tendon is cut from the head of the fibula, but leaving it in fascial continuity with the peroneus longus. The anterior tibial arch may be very difficult to see at this point, and it is important to mark the interosseus membrane here with a suture so as to know how to identify which compartment one is dissecting in subsequently.

In order to identify the artery at this point the peroneus longus muscle is pulled forward. The most medial branch of the peroneal nerve is the anterior tibial nerve, which passes from its association with the muscle to lie in the neurovascular bundle at a level about three centimeters below the facet on the lateral condyle of the fibula. Traction on this nerve identifies the anterior tibial artery, which can then be dissected free up to its juncture with the popliteal and posterior tibial arteries.

The resection of the head of the fibula gives excellent exposure under some circumstances to the distal popliteal artery, but it is much more complicated than the exposures described prior to this. Henry's book, *Extensile Exposure,* is recommended to the reader who is interested in the surgical-anatomical detail of this area.[38]

Four surgical procedures may be done in reconstruction: open endarterectomy, semiclosed endarterectomy, open endarterectomy with full length vein patch, and bypass graft.

OPEN ENDARTERECTOMY

Open endarterectomy was advocated by Wylie[88] and by Barker and Cannon (Fig. 8–3A).[5]

Bazy[7] had introduced minor modifications in the method of J. dos Santos.[26] Wylie's technique,[88] with which we became familiar in 1951, was performed through a single longitudinal arterial incision. Our first report[5] dealt with operations performed entirely with this technique, although in several instances a tunnel dissection was done to remove the atheromatous core under the inguinal ligament. Based on his familiarity with this procedure, which was also performed at the aortic bifurcation so as to avoid a Y-shaped incision there, Cannon[13] developed a blunt dissector which could be used through widely separated arteriotomies to free the atheromatous core (Fig. 8–3C). The first models of this stripper were rather crudely made of piano wire; far more refined models, made of stainless steel, are now available. Application of this loop dissector will be described in a later section of this chapter.

In open endarterectomy, the length of the obstructed segment is exposed after patency of the distal tree has been demonstrated. Once the sartorius has been mobilized, the femoral sheath is opened and the artery is exposed. The artery is mobilized only enough to permit control of the muscular branches and to free the plexus of veins on its surface. The saphenous nerve is mobilized gently and cautiously (Fig. 8–1B).

The muscular branches of the artery must be controlled at this point. Tantalum clips may be placed temporarily on these vessels; small bulldog clamps or double loops of heavy suture (No. 0 silk) may be placed temporarily around them. These branches should be preserved, for they may in certain circumstances supply most of the flow of the superficial femoral system.

Cannon[10] has described electromagnetic flowmeter studies at the level of the proximal superficial femoral artery and the popliteal artery in the presence of an obstruction in the distal femoral artery. Before endarterectomy the flows recorded were 250 ml. and 50 ml. per minute, respectively; after endarterectomy the proximal flow recorded was 850 ml. per minute and the distal popliteal flow, 250 ml. per minute. The latter figure approximates the flow supplied by a simple graft bypass. The difference between the proximal and distal recordings—600 ml. per minute—indicates the volume of flow into muscular and genicular branches.

A finger or a curved clamp is placed behind the vessel at the lower boundary of the occluded area to flatten the opened artery (Fig.

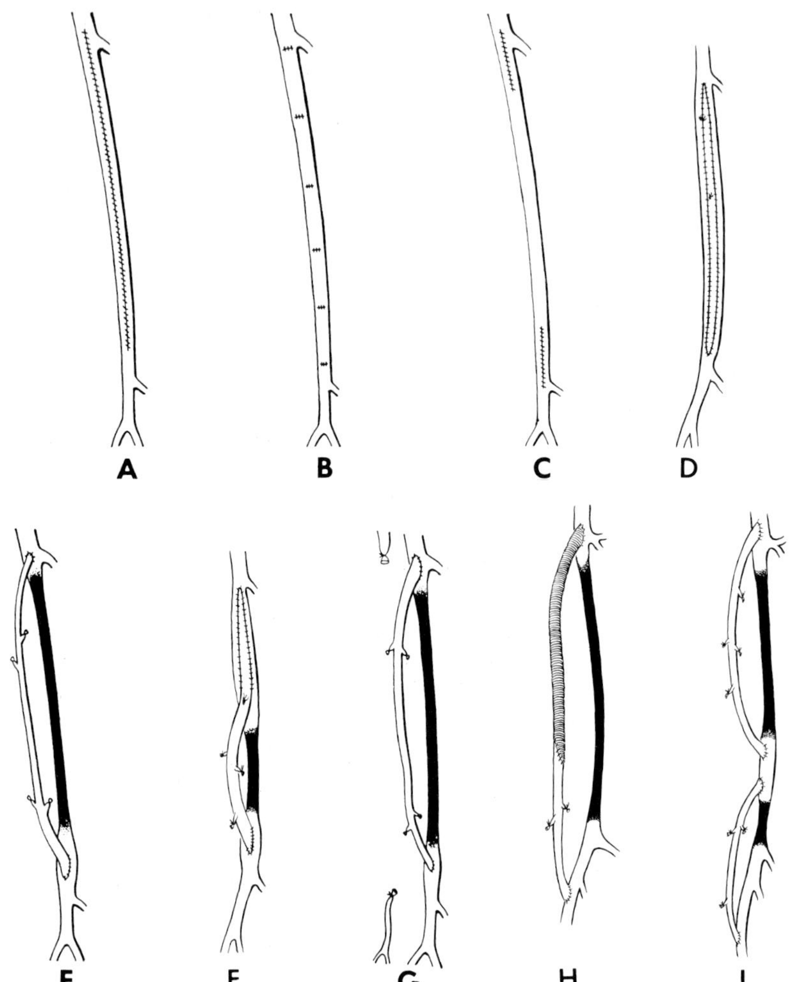

Figure 8–3. Schematic representation of various forms of femoral artery repair. *A,* Full length open endarterectomy. *B,* Endarterectomy through multiple short transverse arteriotomies. *C,* Two longitudinal arteriotomies for endarterectomy, using the loop dissector. *D,* Full length endarterectomy closed with open patch and endarterectomy. Saphenous vein is the preferred source of the patch if available, but Dacron may also be used. *E,* Full length bypass using a reverse segment of the saphenous vein. Other tubular substitutes can be used as indicated in the text, but the saphenous vein is preferable. *F,* Partial bypass using the tube for the lower part of the reconstruction. In the upper part of the reconstruction the same tube is used as a patch on the open endarterectomy. *G,* Full length bypass using *in situ* saphenous vein. *H,* Composite Dacron vein graft. *I,* Sequential graft.

7–6, p. 142). The distal tip of the atheroma is elevated with a Freer dissector and the plaque dissected upward. If any significant area of atheroma remains in the intima, mattress sutures placed and tied from the external surface of the vessel should be used to secure the edge of undissected intima to the media (Fig. 7–7). If additional plaques extend further, wider exposure and dissection must be considered. A disease-free area may be found; however, it may occur only in much smaller vessels, requiring such an extensive intimectomy as to affect adversely the possibility that blood flow will be adequate through the reconstructed segment. An effective compromise might be to use a vein patch to widen the terminus of the intimal excision just enough to assure continuation of flow into an endothelialized tree that has already shown its ability to support flow without clotting at rates even lower than will follow successful reconstruction.

The largest rubber catheter that will easily pass should be placed in the distal artery, and dilute heparin (10 units per ml.) administered. Gentle dilatation with coronary or Bâkes dilators may be performed to make repair easier. Martin[55] has described a cervical dilator in which a longitudinal slot has been cut in order to facilitate placement of sutures in the dilated artery.

Dissection of the atheroma upward is now done. The arterial wall is incised with scissors. The incision must be kept in the most accessible surface of the vessel to facilitate repair. The tip of the scissors may lie in the lumen of the vessel, or it may lie in the plane between intima and media and cut only the media.

The atheromatous sequestrum is lifted gently from the wall and freed from the media by blunt dissection. All layers of atheroma must be removed so that only a smooth layer remains. Darling and Linton[22] have stressed the importance of removing all circular muscle fibers (Figs. 10–1, 10–2). It is of great importance that all rough surfaces be removed that might nurture thrombosis. The surgeon naturally hesitates to dissect so deeply into the deeper (more peripheral) layers of the medial wall lest the wall be too thin to support arterial pressure, but most of the structural strength lies in the fibrous adventitia.

The inexperienced endarterectomist often fears he has dissected too deeply, forgetting that the normal arterial wall is exceedingly thin. Preservation of the fibrous adventitia provides autologous external support for the endarterectomized vessel; hence the surgeon must avoid extensive preliminary dissection that removes this adventitia.

In most instances the disease requires endarterectomy along the full length of the superficial femoral artery. Only rarely will truly circumscribed lesions be encountered in which this long dissection is not required.

The upper limit of dissection then will usually lie in the common femoral artery. Occluding clamps are placed on the common femoral and deep femoral arteries as the level is approached at which a patent lumen connects with the proximal arterial system.

At times it may seem logical to dissect the intimal atheroma from below without opening the proximal common femoral bifurcation.

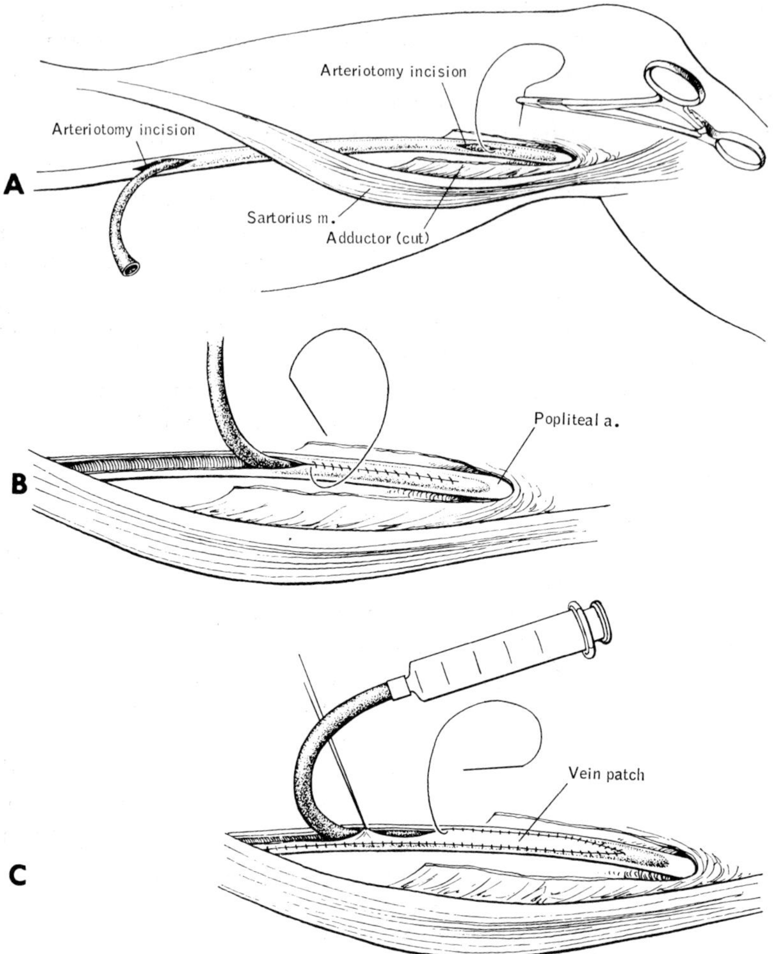

Figure 8–4. *A,* Femoral endarterectomy by use of the loop stripper into two discrete arteriotomies. Stent of rubber catheter is led out through the upper arteriotomy, which is more accessible, and is usually in a larger caliber vessel. This placement also allows heparin to be dripped into the distal tree during the repair. *B,* Repair of the full length open endarterectomy performed over the catheter, which is used as a stent. The repair begins from below and proceeds proximally for the reasons already indicated. *C,* Repair of full length open endarterectomy, using the vein patch. The repair is performed from below and proceeds proximally. Stay sutures help to hold the vein patch in position over the rubber catheter stent.

This procedure may well be justified if prior arteriography has shown all areas of atherosclerosis to lie well below the origin of the superficial femoral artery, and if the atheroma is freed below that level. Commonly, atherosclerosis does involve the origin of this artery, and it is usually best to be certain by direct exposure that this orifice is clear and that no intimal flap remains to hinder flow into the *deep femoral artery.*

As a rule, after the occluding clamps have been placed across the proximal common femoral artery and the deep femoral artery, the longitudinal arteriotomy is extended into the common femoral segment. If possible, the intima is amputated above the level of area of greatest thickening. Reattachment of the proximal flap of intima to the media is not crucial; if the intima is divided below the profunda femoris, however, great care must be taken to repair the proximal portion of the superficial femoral artery. There is often a minor isthmus at this point (Fig. 2–18, p. 34), if arteriotomy must be done through this isthmus, the use of a narrow patch graft of vein may be justified in order to assure closure without stenosis.

As the dissection progresses upward several major femoral muscular branches are encountered which cause much reflux bleeding. These must be carefully dissected and secured temporarily with a heavy loop of suture or a small bulldog clamp.

Repair of the arteriotomy should begin distally (Fig. 8–4A, B). The largest catheter that can be inserted into the distal tree may be considerably smaller than the caliber of the femoral artery above the level of origin of the genicular arteries. It may be desirable, therefore, to substitute a larger one as soon as the first few inches have been sutured, so that the repair may be completed over the largest possible stent. Use of a straight needle expedites the repair (see Figure 7–11 and page 144). Before the stent is removed, clots are flushed from the upper tree by momentary release of the proximal occluding clamps; reflux and freedom from clots should be demonstrable in the distal system.

A systemic level of heparin should be established as soon as arterial repair is begun, with intravenous administration of 2500 to 5000 units of heparin (25 to 50 mg.). As the catheter stent is removed, dilute heparin is flushed through the repaired segment. Apparent leaks in the suture line need not be treated at this time unless they are gaping, as intraluminal pressure will serve to tighten the arterial sutures, and the more viscous blood will quickly clot in small suture leaks. When closure of the arteriotomy is complete, the distal clamps are removed first, so as to allow residual air to be flushed out along the suture line and demonstrate major leaks in the reconstructed vessel. With removal of proximal clamps and loops of the suture on the muscular branches, restoration of flow is completed.

Beales, Cohn, Martin, Kiely, and others have recognized that serious involvement of the deep femoral system is an accompaniment of advanced stages of arterial disease.[8, 14, 48, 55] Endarterectomy or patch arterioplasty as far as the second or third major branch in the descending branch of the deep femoral artery can be added to superficial femoral artery reconstruction. At times, however, this is more important as the only procedure that may be done when distal disease in the main popliteal and tibial systems is too extensive to allow reconstruction. This operation may even be done under local anesthesia and may be applied to very poor risk patients. It has been applied in particular to some patients who urgently need some repair, but who at the immediate moment may not be suitable candidates for general anesthesia and full femoral popliteal reconstruction. (See page 205.)

SEMICLOSED ENDARTERECTOMY

Because of the extensive dissection and the long arterial suture line necessitated in open endarterectomy, Cannon[12] modified the technique with a loop dissector that often allows complete femoropopliteal endarterectomy through two widely separated incisions and arteriotomies (Fig. 8–3C). Other surgeons have modified this loop dissector further; fundamentally, the techniques are similar, however, and those to be described are particularly applicable to Cannon's original stripper, modified only in being made of a heavier gauge of metal and having a blunter leading edge. This instrument is less likely to be deformed by a calcific plaque. It has greater application as a blunt dissector, rather than a sharp one, and it is less likely to tear the medial wall (Fig. 7–4A).

The initial steps are the same as in the open technique (p. 183). The distal portion of the obstructed area is identified and the adequacy of outflow into the distal tree is demonstrated. The distal intima is similarly handled, being sutured to the media, if necessary, and with a catheter placed in the distal tree for use as a stent to allow access to the distal tree for heparinization or arteriography.

Regardless of level, the short distal arteriotomy is made just long enough to permit grasping the intimal core and dissecting upward with a Freer elevator between media and intima. Once a clear plane is established, a loop dissector is introduced. The leading tip of the dissector is usually easily introduced into the superficial part of the circumference, and with a thrusting, twisting motion—always gently done—the core is gradually mobilized. Frequently the loop may be passed the full length of the artery in the first attempt, but if any significant difficulty is encountered in passing the stripper upward, the area of obstruction must be exposed. The stripper may be engaged at a branch and mobilized from the outside without incising the artery. One should not hesitate to perform arteriotomy if there is any question.

The helical stripper designed by LeVeen[52] (Fig. 7–4B) is said to have the merits of easier insertion, less likelihood of penetrating the arterial wall, and to be less likely to cause complications postoperatively if the arterial wall is torn. The helical stripper is introduced the full length of the artery, *then* withdrawn with the core, dissecting as it is withdrawn.

When dissection with the loop has been carried as far as necessary (usually to the common femoral artery), a short arteriotomy is made and the intimal core is divided and removed. The upper edge of the intima usually need not be reattached with suture.

The core which has been withdrawn should be inspected carefully to be certain its surface is free of flaps of intima that match other intimal flaps hidden in the tunnel that may be the site of later obstruction and thrombosis. Passage of a rubber catheter through the dissected segment may indicate a clean dissection. A sound may be introduced[52] to verify this. A pledget of gauze of appropriate size may be pulled through the dissected segment to remove any loose fragments of intima. Arteriograms should be used to demonstrate adequacy of dissection.

Blind stripping from a proximal arteriotomy *downward* should rarely be risked. If the atheromatous core is "ripe," that is, if it is firm, rubbery, and homogeneous, and dissects easily, the stripper easily passes distally. The core may be dislodged and returned into the wound with a discrete point at the distal limit. If the distance to which the stripper has been passed corresponds to the area of disease demonstrated by arteriogram, if a catheter of appropriate size can be passed into the open segment *below* the level of termination of endarterectomy, and if flow into the catheter seems unimpeded, the dissection may be adequate. Arteriographic proof is essential. Unless this distal segment has been visualized directly, however, it is not certain that the transition is smooth. Lack of a smooth transition is one of the common reasons for failure of endarterectomy. Unwise attempts of the inexperienced surgeon to end the operation without being certain about the condition of the remaining segment are apt to end in failure. Review of our experience with blind distal endarterectomy indicated that in only four of 15 instances did the patient leave the hospital with distal pulses palpable, and on later follow up only two stayed open for over a month.[4]

GAS ENDARTERECTOMY

Gas endarterectomy, as introduced by Sawyer, is a valuable technique for performing semiclosed endarterectomy[69, 72] (see Fig. 7–5, p. 140). The distal limit of the occlusive disease is identified exactly as in the prior discussion. Before opening the artery, however, the limit of proximal dissection must also be identified and the vessel doubly clamped. The gas, under carefully controlled pressures, is then introduced by needle between the media and the atheromatous sequestrum, and the gas performs the dissection rapidly and atraumatically. The major hazard is from rupture of the media with poorly monitored gas pressures. The distal site is opened and the distal intimal flap carefully trimmed or sutured in place if necessary. The lower of the two upper clamps is then removed, and the atheromatous sequestrum is dissected free of any remaining attachments and removed. Closure of the short arteriotomies is performed if possible without a patch, but if serious narrowing is present a narrow patch of autologous vein or Dacron coated with velour may be used.

OPEN ENDARTERECTOMY WITH VEIN PATCH

Dissatisfaction with semiclosed endarterectomy by means of loop strippers has led many surgeons to abandon this procedure and to turn to other methods.[22, 29] Their dissatisfaction arose from operative failures due to inadequate removal of all plaques from the tunnel or to leaving flaps of nearly normal intima. Further, according to Poiseuille's law (p. 41), which is applicable to the situation, minor increases in the diameter of the vessel might greatly increase the flow, if other factors of perfusion gradient, peripheral resistance, viscosity, etc., remained constant. Edwards[29] introduced the full-length vein patch because of the difficulty in maintaining flow through a long, narrow, endarterectomized segment (Fig. 8–3D). He performed open endarterectomy to be *certain* of removing all intimal debris, then split the carefully mobilized saphenous vein and sutured its full length into the long arteriotomy.

The potential flow that could be supplied through the patched artery is great. For instance, if an artery 5 mm. in diameter is patched with a saphenous vein 5 mm. in diameter, a vessel is created which is $3.1416 \times (5 \times 2)$ mm. in circumference, or 1 cm. in diameter, assuming there is no constriction created by the suture line and no dilatation of the wall. Thus the *potential* augmentation of flow is of the magnitude of 16:1, or $5^4 : 2.5^4$ or 625:39. Obviously, this is more than all the muscular branches and the entire distal outflow tract can accept, since flow is primarily determined by peripheral resistance. Thus, two theoretical drawbacks quickly become apparent.

First, the velocity of flow may be diminished by almost this same factor. Indeed, Edwards' cinearteriographic studies[29] demonstrated that flow proceeded through the reconstructed femoral artery at the rate of about 1.5 to 2 cm. per second, requiring 20 seconds to traverse the thigh. As a result, clotting became a hazard. In Edwards' series there was a failure rate of 20 per cent (and our experience with a smaller group of patients is similar); sudden occlusion occurred in a limb that seemed to be improving. The following example illustrates this phenomenon.

L.D., a 56-year-old male, was admitted for the treatment of a severely ischemic extremity. Lumbar sympathectomy and femoral endarterectomy were performed, and a full-length vein patch was applied in closure to a 35 cm. segment of femoropopliteal vessel. Postoperatively, the patient showed marked improvement, with excellent color, warm skin, and strong pedal pulses. Two weeks postoperatively, however, his leg suddenly became painful and blue as he stood, but did not swell. He declined further surgery and made a gradual recovery, but his pulses never regained their vigor. Oscillometric excursions, which had been 6 to 8 units in the calf, decreased to ½ to 1 unit, but a year later increased to 2 to 3 units. The patient now walks with little limitation, being able to walk more than a mile a day without experiencing claudication.

Although the exact mechanism was not determined in this case, it is assumed that a loose clot migrated from the femoral vessel and became fragmented in the distal tree. There was nothing palpable in the thigh that might suggest the presence of an aneurysm.

The second theoretical drawback is the possibility of development of a true aneurysm. In this type of reconstruction, application of Laplace's ($T = pd$, where $T =$ the tension on the wall, $p =$ the intraluminal pressure, and $d =$ the diameter) indicates how an aneurysm might occur in the dilated vessels. Although we have had no clinical experience with this situation, it does occur in dogs in which the fresh autologous femoral artery is placed as a patch on the opposite femoral artery, doubling its diameter. The dilated vessel so created commonly ruptures within a week or two.

It is essential that the reconstructed segment be of the correct size. In open endarterectomy the use of a patch is often unnecessary; however, if the segment of reconstructed artery is *too narrow* and *too long* then the poiseuillian formula is applicable. These terms — *too narrow* and *too long* — can be only arbitrarily defined at this time, but the author recommends the use of a vein patch to restore a lumen about the diameter of a No. 14 to 16 Fr. catheter (4.5 to 5.1 mm. in diameter) if the lumen is narrower than a No. 10 Fr. (3.2 mm.) for a length of more than 7 to 8 cm., or narrower than a No. 12 Fr. (3.8 mm.) for longer distances. Edwards[29] has recommended the use of a No. 18 Fr. catheter as being of proper size. It is possible, therefore, to remove a shorter segment of vein than the length of the artery that is to be patched, for the vein can be split into two strips.

Such a margin of safety obviates the need for minute suturing. Not only can larger sutures be placed more quickly but they also assure ample protection against leakage. This margin of safety, however, should not provide an excuse to use careless or lax technique.

FEMORAL BYPASS GRAFTS

As noted in the introduction to this chapter, femoral bypass grafts have become substantially the standard operation for repair of vascular occlusions below the inguinal ligament. This is particularly true for those occlusions which require restoration of flow to a level well below the knee. Morris[58] and Tyson,[84, 85] were among the early advocates of very long grafts below the knee. Although there is much argument as to the long term and overall merit of these grafts, the actual flow measured in many of the femoral-tibial grafts was of the same magnitude as that measured in femoral popliteal grafts.[9] Hence the initial apprehensions that the outflow tract would be insufficient to provide long term patency rates has not necessarily been borne out. On the other hand, Kaminski[47] and his associates have noted that the anatomical appearance of the outflow tract has a better parallel with ultimate success as far as protracted limb salvage is concerned than does the actual intraoperative flow measurement.

Imparato[43] and his associates point out that tibial arterial reconstruction is usually successful if at least the anterior or posterior tibial artery was patent from below the level of the midcalf, with filling of at least a portion of the pedal arch. If only the peroneal artery was patent and there was no filling of the pedal arch the immediate failure rate was more than 80 per cent.

The reconstructions to the level of the malleolus were necessary when occlusions of the tibial arteries extended beyond the mid-calf. If a pedal arch was involved by occlusive disease, so that it was not complete from one malleolus to the other, reconstruction universally failed within minutes to hours, whereas if the arch was complete immediate patency was frequent.

Among the first successful operations for the relief of occlusive disease were those reported by Holden[41] who in 1949 replaced a segment of obstructed artery with a length of superficial femoral vein. Shortly thereafter, Julian[45] reported on a series of cases so treated. Kunlin[49] introduced the bypass procedure in 1951 and it was popularized by Linton (Fig. 8–3E).[53] Various materials have been used for grafting: femoral veins, saphenous veins, arterial homografts, plastic prostheses arterial heterografts (bovine carotids)[65] and collagenized implanted Dacron tubes,[60, 73, 74] to name but a few.

The use of femoral vein has been largely discarded because the vein is considerably larger and thinner walled than is desirable, dissection of it is an extensive procedure, and once it has been sacrificed there is considerable interference with venous return.

Arterial homografts were technically easy to use and were of appropriate size, but most showed marked degenerative changes with passage of time.[79] The degenerative changes and the difficulties in procurement and sterilization have led to abandoning their use.

Fabric prostheses are, of course, always available in any size, are strong, and can easily be sterilized. Their defects, however, balance their advantages, and their use is not recommended when other means of replacement can be used; nevertheless, several groups[17, 23, 24, 42, 68] have reported results sufficiently good to warrant the use of fabric if no other material is suitable. Of primary concern is the slow rate of maturation in some instances: the slow rate at which the graft is penetrated by granulation tissue and a firmly adherent lining similar to endothelium is established. The fragility of this lining, the persistence of granulating surfaces within a synthetic tube, and the ten-

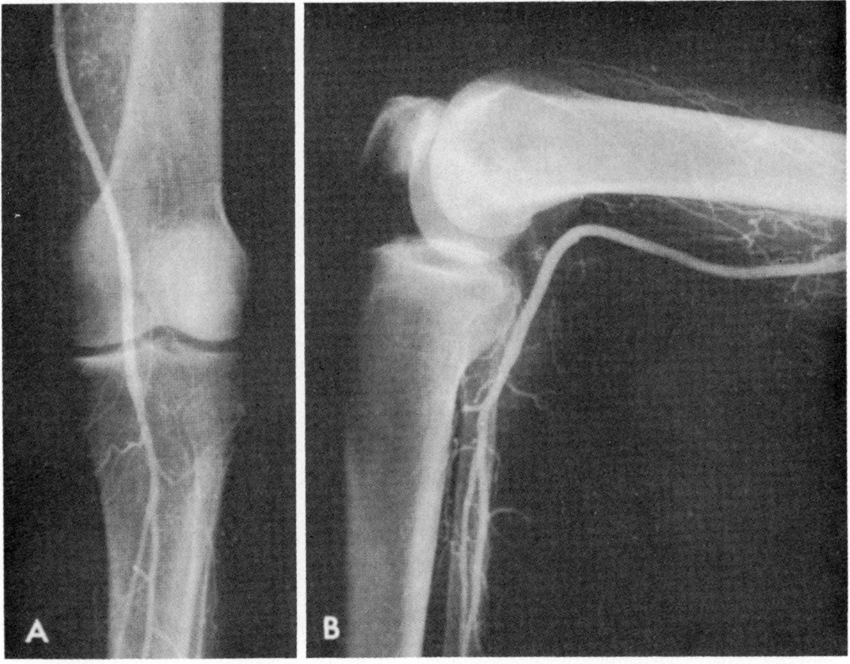

Figure 8–5. Arteriogram of a 61-year-old patient who had a 41 cm. saphenous vein autograft placed from the left common femoral artery to the distal popliteal artery because of obstructive arteriosclerosis of the femoral artery. This postoperative arteriogram was obtained at 18 months. *A,* Anteroposterior view of graft with the leg in extension. *B,* Same patient, lateral view, with knee in flexion. Note the smooth curve of the reconstructed area without any angulation of the graft. The patient had adequate pulses for at least 3½ years after operation. (Courtesy Dr. Robert Linton and the New Eng. J. Med.)

dency of the prostheses to stiffen and kink upon flexion all act to produce a rate of late failure that is excessive. The stiffening caused by growth of fibroblasts into the graft causes considerable kinking, with consequent risk of occlusion, if it crosses the knee. Darling and Linton[22] have pictured this well (Figs. 8–5 and 8–6). Others believe that the flexion deformity is only transient and does not result in serious deformity of lasting consequence.[78]

The addition of a velour surface to either the external or internal surface of the Dacron graft has offered an improvement in plastic prostheses. Fibroblastic invasion is greatly promoted by the velour surface, and Sauvage has demonstrated that such grafts frequently develop a truly adherent neointima, which may be better able to resist damage from flexion than other plastic tubes.[68] On the other hand,

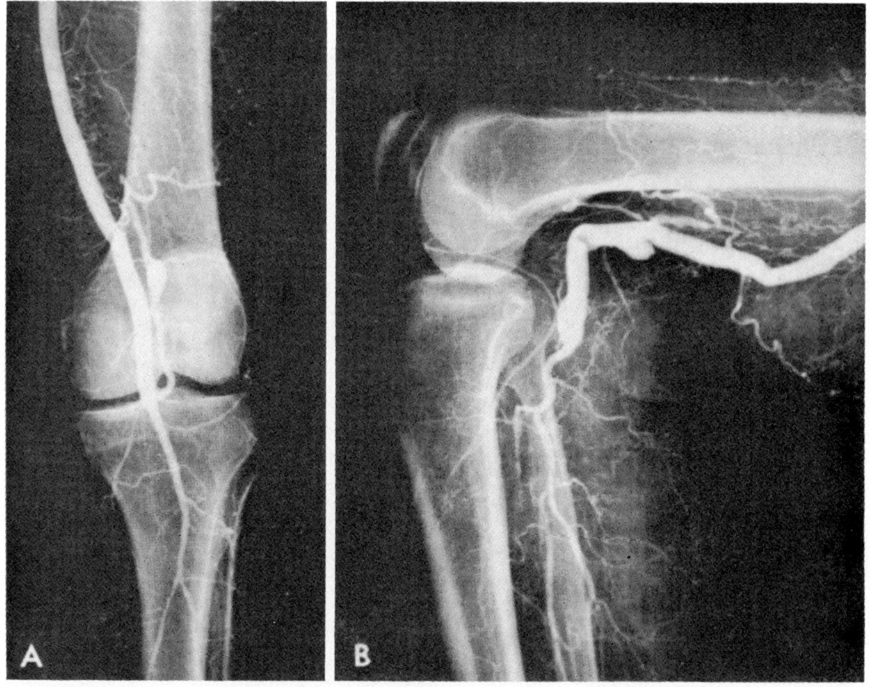

Figure 8–6. Arteriogram of a 55-year-old patient in whom a Teflon-Dacron graft, 46 cm. long and 13 mm. in diameter, had been placed from the left common femoral artery to the distal popliteal artery because of obstructive arteriosclerosis in the femoral artery. This arteriogram was done slightly more than 4 years after operation. *A,* Anteroposterior view showing the smooth contour of the graft in extension. *B,* Lateral view of the graft in flexion. Note buckling and kinking of the graft near its site of attachment. Despite the buckling and kinking, the patient had an adequate pulse at this time, and maintained sufficient pedal pulsation for at least 2 more years. (Courtesy Dr. Robert Linton and New Eng. J. Med. *270:*609, 1964.)

there is a possibility that the intima may be at least as susceptible to atherosclerosis as the original vessel.

Stoney, Albo and Wylie[76] advocate the use of autologous arteries at sites of recurrent flexion, and autologous vein can be used similarly.[22] The composite graft may be used when the length of the reconstruction dictates the use of a fabric prosthesis (Figs. 7–19, 8–3F, H).

The most acceptable grafting material currently available is the autologous saphenous vein.[15, 16, 17, 18, 22, 29, 35, 49, 53, 56, 64, 65, 81] It is usually available, and of sufficient length and width. Its media is sufficiently fibrous to resist arterial pressure well and to tolerate transplantation as a free graft. The frequency with which it is being used necessitates a note of caution regarding indiscriminate resection of the long saphenous system for minor varicosities. The greater incidence of femoral arteriosclerosis in males makes one question the wisdom of vein stripping in males. Certainly, the finding of diminished popliteal or pedal pulses, diminished oscillometric readings in the calf, or claudication should constitute an absolute contraindication. Family history of claudication, gangrene, or diabetes should also invoke caution. Varicose veins should not be made the "scapegoat" for ill-defined symptoms in the leg at any time; arterial symptoms especially must not be mistaken for venous symptoms.

A compromise between full saphenous stripping and no operation at all may be offered: high ligation and division of the saphenofemoral junction, with low ligation at the knee and stripping and excision of the offending veins in the calf.

Technical Considerations

The initial step, as in femoral endarterectomy, is the identification of an open segment of artery distal to the site of major obstruction which is suitable for distal anastomosis. In some cases, such a site may have been defined clearly by previous arteriography, but in others exploration of the popliteal artery by means of a medial midlateral incision (p. 179) and distal angiography[3] is necessary.

A saphenous vein graft may be successful with only a minimal outflow tract, for the endothelial lining of the vein has a good chance of being preserved so it can support arterial flow at low rates without thrombosis, especially if the vein is handled carefully. Reichle and his associates,[63] however, have recently demonstrated with the electron microscope that even in vein grafts successful after 14 months, large areas of the graft were denuded of endothelium, and blood was flowing successfully over large areas of collagen. In Dacron grafts, flow continues over a network of fibrin.

To take a hint from the renal transplantationists, it might be well to preserve the vein until it is ready for use in Simmons' solution or similar fluid. Sacks and his associates[67] recently used a similar solution with an electrolyte composition substantially that of the intracellular fluids, but rendered in addition hypertonic with mannitol with great success in ex-vivo bench work on autotransplanted kidneys.

As a rule, the entire femoral segment is bypassed, just as in femoral endarterectomy the entire femoral artery is usually freed of atheroma. The adequacy of the inflow tract must be proved as certainly as the adequacy of the outflow. Prior to operation the excellence of the femoral pulses, freedom from bruits, and arteriography combine to give assurance of adequate input. At operation the direct measurement of intra-arterial pressure comparable to arterial aortic pressure assures adequacy.

The proximal femoral artery should be exposed through a longitudinal incision. If the superficial femoral artery is completely occluded, the origin of the prosthesis should be the common femoral artery. If some proximal branches in the superficial femoral artery are patent, they may be made to function longer by using the prosthesis as a patch to widen the origin of the superficial femoral artery (Fig. 8–7). Several authors have indicated the likelihood that a femorotibial graft may succeed at least as well as a femoropopliteal graft.[9]

If a plastic fabric is to be used, it is simply cut obliquely and the edge is cauterized to prevent raveling. A square toe to prevent narrowing at the end can now be fashioned. If a vein is used it is cut longitudinally for a short distance, and the corners are cut so as to produce a bell-shaped configuration.[50, 53] Thus, the effect is similar to that of the square cut on the toe of the plastic prosthesis (Fig. 8–7).

The manner of removal of the vein is critical. It is easy enough to remove the vein if the entire leg is opened with a single long incision, but even then the vein must be handled very little and with the lightest possible touch (Fig. 8–2). Undue trauma to the vein may well provoke later thrombosis. Undue distention must be avoided.

When the placement of the graft is to be done through two widely separated arteriotomies and separate skin incisions, it is necessary to dissect the vein through a series of small incisions along its course.

The vein may be used in any of several ways. Hall,[36] Connolly[15, 16] and Rob[56, 64] have advocated leaving the vein *in situ*, and destroying the valves as is illustrated in Figure 8–3G. Major branches must be ligated. The vein is left superficial and very vulnerable to trauma of any kind. There is only a slight possibility that arteriovenous fistulas will develop, and if they do, they will not necessarily aggravate the situation, because such fistulas have been advocated as a means of maintaining patency in a reconstructed artery. The fistula can easily be localized and treated. The size and configuration of any major branches should be evaluated by phlebography preoperatively.

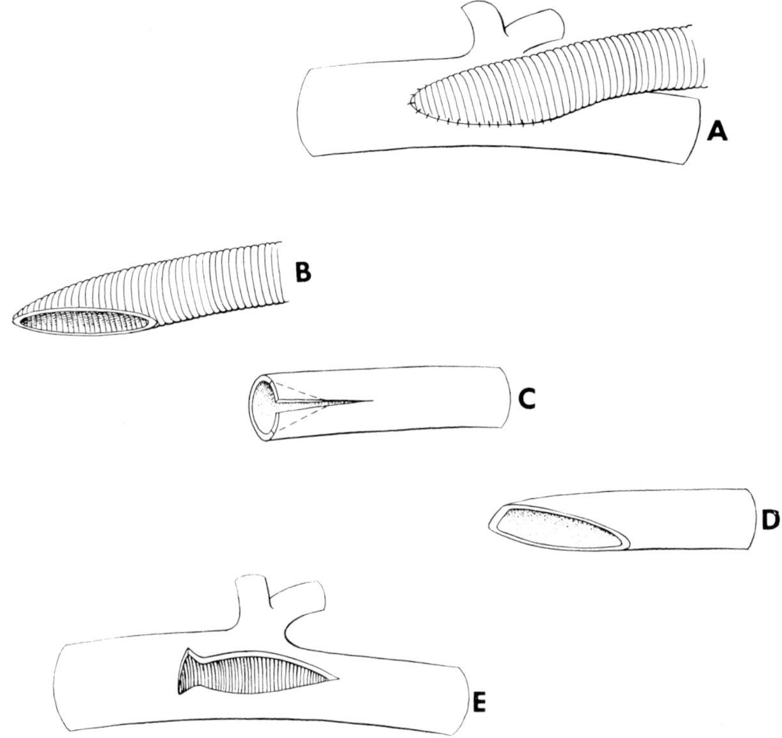

Figure 8–7. A, Placement of a bypass graft, in this case a crimped plastic tube, at the origin of the superficial femoral artery so as to widen the orifice and allow greater possibility of flow into the proximal superficial femoral artery. B, Shape of the graft when cut obliquely. The toe comes to a sharp point. C, D, Tailoring of the vein graft as originally described by Linton (Surgery 38:817, 1955). The plastic graft may be cut to the same square-toe shape. E, T-shaped arteriotomy recommended by Taylor (personal communication) to accept the square-toed graft and to minimize the hazard of narrowing at the site of attachment. (See text, and Figure 7–19.)

Destruction of the valves with a Zollinger intraluminal vein stripper occasions minimal trauma to the endothelium,[15] whereas use of an arterial stripper is apt to cause greater trauma.

In spite of the potentially increased chance of pressure on the vessel in its superficial bed causing thrombosis, the greater viability of the vein that has not been dissected from its bed may decrease the chance of early thrombosis.[64, 81]

Use of *in situ* saphenous vein appears to be especially applicable to poor-risk patients, because there is a good possibility of early function, and the operation usually can be performed under local anesthesia.

Most surgeons who are using the saphenous vein for a graft dissect it entirely from its bed and tie off any branches directly. Some believe it is simpler to use the larger (central) end for anastomosis with the larger (proximal) artery, placing the smaller end of the vein on the smaller artery. In this case, also, the valves must be destroyed so they cannot serve as an impediment to flow. It may, however, be preferable hemodynamically to have the larger vein serve as a widening patch on the smaller artery, and the smaller end serve as a narrower patch where less width is needed. Since this graft is a simple shunt, the flow into one end is equal to the flow out of the other, and the position of the vein will not of itself alter the flow, but only the velocity of flow.

The author's preference, particularly when a tunnel is to be used in which visualization of the bypass will be difficult, is as follows. The lower end of the vein is dissected free and divided at such a level that the length of vein from the site of division up to the saphenofemoral junction will be sufficient. As a rule this procedure entails division of the vein *below* the level at which a patent popliteal artery exists and is suitable to anastomose to the lower end of the bypass.

The vein may then be dissected upward but left attached to the saphenofemoral junction (Fig. 8–8). The branches of the vein are divided and tied with transfixing sutures of fine nonabsorbable suture material. If small branches are inadvertently avulsed, the hole in the vein wall can best be closed by a longitudinally placed mattress suture that does not produce any narrowing from a purse string effect. The free (distal) end of the vein is now joined to the artery and a temporary arteriovenous shunt is established which will enable the surgeon to distend the vein and locate bleeders, and especially enable him to divide the fine oblique strands of adventitia that constrict the vein graft occasionally. Division of these fibers at critical points affects the diameter and consequently flow through the shunt. By keeping the vein attached to the artery, mishaps are prevented such as placing the vein in the wrong direction or sending it to the laboratory as a specimen. This method may allow "preservation and storage" of the vein in contact with circulating blood and may be the best means of preserving the venous endothelium.

The temporary arteriovenous shunt must not allowed to function for too long a time. Most patients tolerate it well for the few minutes necessary for the preparation of the vein, but one elderly patient demonstrated an alarming tachycardia which was relieved by cross-clamping the arterial input. Root and Cruz[65] recently described the combination of reconstruction with formation of a permanent arteriovenous fistula to correct those situations in which runoff seems inadequate. Despite the objection on theoretical grounds that the ischemia in the distal part of the leg might increase if the shunt diverted too much arterial blood into the venous system, no such instances were found in

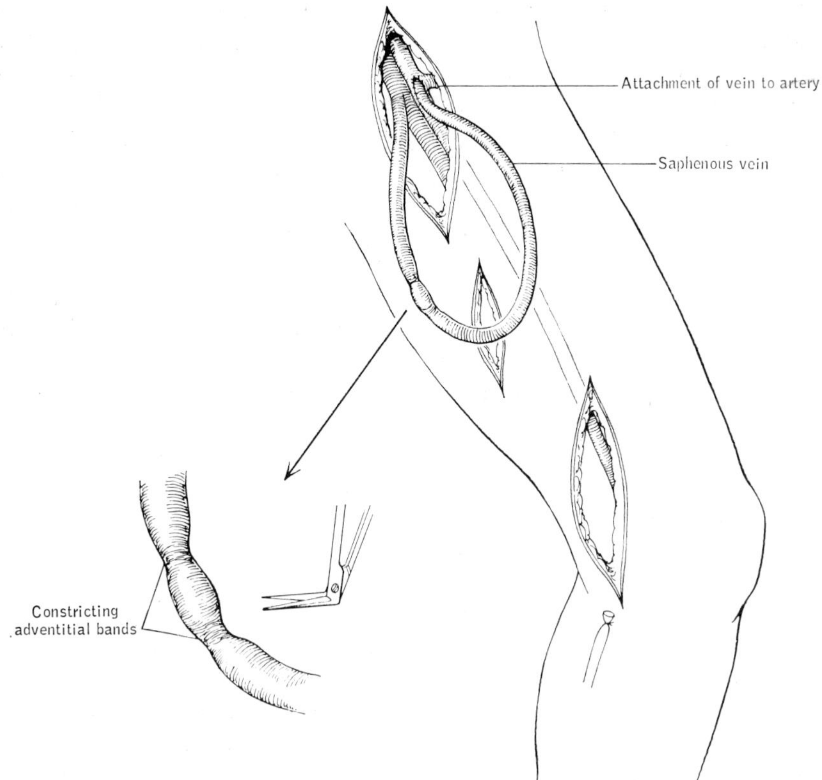

Figure 8–8.   Steps in attachment of saphenous vein, using reversal technique. The distal end of the vein has been divided and the vein has been dissected free from its bed. The distal end of the vein is attached to the artery and flow is established through the vein to distend it with blood. This is a temporary arteriovenous fistula. Constricting adventitial bands can now be seen and can readily be cut with sharp scissors to allow the vein to distend to its maximal diameter. The upper end will then be detached, and the vein will be emptied of blood and reattached to the distal femoropopliteal artery at the site previously chosen.

their series of small shunts. Generalized hemodynamic changes such as cardiac failure were not seen. The known location of the shunt makes it possible to obliterate it, if needed. This procedure deserves further evaluation. It might be added that a similar procedure was advocated in 1914 (without other vascular reconstruction) but was discarded.[37]

The vein is now divided at the saphenofemoral junction, irrigated until free of blood, led through the appropriate tunnel, and anastomosed to the distal artery. One of the disadvantages of this technique lies in the necessity of performing the venoarterial anastomosis deep in the wound with the vein under tension and not free to be displaced from side to side—a maneuver which often makes such an anastomosis easier. If this immobility poses too many technical difficulties in performance of this critical anastomosis, then the upper segment of the vein may be divided just below its site of femoral attachment, the saphenopopliteal anastomosis performed, and the saphenous vein reanastomosed by simple end-to-end suture. Initial anastomosis to the popliteal site is an alternative, but the pressure in the popliteal artery would not ordinarily be sufficient to allow as satisfactory preparation of the vein. This use of the vein as a temporary arteriovenous shunt is not advocated for repairs in the tibial level.

The preferred site of the tunnel for the vein is under the deep fascia, passing under the sartorius muscle similarly to the femoral artery in the normal state. Placed here, it is free from superficial mechanical encroachment, is in a healthy bed, is away from superficial wound infections, and is protected mechanically by the sartorius muscle. This tunnel may be dissected under direct vision, or it may be made blindly with a large olive-tipped dissector.

Following any reconstruction of the femoral artery there was particular reference to a reconstruction following autogenous vein bypass procedures. Porter and others[62] have incriminated operative disruption of the inguinal lymphatics and, to a lesser degree, possibly popliteal lymphatics by removal of the ipsilateral vein at the time of operation. It is this author's observation that the extent of edema often parallels the extent of ischemia prior to operation. Porter could not, however, establish any correlation between the severity of preoperative ischemia and postoperative edema in the absence of inguinal lymphatic disruption. The third possibility which is not in any way an exclusive explanation with regard to the two previous proposals, is that in the presence of severe ischemia of arterial origin there is often smoldering, deep venous thrombosis, in which symptoms may be aggravated by restoration of a high rate of flow to the leg.

Alternative Procedures

The author's choice of reconstructive technique in the absence of a good ipsilateral saphenous vein has altered since 1966. In the following paragraphs will be presented in rough order of choice some comments about the other procedures that may be used.

The contralateral saphenous vein is probably the wisest choice, provided that it is not necessary for reconstruction of the contralateral artery. For instance, the more extensively diseased artery may require the use of the only available good vein, and the less seriously diseased artery may be treated by some other means.

If for some reason the contralateral vein is unavailable, another vein, such as the cephalic, as advocated by Kakkar,[46] Stipa[75] and others, may allow solution of the problem.

The newer plastic prostheses, in particular the velour-covered grafts, may function very well in relatively high flow situations. There is ample precedent for the use of plastic fabric tubes in the experience of DeBakey,[23, 24] Humphries,[42] and Sauvage.[68] The plastic prostheses offer many advantages but, on the other hand, some surgeons have believed them unsatisfactory because of the high rate of late failure. If other measures are not suitable and there is urgency with regard to time, the use of a fabric tube may be appropriate as long as one is willing to accept the higher risk of late occlusion. For example, a plastic tube might be most effective in restoring flow to a limb in which there is advanced distal ischemia, in a patient whose general condition is poor and who cannot tolerate any delay. Necrotic ulcers, gangrenous toes and similar conditions must be treated but in some patients can be expected to heal only after proper vascular treatment. If a plastic tube can be placed one may anticipate healing of such necrotic lesions and, although one might anticipate that failure of the graft at a later date might provoke recurrence of necrosis, this may not occur.

The current availability of long bovine carotid heterografts in diameters small enough to allow good anastomoses to the distal artery makes this material an excellent choice.[66]

The ipsilateral superficial femoral vein can also be used, but the dissection is often unnecessarily traumatic, the caliber is often too great, and its removal may be associated with serious secondary affects. In addition, there is information from Vietnam suggesting that ipsilateral vein removal may endanger vascular reconstructions, at least in the face of trauma, not only because of decreased venous return per se but also because of decreased femoral artery flow.[40]

The construction of a tube from nonvascular tissue such as fascia lata is mainly experimental and should be considered only as a last resort. On the other hand, Eiken,[31] Parsonnet[60] and Sparks [73, 74] have been working with tubes created by autologous collagen around mandrils of silastic rubber placed in the tissue. The initial tubes seemed to be too weak to allow proper support on intraluminal pressure, and currently the method is modified to allow a plastic fabric sheath to be placed around the tube. The tube and plastic sheath form a new artery in which the plastic fabric is incorporated in the collagenous wall of the artery. When the graft has matured, and this may take six weeks, the edges of the tube are dissected free, the mandril withdrawn and the neoartery anastomosed to the host artery by standard techniques. Tubes smaller than 5 millimeters are not very satisfactorily maintained under these techniques but, according to Parsonnet, the smaller tubes fail at the region of the suture line and not in the center of the graft. Infrequently, when one can delay the definitive operation for six weeks, a graft of this kind may be used, hence the clinical applicability of this method may be somewhat limited, but under circumstances allowing the time, the procedure deserves further evaluation.

The use of saphenous vein homografts offers another possible alternative although clinical experience is limited.[61, 82]

As a general principle, Taylor[81] has recommended simultaneous local amputation and revision of wounds or unhealed amputations at the time of reconstruction in order to accomplish healing as expeditiously as possible lest subsequent failure of the reconstruction occur.

The plastic is, however, particularly hazardous in the presence of sepsis, and septic areas in the distal extremities should be drained meticulously before inserting a plastic prosthesis. The graft must also be employed with full recognition that infection developing at the site of reconstruction would usually necessitate removal of the graft and possible amputation of a leg.

The author's choice of plastic prostheses are, in order: the Sauvage velour graft, the Wesolowski graft, the woven microcrimped DeBakey Dacron graft, and the Szilagyi-Sidebotham Helanca graft. From one point of view it is desirable to insert as little foreign matter as possible, but the difference between the finest Szilagyi graft and the heaviest knitted tube is not great. The quality of elasticity is helpful during placement, but most of the fibers ultimately become elongated and are subject to kinking unless the graft is inserted under maximal tension, or inserted in such a way as to allow quite generous arcing curves. Neither elasticity nor crimping guarantees total freedom from kinking on flexion and extension in long term use. The matter of strength in the graft is important. At 10 years some of the finer Dacron grafts begin to lose a serious amount of tensile strength. In many ways, however, the choice of one graft material over the other is a matter of personal preference. The only objective information about the greater value of one is that provided by Sauvage, indicating that at least experimentally and in some clinical circumstances the external velour surface does provide complete endothelialization. The Sparks-Parsonnet collagenized Dacron tube deserves consideration here if time allows its use.

If one chooses not to place a plastic graft then one might attempt endarterectomy just so long as the attempt does no harm locally and does not prolong the operation in a poor-risk patient. Such a choice is now described.

K.M., a 64-year-old woman, was operated upon because of impending gangrene of the leg. Because of her feeble condition and preoperative arteriographic demonstration of a poor popliteal runoff, it was decided to use an *in situ* saphenous vein bypass. At operation, however, the vein was not of an entirely satisfactory caliber, and the popliteal artery itself was atherosclerotic throughout. During attempts to perform local endarterectomy so as to provide a satisfactory vessel for anastomosis, the popliteal atheroma was freed in one piece and a vigorous backflow was obtained. Operative angiograms indicated satisfactory runoff, much better than had been anticipated on preoperative arteriography. Because the atheroma had been mobilized so readily, the surgeon passed a loop dissector upward and found that it could be passed easily to the level of the common femoral artery. The operation was completed quickly with a short incision in the groin and removal of the sequestrum through a short incision in the common femoral artery. Excellent flow was restored and a good pulse promptly returned to the foot.

Sometimes vein bypass and vein onlay patch and endarterectomy are combined (Fig. 8–4C);[18] in fact, Edwards[30] argues that if the endarterectomy is over 6 inches in length the combined procedure is superior. Endarterectomy is particularly suitable in regard to restoration of flow into major collaterals. Bypass around a joint is subject to repeated flexion of the joint, and endarterectomy is preferable in this area. A vein graft is more satisfactory than is the plastic prosthesis in an area of flexion; nevertheless it is sometimes possible to use a vein as the origin for the bypass in the upper thigh, lead it down into the lower thigh as a bypass under the sartorius muscle, and apply it to the distal femoropopliteal segment to restore flow into the major genicular collaterals and into the upper popliteal artery. The distal portion therefore serves as a vein patch. This combined procedure requires less operating time than endarterectomy and vein patch, performed separately, yet is adequate provided the vein is of sufficient size. If the vein is too narrow, it too can be patched (Fig. 8–9), simply increasing the operative time to what would be needed to perform a full open endarterectomy and vein patch. When there is a defect in the femoral artery and bypass is mandatory, a secondary patch may be applied to widen the saphenous vein. The case report material below illustrates this point.

The patient was a 59-year-old man, who was vigorous and active except for symptoms referable to his legs. Arteriogram revealed aortic and iliac arterial stenosis; occlusion was almost complete on the right side. There was extensive left femoral occlusion, but the distal popliteal artery was patent. Aortoiliac reconstruction was performed by endarterectomy and bilateral lumbar sympathectomy without difficulty, but as there still appeared to be serious limitation resulting from the occlusion in the left femoral artery, the thigh was opened. Endarterectomy was undertaken, but the stripper could not be passed for more than a few centimeters down the superficial femoral artery. The artery was opened at the knee and the stripper could be passed up for perhaps 5 inches, but then met a firm obstruction. The artery was exposed, and it was evident that a severe inflammatory process had destroyed the normal planes of dissection. Bypass appeared to be necessary. The saphenous vein was dissected out and placed as a patch graft on the distal common femoral and proximal superficial femoral arteries. It was then led as a bypass under the sartorius muscle and joined as a patch graft onto the distal femoral and proximal popliteal arteries. The mid-segment of this vein was exceedingly small, and although flow seemed satisfactory at first, it failed within minutes. The only defect apparent was the extremely narrow junction of the upper segment of vein patch and the bypass. Additional saphenous vein was available; the vein bypass was split longitudinally and a segment of saphenous vein was inserted to widen the vessel (Fig. 8–9). There was now ample flow through the reconstructed vein.

If it becomes necessary to use a prosthetic graft for a long stretch in the leg, short segments of vein may be available from other areas. Short segments of saphenous vein attached to the distal host artery and passing across the crease of the knee joint combined with the Dacron tube may provide a very useful composite graft.[54]

Another alternative, when no single vein is long enough to bridge the entire length of the leg, involves the utilization of sequential bypasses as described by De Laurentis.[25] Here a short graft may bridge from femoral to midpopliteal artery, for instance, and an-

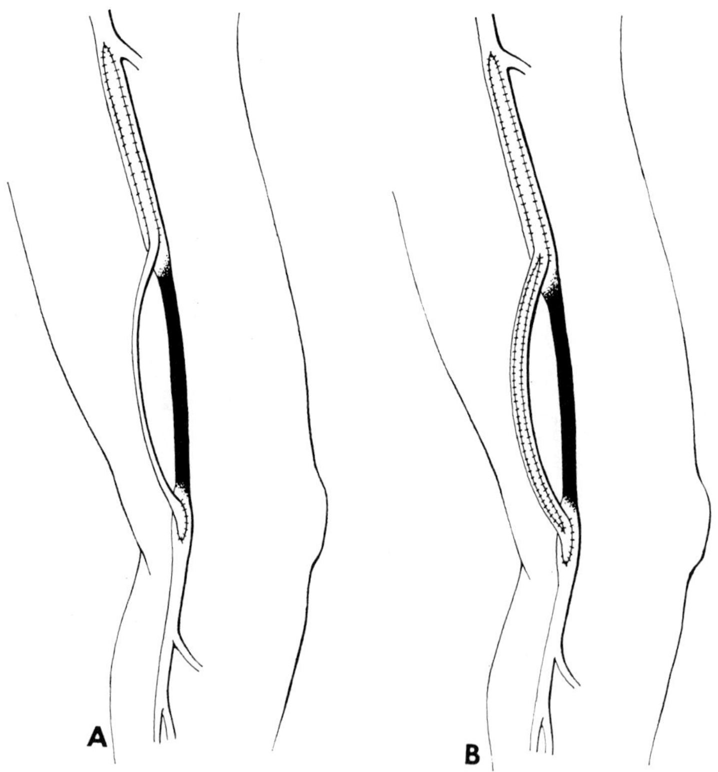

Figure 8–9. *A,* Saphenous vein was used partly as an onlay patch in the upper part of the reconstruction where endarterectomy was performed. *B,* In the lower portion the vein was used as a bypass graft but was too small to support adequate flow. A further length of saphenous vein was available and was used. It was used here as a patch to widen the vein and as a patch on the bypass graft itself.

other shorter graft from the distal popliteal to one of the tibial branches. Under these circumstances it might be possible even to use a fabric tube as the upper segment. Use of this sequential bypass might avoid problems seen in such patients as the one described below.

T.A., a 72-year-old man, was admitted because of gangrenous patches of skin over several areas in the leg and several gangrenous toes. Arteriogram indicated that there was some flow into the superficial femoral artery but, with the exception of a mere trickle at the popliteal segment, the first artery of consequence appeared near the ankle. A long graft was carried from the upper superficial femoral artery to the dorsalis pedis artery. The graft functioned very well. The ulcers in the distal half of the leg healed, and the foot became hot and the toes healed. Gangrene proceeded, however, in the muscles of the calf of the upper part of the lower leg, forcing ultimate amputation through the low thigh and a functioning venous graft, although the foot healed and remained well until the time of amputation.

ISOLATED PROFUNDOPLASTY

As previously indicated on page 188, Beales,[8] Martin,[55] Kiely,[48] Miller,[57] Cohn[14] and others have recognized the importance of repair of the profunda femoris artery when no other suitable reconstruction can be performed because of lack of an outflow tract. The artery is exposed through an incision over the femoral triangle and carefully dissected distally as far as is necessary. If the artery is very large simple endarterectomy is all that need be performed, and this may be carried down as far as the second or third major branch of the deep femoral artery. If the artery is narrow, the placement of a patch to widen the artery may be a better procedure, whether it be associated with endarterectomy or not. This may allow excellent flow into the proximal branches arising from this segment. Great care must be taken to be sure that the actual orifice from the common femoral artery is widely patent, and at times it is advisable to place a patch in this area to be sure of that widening.

Of great aid in the performance of this operation is accurate demonstration of the extent of the disease in the deep femoral artery itself. This can be done if the superficial femoral artery is partially patent, and therefore overlying the orifice of the deep femoral if an oblique view is taken to open out the angle between the two vessels according to the techniques described by Beales[8] and by Martin.[55]

PERCUTANEOUS TRANSLUMINAL ARTERIAL DILATATION

Under some circumstances a major surgical operation necessary to correct a very minor stenosis in a superficial femoral artery seems much too large for the benefit to be gained. This is particularly true if the patient has some other complicating disease limiting major anesthesiology techniques. Dotter's[27, 28] technique for percutaneous dilatation of such vessels has caused great interest. A stiff catheter capable of dilating a narrowed atherosclerotic cleft is passed forcibly through the stenotic area after the catheter has been inserted in the artery under angiographic control through a percutaneous femoral puncture. Longer segments are difficult to dilate, as are totally occluded segments, although Dotter has had some success in this, perhaps because of his greater experience.

The procedure must be done with extreme care because of the risk of dislodging a plaque. The surgeon finds it difficult to be sure that all intimal fragments are clearly dissected free or else sutured in place, even when the artery has been widely opened at operation. If any arterial debris remains in the lumen, thrombosis is likely to follow. Simple manipulation of the artery from the outside is apt to dislodge a plaque, and even soft catheters passing down the lumen of an artery may easily pass under a plaque and cause a total obstruc-

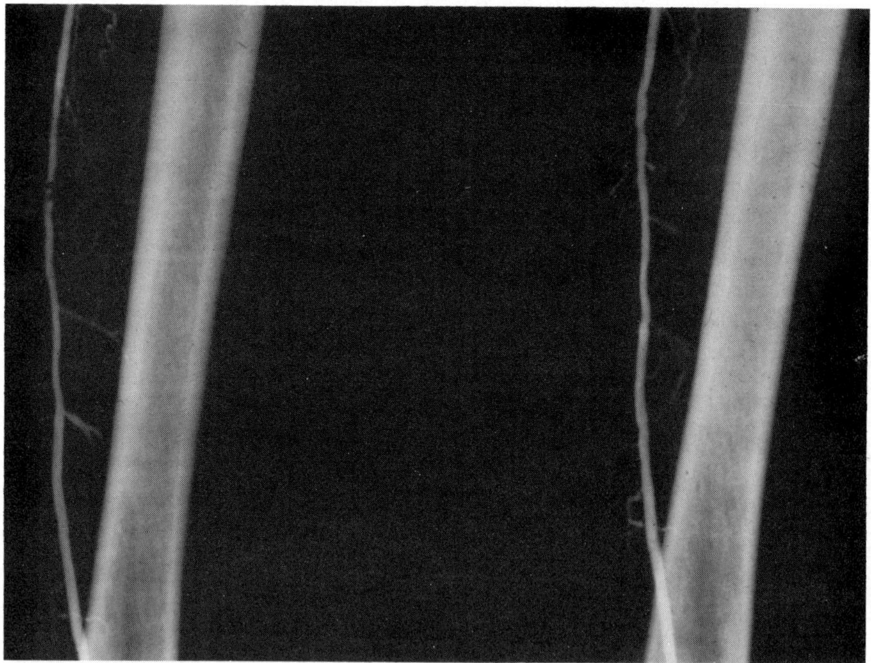

Figure 8–10. The left-hand figure shows a short stenosis in the midportion of the superficial femoral artery in a 51-year-old man who was a poor surgical candidate. Following Dotter dilatation an arteriogram was performed. The dilatation of the vessel is shown in right-hand figure. This represents the ideal candidate and the ideal result for the Dotter technique.

tion of the artery. It is, therefore, of greatest importance that this procedure be done by someone who is trained and skilled in its use, and that it be done under optimal conditions of fluoroscopic control. It is undoubtedly a technique which should be explored by more surgeons in cooperation with the radiologists, because when properly done in the correct patients it can produce considerable relief at the expenditure of minimal risk (See Fig. 8–10).

SUMMARY

Treatment of femoral artery obstruction is more difficult than treatment of aortic or iliac occlusion. This is so because the smaller vessel is occluded over a longer distance, with consequent decreased rate of flow, and because in femoral disease there is a greater risk of more diffuse systemic involvement. The treatment of obstructions of the femoral arteries requires greater experience and skill than does the treatment of obstructions in the larger and more proximal vessels. These comments with regard to femorotibial reconstructions are even more cogent.

REFERENCES

1. Assefi, I., and Parsonnet, V.: An arterial prosthesis composed of an autogenous fibrocollagenous tube with incorporated polypropylene mesh. J. Newark, Beth Israel Hospital *15*:161, 1964.
2. Barcroft, H., and Swan, H. J. C.: *Sympathetic Control of Human Blood Vessels.* London, Edward Arnold, Ltd., 1953.
3. Barker, W. F.: Distal angiography as an aid in endarterectomy. Surgery *36*:233, 1954.
4. Barker, W. F.: Complications in arterial surgery. *In* Dale, W. A. (Ed.): *Management of Arterial Occlusive Disease.* Chicago, Year Book Medical Publishers, 1971.
5. Barker, W. F., and Cannon, J. A.: An evaluation of endarterectomy. Arch. Surg. *66*:488, 1953.
6. Barner, H. A., DeWeese, J. A., and Schenk, E. A.: Fresh and frozen homologous venous grafts for arterial repair. Angiology *17*:389, 1966.
7. Bazy, L., Huguier, J., Reboul, H., and Laubry, P.: Technique des "endartériectomies" pour artérites oblitérantes chroniques des membres inférieurs des iliaques et de l'aorte abdominale inférieure. J. Chir. *65*:196, 1949.
8. Beales, J. S. M., Adcock, F. A., Frawley, J. F., Nathan, B. E., McLachlan, M. S. F., Martin, P., and Steiner, R. E.: The radiologic assessment of disease of the profunda femoris artery. Brit. J. Radiol. *44*:854, 1971.
9. Bernhard, V. M., Ashmore, C. S., Rodgers, R. E., and Evans, W. E.: Operative blood flow in femoral-popliteal and femoral-tibial grafts for lower extremity ischemia. Arch. Surg. *103*:595, 1971.
10. Cannon, J. A.: In discussion of paper by Dale, W. A., DeWeese, J. A., and Scott, W. J. M.: Autogenous venous shunt grafts. Surgery *46*:145, 1959.
11. Cannon, J. A. *A Current Technique of Aortoiliac and Femoropopliteal Endarterectomy for Obliterative Atherosclerosis.* Springfield, Ill., Charles C Thomas, 1965.

12. Cannon, J. A., and Barker, W. F.: Successful management of femoral arteriosclerosis by endarterectomy. Surgery 38:48, 1955.
13. Cannon, J. A.: Surgical judgement in vascular surgery. Arch. Surg. 103:521, 1971.
14. Cohn, L. H., Trueblood, W., and Crowley, L. G.: Profunda femoris reconstruction in the treatment of femoral popliteal occlusive disease. Arch. Surg. 103:475, 1971.
15. Connolly, J. E., and Harris, E. J.: Autogenous in situ saphenous bypass for femoro-popliteal occlusive disease; a follow up study. Am. J. Surg. 110:270, 1965.
16. Connolly, J. E., Harris, E. J., and Mills, W. Jr.: Autogenous in situ saphenous vein for bypass of femoro-popliteal obliterative disease. Surgery 55:144, 1964.
17. Crawford, E. S., DeBakey, M. E., Cooley, D. A., and Morris, G. C. Jr.: Use of crimped, knitted dacron grafts in patients with occlusive disease of the aorta and of the iliac, femoral and popliteal arteries. In Wesolowski, S. A., and Dennis, C.: *Fundamentals of Vascular Grafting*. New York, McGraw-Hill Book Co., Inc., 1963.
18. Dale, W. A.: *Autogenous Vein Grafts*. Springfield, Ill., Charles C Thomas, 1959.
19. Dale, W. A.: Autogenous venous grafts. In Wesolowski, S. A., and Dennis, C.: *Fundamentals of Vascular Grafting*. New York, McGraw-Hill Book Co., Inc., 1963.
20. Dale, W.: Grafting small arteries: experience with 19 shunts below the knee. Arch. Surg. 86:22, 1963.
21. Darling, R. C., and Linton, R. R.: Aortoiliofemoral endarterectomy for atherosclerotic occlusive disease. Surgery 55:184, 1964.
22. Darling, R. C., and Linton, R. R.: Management of the late failure of arterial reconstruction of the lower extremities. New Eng. J. Med. 270:609, 1964.
23. DeBakey, M. E., Crawford, E. S., Morris, G. C. Jr., and Cooley, D. A.: Surgical treatment of chronic occlusive disease of the aorta and major arterial. In Lewis, D. D. W.: *Practice of Surgery*. Hagerstown, Md., W. F. Prior Co., 1949.
24. DeBakey, M. E., Jordan, G. L. Jr., Abbott, J. P., Halpert, B., and O'Neal, R. M.: The fate of dacron vascular grafts. Arch. Surg. 89:757, 1964.
25. De Laurentis, D. A., and Friedmann, P.: Sequential femoropopliteal bypasses: another approach to inadequate saphenous vein problem. Surgery 71:400, 1972.
26. dos Santos, J.: Sur la Désobstruction des thromboses artérielles anciennes. Mém. Acad. Chir. 73:409, 1947.
27. Dotter, C. T., and Judkins, M. P.: Transluminal treatment of arteriosclerotic obstruction: description of a new technique, and a preliminary report of its application. Circulation 30:654, 1964.
28. Dotter, C. T., and Rosch, J.: Transluminal angioplasty—the catheter treatment of peripheral arterial obstruction. *In* Dale, W. A. (Ed.): *Management of Arterial Occlusive Disease*. Chicago, Year Book Medical Publishers Inc., 1971.
29. Edwards, W. S.: Personal communication.
30. Edwards, W. S.: Composite reconstruction of the femoral artery with saphenous vein after endarterectomy. Surg. Gynec. Obstet. 111:651, 1960.
31. Eiken, O., and Norden, G.: Bridging small artery defects in the dog with in situ performed autologous connective tissue tubes. Acta Chir. Scand. 121:90–102, 1960.
32. Elkin, D. C.: Exposure of blood vessels. J.A.M.A. 132:421, 1946.
33. Elkin, D. C., and Kelly, R. P.: Arteriovenous aneurysms: exposure of the tibial and peroneal vessels by resection of the fibula. Ann. Surg. 122:529, 1945.
34. Garrett, H. E., Kotch, P. I., Green, M. T., Jr., Diethrich, E. B., and DeBakey, M. E.: Distal tibial artery bypass with autogenous vein grafts. Analysis of 56 cases. Surgery 63:90, 1968.
35. Gutelius, J. R., Kreindler, S., and Luke, J. C.: Comparative evaluation of autogenous vein bypass graft and endarterectomy in superficial femoral artery reconstruction. Surgery 57:28, 1965.
36. Hall, K. V.: The greater saphenous vein used in situ as an arterial shunt after vein valve extirpation. Acta Chir. Scand. 128:365, 1964.
37. Halstead, A. E., and Vaughan, R. T.: Arteriovenous anastomosis in the treatment of gangrene of the extremities. Surg. Gynec. Obstet. 14:1, 1912.

38. Henry, A. K.: *Extensile Exposure*. 2nd Ed. Baltimore, Williams and Wilkins Company, 1957.
39. Hines, E. Jr., and Barker, N.: Arteriosclerosis obliterans: clinical and pathologic study. Am. J. Med. Sci. *200*:717, 1940.
40. Hobson, R. W., Howard, E. W., Wright, C. B., Collin, G. J., and Rich, N. M.: Pathophysiology of venous ligation: significance in combined arterial/venous injuries. Surgery *74*:824, 1973.
41. Holden, W. D.: Reconstruction of the femoral artery for arteriosclerotic thrombosis. Surgery *27*:417, 1950.
42. Humphries, A. W., deWolfe, V. G., Young, J. R., and LeFevre, F. A.: Evaluation of the natural history and the results of treatment in occlusive arteriosclerosis involving the lower extremities in 1850 patients. *In* Wesolowski, S. A., and Dennis, C.: *Fundamentals of Vascular Grafting*. New York, McGraw-Hill Book Co., Inc., 1963.
43. Imparato, I. M., Kim, G. E., Madayag, M., and Haveson, S.: Angiographic criteria for successful below knee arterial reconstruction. Surgery *74*:830, 1973.
44. Julian, O. C.: In Wesolowski, S. A., and Dennis, C.: *Fundamentals of Vascular Grafting*. New York, McGraw-Hill Book Co., Inc., 1963.
45. Julian, O. C., Dye, W. S. Jr., Olwin, J. H., and Jordan, P. H.: Direct surgery of arteriosclerosis. Ann. Surg. *136*:459, 1952.
46. Kakkar, V. V.: The cephalic vein as a peripheral vascular graft. Surg. Gynec. Obstet. *128*:551, 1969.
47. Kaminski, D. L., Barner, H. B., Dorighi, J. A., Kaiser, G. C., and Willman, V. L.: Femoral-tibial bypass grafting. Arch. Surg. *104*:527, 1972.
48. Kiely, P. E., Lumley, J. S. P., and Taylor, G. W.: Extended endarterectomy of the profunda femoris artery. Arch. Surg. *106*:605, 1973.
49. Kunlin, J.: Le traitement de l'ischémie artéritique par la greffe veineuse longue. Rev. Chir. Paris *70*:206, 1951.
50. Lazzarini-Robertson, A. A., Jr.: Hemodynamic principles and end-to-side vascular anastomoses. Arch. Surg. *82*:384, 1961.
51. LeFevre, F., Corbacioglu, C., Humphries, A., and deWolfe, V.: Management of arteriosclerosis obliterans of the extremities. J.A.M.A. *170*:656, 1959.
52. LeVeen, H. H.: Technical features in endarterectomy. Surgery *57*:22, 1965.
53. Linton, R. R.: Some practical considerations in surgery of blood vessel grafts. Surgery *38*:817, 1955.
54. Linton, R. R., and Wirthlin, L. S.: Composite Dacron and autogenous vein-femoral popliteal bypass graft. A preliminary report. Arch. Surg. *107*:748, 1973.
55. Martin, P., Frawley, J. F., Barabas, A. P., and Rosengarten, D. S.: On the surgery of the profunda femoris artery. Surgery *71*:182, 1972.
56. May, A. G., DeWeese, J. A., and Rob, C. G.: The arterialized in situ saphenous vein. Arch. Surg. *91*:743, 1965.
57. Miller, T., Niazmand, R., and Barker, W. F.: Femoral artery reconstruction under local anesthesia. Maximal results from minimal risks. Am. J. Surg. *122*:513, 1971.
58. Morris, G. C. Jr., DeBakey, M. E., Cooley, D. A., and Crawford, E. S.: Arterial bypass below the knee. Surg. Gynec. Obstet. *108*:321, 1959.
59. Nicholas, G. G., Barker, C. F., Berkowitz, H. D., and Roberts, B.: The effect of reconstructive surgery distal to the popliteal trifurcation on the natural history of arterial occlusive disease. Arch. Surg. *107*:652, 1973.
60. Parsonnet, V., Alpert, J., and Brief, D. K.: Autogenous polypropylene-supported collagen tubes for long term arterial replacement. Surgery *70*:935, 1971.
61. Perloff, L. J., Reckard, C. R., Rowlands, D. T., Jr., and Barker, C. F.: The venous homograft, an immunological question. Surgery *72*:961, 1972.
62. Porter, J. M., Lindell, T. D., and Lakin, P. C.: Leg edema following femoral popliteal autogenous vein bypass. Arch. Surg. *105*:883, 1972.
63. Reichle, F. A., and Stewart, G. J.: A transmission and scanning electron microscope study of linings of Dacron and autogenous vein bypass grafts. Surgery, *74*:945, 1973.
64. Rob, C. G.: In Wesolowski, S. A., and Dennis, C.: *Fundamentals of Vascular Grafting*. New York, McGraw-Hill Book Co., Inc., 1963.

65. Root, H. D., and Cruz, A. B. Jr.: Effects of an arteriovenous fistula on the devascularized limb. J.A.M.A. *191*:645, 1965.
66. Rosenberg, D. M. L., Glass, B. A., Rosenberg, N., Lewis, M. R., and Dale, W. A.: Experience with modified bovine carotid arteries in arterial surgery. Surgery 68: 1064, 1970.
67. Sacks, S. A., Petritsch, P. H., and Kaufman, J. J.: Canine kidney preservation using a new perfusate. Lancet *1*:1024, 1973.
68. Sauvage, L. R., Berger, K., Wood, F. J., Nakagawa, Y., and Mansfield, P. B.: An external velour surface for porous arterial prostheses. Surgery 70:940, 1971.
69. Sawyer, P. N., Pasupathy, C. E., Fitzgerald, J., Kaplitt, M. J., Costello, N., Keates, J. R. W., O'Malley, G., and Lapousky, A.: Six year follow-up study in the use of gas endarterectomy. Surgery 72:837, 1972.
70. Schilling, F. A., Shurley, H. M., Joel, W., Richter, K. M., and White, B. N.: Fibrocollagenous tubes structured in vivo. Arch. Pathol. *71*:5, 1961.
71. Shepherd, J. T.: *Physiology of the Circulation in Human Limbs in Health and Disease.* Philadelphia, W. B. Saunders Co., 1963.
72. Sobel, S., Kaplitt, M. J., and Sawyer, P. N.: Gas endarterectomy. Surgery 59:517, 1966.
73. Sparks, C. H.: Die-grown reinforced arterial grafts: observation in long term animal grafts in clinical experience. Ann. Surg. *172*:787, 1970.
74. Sparks, C. H.: Silicone mandril method for growing reinforced autogenous femoral-popliteal artery grafts in situ. Ann. Surg. *177*:293, 1973.
75. Stipa, S.: The cephalic and basilic veins in peripheral arterial reconstructive surgery. Ann. Surg. *175*:581, 1972.
76. Stoney, R. J., Albo, R. J., and Wylie, E. J.: False aneurysms occurring after arterial grafting operations. Amer. J. Surg. *110*:153, 1965.
77. Stoney, R. J., James, D. R., and Wylie, E. J.: Surgery for femoral popliteal atherosclerosis. A reappraisal. Arch. Surg. *103*:548, 1971.
78. Szilagyi, D. E.: In Wesolowski, S. A., and Dennis, C.: *Fundamentals of Vascular Grafting.* New York, McGraw-Hill Book Co., Inc., 1963.
79. Szilagyi, D. E., McDonald, R. T., Smith, R. F., and Whitcomb, J. G.: A study of the biologic fate of human arterial homografts. Arch. Surg. 75:506, 1957.
80. Szilagyi, D. E., Smith, R. F., Elliott, J. P., and Vrandecic, M. T.: Infection in arterial reconstruction with synthetic grafts. Ann. Surg. *176*:321, 1972.
81. Taylor, G. A.: personal communication.
82. Tice, D. A., and Santoni, E.: The use of saphenous vein homografts for arterial reconstruction. Surgery 67:493, 1970.
83. Tomatis, L. A., Fierens, E. E., and Verbrugge, J. P.: Evaluation of surgical risk in peripheral vascular disease by coronary angiography: a series of 100 cases. Surgery 71:429, 1972.
84. Tyson, R. R., and De Laurentis, D.: Femoro-tibial bypass. Circulation 33:183, 1966.
85. Tyson, R. R., and Reichle, F. A.: Femorotibial bypass. Ann. Surg. *170*:429, 1969.
86. Van de Water, J. M., and Gaal, P. G.: Management of patients with infected vascular prostheses. Am. Surgeon *31*:651, 1965.
87. Vollmar, J., Trede, M., Laubach, K., and Forrest, H.: Principles of reconstructive procedures for chronic femoropopliteal occlusions: report on 546 operations. Ann. Surg., *168*:215, 1968.
88. Wylie, E., Kerr, E., and Davies, O.: Experimental and clinical experiences with use of fascia lata applied as graft about major arteries after thromboendarterectomy and aneurysmorrhaphy. Surg. Gynec. Obstet. 93:257, 1951.

Chapter Nine

TREATMENT OF COMBINED AORTOILIAC FEMOROPOPLITEAL LESIONS

The two preceding chapters have detailed the exposures and techniques which are useful in performing surgery on either the aorta and the iliac arteries, or on the femoral popliteal and tibial branches. The techniques for combined aortoiliac and femoropopliteal lesions are the same.

MAGNITUDE OF COMBINED LESIONS

Combined aortoiliac femoropopliteal lesions are considered apart from others because of the increased severity of disease, the more extensive operation, and the complications. The extent of the lesion necessitates longer and more complicated operation with greater tissue dissection; the more diffuse arterial involvement implies that the patient's status is more fragile and that any type of operation involves a greater mortality risk. The older age of the patient parallels the more extensive, diffuse disease (Table 5–1). Furthermore, such extensive lesions invariably require exposure in the groin, and the groin has been implicated by Szilagyi[7] as one of the critical sites in which arterial infections arise.

Several possible variations and combinations of technique may be utilized. These are summarized in Table 9–1, which summarizes our experience in the early years, 1955–1961. There were 12 acute

Table 9–1. Summary of Operative Procedures for
Combined Lesions (1955–1961)

Unstaged Procedures	43	
Aortofemoral graft (with resection of aortic aneurysm) plus partial superficial endarterectomy	6	
(no early failures)		
Aortofemoral bypass grafts with common femoral endarterectomy	6	
(acute failure and death)		1
Aortofemoral bypass graft with superficial femoral endarterectomy	3	
(acute failure)		1
Aortofemoropopliteal bypass graft	2	
(acute failure, one side)		1
(operative death)		1
Aortoiliac femoral endarterectomy	25*	
(acute failures, one death)		2†
(operative deaths)		4
Iliofemoral endarterectomy	1	
(failure)		1
	43	11
Staged Operations	15	
Staged operations completed	4	
H.D. (1) Aortoiliac and right superficial femoral endarterectomy followed by (2) right external iliac and left superficial femoral endarterectomy.		
E.G. (1) Aortoiliac and right superficial femoral endarterectomy followed by (2) left superficial femoral endarterectomy (second side failed early).		
C.Z. (1) aortoiliac endarterectomy followed by (2) left external iliac to superficial femoral endarterectomy.		
E.T. (1) Aortoiliac and left superficial femoral endarterectomy followed by (2) right superficial femoral endarterectomy.		
Staged operations planned but only one stage completed	11	
Aortofemoral grafts; femoral disease not treated—	5	
early failure (one arm of graft, on side of femoral occlusion);		1
late failure (one arm of graft, on side of femoral occlusion)		2
Aortoiliac or aortoiliac-common femoral endarterectomy	3	
early failure		1
Distal reconstruction without proximal operation		
Femoropopliteal endarterectomy	2	
Failure		1†
Failure (and death)		1
Femoropopliteal venous bypass	1	
	11	6

*Two patients had composite vein patch procedures (Fig. 8–3*E*).

†Two patients listed as acute failures were reoperated upon and successfully restored for 1½ and 3 years, respectively (to last follow-up date).

failures (involving at least one leg), with three deaths. Five other patients died during surgery or in the early postoperative period. The survivors have been followed up to 9 years (four patients), with an average survival of over 3 years. The long survivals in this group present a challenge to the surgeon to undertake reconstruction; an improved mortality rate and acute success rate must be sought.

As a rule, we have been cautious about applying aggressive surgical treatment in the presence of extensive arteriosclerotic lesions or advanced disease of another nature elsewhere in the body. This caution results from our earlier experience with arterial reconstruction, an example of which is presented.

I.M., a 63-year-old man who had no symptoms of hypertension or myocardial disease, entered for treatment of bilateral hip and thigh claudication. Bilateral lumbar sympathectomy and endarterectomy from the aortic to the popliteal artery was done. The operation was lengthy, requiring more than 6 hours, but there were no episodes of hemorrhage or significant hypotension.

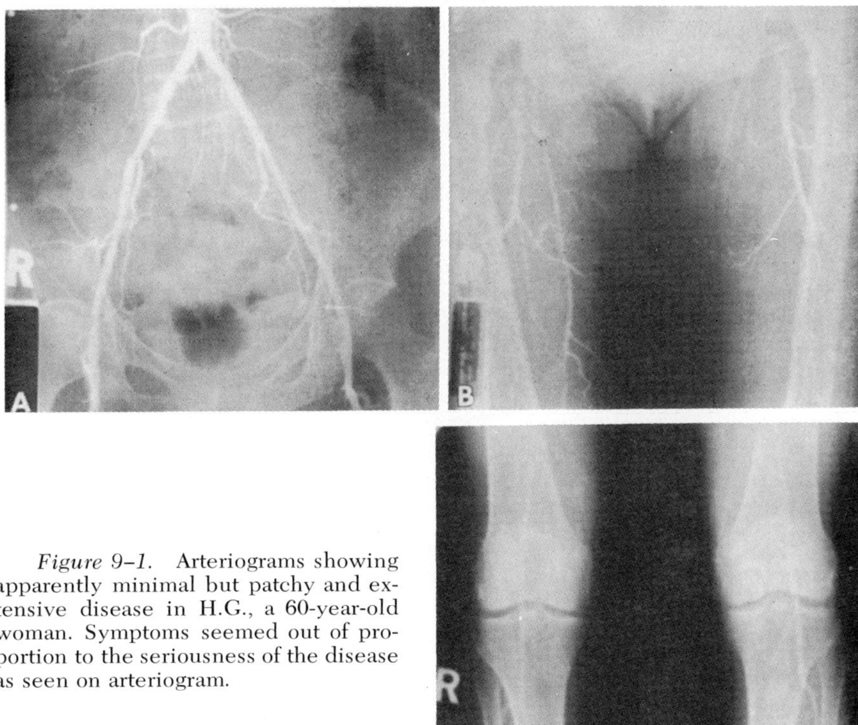

Figure 9–1. Arteriograms showing apparently minimal but patchy and extensive disease in H.G., a 60-year-old woman. Symptoms seemed out of proportion to the seriousness of the disease as seen on arteriogram.

The patient made a prompt and uneventful recovery and was discharged from the hospital 10 days later, having strong bilateral pedal pulses. A few days after discharge he was found dead, having had a massive myocardial infarction.

As a rule, endarterectomy or bypass in one stage from aorta to popliteal artery carries a serious risk to the patient. The kind of operation often encountered is represented by the following cases, the first of which represented our first successful endarterectomy.

J.W., a 56-year-old woman with a history of previous myocardial infarction, entered for treatment of claudication in the left hip and thigh and early gangrenous changes in the left toes. In October, 1951, endarterectomy was performed from aortoiliac to the middle segment of the left superficial femoral artery, as well as bilateral lumbar sympathectomy. A small aortic aneurysm was endarterectomized, plicated, and wrapped in fascia lata. The patient maintained strong pedal pulses until her death 9½ years later, during which time she had two major strokes and an episode of occlusion of the right superficial femoral artery.

H.G., a 60-year-old woman, was admitted because of claudication in the hip and calf bilaterally which restricted her walking to less than a block. No pulses could be detected in her legs or feet; and there were no trophic changes. Arteriograms revealed extensive patchy incomplete occlusion of the aorta and the iliac and femoral system (Fig. 9–1). Bilateral lumbar sympathectomy and endarterectomy of the aorta and the iliac and common femoral arteries were done. The degree of obstruction and the pathologic changes in the vessels were much more severe than had been apparent on arteriography. The procedure had gone well and the surgeon therefore undertook blind stripping into the superficial femoral arteries; he removed a core that had a texture like firm rubber the size of which was consistent with what had been seen on roentgenography (Fig. 9–2). The specimen had a smooth pointed tip that suggested it was completely removed.

The operation lasted 5 hours, and 2 units of blood were transfused. The patient made a prompt and uneventful recovery; she was discharged on the seventh day. At last report, 9 months later, she is in excellent health, having adequate pedal pulses, normal oscillometric excursions, and complete relief of claudication.

The introduction of a Dacron bifurcation graft which might allow, in one operation, sequential anastomoses from aorta to femoral system to popliteal system had seemed to make the lengthy operative obstructions seem far less formidable.[4] The results, however, have not been as satisfactory as had been anticipated.[2, 3] Early in our experience, with seven patients undergoing this procedure there was only one patient in whom the pedal pulses were preserved for a year, and the mortality risk seemed excessive.

On the basis of this experience we have restricted the arterial reconstructions involving the great distances from the iliac system to the femoral system and then into the popliteal or tibial system to staged procedures wherever possible. One of the few exceptions to this has been the circumstance in which it has been unequivocally

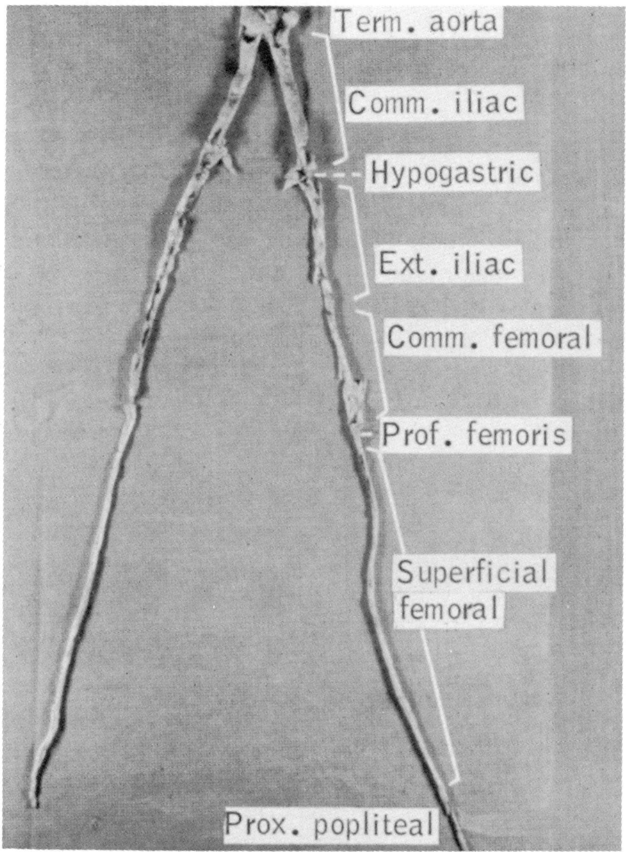

Figure 9–2.   Specimen (restored) after removal by endarterectomy on patient H.G., whose arteriograms are shown in Figure 9–1. Operation resulted in complete relief of symptoms.

necessary to extend the operation to an open outflow tract in the distal leg in order to keep an aortofemoral reconstruction open and keep a limb alive. As a rule this circumstance does not occur in the usual forms of occlusive disease. It is probable that the effectiveness of the deep femoral system as a collateral station allows one to restore flow into the deep femoral system with great success. There are many circumstances, for instance, in which restoration of flow into a large profunda femoris system allows clear return of excellent pressures at the ankle as well as palpable pulses, with total relief of symptoms. This is characterized by the following case report.

M.D., a 57-year-old woman, was admitted to the hospital because of serious claudication limiting her walking distance to 50 feet. Arteriography indicated that she had extensive atherosclerosis of the aortoiliac bifurcation and bilateral superficial femoral artery occlusion. Both profunda femoris arteries filled from the iliac system; also, they were very large in size and through quite large collaterals refilled the popliteal system (similar to those shown in Fig. 9–3). On this basis the patient underwent an aortoiliac endarterectomy and bilateral lumbar sympathectomy. On discharge, her symptoms were completely relieved and she had bilaterally palpable pedal pulses.

We now prefer, therefore, in such extensive lesions to perform a separate proximal aortoilac or aortofemoral bypass graft. We have no hesitation in carrying the reconstruction below the inguinal ligament,[6] although certain precautions should be undertaken in these circumstances. These precautions include the greatest attention to aseptic detail, the use of antibiotics begun before operation and maintained for at least five days afterward, and the use of Teflon-coated Dacron suture or polypropylene sutures in the groin. The square-toed graft described in previous chapters has been a major contribution toward elimination of the femoral "detachment-anastomotic aneurysm." Furthermore, wherever there is not a good layer of subcutaneous tissue under which the graft can be buried, it is our practice to detach the upper portion of the sartorius from the anterior superior iliac spine and mobilize it medially to cover the arterial anastomosis.

We have been careful wherever possible to be sure that we could restore arterial flow into the profunda femoris artery, and have used whatever plastic reconstructive procedures seem necessary to improve the outflow from the common femoral artery into the deep femoral system.

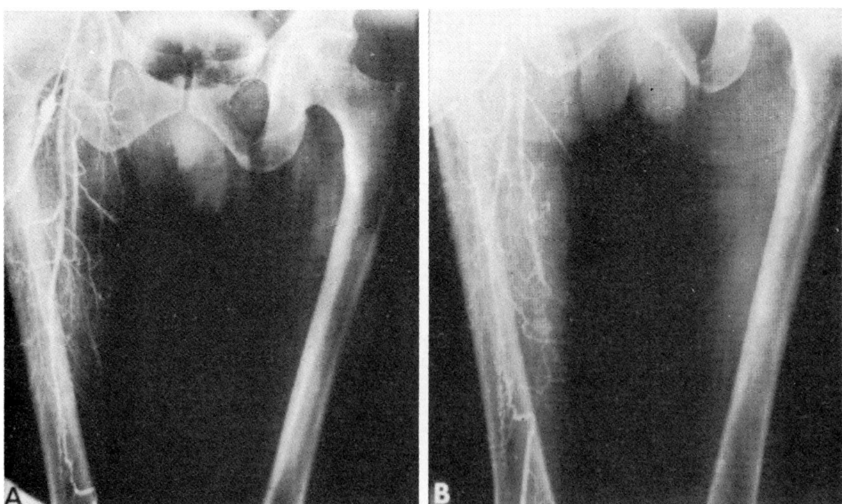

Figure 9–3. Arteriogram showing extensive and functionally excellent collateral branches bypassing an obstruction of the femoral artery. This patient, a 65-year-old male, also had a proximal aortoiliac obstruction. After the proximal aortoiliac lesion was treated by placement of a bypass graft of Dacron, pulses were restored to the foot through this collateral network.

The logic of the sequence of proximal operation before distal operation, if only one stage is to be attempted initially, derives from the presumed ability to restore a high inflow pressure into the level where the second reconstruction may begin, thus improving the chance of success in the second procedure. In addition, lumbar sympathectomy performed at the initial operation will be successful to a certain degree in reducing peripheral resistance in the lower extremity and augmenting the chance of a good differential pressure through the second anastomosis, which speaks in favor of a successful result. Lumbar sympathectomy may also accomplish a partition of blood toward the skin in these patients and may achieve a physiological dilatation of the saphenous vein, making it possibly a better substance for reconstruction.

Ordinarily, the patient will be given several months for an evaluation of his status after the proximal reconstruction before even considering more distant femoral, or femoropopliteal–tibial, reconstructions.

In the initial edition of this book we described a patient who had an aortoiliac femoral endarterectomy and who had at the same time a very quick pass with an intraluminal stripper down the superficial femoral artery. This patient was one of the few who had lastingly good results from the blind proximal stripping, which under most circumstances has resulted in prompt thrombosis beyond the level at which the artery could be identified (see page 189).

One special occasion, however, which may require immediate femoropopliteal reconstruction at the same time as aortoiliac reconstruction is that which occurs because of acute thrombosis of a popliteal aneurysm. This may result from the low flow state during proximal arterial occlusion for reconstruction for either occlusive or aneurysmal disease. If this is recognized as a risk, the greatest protection can be achieved by placing catheters in the distal arterial tree at the operative site at the time of operation, and using them to provide intermittent instillation of liberal amounts of a dilute heparin solution, such as 10 ml. every 10 minutes of a solution which contains 1000 units of heparin per 500 ml. of solution. Solitary injections of a single larger dose of heparin distally at the initiation of the arterial dissection have been much less successful as protection against this type of distal thrombosis.

There are exceptions to the rule that the proximal stage should always be performed first. The following case represents a successful outcome of the opposite sequence, but the success was probably based on the fortuitous fact that iliac stenosis progressed much more slowly than we would ordinarily expect it to today.

G.K., a 60-year-old man, was admitted with the complaint of claudication, primarily referable to his right calf, but also affecting the left calf. Good femoral pulses were palpable, but a loud bruit was heard in the left groin. Bilateral lumbar sympathectomy was performed, and despite the presence of palpable areas of plaque in the left common iliac artery, there was a patent channel in the iliac arteries and complete occlusion of the right superficial artery, both indicated by arteriography. There were areas of stenosis in the left superficial femoral artery. A reversed saphenous vein graft was placed as a bypass in the right thigh. Pulses were weak at first, but became stronger over the next few weeks. Seven years later the patient remained free of significant claudication in his right calf, although pain in the left hip developed if he hurried. Some myocardial insufficiency and cerebrovascular symptoms developed, although he had no myocardial infarction or cerebrovascular accident. No extracranial carotid lesions were demonstrable. During the seventh year after operation occlusion of the stenotic iliac artery was manifested by a decrease in oscillometrics, absence of the femoral pulse, and disappearance of the bruit in the left groin. Claudication worsened only slightly, but 10 years after the original operation there has been no further deterioration.

The patient just described was not considered for combined aortoiliac femoropopliteal reconstruction despite the femoral bruit. The stenotic lesion in the iliac artery did not progress to occlusion for 7 years, and in view of the patient's minor leg symptoms coupled with the more severe cardiovascular symptoms, no additional surgery is contemplated.

IMPORTANCE OF OTHER SITES OF INVOLVEMENT

Areas other than the aortic, iliac, femoral, and popliteal arterial systems may be involved.[5] The coronary arteries are frequently affected, and occasionally the extracranial carotid tree is. A case in point is that of the patient described in Chapter Five. Severe extracranial carotid or vertebral disease may be treated prior to peripheral repair as otherwise hypotension might ensue that would result in a cerebrovascular catastrophe although this dictum has recently been challenged by Treiman and his associate,[8] who found no reason to operate on patients with carotid bruits that had occasioned no symptoms. The presence of permanent cerebral impairment due to disease of the large or small vessels is a definite contraindication to major reconstruction. Under such circumstances only the minimal procedures aimed at salvage of the endangered extremity are justified, and relief of claudication should not be attempted.

REFERENCES

1. Barker, W. F.: *Surgical Treatment of Peripheral Vascular Disease.* New York, McGraw-Hill Book Co., Inc., 1962.

2. Darling, R. C., and Linton, R. R.: Management of the late failure of arterial reconstruction of the lower extremities. New Eng. J. Med. *270*:609, 1964.
3. Darling, R. C., and Linton, R. R.: Aortoiliofemoral endarterectomy for atherosclerotic occlusive disease. Surgery *55*:184, 1964.
4. DeBakey, M. E., Crawford, E. S., Cooley, D. A., and Morris, G. C., Jr.: Surgical considerations of occlusive disease of the abdominal aorta and iliac and femoral arteries; analysis of 803 cases. Ann. Surg. *148*:306, 1958.
5. Humphries, A. W., de Wolfe, V. G., Young, J. R., and LeFevre, F. A.: Evaluation of the natural history and the results of treatment in occlusive arteriosclerosis involving the lower extremities in 1850 patients. In Wesolowski, S. A., and Dennis, C.: *Fundamentals of Vascular Grafting.* New York, McGraw-Hill Book Co., Inc., 1963.
6. Moore, W. S., Cafferata, H. T., Hall, A. D., and Blaisdell, F. W.: In defense of grafts across the inguinal ligament: an evaluation of early and late results of aorto-femoral bypass grafts. Ann. Surg. *168*:207, 1968.
7. Szilagyi, D. E., Smith, R. F., Elliott, J. P., and Vrandecic, M. T.: Infection in arterial reconstruction with synthetic grafts. Ann. Surg. *176*:321, 1972.
8. Treiman, R. L., Foran, R. F., Shore, E. H., and Levin, P. M.: Carotid bruit. Significance in patients undergoing an abdominal aortic operation. Arch. Surg. *106*:803, 1973.

Chapter Ten

RESULTS OF ARTERIAL RECONSTRUCTION FOR CHRONIC OCCLUSION

PROCESS OF HEALING

The optimal local results of an arterial reconstruction would be restoration of physiologic quantities of blood through a vessel which is not subject to abnormal degeneration, and is not apt to undergo thrombosis. Flow through the segment should be substantially laminar. Although desirable, it is not necessary to restore flow through all of the small branches arising from the reconstructed segment of artery. These results should be accomplished with the least possible hazard to the patient's life and limb and should be long-lasting.

The mechanisms of healing may vary according to the reconstructive procedure, and must be discussed separately.

Endarterectomy

In *endarterectomy,* the medial wall of the artery is denuded, deep to the internal elastic lamella (Figs. 10–1 and 10–2). Our earlier studies[3] suggest that if heparinization is used to control the deposition of red clot, then a thin layer of fibrin and platelets is deposited on the raw medial wall. From islands of intact endothelium at the orifice of branches and from the intact intima at the end of the segment, endothelium grows rapidly over the layer of fibrin and platelets. Endothelial cover is complete in 2 to 4 days. Islands of red clot at the site of rough spots or irregularities usually must be organized by the ingrowth of granulation tissue before endothelization occurs. There is ingrowth of granulation tissue at the suture line in the vessel; endothelium derived from the buds of granulation tissue helps cover this area (Fig. 10–3).

Wylie[85] had orginally suggested that circulating totipotent cells adhered to the endarterectomized wall and became transformed into endothelial cells, achieving endothelial cover in the same brief interval, and this thesis was supported by Jordan,[42] Lazzarini-Robertson[49] and more recently by Kennedy and Weissman.[47]

Jordan suspended a fragment of Dacron in a pig's aorta by fine guy sutures and observed the development of all types of cells normally found in the wall of blood vessels. Lazzarini-Robertson transfused male animals with blood from female donors shortly after insertion of a fabric graft and was able to show that many of the cells in the new endothelial lining had female sex characteristics in the chromosomes.

Kennedy and Weissman demonstrated by means of fluorescent antisera that some host cells, but mostly donor cells, could be iden-

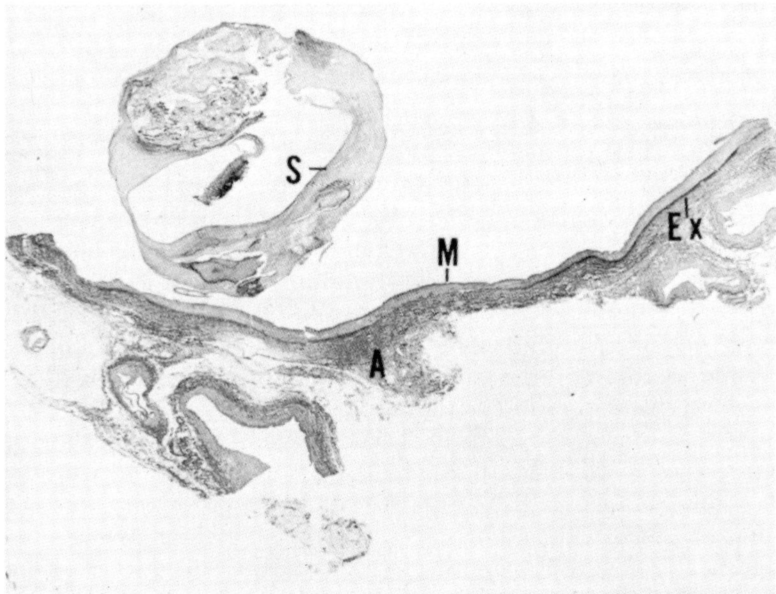

Figure 10–1. Photomicrograph of a smoothly endarterectomized wall in the presence of a markedly atheromatous sequestrum. Specimen was prepared following removal of the femoral artery at autopsy from a patient who had died of other causes. Endarterectomy was performed on the specimen, and the artery was opened out by a longitudinal incision. The sequestrum and the vessel wall were then fixed and mounted in normal anatomical relationship. Remaining artery is composed of the external elastic membrane (Ex) and the adventitia (A). Atheromatous core or sequestrum is shown at (S). Elastic tissue stain.

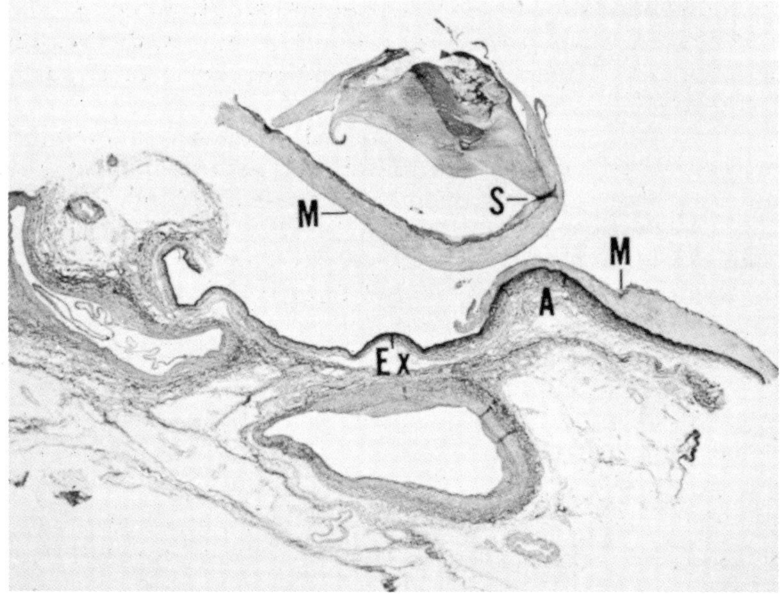

Figure 10–2. Endarterectomized wall, with irregular dissection. Specimen was prepared as in Figure 10–1. Plane of dissection, however, could not be cleanly established, as is evident in ragged remaining wall, which in this instance is chiefly only elastic membrane (Ex) and adventitia (A). There is some remaining media (M) at right. The sequestrum (S) contains a thick strip of media. This layer of dissection is not necessarily incorrect; the problem arises because of the mechanical irregularity which is very unfavorable if such strips are not recognized. Elastic tissue stain.

tified in the intima in cardiac allografts, thus agreeing with the concept that the new intimal cells come from two sources.[47]

Irregularities in the raw surface of the vessel that has been endarterectomized may create areas of granulation tissue and subsequent cicatricial narrowing such as was observed by Warren[81] and by others. We have observed endarterectomy in the muscular arteries of dogs to result in necrosis of the smooth muscle of the artery wall. Such necrosis might lead either to dilatation and aneurysm or to cicatricial stenosis. The normal smooth wall that is usually seen after healing is demonstrated in Figures 10–3 and 10–4. The excellence with which this healing persists is shown in Figure 10–5A, an aortogram taken 5 years after aortoiliac endarterectomy. Unsatisfactory results are indicated in the postoperative arteriogram shown in Figure 10–5B. Restoration of flow to many of the small branches is anticipated, unless the atheroma extends well into the branch—an unusual circumstance. Figure 10–6 illustrates healing of the intimal surface of the aorta 6 weeks after operation, with restoration of the channel into the orifice of small collaterals.

In addition, Imparato and his associates have recently pointed out that one can observe a fibrous proliferation in many reconstructions, where both endarterectomies and venous grafts have been performed, in which fibrous plaques develop that are very similar morphologically to the fibrous plaques in fibroatheromatous lesions.[40] They believe that these are related to hemodynamics, either acceleration or deceleration of flow, and alterations in blood vessel geometry, although the plaques do not seem to occur so commonly in the major vessels such as the aortic and iliac system. He postulates that part of their origin may be related to bursts of sonic energy of between 40 and 80 Hz which are found to occur at the sites at which subsequently lesions will be found in experimental animals.

Grafts

Grafts heal by different mechanisms. Arterial homografts from small vessels such as the femorals undergo considerable degenerative change and are not suitable for reconstruction.[37, 75, 76]

Arterial homografts from the larger more fibrous and elastic vessels such as the aorta may also undergo degeneration, but in general are long-lasting. The author has had experience with two cases in which replacement following aortic aneurysm has yielded satisfactory results for over 10 years. Szilagyi has carefully evaluated 53 aortoiliac

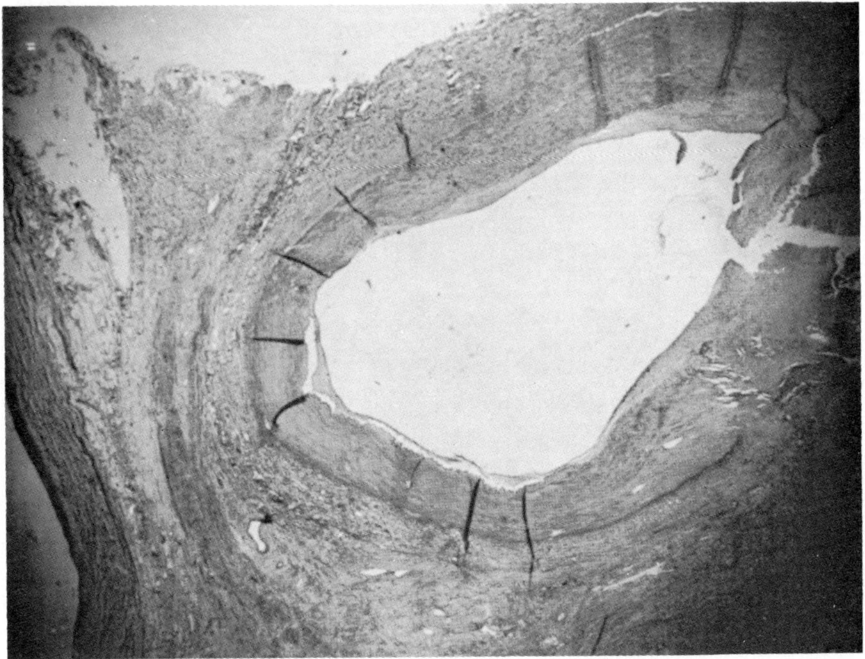

Figure 10–3. Cross section of popliteal artery in patient who died of a ruptured aneurysm 6 weeks following successful endarterectomy of femoral popliteal artery. Intima is thin and fibrous, but is thicker at site of arteriotomy. Here granulation tissue is growing in from the outside of the wall. Media is fairly well preserved. There is considerable perivascular fibrosis. Fragments of silk suture are seen in this section. Hematoxylin eosin stain.

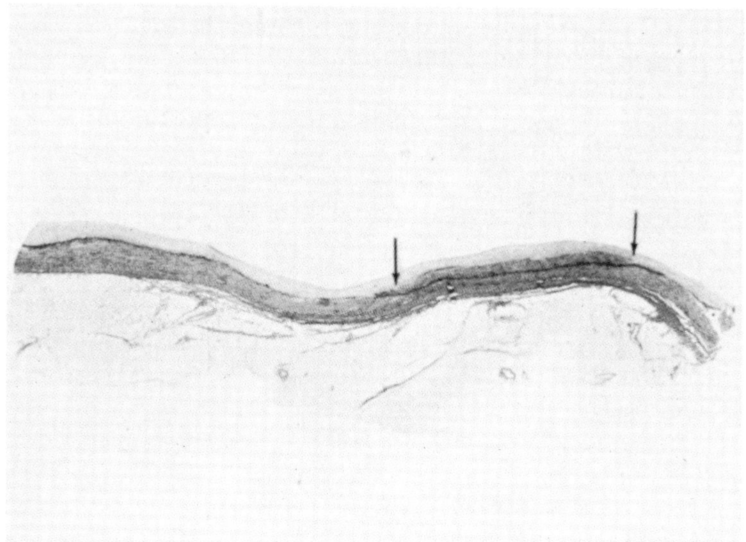

Figure 10–4. Cross section of iliac arteries of patient who died from a pulmonary embolus 6 weeks following successful aortoiliac femoral endarterectomy. The artery has been opened. The adventitia and external elastic membrane are coated with a layer of re-endothelialized fibrous tissue. Remnants of smooth muscle may be seen between the arrows. Elastic tissue stain.

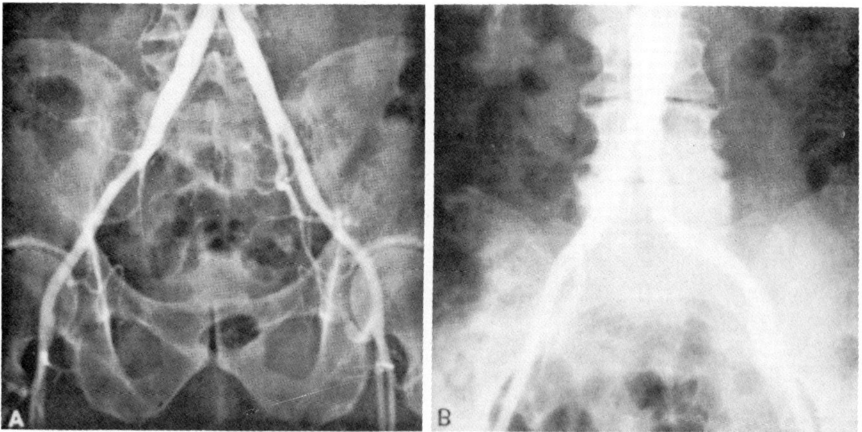

Figure 10–5. *A,* Arteriogram done 5 years following endarterectomy in a 62-year-old man. The wall of the reconstructed area is of good caliber and is not dilated. There is a smooth transition from endarterectomized area and normal vessel. *B,* Arteriogram done 2 years after endarterectomy in a 57-year-old woman. Patient had recurrence of symptoms. There is a ragged intraluminal mass which consists of atheroma, fibrous tissue, and fresh clot. Above and below the mass there is the suggestion of early aneurysm formation.

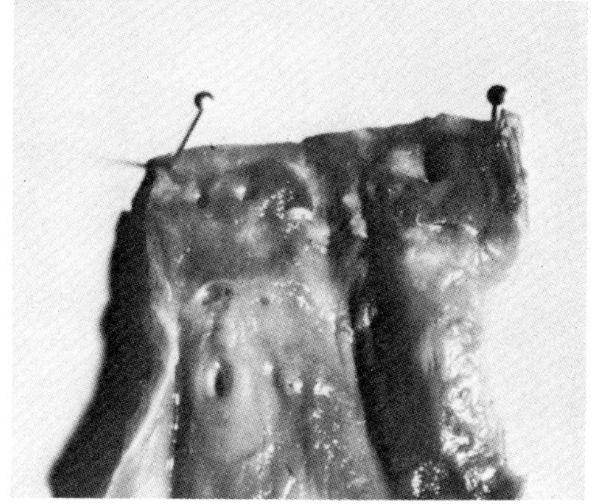

Figure 10–6. Section of aorta which was divided just above the upper level during endarterectomy. Vessel has been opened longitudinally. Transition between the intact vessel and endarterectomized area appears as an irregular line just below the level of transection. The wall is smooth and glistening below this line. The orifices of lumbar and other small arteries are clearly opened. Same patient as in Figure 10–4.

and nine femoral arterial allografts.[76] His evaluation confirms the concept that the late results of the femoral grafts are very poor. Although 18 of the aortoiliac grafts were open at the 15 year mark, 14 of them developed aneurysms and three patients lost their lives due to complications of the secondary aneurysms in the grafts. In spite of the early satisfactory appearance of these allografts, the collagen they contained served as an unpredictably durable framework for invasion by the host tissues.

Arterial autografts perform very well with minimal structural alteration, but they are not readily available. The endothelium remains almost intact.

Venous autografts also seem to heal with minimal alteration of the endothelial surface,[78, 83] but recent studies by Reichle indicate that, even in grafts which have functioned for 14 months, the base over which blood is flowing is composed of areas of raw collagen fibrils and not intact endothelial cells.[63] Revascularization of the graft is prompt, however, and it is generally true that the venous graft preserves its structural strength. On the other hand, the author recently has observed bilateral aneurysms developing in vein grafts which had been used ten years previously to replace popliteal aneurysms. DeWeese recently presented a series of vein grafts in which aneurysms had developed. Venous dilatation also occurs late in the history of vein grafts used for aortorenal reconstructions.[26] Venous autografts still remain the primary choice for arterial reconstruction (except in the abdomen or in the leg when only a very short segment is involved). An experience with the venous homograft has recently been reviewed by Ochsner, DeCamp and Leonard,[29, 58] and Perloff and his associates have evaluated the immunological reactions of the venous homograft.[60] These authors found that minimal evidences of rejection which

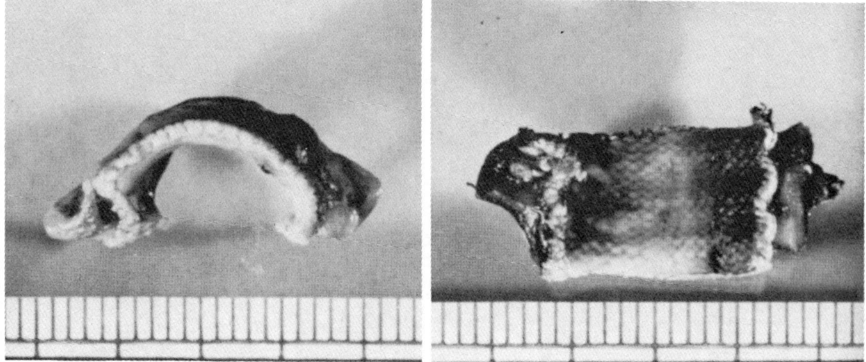

Figure 10–7. *A*, Cross section and *B*, Face, tubular graft after more than 1 year. The lining is smooth, glistening, and transparent, although there are a few small areas of granulation tissue. After DeBakey.

might be recognized in the experimental situation did not seem to alter the efficiency or the durability of the grafts. The role of immunology has not been well evaluated in the clinical situation, however.

Heterografts consisting of bovine carotid arteries which have been treated with the proteolytic enzyme ficin and then mildly tanned have been introduced by Rosenberg and his associates. The healing of these tubes occurs with gradual incorporation into the tissues and a formation of a compacted fibrin lining.[65, 68]

The maturation of *fabric prostheses* is a relatively slower process. The material provides the basic tensile strength. If the interstices in the fabric are large enough to allow it, the graft usually becomes fixed in the tissues by ingrowth of fibrous tissue from the bed in which the prosthesis has been placed. Blood flows through the tube fast enough to keep the lining free of clot; any clot that develops within the wrinkles, pores, and depressions of crimped or noncrimped fabrics is soon deprived of extra clotting factors by dilution. Some clots are absorbed, but most remain to be organized by the granulation tissue that grows into the fabric wall[16, 22, 24, 62, 66] and forms a thin, smooth, glistening lining (Fig. 10–7).

When a prosthesis is not incorporated into the bed, it remains encased in a pseudocyst-like cavity from which it can be lifted easily. This occurs with any fabric in the presence of infection, but also commonly with Teflon prostheses in the absence of infection. Teflon is chemically inert and provokes no reaction in the host nor significant clotting in the blood flowing through it. The nonwettability of the fabric requires that it be woven so tightly that no blood can leak through the interstices. The porosity of the fabric is so low that it cannot be pervaded by fibroblasts and the lining membrane cannot become adherent to the graft wall. A loose membrane may be built up on the lining of the prosthesis much as occurs in the lining of Lucite tubes, as described by Hufnagel.[35] This loose membrane is easily dislodged to become a mechanical source of obstruction and impediment to flow.

More porous fabrics of either knitted or woven Dacron are only slightly more reactive. They are suitably incorporated into the body's fibroblastic reaction, and invading fibroblasts mature or organize islands of mural clot to allow ultimate complete endothelialization. Undoubtedly some endothelial growth extends from the site of attachment to an artery lined with intima.[62] The work of Dale and Lewis on vascular patch grafts illustrates this phenomenon.[19] Jordan[42] and Lazzarini-Robertson[49] have demonstrated the ability of circulating cells in the bloodstream to form endothelium *de novo*. In addition, granulation tissue pervading the fabric can carry endothelial buds to the inner surface to allow endothelium to spread from multiple sites simultaneously.

In prostheses in which flow has been slow or maturation delayed, a thick, granular, amorphous layer may form which is only loosely adherent to the wall and is easily separated from it. Ultimately, if it does not break away or cause thrombotic occlusion, it becomes organized or absorbed, neither of which occurs quickly. This situation represents the major disadvantage of fabric prostheses. A typical case is described.

C.T., a 64-year-old male, was operated upon for aortoiliac atherosclerosis. Because the narrow external iliac arteries as well as the aortic bifurcation and common iliac arteries were atherosclerotic, a bypass prosthesis of knitted Dacron was placed from the distal aorta to the common femoral arteries. A favorable outcome was manifested by complete relief of symptoms and return of excellent pedal pulsations. Nine months later symptoms recurred in the left leg, with a sudden exacerbation. The patient entered with a cold, pulseless, but viable left leg, and with excellent vascularization of the right leg. Exploration demonstrated a prosthesis so adherent that it was difficult to remove. The left arm of the graft was filled with adherent, organizing, granular debris. There was no kink or twist, and the thrombosis did not extend into the right arm of the prosthesis or into the femoral artery. A new limb of Dacron was inserted, and flow was effectively re-established. The patient remains healthy 4 years later. No adequate explanation for the complete occlusion of the arm of the prosthesis was ever obtained.

The newer prostheses such as the velour coated graft of Sauvage offer a vastly improved rate of healing with more prompt incorporation and a true neointima without the fibrous compaction that characterizes most Dacron grafts. This has been demonstrated both in experimental animals and in the human patient.[66]

One aspect of the healing process that deserves mention has been described by Callow.[9] Placement of a graft bypassing stenotic lesions in experimental animals brought about complete thrombosis of the stenotic segments. It has been suggested that placement of the bypass graft into an open segment of vessel lying below an area of stenosis from which collateral vessels arise would promote retrograde flow into the collaterals. In some patients there is apparently prompt thrombosis of the bypassed vessel but in others there is sufficient retrograde and antegrade flow to maintain the original channels in a patent status for many years.

Patches composed of the materials described heal by similar mechanisms. Fabric patches are incorporated even more quickly than tubular segments because of the ready access to the fabric surface by endothelium from the vessel being repaired.[19] Even if the patch is used on an endarterectomized vessel, endothelium from the vasa vasorum and the granulating suture line is available for cover.

One of the deficiencies of fabrics is their incorporation into scar and subsequent stiffening which causes kinking (Figs. 8–5 and 8–6) and either temporary obliteration and thrombosis or dislodgment of the loosely adherent lining. According to Szilagyi,[72] however, the kinking that is seen on marked flexion disappears on extension with persistence of only minor wrinkling, rather than true indentations.

CLINICAL RESULTS

In the earlier series 188 operations were performed on 184 patients.[2, 4, 11, 13] The summary of these results is presented in Table 10–1. For comparison, similar figures for 119 patients from the current period are presented in Table 10–2.

Types of Operation

The preference for thromboendarterectomy is reflected in the frequent use of this operation in the early series, but its persistent popularity shows up in the aortoiliac reconstructions in the current group.

In the latter series, Dacron prostheses came into more common use because of several factors: more surgeons were operating in this service without a strong emotional attachment to the operation of thromboendarterectomy; some of the surgeons operating were not well trained in the performance of thromboendarterectomy; and more older patients with more aneurysmal changes appear in the second group. Furthermore, the surgeons were more inclined to use prostheses with more liberal indications when significant disease appeared in the external iliac system.

Table 10–1. Operative Results by Procedure and Site—
Original Series (1955–1961)

| | | | Reconstruction | | |
Site and Operation	No.	Operative Deaths	Initial Success	Initial Failure†	Late Failures
Aortoiliac endarterectomy	72	1	71	0	12‡
Aortoiliac graft	9	0	9	0	2§
Femoral endarterectomy	34	2*	29	5*	7
Femoral bypass graft	11	1*	8	3*	1
Combined aortoiliac femoral endarterectomy	40	3*	30	8¶	6
Combined aortoiliac femoral bypass graft‖	22	2*	19	3*	3
	188	9	167	19	31

*Operative deaths are those specifically related to the operative procedure, although occurring months later (Table 10–4).

†Includes operative deaths.

‡One patient whose reconstruction thrombosed on the day of operation had a successful immediate reoperation followed by late (16 months) failure.

§Patient died of aortoenteric fistula 3½ years postoperatively.

¶Patient had an acute thrombosis and immediate reoperation with successful (18 months) reconstruction.

‖The majority of suprainguinal prostheses were Dacron. The majority of grafts distal to the inguinal ligament consist of autologous veins.

The second series indicates that aortoiliac reconstruction continues to have excellent results. One death followed reconstruction by means of a graft but should not be specifically related to the type of operation. The patient had a combined aortoiliac and bilateral renal reconstruction and died of acute renal failure and pancreatitis.

Table 10–2. Operative Results by Procedure and Site—
Current Series

Site and Operation	Total	Operative Death (%)	Initial Success of Reconstruction (%)	Initial Failure of Reconstruction (%)
Aortoiliac endarterectomy or graft	43	1 (2)	41 (95)	1 (2)
Femoropopliteal endarterectomy or graft (or femorotibial)	13	2 (15)	6 (46)	7 (54)
Aorto–common femoral reconstructions	28	1 (4)	27 (96)	0
Aorto–superficial femoral reconstructions	29	4 (14)	18 (62)	11 (38)
Miscellaneous: second stage of aortofemoral operation, distal stage only in presence of advanced proximal disease, etc.	6	1 (17)	1 (17)	4 (73)

The scant number of femoral reconstructions and the very poor results in the series tabulated here reflect the pessimism expressed by Stoney, James and Wylie,[71] and by Cannon[10] at the time these procedures were performed. The operation was being applied to only the most dismal candidates for operation, and the results reflect the poor choice of patients. The series also represents the failure at the time to recognize that bypass reconstructions into the distal vessels of the leg well below the knee not only can be done but often can be accomplished with better flow rates and better clinical results than the operations that are held to the region of the knee.[5, 33, 51, 52, 79] Because of the experience with the poor results from endarterectomy carried into the tibial vessels, many had been hesitant to extend grafts below the knee.

In a sense reflecting the same phenomenon — that is, success when the entire segmental disease can be bypassed into patent distal vessels — is the remarkably good result seen when the aortoiliac reconstruction is carried into the femoral artery rather than when the operation is falsely compromised because of the fear of crossing the inguinal ligament.

Moore and his associates have decried the tendency of the surgeon to hesitate to extend the reconstruction into the groin, and point to excellent results;[54] nonetheless, the groin does represent the area of danger in which infections are most likely to develop,[77] and appropriate precautions should include meticulous hemostasis and lymphostasis; coverage of the reconstruction with as many layers of tissue as possible, including the sartorius muscle if necessary; and the use of prophylactic antibiotics.

On the other hand, if the reconstruction is carried into the superficial femoral artery (as opposed to the common femoral), results begin to diminish. In this series many of these failures represented an attempt to do blind distal endarterectomy far below the limit of the exposure of the vessel. In this series there were seven patients in whom attempts were made to extend the operation by this means; only two of the patients left the hospital with distal pulses.

The more rational approach to combined aortoiliac and femorotibial disease seems to be a major reconstruction into the external iliac, common femoral or even deep femoral artery as a first stage. Many patients who have this first stage done require nothing further; if, however, after a period of time it becomes apparent that more is necessary the appropriate femoropopliteal or femorotibial reconstruction can be carried out with a lesser overall risk. Lumbar sympathectomy performed at the first stage increases the likelihood that the second stage will be unnecessary.

The durability of the autologous vein is reflected in the fact that at least two patients from the earlier series who had vein grafts placed still have patent reconstructions at 17 to 19 years.

The figures reported here for femoral reconstruction, whether for reconstructions into the open popliteal segment, an isolated popliteal segment, or a patent tibial artery, are to be considered neither satisfactory nor representative of the excellence of results obtained either by other authors (see Table 10–10) or, in more recent years, by the author and the resident staff at the Hospital of the University of California at Los Angeles. Although femoral artery reconstructions may never reach the level of excellent results shown by reconstructions of the aorta, iliac, and common femoral arteries, it is nonetheless an eminently successful operation when performed for serious indications, and when the ominous mortality rate that will be encountered in the patients who have good local results is recognized.

Among the operations listed as miscellaneous are several extra-anatomic bypass operations such as the axillofemoral and the femoro-femoral grafts. Moore and his associates have noted the importance for the durability of the axillofemoral bypass of performing the operation as an axillary *bilateral* femoral bypass.[55] This principle, however, depends upon the presence of obstruction in both iliac systems, for without a good pressure gradient across which flow can be well maintained, either the segment between the axilla and the graft bifurcation or the segment between the better femoral artery and the graft bifurcation will fail promptly. In any case, if there is one good femoral artery with reasonable proximal inflow, then the choice would be for a femorofemoral crossover graft.[80] One of the unsuspected problems that may be encountered if one fails to observe this principle of placing a graft across an area of pressure drop is exemplified by the following case report.

A 45-year-old woman had had an aortoiliac endarterectomy for localized iliac occlusions four years previous to her admission with an acute thrombosis of the left limb of the reconstruction. In retrospect, she had had some left iliac claudication manifesting itself, as well as a gradual diminution of pressures in the left leg in the preceding year. A femorofemoral graft of knitted Dacron was placed and, before completing the left femoral suture line, a Fogarty catheter was passed down the leg, and then up the left iliac artery. To the surgeon's surprise and temporary pleasure, a considerable amount of thromboatheromatous debris was removed, and a vigorous flow of blood followed down from the aorta. The suture line was completed. The situation now had been created in which there was no longer any significant pressure gradient across the site of placement of the graft, nor had a perfect reconstruction been completed in the left iliac system. The Dacron graft therefore ceased to pulsate within 24 hours, and, furthermore, the left iliac artery also thrombosed within a week, leaving the patient exactly as she had been on admission. The femorofemoral graft was then replaced, but on this occasion no attempt to restore flow down the iliac artery from above was even considered. The patient now has a well functioning femorofemoral graft two years later.

Table 10–3A. Number of Patients with Good Results at Time of Last Follow-up — Original Series

	Years									
Site and Procedure	1	1–2	2–3	3–4	4–5	5–6	6–7	7–8	8–9	9–10
Aortoiliac endarterectomy	26	10*	8	3	1	6	2*		1	2
Aortoiliac graft	4	1	2							
All aortoiliac procedures combined	30	11	10	3	1	6	2		1	2
Femoropopliteal endarterectomy	12	3	4	1				2		
Femoropopliteal graft	4*	1	1					1		
All femoropopliteal procedures combined	16	4	5	1				3		
Aortoiliofemoropopliteal endarterectomy	12†	2	3			2		3	1	2
Aortoiliofemoropopliteal graft	8*	3*	2		1	1		1		
All aortoiliofemoro-popliteal procedures combined	19	5	5		1	3		4	1	2
Total	$\frac{19}{65}$	$\frac{5}{20}$	$\frac{5}{20}$	$\frac{}{4}$	$\frac{1}{2}$	$\frac{3}{9}$	$\frac{}{2}$	$\frac{4}{7}$	$\frac{1}{2}$	$\frac{2}{4}$

* = Death.
†Four deaths in this group.

Length of Follow-up

Length of follow-up is shown in Tables 10–3A, 10–3B, and 10–4 for the original series and in Tables 10–5A, 10–5B, and 10–6 for the second series. The second series of tables is constructed with slightly different categorizations because of the different philosophical approaches to similarly named operations, but the attempt is made to present the data so it can be most nearly comparable. Tables 10–4 and 10–6 present the results in terms of what Stokes calls the "accumulative patency rate."[69] This rate is based on the number of failures occurring in any given period and the number of patents "at risk" in that period. The category, "at risk," includes all patients who have been followed during this period, even though they may subsequently experience a failure, but excludes those whose follow-up was terminated earlier, whether from failure, death, or other causes. The percentage of good results continuing from one interval into the next is reduced for each period by the fraction represented by the failures during this subsequent period as the numerator and the total cases followed through this subsequent period as the denominator. The accumulative patency rates are compared in Figures 10–8, 10–9 and 10–10.

Table 10–3B. Time of Failure of Initially Successful
Operative Procedure — Original Series

| | Years | | | | | | | | | |
Site and Procedure	0–1	1–2	2–3	3–4	4–5	5–6	6–7	7–8	8–9	9–10
Aortoiliac endarterectomy	4	3	2	1		1		1		
Aortoiliac graft					1	1				
All aortoiliac procedures combined	4	3	2	1	1	2		1		
Femoropopliteal endarterectomy	3	2*		1			1			
Femoropopliteal graft	1									
All femoropopliteal procedures combined	4	2*		1			1			
Aortoiliofemoropopliteal endarterectomy	1*	2	1			1	1			
Aortoiliofemoropopliteal graft		1								
All aortoiliofemoropopliteal procedures combined	1*	3	1			1	1			
Total	9*	8*	3	2	1	3	2	1		

* = Amputation.

Table 10–4. Cumulative "Patency Percentages" —
Original Series

| | | Years | | | | | | | | | |
Site and Procedure	Initial Success	0–1	1–2	2–3	3–4	4–5	5–6	6–7	7–8	8–9	9–10
Aortoiliac endarterectomy	99	93	86	80	76	76	70				
Aortoiliac graft	100	100	100	100	50						
All aortoiliac procedures combined	99	94	88	83	78	74	63	63	47	47	47
Femoropopliteal endarterectomy	78	70	60	60	48	48	48	32	32		
Femoropopliteal graft	83	72	72	72	72	72	72	72	72		
All femoropopliteal procedures combined	79	69	62	62	50	50	50	38	38		
Aortoiliofemoropopliteal endarterectomy	81	72	62	62	56	56	56	48	48	48	
Aortoiliofemoropopliteal graft	85	80	71	71	71	71	71	71	71		
All aortoiliofemoropopliteal procedures combined	82	73	65	65	60	60	60	57	57	57	
Endarterectomy, all sites	89	81	74	71	64	64	62	54	49	49	49
Grafts or combined procedures, all sites	88	82	78	78	78	65	49	49	49		
All cases	89	82	75	73	67	65	60	54	50	50	50

Table 10–5A. Number of Patients with Good Results at Time of Last Follow-up — Current Series

	Years			
Procedures	0–1	1–2	2–3	3–4
All aortoiliac reconstructions	23	20	16	11
All femoropopliteal or tibial reconstructions	12	6	5	4
Aortoilio-common femoral procedures	19	11	7	4
Aorto–superficial femoral procedures	12	10	7	3
Miscellaneous	6	–	–	–

Table 10–5B. Time of Failure of Originally Successful Operative Procedure — Current Series

	Year of Failure			
Procedure	0–1	1–2	2–3	3–4
All aortoiliac procedures	5	3	1	3
All femoropopliteal or tibial reconstructions	3	–	–	–
Aorto-common femoral procedures	1	–	1	–
Aorto–superficial femoral reconstructions	–	1	1	1
Miscellaneous	1	–	–	–

Table 10–6. Cumulative "Patency Percentages" — Current Series

		Years			
Procedure	*Initial Success*	0–1	1–2	2–3	3–4
All aortoiliac operations	95	78	68	64	46
Femoropopliteal operations	72	45	45	45	45
Aorto-common femoral operations	100	95	95	81	81
Aorto-superficial femoral operations	62	62	53	43	32
Miscellaneous	83	42	–	–	–

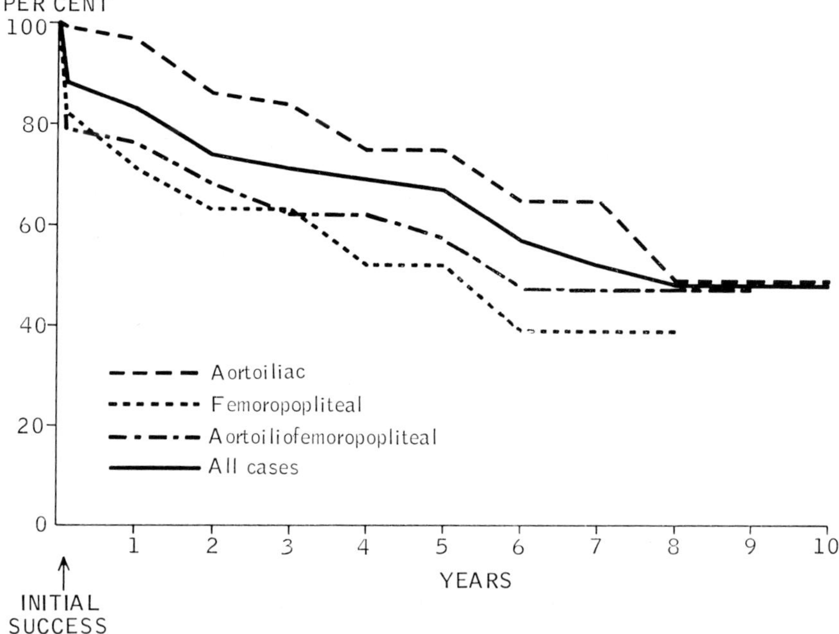

Figure 10–8.   Accumulative patency rates by anatomical site.

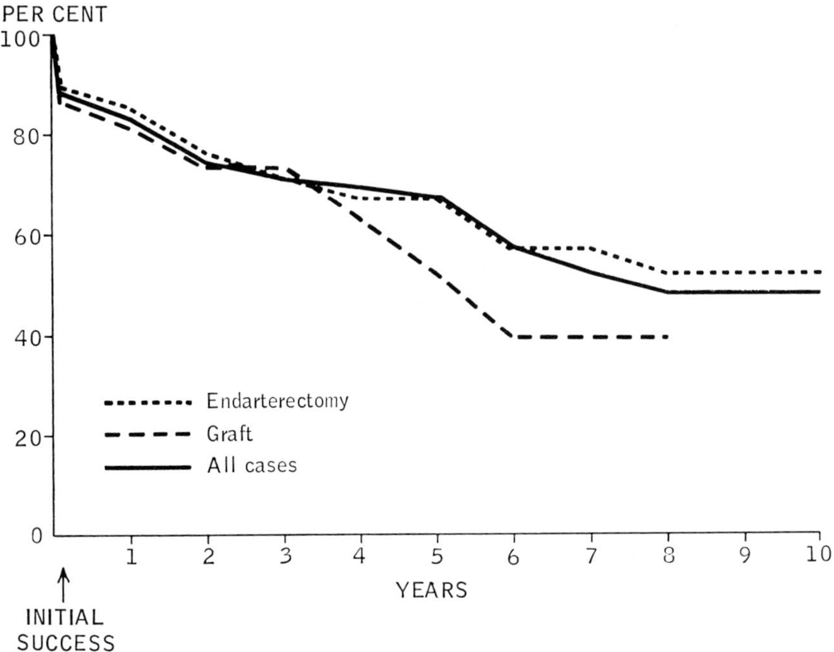

Figure 10–9.   Accumulative patency rates by operative procedure.

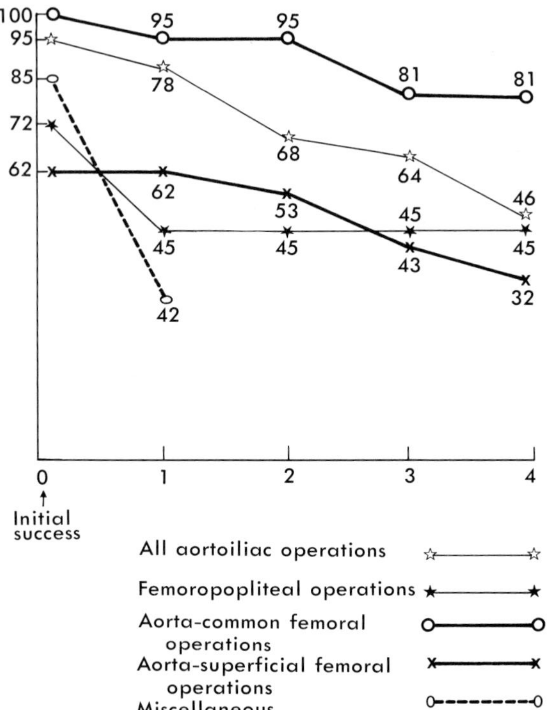

Figure 10–10. Accumulated patency rates by anatomical sites, current series.

From these tabulations and sketches it is apparent that aortoiliac reconstruction is a highly successful operation whether carried out by endarterectomy or by prosthetic bypass. From such small groups it is hazardous to draw extensive conclusions, but in both series it appears that the best results are obtained when the aortoiliac operation truly is extended beyond the limits of the disease. In other words, if the external iliac artery is diseased it should be carefully endarterectomized or a bypass must be placed all the way into the common femoral artery. Attempts to carry the reconstruction into the superficial femoral artery have not met with the success that has followed simple reconstruction into the patent profunda femoris artery. The importance of the deep femoral artery as a collateral for the superficial femoral artery appears greater and greater.

Many of the patients listed as having had a successful graft had plastic prostheses placed from the aorta to the femoral artery and a combination of endarterectomy and vein bypass in the lower leg. Only four patients in the early series also had Dacron prostheses placed in the femoral segment. One patient had an acute failure; his distal tree was acutely occluded, and he died of coronary occlusion and acute hepatic failure. The other three did well initially, but one died at 2 weeks of a pulmonary embolus and one had a thrombosis in the prosthesis of 6 months and died following attempted replacement. The other one remained well at the last follow-up, 26 months later.

Our early experience with the early woven or knitted Dacron prostheses in the thigh was very unpleasant. Of more than 30 Dacron tubes placed in the thigh of patients at the Veterans Hospital in West Los Angeles, only one remained patent for more than a year. It should be noted that these prostheses were used in only the worst-risk patients, both in terms of the general status of the patient and with regard to the local situation in the leg; furthermore none were placed below the knee. Many surgeons had given up the use of the plastic prostheses in the thigh although several groups[23, 36] continued to report good results.

The changing spectrum of femoral artery reconstruction, however, must be mentioned in terms of an addition to the results presented in Table 10–2. In the months since this tabulation was prepared, the author has operated on 10 consecutive patients with femoral artery reconstructions. Six of these patients had extremities which had been operated upon elsewhere and which, following failure of the orginal operation, were seriously ischemic; the other four represented primary operations, two for severe ischemia and two for combined occlusive and aneurysmal disease of the popliteal artery. In only two patients could the patient's own veins be used; both of these were successful. In the remainder, the external velour graft of Sauvage was used, and six of these eight have had excellent results.

The continuing need for the saphenous vein for coronary bypasses should make the peripheral vascular surgeon hesitant about using it as the primary method of reconstruction of a femoral obstruction, especially as other methods of reconstruction such as the newer prostheses and bovine heterografts become more clearly excellent alternatives.

Mortality

The overall mortality in the first series was five per cent for primary operations, but was eight per cent in the second group. The operative deaths are detailed in Tables 10–7A and 10–7B.

Four patients in the current series suffered lethal myocardial infarctions and all had prior history of severe coronary disease; a fifth patient died of a probable myocardial arrhythmia. Two patients died of visceral thromboses, one died of aspiration of gastric contents, a complication that should have been completely preventable.

Table 10–7A. Operative Deaths — Original Series

Site of Disease	Patient	Age, Sex	Remarks
1. Aortoiliac endarterectomy	FR	48M	Died of diffuse sepsis and hemorrhage 5 weeks after operation; flow through endarterectomized segment was adequate
2. Femoral bypass graft	NG	49M	Acute myocardial infarction, thrombosis of Dacron bypass, and acute hepatic necrosis
3. Femoral endarterectomy	AB	78M	Died of shock and probable coronary thrombosis after hemorrhage; thrombosis in endarterectomized segment
4. Combined aortoiliofemoral bypass graft	MM	51M	Pulmonary embolism 2 weeks after successful aortofemoropopliteal bypass procedure
5. Combined aortoiliofemoral endarterectomy and graft	LB	59M	Died of unexplained intestinal hemorrhage 3 weeks after successful combined aortoiliac endarterectomy and grafting procedure from iliac to left femoral artery (autopsy unrevealing)
6. Combined aortoiliofemoropopliteal endarterectomy	JA	45M	Died of sudden dehiscence of aortic suture line 2 days after successful aortoiliac endarterectomy and placement of 4 cm. grafts in superficial femoral artery
7. Combined aortoiliac disease, local femoral endarterectomy	RM	58M	Died of acute bacterial endocarditis after repeated episodes of sepsis and hemorrhage from thrombosed femoral endarterectomy site
8. Combined aortoiliofemoral endarterectomy	TP	58F	Died of coronary occlusion 24 hours after aortoiliac femoral endarterectomy; femoral reconstruction failed
9. Combined aortoiliofemoral endarterectomy	AV	50M	Prompt thrombosis of one side of reconstructed segment in patient with angina. Second thrombosis followed exploration. Died on seventh day from leakage in aorta proximal to suture line

Acute Failures

In the original series, 19 patients suffered acute postoperative thromboses; six were subjected to reoperation which was completely successful in only two instances. There were five deaths in this group; six required amputation (one bilaterally). In the current series there were 17 postoperative thromboses. Death occurred in two patients without amputation. Only three amputations followed these 17 thromboses; these amputations were accepted because of either a poor risk patient or a seriously involved distal tree that was believed to preclude further chance at reconstruction.

Rather than to supply a simple, anecdotal account of these failures, an attempt has been made to classify them into several groups, although the inclusion of patients into specific groups is at times an arbitrary and difficult choice.

Group A

The surgeon is overmatched by either the extent or the severity of the disease; either generalized problems such as acute myocardial infarctions should have precluded the operation, or total lack of adequate distal vessels made reconstruction impossible. There were five such instances in the first series, and two in the current series.

Table 10–7B. Operative Deaths — Current Series

Site of Disease	Patient	Age, Sex	Remarks
1. Aortoiliac bypass with bilateral renal artery graft	AA	67M	Acute renal failure, pancreatitis and aspiration pneumonitis.
2. Femoropopliteal endarterectomy	FM	63F	Acute femoral occlusion with imminent loss of leg, threatened during the course of an acute myocardial infarction; operation failed, with death from the extension of the myocardial infarction.
3. Femoral endarterectomy	KL	63F	Femoropopliteal endarterectomy for gangrene of foot. Unrelieved hypotension during operation culminated in massive myocardial infarction and death on the first postoperative day.
4. Aortoiliac femoral endarterectomy	BP	52F	Aortoiliac operations for ischemic ulcers on the leg. Thrombectomy of the common femoral artery was necessary on day one; popliteal thrombosis on the 9th day could not be corrected. On the 10th day the patient collapsed and died; autopsy revealed no obvious cause.
5. Aortoiliac superficial femoral endarterectomy	AH	61M	Diabetic patient; superficial femoral arteries could not be reopened by distal blind endarterectomy and the entire segment thrombosed with extension to the renal arteries with showers of emboli to the other abdominal viscera.
6. Aortoiliac superficial femoral endarterectomy	JB	63M	Ischemic ulcerations of the lower leg; blind distal endarterectomy failed and there was hemorrhage from the aortic suture line on the 4th postoperative day. The patient died of renal thrombosis and hepatic necrosis. The patient received no postoperative heparin.
7. Iliofemoral graft and femoropopliteal endarterectomy	GK	54M	The patient was a severe hypertensive with an old myocardial infarction who died of a second infarction on the 6th postoperative day in spite of a successful reconstruction.
8. Aortoiliac superficial femoral endarterectomy	CS	66M	Patient had had two prior major myocardial infarctions and developed a massive ininfarction and death on the day after operation. The operation had been conducted without significant blood loss or hypotension.
9. Common and superficial femoral endarterectomy	PG	60M	Operation was performed for sudden severe ischemia of the leg. Patient suffered aspiration in the operating room and became decerebrate, and finally died of pseudomonas pneumonia. Patient had untreated proximal occlusive disease.

Group B

The operation was not well conceived, or it was misapplied. On the basis of *presently* available techniques a different approach or operation would have been used. Six patients were in this category in the first series, one in the current series. This is another way of saying that there are now available techniques which were not applicable at the time of the first series but which might have saved the situation had they been so.

Group C

Technical failures: the failure of an operation which apparently should have had a good result. In some a cause can be assigned and in some it remains hidden. There are seven such patients in the first series and 14 in the current group. In this latter group are included seven patients in whom blind distal stripping on one or usually both legs failed but did not necessarily result in a catastrophe, insofar as a proximal reconstruction into the groins remained successful. Three acute thromboses were successfully treated by thrombectomy and institution of heparin therapy, with long lasting good results and no other modification of the reconstruction. In four patients there was a technical error, and in two of these the error was identified and corrected; in the other two the error was not identified and the thrombosis not successfully treated.

For the most part, the patients in group A of both series were older and more feeble and represent, perhaps, the same philosophical errors that apply to the surgeon who treats the woman admitted with a brain tumor metastatic from a cancer of the breast by a radical mastectomy. Some patients simply have disease that is not appropriately treated by attempts at vascular reconstruction. It is with the failures of groups B and C, however, that the surgeon should be more concerned, for under ideal circumstances there should be almost no patients in these categories.

The surgeon must not allow the patient to dictate the performance of reconstruction in the face of almost hopeless operative risks, as happened in several patients in this group. Techniques of reconstruction must be kept as simple as possible in these patients.

Late Failures

The interval between the initial success and later failures is described in Tables 10–3B and 10–5B. The majority of late failures have occurred through recurrence of the occlusion in an endarterectomized segment (atherosclerosis combined with thrombosis);

through stenosis, mechanical, extrinsic, atheromatous or fibrous in vein grafts; through thrombosis or dislodgement of the compacted fibrin lining of a Dacron graft; or at the end of a reconstructed segment, with either fibrous or atheromatous hyperplasia and secondary thrombosis. Much more infrequent causes of late failure are attachment aneurysms, sepsis, enteric fistula or occlusion by a rare tumor.

A.R., a 50-year-old man, was treated for aortoiliac atherosclerosis by aortoiliac endarterectomy. Five and one half years later he developed signs of recurrent disease. Transbrachial arteriography (Fig. 3–1) indicated areas of segmental stenosis. Their relationship to the previous endarterectomy was not defined until operation, when the atherosclerotic lesion was seen to be in the form of a diaphragm at the site of previous application of occluding clamps to the iliac arteries. Because of the adherence of the ureters at this site, it was deemed wiser to place a bypass prosthesis from the endarterectomized terminal aorta. Acute embolic occlusion of the popliteal artery on the left required surgical correction by means of a Fogarty[30] catheter inserted through the proximal superficial femoral artery. An excellent result has been maintained for eight years.

With the passage of time, even larger segments of the patient population than were earlier reported have shown progression of atherosclerosis in distant sites. Only a few of these patients manifest clearcut lipid disorders that can be recognized or treated; this may only be another way of saying that the subtle lipid changes responsible for atherosclerosis have not yet been identified.

A large proportion—two thirds—of these patients with recurrent atherosclerotic disease have had the recurrent disease treated. One might question such therapy, for one might assume that not only is the patient older than when originally treated but also he is already manifesting the form of aggressive atherosclerosis that suggests there will be further recurrence—and yet the repeated operations on some of these patients produce long-standing satisfactory results.

Szilagyi's discussion of secondary operations in his large experience separates these patients into two groups: the initial and early operations, which are attempts to recover a technical error or shortcoming, and the late operations, which probably represent corrections of recurrences or of new occurrences of the old disease of atherosclerosis.[73]

At times, however, the continued attempts at reconstruction find both the physician and the patient in the psychological trap of being unwilling to accept a failure even at the risk of a series of hazardous procedures which will result in an investment of great risk, effort, pain and logistical assets in the treatment of an ultimately hopeless situation. Such a case is presented here.

S. I. was a 52-year-old man who presented with a history of advanced aortoiliac claudication in 1965. Although he had had a major myocardial infarction in the past, he was subjected to an initially successful aortoiliac endarterectomy and bilateral lumbar sympathectomy. In 1966 he had a Dacron graft placed from the arch of the aorta to his right carotid artery because of transient cerebral ischemia, believed due to common carotid occlusion. This thrombosed later, however, and two years later he underwent a saphenous bypass graft from the left to the right carotid. In 1969 the aortoiliac reconstruction failed and was re-endarterectomized, with the addition of patches on the femoral bifurcation on the left. The left femoral artery subsequently underwent thrombosis, and was replaced with a Dacron graft. In spite of anticoagulation therapy with Coumadin, this graft underwent repeated thromboses and repeated successful thrombectomies. During one episode, however, the aortoiliac system thrombosed as well and, in spite of progressive coronary disease with serious angina pectoris, he underwent an axillo-bilateral femoral graft. This, too, underwent at least one episode of thrombosis and thrombectomy before the patient's heart finally caused his demise. Neither the patient nor his family nor his physicians were willing to accept failure and simple amputations, even though he was disabled by his severe heart disease.

Operations for Advanced Ischemia

Morris treated 315 cases in which gangrene had developed or was impending, with a salvage rate of about 80 per cent: aortoiliac lesions, 91 per cent; femoropopliteal lesions, 77 per cent; and combined lesions, 73 per cent. Of the initial successes, 18 per cent failed later, and patency was again restored in half of these.[56] We have seen very few patients whose extremities were seriously endangered by aortoiliac disease alone.

The series of Morris represents an aggressive attempt to treat gangrene, and was attended by a 6.3 per cent mortality rate. The patients in this series had more extensive disease than the usual candidate for elective surgery of occlusive arterial disease. The duration of the results was not defined.

Harrison[33] treated 216 legs, and reported an over-all acute success rate of 82.9 per cent and a limb salvage rate of 72.3 per cent, using primarily endarterectomy with vein patch or saphenous bypass graft. In half of the cases, the reconstruction was carried into one of the branches of the popliteal artery.

Taylor[78] has described an equally aggressive attack on advanced ischemia which was carried out at St. Bartholomew's Hospital in London. One hundred fifty limbs of 137 patients were treated, the patients ranging in age from 35 to 88 years. Thirty-seven limbs were amputated immediately because of extensive or irreversible gangrene, because of generally restricted activity due to systemic disease such as hemiplegia or arthritis, or because the area of vascular occlusion was unsuitable for reconstruction. Most liberal indications for reconstruction were used; if at least 2 or 2.5 cm. of open posterior tibial or popliteal artery was found, the reconstruction was undertaken. In 59 patients there was at least one artery in the distal tree which was patent throughout, and in this group there were only three early failures. In the group of 54 patients in whom no artery was patent throughout, there were nine acute failures. One year after operation 82 limbs of the initial 150 were surviving (except for local revision of gangrene and minor local amputation). Endarterectomized limbs apparently survived better than those reconstructed with vein grafts, but this situation may be related to the run-off which was probably better in the patients in whom endarterectomy was undertaken. There were only two deaths in this series, both due to early postoperative coronary occlusion. Of special importance in Taylor's series was his prompt conservative amputation and reconstruction of gangrenous areas which was done immediately following the reconstructive procedure. This aggressive approach might well result in a healing process which would not deteriorate if the reconstruction were to fail.

In our original series of 184 cases, only 17 patients had advanced

Table 10–8A.   Results in Patients Who Had Acute
Ischemia — Original Series

Patient	Age, Sex	Artery	Local Result	Outcome
1. MM	59F	Aortoiliac	Good	Survived
2. FR	81M	Aortoiliac	Good	Survived
3. IN	75F	Femoral	Condition of foot improved, but functioning of pulses undetermined	Survived
4. NG	49M	Femoral	Thrombosis, immediate	Died of coronary disease and hepatitis
5. LD	59M	Femoral	Good, but failed at 14 months, reoperation failed; amputation performed	Surviving three years postoperatively
6. JF	60M	Femoral	Prompt failure, transmetatarsal amputation	Survived
7. AB	78M	Femoral	Prompt failure	Coronary disease
8. MH	F	Femoral	Bypass thrombosed, attempted replacement thrombosed immediately	Died, coronary disease
9. EG	70F	Combined	Improved	Survived
10. ES	57F	Combined	Immediate failure; treated and corrected	Survived
11. TL	65F	Combined	Healed gangrenous ulcers	Survived
12. WP	59M	Combined	Healed gangrenous ulcers, functioning of pulses undetermined	Survived
13. LD	56M	Combined	Good	Survived
14. RW	59M	Combined	Femoral segment thrombosed: thigh amputation	Survived
15. CZ	54M	Combined	Healed transmetatarsal; good	Survived
16. JH	62M	Combined	Good	Survived
17. TP	58F	Combined	Thrombosis, reoperation, rethrombosis	Died

ischemia with actual necrosis or impending gangrene and advanced rest pain. There were three deaths and four major amputations (one of which was in a patient who subsequently died). Only two patients of the 81 who had aortoiliac disease could be classified as having advanced ischemia, six of the 43 with isolated femoral artery disease could be so classified, and nine of the 60 with combined aortoiliac and femoropopliteal lesions could be. The results are tabulated in Table 10–8A. Eleven of these 17 patients were clearly improved, although distal pedal pulses could be demonstrated in only six.

The results outlined point up the paradox that commonly faces the vascular surgeon: the more acute the need for reconstruction, the less likely is the reconstruction to be successful, and the greater is the risk to the patient if it fails. The mortality rate is low and the success rate is high in cases of minor occlusion, and the mortality risk increases when amputation is performed.[36, 38]

Taylor's experience[78] suggested that we had been too conservative in offering reconstruction to poor-risk patients. As a result, we have indeed offered some of the more debilitated patients, and those with very restricted run-off beds, reconstructions by means of vein grafts, reversed or in situ, or even long Dacron or bovine carotid heterografts.[14, 15, 17, 64, 65, 68, 79]

In the current series 16 of the 119 patients had acute ischemia as the immediate indication for operation. Ten had an actual ulcer or an area of gangrene, six had advanced and acute or pregangrenous ischemia. Only nine patients had early good local results, and two of these died in the postoperative period. These 16 patients are described in Table 10–8B.

Humphries[38] divided a series of 495 patients who had severe ischemia into three groups on the basis of treatment rendered. These groups are similar—but not identical—in respect to severity of the obliterative disease. One group received no surgical treatment, one group was treated by sympathectomy alone, and the third group was treated by arterioplasty. Improvement of the limb was seen in 24, 40, and 77 per cent of these groups respectively, whereas ultimate amputation was needed in 66, 46 and 22 per cent respectively.

The critically important observation in the entire group of Humphries' patients is the correspondence between amputation and death while still in hospital. In the first group 33 patients who died in hospital had 30 amputations; in the second group 14 died and 14 had amputations; and in the last group 6 died and 3 had amputations. The added stress of toxemia from a dead limb and surgical amputation was responsible for the increased risk.

The percentage of late deaths in all the groups was approximately the same, and represents the anticipated actuarial hazard rather than relationship to the form of treatment.

Table 10–8B. Results in Patients Who Had Acute
Ischemia—Current Series

Patient	Age, Sex	Artery	Local Result	Final Outcome
1. FM	63F	Femoral	Amputation	Survived
2. EW	70M	Femoral	Amputation	Survived
3. FH	64F	Femoral	Thrombosed graft	Survived, no amputation
4. JS	53M	Combined aortofemoral	Good early, failed late	Survived, ulcer healed in spite of later failure
5. JB	64M	Combined	Distal partial thrombosis	Bled, died of hepatic necrosis
6. HL	56M	Combined	Good	Survived
7. BC	55M	Combined	Good	Tolerated local digital amputation for gangrene with no late problems
8. CS	64F	Combined	Good	Survived
9. JM	67M	Combined	Good	Survived
10. HP	59M	Combined	Good	Survived
11. AH	61M	Aortoiliac	Good	Died, acute renal failure
12. AO	69M	Femoral	Amputation	Survived
13. KL	73F	Femoral	Good	Died, postoperative myocardial infarction
14. JJ	65M	Femoral	Failed	Survived, no amputation
15. PG	60M	Combined	Failed	Died, aspiration
16. PH	56M	Combined	Good	Survived

SUMMARY OF RESULTS OF OTHERS

Many reports[1, 2, 4, 11, 18, 20, 23, 29, 32, 34, 36, 38, 43, 48, 51, 56, 64, 72, 81, 82, 84, 85] were cited in the original edition of this book and are summarized in Table 10–9. Each author has used somewhat different criteria in selecting patients. Another bias represents the surgeon's preference, which has often been established early on the basis of the experiences of his learning days, for one surgical technique over another. As a result, the cases that appear to be preoperatively most favorable will probably have been treated by that technique with which the surgeon is most familiar. The present author recognizes his own preference for endarterectomy over grafting procedures, and in most instances of femoropopliteal disease has employed in the original series a grafting procedure only when the disease was far advanced and unfavorable.

Our experience also suggests very strongly that the technical details of grafting are easier to learn than the technical details of endarterectomy. The latter is more exacting and the surgeon must be prepared for failure unless the operation is meticulously carried out. It probably would be wise for the surgeon who is not well trained in the techniques of endarterectomy to adhere to the use of grafting procedures.[31]

A few selected series from more recent dates[8, 17, 25, 27, 28, 39, 41, 45, 46, 50, 52, 53, 59, 61, 65, 67, 68, 74, 79] are presented in Table 10–10. Table 10–9 is published as it appeared in the first edition of this volume so that some comparison may be made by the reader with current techniques and results as they are presented in Table 10–10.

Criteria for Choice of Operation

First, the site of the lesion has great influence on the rate and duration of successful reconstruction.

Second, with respect to localized aortoiliac lesions, either endarterectomy or bypass grafting is satisfactory in more than 95 per cent of patients, and the mortality risk is no more than 1 to 3 per cent in most instances.

Third, in reconstruction of the femoral artery, almost all groups have come to use the saphenous (or cephalic) vein autograft as the primary choice. A few groups are using the modified bovine carotid heterograft.[17, 65, 68] Endarterectomy is still used by a few groups,[67] although for the most part endarterectomy is used in only very localized lesions of the femoral system. The mortality rate for these operations is low unless the operation is performed as an emergency procedure in the face of acute myocardial ischemia. Initial patency rates will vary from 50 to 90 per cent, but the late patency rates will drop off considerably. More important is the figure quoted by DeWeese of a 45 per cent mortality in a five year follow-up.[26] Clearly, the surgeon must think of the overall status of the patient as well as the reconstructibility of the local arterial occlusion.[10, 71] Studies currently appearing indicate that there is no clear-cut relationship between the size of the graft, the apparent status of the outflow tract from an anatomical point of view,[52] or many of the other criteria which had orginally been introduced to govern the choice of operative candidates.[53, 59]

Fourth, the combined aortoiliac and femoropopliteal lesions carry a significant mortality risk but have a surprisingly long duration of good results. The duration of the results requires that the greatest care be taken to reduce the surgical risks to the minimum.

One paradox now being documented is the ominous overall prognosis for the relatively young patient who has major occlusive disease.[6, 57]

Fifth, operations for acute ischemia carry an increased mortality risk, but if properly conducted can be expected to provide long-lasting salvage of more than half the limbs endangered by impending or overt gangrene.

The surgeon bases his choice of procedure not only on the patient's local disease process and general medical status, but also on his own experience and skill in using the several procedures. The author's choice of operations would probably be the following:

A relatively young and otherwise healthy patient with aortoiliac occlusive disease would ordinarily be treated by endarterectomy.

Most patients who have serious involvement of the external iliac system as well will be treated by aortofemoral bypass grafts of Dacron. Only the younger patient who has relatively larger external iliac arteries will be treated by endarterectomy into the common femoral level (larger than a 16 French catheter). There should no longer be serious hesitation in extending the Dacron graft into the groin if mechanical indications require it, for the results will be vastly superior if good flow is obtained. There will be almost no circumstance in which the aortoiliac reconstruction will be extended below the common femoral artery if a good runoff bed is supplied by the deep femoral artery.

Table 10–9. Summary of Results Reported in the Literature (Republished from First Edition)

Author	Cases	Remarks	Operative Mortality (%)	Early Failure Rate (%)	Late Success Rate (%)	Time of Follow-up (yrs.)
		Aortoiliac Series				
Barker	72	Endarterectomy	1.2	1.2	84	1–9
	9	Synthetic prostheses	0	0	79	1–9
DeBakey[23]	179	Endarterectomy	3			1–5
Healey[34]	26	Endarterectomy	11	0	80	1–5
	36	Synthetic prostheses	11	6	61	Not stated
Julian[43]	164	Synthetic prostheses	Not stated	9	91	3–5
Szilagyi[72]	331	Dacron prostheses	Not stated	12	84	Not stated
Whitman[82]	28	Endarterectomy	0	14	75	Not stated
	59	Synthetic prostheses	5	17	60	
Wylie[84]	134	Endarterectomy	1.8	3.2	89	1–12
		Femoral Series				
Austin [1]	31	Nylon bypass		6	55	
	45	Teflon bypass		11	31	
	20	Saphenous vein bypass or replacement		10	75	Up to 89 months (entire series)
	49	Endarterectomy, no patch		8	80	
	10	Endarterectomy, Dacron patch		0	70	
	11	Endarterectomy, vein patch		0	82	
Barker	34	Endarterectomy	6	15	65	1–9
	11	Bypass (saphenous vein used primarily)	9	30	63	1–9
Connolly[14]	27	27 of 37 cases of autogenous *in situ* saphenous vein bypass have been followed 1 to 2 years	0	Not stated	83	1–2
Dale[18]	49	Vein grafts	4	69	60	0–5½
DeBakey[23]	1441	Dacron prostheses	3			
Edwards[29]	150	Synthetic bypass	Not stated	Not stated	25	Not stated
	Not stated	Semiclosed endarterectomy	Not stated	Not stated	"Many failures"	Not stated
	30	Open endarterectomy	Not stated	Not stated	60	Not stated
	51	Open endarterectomy	Not stated	Not stated	75	Not stated
	41	Composite vein bypass and open endarterectomy with vein patch	Not stated	Not stated	85	Not stated

The phrase "not stated" appears in connection with reports in which the applicable figure could not readily be determined.

(*Table continued on following page.*)

Table 10–9. Summary of Results Reported in the Literature (Republished from First Edition) (*Continued*)

Author	Cases	Remarks	Operative Mortality (%)	Early Failure Rare (%)	Late Success Rate (%)	Time of Follow-up (yrs.)
Gutelius[32]	20	Endarterectomy		30	55	Up to
	60	Saphenous vein bypass		18	80	16 mos.
Julian[43]	72	Dacron bypass	Not stated	Not stated	17	3
Laufman[48]	96	Synthetic prostheses	Not stated	Not stated	72	1
					57	2
					46	3
					38	4
Szilagyi[72]	193	Synthetic prostheses	Not stated	25	58	3–5
Wylie[84]	94	Endarterectomy for severe ischemia and severe distal outflow disease	1	1	40	4
					85	4
					97	4
		Combined Aortoiliac Femoropopliteal Reconstruction				
Barker	40	Endarterectomy	5	18	72	0–9
	22	Combined prostheses, vein grafts, and endarterectomy	0	14	64	1–9
Darling[20]	97	Endarterectomy	2	3	98	2–3
	38				100	3–5
Rob[64]	388	Endarterectomy	Not stated	Not stated	81.6	
	133	Autogenous vein (various sites)	Not stated	Not stated	69.9	2 or
	206	Homologous artery graft	Not stated	Not stated	68.4	more
	285	Synthetic prostheses	Not stated	Not stated	48.4	
Harrison[33]	206	Endarterectomy and vein bypass, half extended below distal popliteal	3	Not stated	83	Not stated
Mannick[51] Morris[56]	30	Reversed saphenous vein bypass in femoral obliterative disease	7	18	7	Not stated
		Aortoiliac prostheses, chiefly synthetic		9		Not stated
	+315	Femoropopliteal prostheses, chiefly synthetic	6.3	23		
		Combined aortoiliac and femoropopliteal prostheses, chiefly synthetic		27		

Combined occlusive disease of the superficial femoral artery and the proximal system rarely needs to be treated at one operation. Most patients will develop sufficient collaterals from the profunda femoris to the popliteal system that symptoms will disappear or be thoroughly tolerable. If serious systems do persist, then staged femoropopliteal or femorotibial operations can be performed.

A few patients are seen in whom there is only femoral artery disease, and no evidence of proximal aortic inflow disease. These patients, just as the patients described in the previous paragraph, should be treated only if symptoms are incapacitating, or if tissue loss is threatened. The choice of the method of reconstruction is a technical

Table 10–10. Late Results — Current Series

Author	Cases	Remarks	Operative Mortality (%)	Early Results (%)	Late Results (%)	Follow-up Period (yrs.)
		Aortoiliac cases				
Barker	43	Aortoiliac endarterectomy	2.0	98	81°	4
Butcher	94	Aortoiliac endarterectomy	6.0	96	72°	5
Duncan	125	Aortoiliac endarterectomy	0.8	98	95.4°	5
	152	Aortofemoral endarterectomy	4.6	94	88.5°	5
	45	Aortoiliac grafts	6.6	92	96.3°	5
	87	Aortofemoral grafts	2.3	97	74.3°	5
Eastcott	190	Aortoiliac — operations not specified	4.0	98	72.6	1–16 years (average 4.1)
Humphries	496	Aortoiliac for claudication	4.4	–	74°	5
		Aortoiliac for severe ischemia			48°	5
Inahara	97	Eversion endarterectomy	5.1	95	96°	5
					93°	9
Perdue	223	Mixed aortoiliac, aortofemoral — mostly operations by Dacron graft	2.2	97.4	93.7	Mean follow-up of 36 mos.
Pilcher	69	Endarterectomy, all over 10 year follow-up	1.5	–	69°	10
Sawyer	64	Gas endarterectomy, aortoiliac	3.0	95	66°	5
		Femoropopliteal cases				
Barker	13	Vein bypass; poor risk patients	15	46	45°	4°°
Cutler	31	⎰Heterografts for claudication 0⎱ Heterografts for rest pain or gangrene 0		81	⎰79 ⎱53	Followed up to 10 years
DeWeese	35	Femoral endarterectomy	Not appli-cable	86	54	At end of
	56	Reversed vein (saphenous)		75	63	5 years
Eastcott	151	Reversed vein for claudication	2.1	89)	45	3 year
	87	Reversed vein for severe ischemia		80)	42	average follow-up
Humphries	496	Endarterectomy for claudication	4.4	–	32°	5
		Endarterectomy for severe ischemia			35°	5
Linton	56	Reversed vein (saphenous)	1.0	92	66°	5
Rosenberg	50	Heterografts	10	64	54	At end of 2 years
Sawyer	138	Gas endarterectomy	–	95	65°	5
Stoney	19	Reversed vein Stage I runoff	0	–	76°	6
	52	Reversed vein Stage II and III runoff	8	–	40°	6
Szilagyi	316	Reversed vein	2.5	76.3	64°	5
Mannick	31	Reversed vein to isolated popliteal segment	3.2	71	65	9 months to 4½ years
Miller	156	Reversed vein (mostly femoro-popliteal, some femorotibial)	1.3	95	70°	5
		Femorotibial cases				
Kahn	53	Reversed vein (saphenous limb salvage)	3	68	51	2 years
Kaminski	22	Reversed saphenous vein for gangrene or severe rest pain	0	78	65	3–29 months
Slovin	14	Heterografts	0	14	60°	18 months average
Szilagyi	61	Reversed vein (saphenous)	1.6	78.7	(58° (54°	2 years 3 years
Tyson	48	Reversed vein (saphenous)	0	–	77	Up to 5½ years

°Figures reported according to cumulative patency rate

°°Late figures include late good results after acute revision of early failure. There are many minor differences among these series, and the apparent differences in results depend greatly on patient selection, composition of the series, and method of reporting.

If a figure is not given, it is because it was not clearly defined in the original article.

one which is best left to the individual operator, although previous chapters have endeavored to provide criteria by means of which he can make a rational choice.

All patients will have lumbar sympathectomy performed as an integral part of the procedure.

Postoperatively, judicious use of anticoagulants and dietary control to reduce the atherogenic potential will be integral parts of the patient's over-all care to reduce the hazards of recurrence.

REFERENCES

1. Austin, D. J., Thompson, J. E., Wheeler, C. G., and Patman, R. D.: Arteriosclerotic occlusive disease of superficial femoral and popliteal arteries. Am. J. Surg. *108*:636, 1964.
2. Barker, W. F., and Cannon, J. A.: An evaluation of endarterectomy. Arch. Surg. *66*:488, 1953.
3. Barker, W. F., Cannon, J. A., Zeldis, L. J., and Ah'Tye, P.: Anatomical results of endarterectomy. Surg. Forum *6*:266, 1955.
4. Barker, W. F., and Hart, J. E.: Arterial reconstruction by endarterectomy. Am. J. Surg. *100*:165, 1960.
5. Bernhard, V. M., Ashmore, C. S., Rodgers, R. E., and Evans, W. E.: Operative blood flow in femoro-popliteal and femoral-tibial grafts for lower extremity ischemia. Arch. Surg. *103*:595, 1971.
6. Bouhoutsos, J., and Martin, P.: The influence of age on prognosis after arterial surgery for atherosclerosis of the lower limb. Surgery *74*:637, 1973.
7. Brief, D. K., Alpert, J., and Parsonnet, V.: Crossover femorofemoral grafts: compromise or preference; a reappraisal. Arch. Surg. *105*:889, 1972.
8. Butcher, H. R. Jr., and Jaffe, B. M.: Treatment of aorto-iliac arterial occlusive disease by endarterectomy. Ann. Surg. *173*:925, 1971.
9. Callow, A. D., Aboulafia, E. D., and Balas, P. E.: The restrictive effect of bypass grafts upon the occluded major arterial channel and its collaterals. Surgery *49*:26, 1961.
10. Cannon, J. A.: Surgical judgment in vascular surgery. Arch. Surg. *103*:521, 1971.
11. Cannon, J. A., and Barker, W. F.: Successful management of obstructive femoral arteriosclerosis by endarterectomy. Surgery *38*:48, 1955.
12. Cannon, J. A., Barker, W. F., and Kawakami, I. G.: Femoral popliteal endarterectomy in the treatment of obliterative atherosclerotic disease. Surgery *43*:76, 1958.
13. Cannon, J. A., Kawakami, I. G., and Barker, W. F.: Present status of aortoiliac endarterectomy for obliterative atherosclerosis. Arch. Surg. *82*:813, 1961.
14. Connolly, J. E., and Harris, E. J.: Autogenous in situ saphenous vein bypass for femoropopliteal occlusive disease; a follow-up study. Am. J. Surg. *110*:270, 1965.
15. Connolly, J. E., Harris, E. J., and Mills, W. Jr.: Autogenous in situ saphenous vein for bypass of femoral-popliteal obliterative disease. Surgery *55*:144, 1964.
16. Creech, O.: In Barker, W. F. (Ed.): *Surgical Treatment of Peripheral Vascular Disease.* New York, McGraw-Hill Book Co., Inc., 1962.
17. Cutler, B. S., Thompson, J. E., Patman, R. D., Persson, A. V., and Manfredi, P. D.: The modified bovine arterial graft: a clinical study. Surgery *76*:963, 1974 (in press).
18. Dale, W. A.: In Wesolowski, S. A., and Dennis, C.: *Fundamentals of Vascular Grafting.* New York, McGraw-Hill Book Co., Inc., 1963.
19. Dale, W. A., and Lewis, M. R.: Lateral vascular patch grafts. Surgery *57*:36, 1965.

20. Darling, R. C., and Linton, R. R.: Aortoiliofemoral endarterectomy for atherosclerotic occlusive disease. Surgery 55:184, 1964.
21. Darling, R. C., Linton, R. R., and Razzuk, M. A.: Saphenous vein bypass grafts for femoropopliteal occlusive disease: a reappraisal. Surgery 61:31, 1967.
22. DeBakey, M. E.: In Wesolowski, S. A., and Dennis, C.: *Fundamentals of Vascular Grafting.* New York, McGraw-Hill Book Co., Inc., 1963.
23. DeBakey, M. D., Crawford, E. S., Morris, G. C. Jr., Cooley, D. A., and Garrett, H. E.: Late results of vascular surgery in the treatment of arteriosclerosis. J. Cardiov. Surg. 5:473, 1964.
24. DeBakey, M. E., Jordan, G. L., Jr., Abbott, J. P., Halpert, B., and O'Neal, R. M.: The fate of dacron vascular grafts. Arch. Surg. 89:757, 1964.
25. DeWeese, J. A.: Results of thromboendarterectomy vs. venous bypass grafts. In Dale, W. A. (Ed.): *Management of Arterial Occlusive Disease.* Chicago, Year Book Medical Publishers, 1971.
26. DeWeese, J. A., and Rob, C. G.: Autogenous venous bypass grafts five years later. Ann. Surg. 174:346, 1971.
27. Duncan, W. C., Linton, R. R., and Darling, R. C.: Aortoiliofemoral atherosclerotic disease: comparative results of endarterectomy and Dacron bypass grafts. Surgery 70:974, 1971.
28. Eastcott, H. H. G.: *Arterial Surgery.* London, Pitman Medical Publishers, 1969.
29. Edwards, W. S.: Personal communication.
30. Fogarty, T. J., Cranley, J. J., Krause, R. J., Strasser, E. S., and Hafner, C. D.: A method for extraction of arterial emboli and thrombi. Surg. Gynec. Obstet. 116:241, 1963.
31. Gaspard, D. J., Cohen, L. J., and Gaspar, M. R.: Aortoiliofemoral thromboendarterectomy vs. bypass graft; a randomized study. Arch. Surg. 105:898, 1972.
32. Gutelius, J. R., Kreindler, S., and Luke, J. C.: Comparative evaluation of autogenous vein bypass graft and endarterectomy in superficial femoral artery reconstruction. Surgery 57:28, 1965.
33. Harrison, J. H., and Preez, A. R.: Advanced ischemia. Arch. Surg. 89:817, 1964.
34. Healey, S. J., Wheeler, H. B., Crane, C., and Warren, R.: Reconstructive operations for aortoiliac obliterative disease. Results and reflections from an eleven year experience. New Eng. J. Med. 271:1386, 1964.
35. Hufnagel, C. A.: Permanent intubation of thoracic aorta. Arch. Surg. 54:382, 1947.
36. Humphries, A. W.: In Wesolowski, S. A., and Dennis, C.: *Fundamentals of Vascular Grafting.* New York, McGraw-Hill Book Co., Inc., 1963.
37. Humphries, A. W., Hawk, W. A., DeWolfe, V. G., and LeFevre, F. A.: Clinicopathologic observations on the fate of arterial freeze-dried homografts. Surgery 45: 59, 1959.
38. Humphries, A. W., Young, J. R., DeWolfe, V. G., LeFevre, F. A., and Beven, E. G.: Severe ischemia of lower extremity due to arteriosclerosis obliterans. Arch. Surg. 87:175, 1963.
39. Humphries, A. W., Young, J. R., and McCormack, L. J.: Experience with aortoiliac and femoropopliteal endarterectomy. Surgery 65:48, 1969.
40. Imparato, A. M., Bracco, A., Kim, G. E., and Zeff, R.: Intimal and neointimal fibrous proliferation causing failure of arterial reconstruction. Surgery 72:1007, 1972.
41. Inahara, T.: Endarterectomy for occlusive disease of the aortoiliac and common femoral arteries. Evaluation of the results of eversion endarterectomy. Am. J. Surg. 124:235, 1972.
42. Jordan, G. L., Stump, M. M., Allen, J., DeBakey, M. E., and Halpert, B.: Gelatin-impregnated dacron prosthesis implanted into the porcine thoracic aorta. Surgery 53:45, 1963.
43. Julian, O. C.: Chronic occlusion of the aorta and iliac arteries. Surg. Clin. N. Amer. 40:139, 1960.
44. Julian, O. C.: In Wesolowski, S. A., and Dennis, C.: *Fundamentals of Vascular Grafting.* New York, McGraw-Hill Book Co., Inc., 1963.
45. Kahn, S. P., Lindenauer, S. M., Dent, T. L., Kraft, R. O., and Fry, W. J.: Femoro-tibial vein bypass. Arch. Surg. 107:309, 1973.
46. Kaminski, D. L., Barner, H. B., Dorighi, J. A., Kaiser, G. C., and Willman, V. L.: Femoro-tibial bypass grafting. Arch. Surg. 104:527, 1972.

47. Kennedy, L. J., and Weissman, I. L.: Dual origin in intimal cells in cardiac-allograft arteriosclerosis. New Eng. J. Med. *285*:884, 1971.
48. Laufman, H.: Surgical management of chronic iliofemoral arterial occlusion. Surg. Clin. North Amer. *40*:153, 1960.
49. Lazzarini-Robertson, A.: Discussion cited by Jordan, G. L.: In Wesolowski, S. A., and Dennis, C.: *Fundamentals of Vascular Grafting*. New York, McGraw-Hill Book Co., Inc., 1963, p. 188.
50. Linton, R. R.: Long term results of femoropopliteal autogenous vein grafts. In Dale, W. A. (Ed.): *Management of Arterial Occlusive Disease*. Chicago, Year Book Medical Publishers, 1971.
51. Mannick, J. A., and Hume, D. M.: Salvage of extremities by vein grafts in far-advanced peripheral vascular disease. Surgery 55:154, 1964.
52. Mannick, J. A., Jackson, B. T., Coffman, J. D., and Hume, D. M.: Success of bypass vein grafts in patients with isolated popliteal artery segments. Surgery *61*:17, 1967.
53. Miller, V. M.: Femoropopliteal bypass graft patency: an analysis of 156 cases. Ann. Surg. *180*:35, 1974.
54. Moore, W. S., Cafferata, H. T., Hall, A. D., and Blaisdell, F. W.: In defense of grafts across the inguinal ligament: an evaluation of early and late results of aortofemoral by-pass grafts. Ann. Surg. *168*:207, 1968.
55. Moore, W. S., Hall, A. D., and Blaisdell, F. W.: Late results of axillary-femoral bypass grafting. Am. J. Surg. *122*:148, 1971.
56. Morris, G. C., Jr., Wheeler, C. G., Crawford, E. S., Cooley, D. A., and DeBakey, M. E.: Restorative vascular surgery in the presence of impending and overt gangrene of the extremities. Surgery *51*:50, 1962.
57. Najafi, H., Ostermiller, W. E., Ardekani, R. G., Dye, W. S., Javid, H. J., Hunter, J. A., and Julian, O. C.: Aortoiliac reconstruction in patients 32 to 45 years of age. Arch. Surg. *101*:780, 1970.
58. Ochsner, J. L., DeCamp, P. T., and Leonard, G. L.: Experience with fresh venous allografts as an arterial substitute. Ann. Surg. *173*:933, 1971.
59. Perdue, G. D., Long, W. T., and Smith, R. B. III: Perspective concerning aortofemoral arterial reconstruction. Ann. Surg. *173*:940, 1971.
60. Perloff, L. J., Reckard, C. R., Rowlands, D. T. Jr., and Barker, C. F.: The venous homograft, an immunological question. Surgery 72:961, 1972.
61. Pilcher, D. B., Barker, W. F., and Cannon, J. A.: An aortoiliac endarterectomy case series followed 10 years or more. Surgery 67:5, 1970.
62. Poole, J. C. F., Sabiston, D. C. Jr., Florey, H. W., and Allison, P. R.: Growth of endothelium in artificial prosthetic grafts and following endarterectomy. Surg. Forum *13*:225, 1962.
63. Reichle, F. A., Stewart, G. J., and Essa, N.: A transmission and scanning electron microscopic study of luminal surfaces in Dacron and autogenous bypasses in man and dog. Surgery 74:945, 1973.
64. Rob, C. G.: In Wesolowski, S. A., and Dennis, C.: *Fundamentals of Vascular Grafting*. New York, McGraw-Hill Book Co., Inc., 1963.
65. Rosenberg, D. M. L., Glass, B. A., Rosenberg, N., Lewis, M. R., and Dale, W. A.: Experience with modified bovine carotid arteries in arterial surgery. Surgery, *68*:1064, 1970.
66. Sauvage, L. R., Berger, K., Wood, F. J., Nakagawa, Y., and Mansfield, P. B.: An external velour surface for porous arterial prostheses. Surgery, 79:40, 1971.
67. Sawyer, P. N., Pasupathy, C. E., Fitzgerald, J., Kaplitt, M. J., Costello, M., Keats, J. R. W., O'Malley, G., and Lapovsky, A.: Six-year follow-up study in the use of gas endarterectomy. Surgery 72:837, 1972.
68. Slovin, A. J.: Arterial below the knee bypass grafts. Experience with the modified bovine heterograft. Amer. J. Surg. *128*:58, 1974.
69. Stokes, J. M., Sugg, W. L., and Butcher, H. R.: Standard method of assessing relative effectiveness of therapies for arterial occlusive diseases. Ann. Surg. *157*:343, 1963.
70. Stone, A. M., and Stahl, W. M.: Effect of ethacrynic acid and furosemide on renal function in hypovolemia. Ann. Surg. *174*:1, 1971.

71. Stoney, R. J., James, D. R., and Wylie, E. J.: Surgery for femoropopliteal athero-sclerosis. Arch. Surg. *103*:546, 1971.
72. Szilagyi, D. E.: In Wesolowski, S. A., and Dennis, C.: *Fundamentals of Vascular Grafting.* New York, McGraw-Hill Book Co., Inc., 1963.
73. Szilagyi, D. E., Elliott, J. P., and Ansari, M. A.: Secondary arterial repairs, In Dale, W. A. (Ed.): *Management of Arterial Occlusive Disease.* Chicago, Year Book Medical Publishers, 1971.
74. Szilagyi, D. E., Elliott, J. P., Hageman, J. H., Smith, R. F., and Dall'Olmo, C. A.: Biologic fate of autogenous vein implants as arterial substitutes: Clinical, angiographic and histopathologic observations in femoro-popliteal operations for atherosclerosis. Ann. Surg. *178*:232, 1973.
75. Szilagyi, D. E., McDonald, R. T., Smith, R. F., and Whitcomb, J. G.: A study of the biologic fate of human arterial homografts. Arch. Surg. *75*:506, 1957.
76. Szilagyi, D. E., Rodriguez, F. J., Smith, R. F., and Elliott, J. P.: Late fate of arterial allografts. Observations 6 to 15 years after implantation. Arch. Surg. *101*:721, 1970.
77. Szilagyi, D. E., Smith, R. F., Elliott, J. P., and Vrandecic, M. T.: Infection in arterial reconstruction with synthetic grafts. Ann. Surg. *176*:321, 1972.
78. Taylor, G. W.: Personal communication.
79. Tyson, R. R., and Reichle, F. A.: Femoro-tibial bypass. Surgery *170*:429, 1969.
80. Vetto, R. M.: The treatment of unilateral iliac artery obstruction with a transab-dominal, subcutaneous, femoro-femoral graft. Surgery *52*:342, 1962.
81. Warren, R., and Villavicencio, J. L.: Iliofemoropopliteal arterial reconstructions for arteriosclerosis obliterans; factors influencing late patency. New Eng. J. Med. *260*:255, 1959.
82. Whitman, E. J., and McGoon, D. C.: Surgical management of aorto-iliac occlusive vascular disease. J.A.M.A. *179*:923, 1962.
83. Wyatt, A. P., Rothnie, N. G., and Taylor, G. W.: The vascularization of vein-grafts. Brit. J. Surg. *51*:378, 1964.
84. Wylie, E., Kerr, E., and Davies, O.: Experimental and clinical experiences with use of fascia lata applied as a graft about major arteries after thromboendarterec-tomy and aneurysmorrhaphy. Surg. Gynec. Obstet. *93*:257, 1951.
85. Wylie, E. J.: Personal communication.

Chapter Eleven

CEREBROVASCULAR INSUFFICIENCY

JESSE E. THOMPSON, M.D.

In the twenty-three years since the first successful carotid artery reconstruction for stroke was performed,[13] cerebral revascularization has become accepted therapy for selected patients with cerebrovascular insufficiency. Recent data from the Joint Study of Extracranial Arterial Occlusion indicate that 74 per cent of patients with ischemic stroke syndromes studied have at least one significant stenotic lesion in the extracranial vasculature at a surgically accessible site.[30] Since three fourths of the patients who suffer strokes have warning symptoms in the form of transient ischemic attacks, recognition of the significance of such episodes and their proper treatment prior to the catastrophic event are important factors in stroke prevention.

ANATOMY

The main vessels supplying blood to the brain are the two carotid and two vertebral arteries and their branches (Fig. 11–1). Many variations in the normal anatomy occur, and anomalies at all levels, from the aortic arch to the circle of Willis, are not uncommon. Numerous pathways for collateral circulation are available when any of the principal vessels are occluded.[23, 57]

Extracranial obstructive lesions responsible for cerebrovascular insufficiency are found in the aortic arch at the origins of the innominate, carotid, and subclavian arteries, in the vertebral arteries at their origins and beyond, in the common carotid bifurcations, and in

the first portion of the internal and external carotid arteries (Fig. 11–
2). Obstructions at the carotid bifurcation, which usually involve the
first few centimeters of the internal carotid artery as well, are by far
the most common. In many cases the intracranial vessels are surprisingly free of demonstrable disease. The segmental nature of the cervical lesions makes possible restoration of cerebral blood flow by
surgical means. Multiple-vessel involvement by stenotic plaques in
both the carotid and vertebral–basilar systems is a frequent finding.

PATHOLOGY

Most of the occlusions are caused by intimal atherosclerotic
plaques that partially or completely obstruct the extracranial vessels.

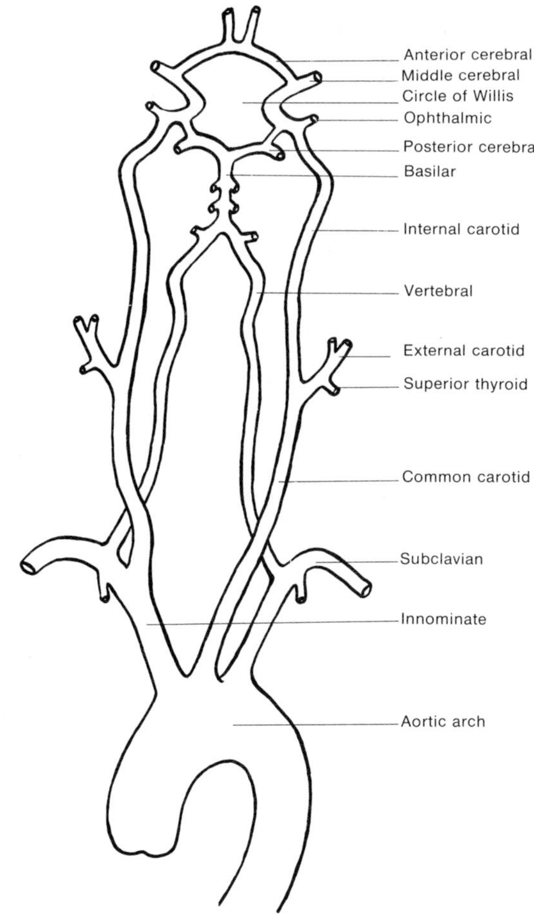

Figure 11–1. Principal arteries and their major branches
which constitute the blood supply to the brain. Many collateral
pathways are available when
one or more of the major vessels
become occluded.

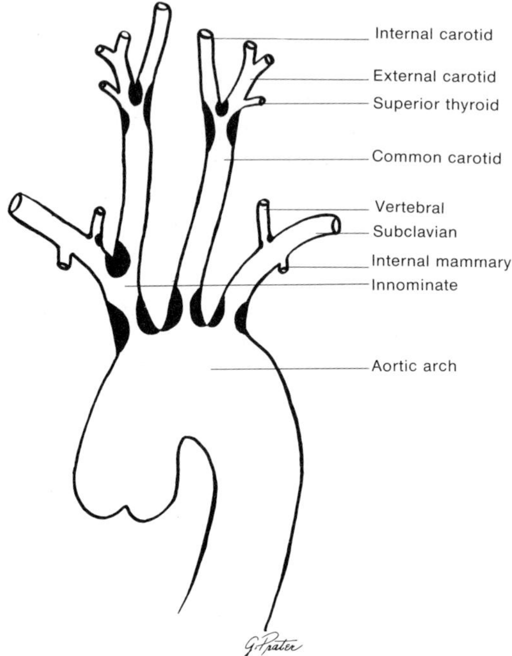

Figure 11–2. Usual extracranial sites of atherosclerotic plaques responsible for cerebrovascular insufficiency.

At times the plaques become necrotic and ulcerated, with deposition of platelets and thrombi on the ulcerated areas (Fig. 11–3). This debris may become dislodged and embolize into the distal circulation. As a plaque enlarges and lumen size diminishes, blood flow decreases. The final episode is thrombosis with complete occlusion of the artery. Thrombosis of the internal carotid artery usually involves its entire extracranial extent. Other lesions which may occasionally be responsible for carotid and vertebral occlusions are aneurysms, arteritis, bony spurs, fibromuscular dysplasia, kinks, and loops.

PATHOPHYSIOLOGY

The basic principles of circulatory physiology important for the vascular surgeon have been discussed in detail in Chapter Three. The factors regulating cerebral circulatory responses in normal and pathologic states have been the subject of much recent review.[2, 22a, 34, 42] Only those salient features related to surgical considerations will be stressed here.

Cerebral blood flow (CBF) is largely determined by the perfusion pressure and the vascular resistance of the brain. Cerebral perfusion

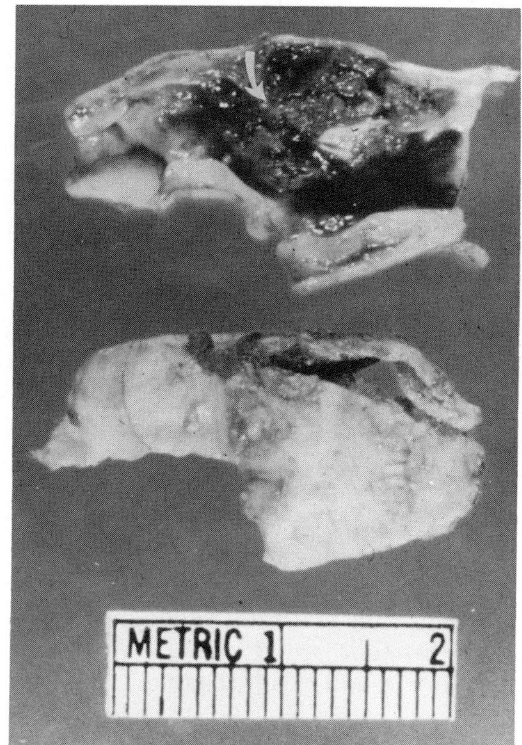

Figure 11–3. Typical atherosclerotic plaque removed by endarterectomy from the carotid artery bifurcation, demonstrating stenosis as well as deposition of thrombotic material on the ulcerated plaque, a source of emboli responsible for preoperative and intraoperative neurological deficits.

pressure is the arterial pressure minus the venous pressure. Under normal circumstances cerebral blood flow is kept relatively constant by means of autoregulation. Although several theories have been advanced to explain autoregulation, the most likely mechanism is through changes in the pH of the extracellular fluid of the central nervous system, by direct action on cerebral arteriolar smooth muscle.[34]

Cerebrovascular resistance is influenced by intracranial pressure, oxygen, and carbon dioxide. Hyperoxia produces cerebral vasoconstriction, but the magnitude of change is small. Hypoxia produces cerebral vasodilatation and increased CBF and will also abolish autoregulation.

The major factor determining CBF is the carbon dioxide in the arterial blood ($PaCO_2$). The CO_2 acts by changing the pH of the extracellular fluid of the brain, which is thought to be the main factor controlling CBF. As $PaCO_2$ is increased (hypercapnia),* cerebrovascular resistance decreases and CBF increases. Conversely, as $PaCO_2$ decreases (hypocapnia), cerebrovascular resistance is increased and CBF decreases.

---

*The word "hypercapnia" is derived from the Greek *kapnos* (smoke), and refers to an increased amount of carbon dioxide in the blood.

Alexander and Lassen[2] recognized that cerebral acidosis, which produces vasodilatation, could be focal as well as generalized. They introduced the term "luxury-perfusion syndrome" to designate the overabundance of blood relative to metabolic needs in regional acidosis of the brain. Cerebral vessels in the involved area show a loss of autoregulation and a lack of responsiveness to changes in $PaCO_2$.

In this syndrome vasodilating agents may cause an "intracerebral steal." This occurs because dilatation of the nonischemic, normally reactive vessels results in a lowered pressure in the collateral circulation, with diversion of blood away from the ischemic area. Vasoconstricting measures, such as hyperventilation, by constricting the reactive vessels and increasing local perfusion pressure, will augment collateral flow into the ischemic area. These observations may have important clinical implications[22] and will be discussed further in the section on methods of cerebral protection (pp. 276–277).

Cerebral arterial insufficiency may take the form of transient attacks of ischemia with reversible neurological dysfunction, or infarction with loss of viability of cerebral tissue accompanied by irreversible changes. In both instances there is reduction in blood supply to the area of brain involved. In one instance it is to a degree and of such duration that recovery ensues, whereas in the other it is more severe and cell death results.[35]

The mechanisms involved in the pathogenesis of both infarction and ischemia are not fully understood. Occlusion with thrombosis in the extracranial or intracranial vessels is the usual cause of infarction but is not found in all cases. Atherosclerotic lesions with or without stenosis are usually present in patients with transient ischemia. Factors necessary to precipitate attacks include (1) distal embolization of thrombi, platelets, or atherosclerotic debris from carotid plaques, or (2) transitory systemic hypotension. The latter may be caused by decreased cardiac output secondary to myocardial infarction, congestive failure or arrhythmias; gastrointestinal hemorrhage; dehydration with extracellular fluid deficit; traumatic shock; and antihypertensive drugs.[40]

Other factors, anatomical and physiological, which have been considered in the pathogenesis of infarction and insufficiency include structural variations in the circle of Willis, the status of the collateral circulation, kinking and compression of vessels in the neck, vasospasm, temporary hypoglycemia, transitory cerebral shunts, anemia, anoxia, and polycythemia. In all probability a combination of factors is necessary.[35, 40, 55]

The concept of total cerebral blood flow, which in disease states is a function of the collateral circulation to the brain, has important therapeutic implications. The main vessels supplying the brain are the two carotid and two vertebral arteries. Recent investigations have established values for normal resting blood flow through each of these arteries. It has been shown in man, without occlusive disease, that the internal carotid arteries carry 85 to 90 per cent of the blood flowing to the brain, while the two vertebral arteries carry the remainder.[45] It is well known that occlusion of one or more of these vessels may occur without significant neurological deficit. Corresponding to the clinical experience is the experimental demonstration that flow in the ipsilateral internal carotid artery may be increased as much as 38 per cent following occlusion of the contralateral common carotid artery.[28] Obstruction to blood flow in any of the four vessels to the brain is followed by a compensatory increase in flow in the other vessels. The functional capacity of the brain, when major vessels are obstructed, is thus largely dependent on the integrity of the compensatory mechanisms responsible for collateral circulation.

Studies of total cerebral blood flow are at times misleading, however, since they may not accurately reflect *regional* cerebral blood flow.[33, 42] In the presence of a single stenotic lesion the measured total flow may be normal, but flow to a focal area may be markedly diminished, with resulting symptoms. The recent development of methods to measure regional cerebral blood flow using radioactive ^{133}Xe and ^{85}Kr isotopes, recording from multiple areas of the brain with collimated scintillation detectors, has made it possible to obtain much new information about events in specific regions of the brain.[2, 22a, 56] The influence of stenotic lesions on regional cerebral blood flow in the individual case must, therefore, be considered along with collateral circulation and total cerebral blood flow.

The anatomical arrangement for cerebral collateral circulation has both extracranial and intracranial components. The various pathways have been described in detail by Fields et al.[23] and by Weibel and Fields.[57] There are numerous extracranial routes connecting the carotid and vertebral systems via ipsilateral and contralateral vessels in the presence of occlusive lesions. The intracranial basis for collateral circulation is provided by the elaborate arrangement of branches constituting the circle of Willis at the base of the brain and to some degree by vessels on the surface of the cerebral hemispheres.

The pattern of collateral circulation for each of the cerebral arteries is clearly defined anatomically. The detail varies widely from one patient to another, however, because of variations in the location of stenotic lesions, the occurrence of multiple lesions, and the presence of anomalies in the vessels supplying the collateral blood supply, especially those of the circle of Willis.

Certain physiological factors are also involved in the development of collateral circulation. Of great importance is the rapidity of occlusion. If occlusion occurs suddenly the compensatory mechanisms may be inadequate, with loss of cerebral function or even frank infarction. On the other hand, if occlusion progresses slowly, the compensatory mechanisms usually provide for adequate collateral cerebral circulation. Cardiac output and systemic blood pressure greatly influence the actual circulation through these collateral pathways.[23]

Clinical experience with arteriography and vascular surgery has elucidated many mechanisms involved in cerebral circulation. In the presence of a totally occluded internal carotid artery, arteriograms show that cross circulation *via* the circle of Willis often is sufficient to supply both hemispheres. In patients with one carotid artery totally occluded and the other severely stenosed, restoration of flow in the single stenosed artery will relieve symptoms. Also pertinent is the observation that patients with neurologic deficits may have occlusive lesions situated in the carotid artery on the ipsilateral or paradoxical side relative to the clinical picture. Removal of such inappropriate occlusions has relieved the neurologic deficits. Not infrequently, symptoms of vertebral-basilar disease seen in patients with both vertebral and carotid lesions are relieved when carotid blood flow only is restored by endarterectomy.

Germane to any discussion of critical levels of total cerebral blood flow is the question of reversibility of neurologic deficits. It has been observed that certain patients with strokes who appeared to have irreversible deficits have had remarkable recoveries following restoration of cerebral circulation.[47] In some cases, therefore, the severe depression of cerebral function which occurs is due to ischemia rather than infarction. Recovery is possible with reversal of the neurologic deficit. This phenomenon has been observed in a number of patients with varying degrees of return of function, some to normal and some with residual deficits, but all with improvement dating from surgical revascularization.

There are significant surgical implications from the foregoing discussion. It is important to preserve and to restore flow in the external carotid as well as in the internal carotid artery since the former is an important source of extracranial collateral circulation. The treatment of stenoses prior to the occurrence of total occlusion, with possible failure of compensatory mechanisms, likewise deserves serious consideration for the prevention of catastrophic events. Several sources of primary or collateral circulation are more effective in restoring or maintaining adequate cerebral blood flow than is a single source.

Anatomical alterations, developmental and pathological, and physiological mechanisms are both involved in cerebrovascular insufficiency. They are responsible for a diversity of clinical manifestations and for the great variation in the rate and degree of recovery from neurologic deficits.

SIGNIFICANCE OF STENOTIC LESIONS

The question arises as to the functional significance of occlusive lesions seen on arteriograms of the extracranial vessels supplying the brain. A lesion which is significant on the x-ray may not be accompanied by clinical manifestations. Most of the significant carotid lesions show a reduction in diameter of the internal carotid artery of 50 per cent or more as measured on the arteriogram (Fig. 11–4). Stenoses of lesser degree are of greater significance if the opposite carotid or the vertebral arteries are also compromised, or if multiple stenotic lesions are present. A stenosis of any degree may be significant if its appearance suggests the deposition of platelet thrombi or the presence of an ulcerated plaque, which may be sources of cerebral emboli (Fig. 11–5).

Crawford et al.[15] made intra-arterial pressure measurements at the time of operation and reported that carotid lesions causing 47 per cent reduction or more of the internal carotid artery diameter resulted in significant pressure gradients.

Brice et al., in experimental studies,[12] concluded that to impair

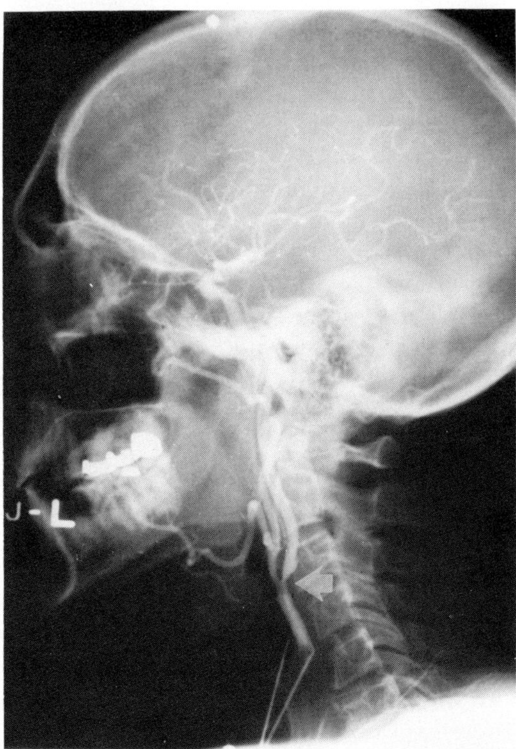

Figure 11–4. Left carotid arteriogram showing a significant stenosis in the internal carotid artery of a male patient with transient ischemic attacks.

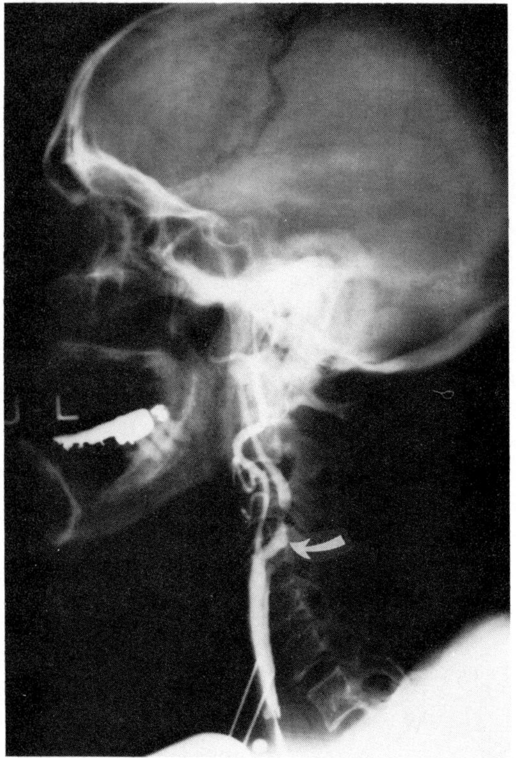

Figure 11–5. Left carotid arteriogram showing an irregular, bulky, stenotic plaque in the internal carotid artery. This lesion gives rise to emboli which may cause transient ischemic episodes.

blood flow through a carotid artery the stenosis must be severe. They stated that the cross sectional area of the artery had to be reduced to at least 5 sq. mm. before significant reduction in blood flow occurred. It should be stressed that the absolute cross-sectional diameter of the carotid artery rather than the relative size of the narrowing is the important factor governing blood flow, other factors being constant.

Clinical studies of carotid and vertebral blood flow using various techniques have been reported.[38, 45] It is difficult to draw conclusions regarding the significance of individual lesions because of the multiplicity of factors involved. Reductions in cerebral blood flow have been observed in patients with cerebral atherosclerosis with and without infarction and with transient and permanent neurologic deficits.

Using intra-arterial pressure recording and the electromagnetic flow meter, De Bakey et al.[17] demonstrated that immediately following removal of a tightly stenotic carotid plaque the pressure gradient dropped from 80 mm. Hg to zero and the rate of carotid blood flow increased nine-fold from 23.6 ml. per minute to 208 ml. per minute.

With the Kety-Schmidt technique, Adams et al.[1] found that patients with aortic arch and multiple carotid and vertebral occlusions who had incapacitating cerebrovascular insufficiency also had significant reductions in total cerebral blood flow. These values were restored to normal by the appropriate endarterectomy. Many patients with occlusive lesions who were asymptomatic and neurologically negative had "normal" values for total cerebral blood flow.

Engell, using the ^{133}Xe technique, found that preoperative pressure gradients across stenotic carotid plaques disappeared following endarterectomy. In a group of 16 patients with normocapnia and stable arterial blood pressure, mean internal carotid pressure increased from 99 to 107 mm. Hg, while internal carotid flow rose by 80 per cent, and regional cerebral blood flow increased by 16 per cent. The amount of brain tissue supplied from the carotid artery increased by 53 per cent.[22a]

CLASSIFICATION OF PATIENTS

The clinical syndromes of cerebrovascular insufficiency vary from a few minor symptoms to catastrophic stroke with paralysis and coma. Manifestations may be related to the carotid system, to the vertebral-basilar system, or to a combination of the two systems. The most common extracranial occlusive lesions amenable to surgical therapy are found in the carotid system.

Patients with carotid occlusive disease have symptoms which include headaches, dizziness, blackout spells, and buzzing noises in the head and ear, as well as mental deterioration and loss of memory. There may be transient monocular blindness on the ipsilateral side of a carotid occlusion or homonymous visual field defects. There may be numbness, weakness, or paralysis of an extremity or of one entire side of the body. Dysphasia or aphasia occurs if the dominant hemisphere is involved. Coma and convulsions also occur. In some patients symptoms are minimal to absent and the only suggestion of occlusive disease is the finding of a bruit over the carotid artery in the neck.[25, 39, 51, 55]

The symptoms and signs of vertebral-basilar insufficiency include vertigo, headaches, bilateral visual disturbances, dysarthria, dysphagia, disorders of equilibrium, impairment of consciousness, and drop attacks. There may be monoparesis or paralysis shifting from side to side and involving any or all of the extremities. Sensory defects on both sides of the body, cranial nerve paralyses, and cerebellar signs with ataxia also occur.[35]

Lesions of the great vessels of the aortic arch may give the clinical picture of either carotid or vertebral-basilar disease.

It is important to classify patients with cerebrovascular insufficiency into specific clinical categories. In this way the proper selection of patients for operation may be made and the results of different methods of therapy within the same categories compared. In the past confusion has existed because of the lack of a standard classification. A detailed clinical classification proposed by a Committee on Nomenclature under the Joint Council Subcommittee on Cerebrovascular Disease of the National Institute of Neurological Diseases and Blindness includes patients who (1) are asymptomatic, or have (2) transient ischemic attacks with or without prior stable neurologic deficits, (3) persistent neurologic deficits with or without prior transient ischemic attacks, (4) actively changing neurologic deficits with or without prior transient ischemic attacks or stable deficits, (5) general cerebral dysfunction, or (6) manifestations without neural deficit.[11]

For purposes of surgical considerations related to carotid endarterectomy, the writer has chosen to classify patients into four clinical groups, which take into account all categories listed above. These are: (1) frank stroke, (2) transient cerebral ischemia, (3) chronic cerebral ischemia, and (4) asymptomatic carotid bruit.[47]

Frank Stroke

This group includes all patients with a neurologic deficit at the time of operation, whether improving, progressively worsening, or stable. All degrees of severity may be present, ranging from mild residual deficits to profound strokes with hemiplegia, aphasia, and coma. The so-called reversible ischemic neurologic deficit (RIND) is included in this group and is not classified as a transient ischemic episode because recovery requires more than twenty-four hours. A few patients with old, stable strokes also are included.

Transient Cerebral Ischemia

This group includes patients with focal attacks of neurologic dysfunction and transient symptoms of generalized cerebral ischemia lasting minutes or hours, but without residual neurologic deficit at twenty-four hours. Focal attacks include ocular, speech, sensory, and motor disturbances. Features of generalized ischemia include dizziness, blackout spells, headaches, and other nonlocalizing symptoms.

Chronic Cerebral Ischemia

Patients in this category exhibit obvious cerebrovascular insufficiency with loss of memory, impaired mentation, or overt motor or mental deterioration. These patients are not numerous and are difficult to classify but, logically, cannot be placed in any other group.

Asymptomatic Bruit

In this group are patients without neurologic symptoms who are found to have carotid bruits during routine auscultation of the neck, and who upon subsequent arteriography show significant occlusive carotid plaques. These cases may be considered prophylactic.

Over the years this classification has proved to be a convenient one for assessing surgical indications and for evaluating the long-term results of operation.[52]

DIAGNOSTIC METHODS

In the workup of a patient with obvious or suspected cerebrovascular insufficiency, the complete history and physical examination should emphasize the salient features of the clinical syndromes outlined above. A history of diabetes, hypertension, or heart disease is particularly important.

The status of the carotid, superficial temporal, subclavian, and radial pulses should be carefully noted. An absent or diminished carotid pulsation in the neck aids in localizing lesions to the aortic arch area. Blood pressure readings in the two arms are helpful in the diagnosis of subclavian occlusions. It is especially important to listen for murmurs over the carotid artery in the neck, over the globe of the eye, in the supraclavicular region, and over the heart. A bell stethoscope is most useful for auscultation of these murmurs. Complete neurological examination must be done.

External compression of the carotid artery in the neck may give helpful information but this test should be used with great caution. Pressure on the involved carotid may induce an episode of cerebral dysfunction or an actual stroke if atherosclerotic fragments are dislodged. Compression of the uninvolved carotid may also cause an ischemic episode if severe contralateral stenosis exists. A sensitive carotid sinus can confuse the picture by inducing hypotension, bradycardia, and unconsciousness. It is usually differentiated from atherosclerotic occlusion by the amount of pressure used in palpation and by the site of application of pressure to the neck. At times the two conditions coexist.

X-rays of the skull and chest are routinely obtained as is an electrocardiogram. An electroencephalogram is frequently done. Lumbar puncture may be performed to help substantiate the diagnosis and to rule out hemorrhagic or expanding intracranial lesions. Ophthalmodynamometry is occasionally used. Brain scan may be used as a diagnostic aid but, so far, has not been helpful in separating ischemia from infarction in transient episodes, those cases most suitable for surgical therapy. The duration and severity of the actual stroke syndrome correlate poorly with brain scan findings.[43]

The differential diagnosis of ischemic stroke includes expanding lesions such as brain tumor and subdural hematoma, intracerebral hemorrhage, cerebral embolism, subarachnoid hemorrhage, Meniere's disease, Stokes-Adams attacks, carotid sinus sensitivity, insulin reactions, hypertensive encephalopathy, and psychosis. All of the diagnostic studies listed above, together with pneumoencephalograms and arteriography, are necessary at times to resolve difficult problems.

Cerebral Arteriography

Following the studies outlined above, one should proceed directly to cerebral arteriography, since definitive evaluation is made only by this means. Four-vessel study should be considered in every case but need not be routinely carried out unless indicated. Carotid arteriograms should be done routinely with visualization of the intracranial as well as the cervical vessels. If the clinical findings are suggestive of vertebral-basilar as well as carotid insufficiency, one may perform a unilateral vertebral study. If this vertebral artery is normal, the other need not be visualized. If it is absent, occluded, or stenosed, the other vertebral must be checked.

Many satisfactory techniques for arteriography are now available.[30, 57] Local or light general anesthesia may be used. Direct carotid arteriography is performed using 50 per cent sodium diatrizoate (Hypaque) as the contrast medium. The common carotid arteries are punctured low in the neck, percutaneously, with 18-gauge thin-walled spinal or 18-gauge Cournand needles. Ten ml. of Hypaque is injected into each artery. Anteroposterior and lateral films of the head and neck are taken serially and simultaneously with the biplane Schönander x-ray unit.

Bilateral carotid artery visualization must be done in every case because of the high incidence of bilateral disease. The intracranial vessels must be seen in order to determine the presence or absence of contralateral filling through the circle of Willis, and to rule out other intracranial pathology such as brain tumor or subdural hematoma.

Arteriograms may be obtained utilizing a percutaneous retrograde brachial technique to visualize the subclavian, vertebral, and basilar arteries. Injection into the right brachial artery visualizes the right carotid system as well. Occasionally, therefore, one may perform a right retrograde brachial and a left carotid arteriogram and obtain a three-vessel study by means of only two injections.

Another satisfactory technique of vertebral arteriography utilizes bilateral infraclavicular subclavian artery catheterization.

For visualization of the innominate, left common carotid, and left subclavian arteries as they arise from the aortic arch one may employ several methods, depending upon the clinical situation and the vessels to be studied. Retrograde catheter techniques through the femoral, brachial, or axillary arteries are those most commonly used. The retrograde femoral approach is being employed with increasing frequency to visualize not only the aortic arch vessels but also the extracranial carotid and vertebral arteries and the intracranial vasculature.

Knowledge of the complications related to cerebral arteriography and methods by which they may be prevented is mandatory if one is to obtain acceptable clinical results. Complications include airway and cardiac problems, hematomas, arterial thrombosis, false aneurysms, pneumothorax, extravasation of contrast material, seizures, and production or aggravation of neurologic deficits.[54]

The complications listed above may be prevented in various ways. Care in the technical performance of the arteriographic procedure is of great importance. Carotid punctures should be made low in the neck to avoid piercing bifurcation plaques. Prolonged procedures of more than one hour's duration with multiple carotid punctures should be avoided. If technical difficulties are encountered, it is better to abandon the procedure and return on another day. Light general anesthesia with halothane is quite safe and is particularly useful for the apprehensive or uncooperative patient. The use of safe contrast material such as 50 per cent Hypaque or 60 per cent meglumine diatrizoate (Renografin) is most important. Hypotensive episodes may be avoided by the administration of 500 to 1000 ml. of lactated Ringer's solution during and after the procedure. Occasionally phenylephrine is necessary to maintain blood pressure at normal levels. Suction apparatus and oxygen must be available in the x-ray department and recovery areas to prevent hypoxia.

Unless the diagnosis of ischemic stroke is in question, it is best to avoid cerebral arteriography during the acute phase of completed, progressing, fluctuating, or improving strokes. It is preferable to delay such procedures until a stable situation ensues, at which time arteriography usually can be performed safely. If there is some question as to the presence of subdural hematoma, intracranial aneurysm, intracerebral hemorrhage, or brain tumor, arteriography is justifiable in the acute situation.

If total occlusion of a stenotic carotid artery, due either to thrombosis or dissection, results from the arteriographic procedure, emergency surgical intervention for restoration of cerebral blood flow becomes necessary.

Although the list of complications related to cerebral arteriography is an imposing one, their incidence nationwide is quite low and has continuously decreased with increasing experience of those performing the procedures. Hass et al.[30] in a report of the Joint Study of Extracranial Arterial Occlusion, in which 4748 patients were studied, gave the overall mortality from cerebral arteriography as 0.7 per cent. An additional 0.5 per cent sustained permanent hemiparesis, making the grave complication rate 1.2 per cent. They conclude that the major complications of direct carotid arteriography are related to advanced disease of vessels on the ipsilateral side, while those from brachial procedures appear to be related to progressive brain stem dysfunction, number of injections, and total amount of contrast material used.

The incidence of minor complications has also been reported by Hass et al.[30] With direct carotid puncture, the overall minor complication rate was 5.3 per cent; with brachial injection, with or without catheter, it was 7.1 per cent; and with subclavian injection it was 5.5 per cent. For retrograde aortic injection, both femoral and axillary, the overall minor complication rate was the highest for any group, being 14.3 per cent. These complications were more likely to occur with the use of a catheter than with a needle alone. Hass et al.[30] state that "many of the complications encountered early in the study are no longer occurring, presumably due to increased experience and technical improvements." The figures quoted above include combined statistics of a number of operators with varying amounts of experience in a number of institutions. For a single experienced operator doing arteriography routinely, mortality and complication rates are considerably lower than those quoted. In our own institution, mortality from arteriography in the hands of the most experienced operators during a ten-year period has been less than 0.1 per cent, and the grave complication rate (neurologic deficits) 0.2 per cent.[54]

In summary, cerebral arteriography, when performed properly, is safe, and is essential for studying patients with suspected cerebrovascular disease. Its liberal though judicious employment is to be encouraged if remediable extracranial occlusions are to be diagnosed precisely and treated properly.

TECHNIQUE OF CAROTID ENDARTERECTOMY

The most common operation used in the treatment of cerebrovascular insufficiency is carotid endarterectomy. Technical considerations are of the utmost importance in this operation since the limits of tolerance to temporary occlusion of the blood supply to the brain may be quite narrow. Safety factors must be employed which will eliminate in most instances the occurrence or aggravation of neurologic

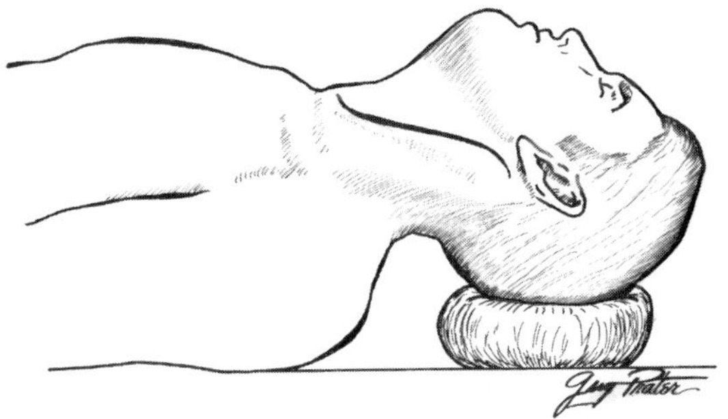

Figure 11–6. Location of the incision employed for endarterectomy of the carotid artery in the neck. The head is on a rubber ring with the neck extended slightly.

deficits. Any method of carotid endarterectomy should carry low mortality, few complications, satisfactory immediate and long-term anatomical results, and good functional results relative to cerebrovascular insufficiency. The technique to be described has evolved over a period of 17 years and has proved safe and reliable.

Operation is performed under light general anesthesia. The head is turned away from the side to be operated upon and placed on a rubber ring. The shoulders are elevated slightly using a folded sheet but no undue extension of the neck is allowed. An oblique incision is made along the anterior border of the sternocleidomastoid muscle, curving medialward at its lower end, centered over the bifurcation of the common carotid artery, and curved slightly inferior to the lobe of the ear at the upper end (Fig. 11–6). Adequate exposure of the common carotid and of the internal and external carotid divisions is essential (Fig. 11–7). The carotid sinus area is infiltrated with 1 per cent lidocaine. The artery is freed completely, including division of the carotid sinus plexus. One must avoid injury to the mandibular branch of the facial nerve and the vagus and hypoglossal nerves. Though rarely necessary, the superior thyroid artery may be ligated and divided to facilitate dissection and exposure. An umbilical tape is placed around

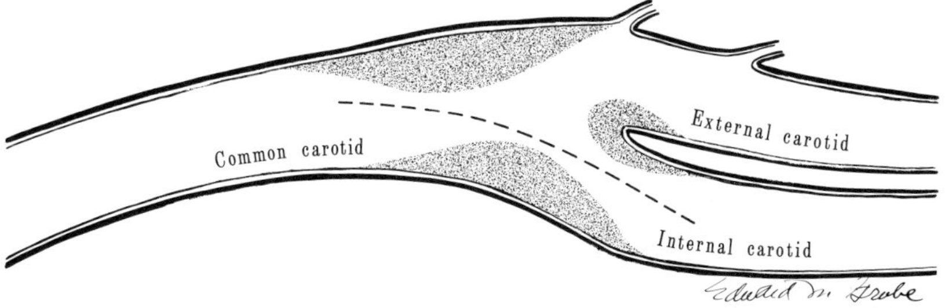

Figure 11–7. Usual site of atherosclerotic plaque at bifurcation of common carotid artery extending into the origins of internal and external carotid arteries. The location of the linear arteriotomy for endarterectomy is indicated. (From Thompson, J. E.: *Surgery for Cerebrovascular Insufficiency (Stroke).* Courtesy of Charles C Thomas, Publisher, Springfield, Illinois, 1968.)

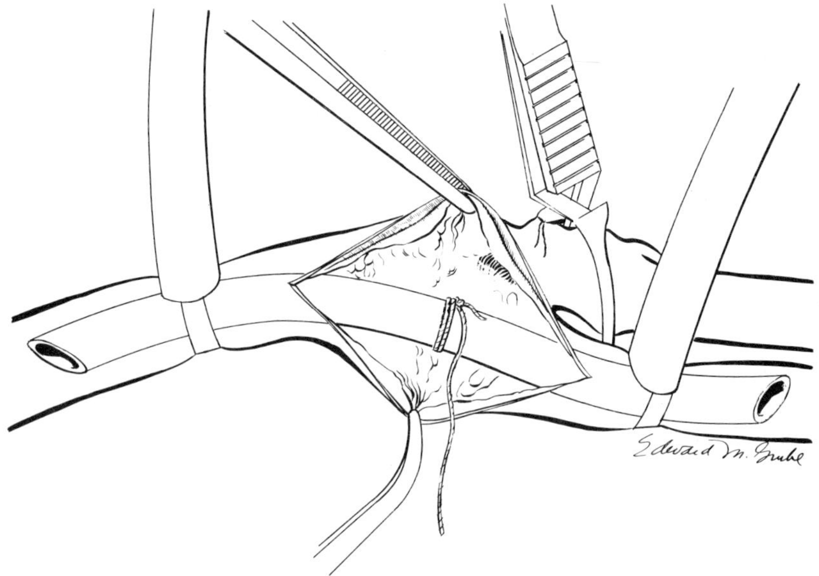

Figure 11–8. The artery has been opened through the full extent of the plaque and a No. 10 French plastic catheter is in place as a temporary inlying bypass shunt. (From Thompson, J. E. *et al.:* Ann. Surg. *163:*751, 1966.)

the external carotid artery. Umbilical tapes are then placed around the common and internal carotid arteries and segments of No. 16 French rubber catheter threaded over the tapes to act as tourniquets (Fig. 11–8).

The occluding plaque is usually located at the bifurcation of the common carotid and extends only a short distance into the internal carotid. The distal internal carotid is ordinarily soft and thin-walled and is freed up for at least one centimeter beyond the palpable distal end of the plaque. Utmost gentleness is used throughout manipulation and the artery is simply palpated, never squeezed, since platelet thrombi or atherosclerotic debris may break off and embolize intracranially.

When satisfactory exposure is obtained, the external carotid is occluded with a bulldog clamp and heparinized with a solution containing one mg. of heparin per ml. The common carotid is then clamped proximally with an angled vascular clamp. The distal internal carotid is occluded with a bulldog clamp and a linear arteriotomy made from the common carotid into the internal carotid beyond the distal extent of the plaque. It is important that the internal carotid be opened beyond the plaque and that the entire extent of plaque be visualized in order to facilitate the succeeding steps of the operation. A plastic catheter shunt is then inserted into the distal internal carotid and the artery allowed to backflow. The proximal end of the plastic shunt is then placed into the common carotid lumen and the umbilical tapes with rubber tourniquets are made snug. Cerebral blood flow is thus restored through the shunt (Fig. 11–8). This step of the operation usually requires from 45 to 90 seconds. The average size shunt which fits the distal internal carotid is a No. 10 French plastic catheter, about 9 cm. in length. A No. 8 or No. 12 catheter may be used as a shunt if the artery is smaller or larger than usual. The internal diameter of the No. 10 catheter used is 2.5 mm. With normal levels of blood pressure a No. 10 plastic shunt used as described carries approximately 125 ml. of blood per minute. Experience has shown that this is adequate flow through the occluded artery during the period required for endarterectomy.

With the intraluminal shunt in place one may endarterectomize the vessel without undue haste. The appropriate plane is entered with a fine-pointed clamp and the plaque dissected from the common carotid, the bifurcation, first portion of the external carotid, and that portion of the internal carotid containing the plaque. The distal end of the plaque in the internal carotid usually feathers off quite smoothly leaving only thin intima above, which should not be disturbed (Fig. 11–9).

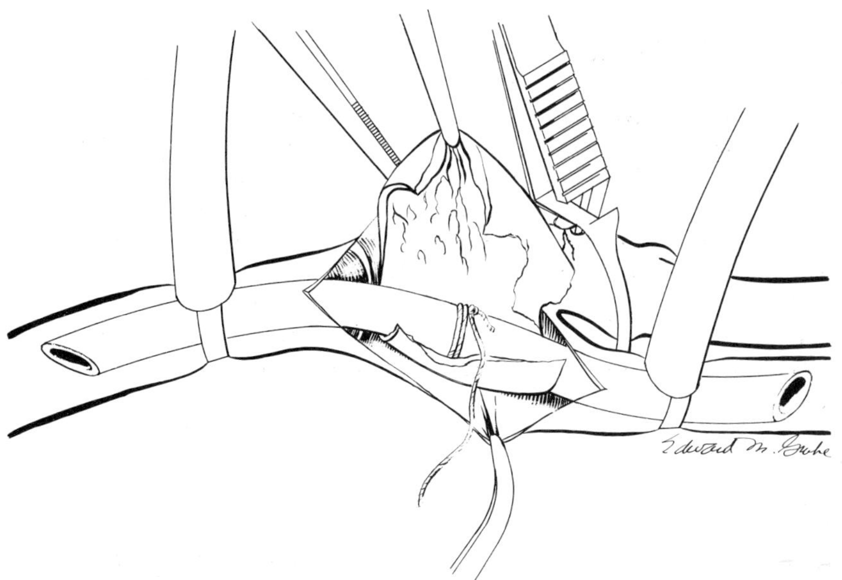

Figure 11–9. The plaque is being removed by endarterectomy from the common carotid, the origin of the external carotid, and the internal carotid. The plaque usually feathers off into thin intima in the distal internal carotid. If it does not, it is secured with a few fine, interrupted sutures. (From Thompson, J. E.: *Surgery for Cerebrovascular Insufficiency (Stroke).* Courtesy of Charles C Thomas, Publisher, Springfield, Illinois, 1968.)

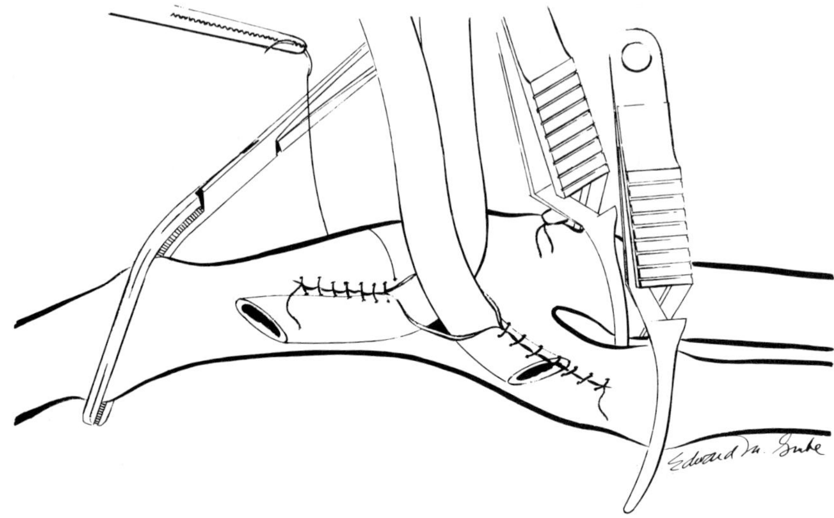

Figure 11–10.   Closure of the arteriotomy is begun at both ends with 6-0 polyester arterial sutures. Clamps are applied, the shunt is removed, and heparin is injected prior to placing the final four or five stitches. The vessels are flushed out prior to final closure. (From Thompson, J. E.: *Surgery for Cerebrovascular Insufficiency (Stroke).* Courtesy of Charles C Thomas, Publisher, Springfield, Illinois, 1968.)

Small bits of debris may be lifted out with forceps or flushed out with saline. It is of the utmost importance that the distal extent of the endarterectomy be visualized so that no large pieces of intima are left to dissect distalward and produce a postoperative occlusion. Occasionally, it is advisable to secure the distal intima with a few interrupted sutures to prevent dissection. It is also important to endarterectomize carefully the origin of the external carotid since this artery is an important source of collateral blood supply to the brain.

The arteriotomy is then closed with running sutures of 6–0 polyester, beginning at each end. Immediately prior to placing the final three or four sutures, the common carotid and internal carotid are clamped and the shunt removed (Fig. 11–10). The vessels are then flushed. The final sutures are quickly placed and tied. At this point, the internal carotid is allowed to backflow and is then reclamped. The clamps are removed from the common and external carotids and flow restored into the external carotid, allowing any debris or air to be flushed into it rather than into the internal carotid. The clamp is then removed from the internal carotid and flow restored to the brain (Fig. 11–11). The occlusion time during this final step is usually about two minutes.

If one is concerned about completeness of endarterectomy or quality of pulsation in the internal carotid following restoration of flow, arteriograms may be performed on the operating table. Some surgeons perform this step routinely,[7] but the writer has not found its routine use necessary.

It is rarely necessary to use a patch graft for closure of the arteriotomy (Fig. 11–11). Long-term results, including the appearance of the artery on postoperative arteriograms, have borne out the fact that this type of closure is quite satisfactory.[52] The neck wound is then closed anatomically in two layers with interrupted sutures of fine cotton, and a small rubber drain is brought out the lower end of the wound, to be removed twenty-four hours postoperatively. The operation as described requires from one to two hours to perform. Bilateral operations, when necessary, are done in separate stages about a week apart to avoid complications of laryngeal edema, transient hypoglossal paresis, and cerebral edema.

For totally occlusive lesions, in contrast to stenotic ones, a shunt is not necessary during endarterectomy. When a thrombus is present in the distal internal carotid, thrombectomy is performed with endarterectomy forceps or small balloon catheters.

It is important that adequate levels of blood pressure be maintained during operation and in the immediate postoperative period. The most satisfactory way to achieve this is to administer 500 to 1000 ml. of lactated Ringer's solution during the operation and postoperatively. Vasopressors are occasionally necessary even when adequate fluids have been given. Routine postoperative heparinization is not used.

In summary, the salient features of this technique of carotid endarterectomy include general anesthesia, the routine use of an intraluminal shunt, the meticulous removal of the plaque under direct view, and the maintenance of adequate blood pressure levels using balanced salt solution.

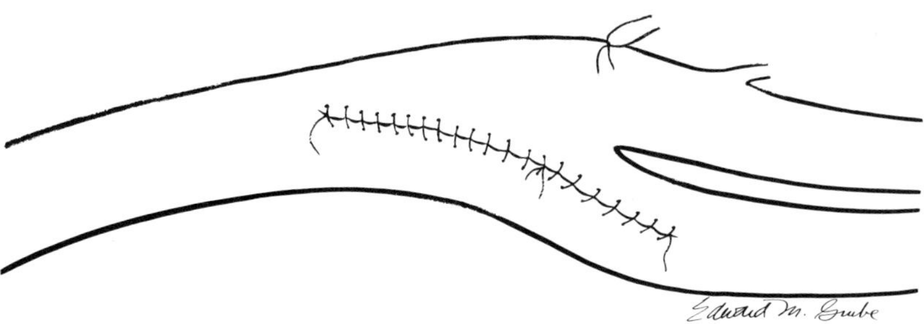

Figure 11–11. Appearance of the artery following final closure. Flow is restored first into the external carotid and finally into the internal carotid. A patch graft is rarely necessary unless the artery is unusually narrow. (From Thompson, J. E.: *Surgery for Cerebrovascular Insufficiency (Stroke).* Courtesy of Charles C Thomas, Publisher, Springfield, Illinois, 1968.)

Complications

Complications associated with carotid endarterectomy which have been seen by the author or have been reported in the literature are listed in Table 11–1.[9, 54] Although the list is rather lengthy, if one is meticulous with details of intra- and postoperative management, the actual incidence of complications is quite low. The most serious complication, the occurrence of neurologic deficits, should be less than 2 per cent. The incidence of all the remaining complications should not total more than 3 per cent. These matters are discussed in more detail in the following sections, dealing with methods of cerebral protection during operation and management of acute strokes.

Two complications deserve special mention. False aneurysm formation in the endarterectomized segment of the carotid artery has occurred following the use of Dacron patch grafts for arterial reconstruction which have been sewn in place with silk sutures. The silk deteriorates with time, the suture line disrupts in varying degrees, and false aneurysms form. Arterial silk was routinely employed before

Table 11–1. Complications of Carotid Endarterectomy

I. Related to anesthesia, general or local
  A. Cardiac problems
  B. Airway problems
  C. Hypotension
II. Related to cervical wound
  A. Infection
  B. Hematoma
  C. Nerve pareses
    1. Vagus
    2. Hypoglossal
    3. Marginal branch of facial
  D. Parotitis
  E. Tracheal obstruction
III. Related to carotid artery
  A. Disruption
  B. False aneurysms
  C. Carotid-cavernous A-V fistula
  D. Infection of Dacron graft
IV. Production or aggravation of neurologic deficits
  A. Intraoperative causes
    1. Embolism
    2. Cerebral ischemia
  B. Postoperative causes
    1. Thrombosis of endarterectomized segment
    2. Hypotension
    3. Intracerebral hemorrhage or edema
    4. Hypertension
V. Miscellaneous
  A. Postoperative headache
  B. Cerebral edema

satisfactory polyester sutures, which do not deteriorate, were developed. The author has seen seven instances of this complication, in patients operated upon early in his series. All were successfully repaired. It is now clear that patch-graft reconstruction is only rarely necessary in carotid endarterectomy. If the artery is very small, a patch of autologous vein or Dacron may be used, sewn in place with Dacron sutures.

Procedures for repair of these false aneurysms vary with the individual circumstances.[54] If the disruption is localized, the sac and old Dacron patch may be trimmed away and the defect reconstructed using a patch graft of autologous vein or Dacron, and Dacron sutures. If the disruption is extensive, segmental replacement may be required. A tubular prosthesis of either saphenous vein or 8 mm. Dacron is satisfactory. Since repair of false aneurysms may require clamping of the carotid artery for considerable periods of time, adequate cerebral protection must be employed to avoid neurologic complications. The simplest means is a temporary inlying shunt.

The second complication is postoperative hypertension, which is not uncommon in the first 24 hours following carotid endarterectomy. Excessively high levels of blood pressure may be deleterious and must be treated aggressively to avoid intracerebral hemorrhage. The pressure should be kept below 200 mm. Hg. Repeated small doses of meperidine (Demerol) (25 mg.) or chlorpromazine (Thorazine) (1 mg.) are usually sufficient, since blood pressure ordinarily reverts to satisfactory levels spontaneously within eight to twelve hours postoperatively. If the hypertension is refractory, one should not hesitate to employ promptly an intravenous drip of 500 mg. of trimethaphan camphorsulfonate (Arfonad) in 500 ml. of 5 per cent dextrose in water, which lowers blood pressure within minutes. Intermittent injections or a properly titrated constant drip of this solution will keep the pressure at appropriate levels until either spontaneous resolution occurs or other longer acting hypotensive agents take effect.

Cerebral Protection During Carotid Endarterectomy

The chief hazard involved in carotid endarterectomy is the production of neurologic deficits not present preoperatively or the aggravation of previously existing ones.[9] Many of these are episodes of transient weakness lasting a few hours or a few days with complete clearing, while others remain as permanent deficits, either mild or severe. Because of the consequences involved no undue risks should be taken during carotid surgery, especially in patients with transient cerebral ischemia and asymptomatic bruits (see Table 11–1).

A common cause of neurologic deficits related to the operative procedure itself is cerebral embolization from necrotic atherosclerotic plaques. Excessive manipulation or rough handling of the carotid artery is responsible for such emboli. This is avoided by gentleness in dissection and by delaying until the final step the placing of a tape around the area of the plaque. Improper flushing of the vessels following closure of the arteriotomy may also result in cerebral embolization of debris.

The second cause of operation-related deficits is cerebral ischemia. Although most patients requiring carotid surgery can tolerate temporary clamping of the artery without deleterious effects, a few require some form of cerebral protection if strokes are to be prevented and aggravation of neurologic deficits is to be avoided. That cerebral protection in the latter group is necessary and beneficial has been amply demonstrated.[50] Patients with severe vascular disease and multiple large-vessel occlusions are least tolerant of carotid clamping.

Several methods to determine the adequacy of cerebral blood flow during carotid clamping have been described. These include temporary occlusion under local anesthesia while checking the neurologic status;[46] observation of the adequacy of retrograde blood flow from the opened internal carotid;[18] determination of blood pressure in the occluded distal internal carotid;[41] monitoring of blood gases, especially jugular venous oxygen saturation;[33, 36, 59] and electroencephalography.[29]

Recent studies suggest that the determination of internal carotid artery back pressure with the artery clamped proximally, the so-called stump pressure, is probably the most reliable method at present for determining the necessity of added cerebral protection at the time of surgery. Various levels of stump pressure have been advocated as being critical. Clinical as well as laboratory data indicate that pressures of 50 to 55 mm. Hg or higher represent adequate cerebral collateral. At lower levels a shunt should be used.[22a, 30a]

Techniques which render cerebral protection during carotid surgery include general anesthesia,[58, 59] hypothermia, induced hypertension, hypercapnia, hypocapnia,[22] temporary intraluminal bypass shunts, and various combinations of these. General anesthesia is reported to increase the tolerance of the brain to ischemia and to reduce cerebral metabolic requirements for oxygen. In addition, when halothane is the agent employed it is said to induce cerebral vasodilatation and to elevate the threshold for unfavorable effects of carbon dioxide.[59]

Hypercapnia reduces cerebral resistance and increases total cerebral blood flow. Although Lyons et al.[36] and White et al.[59] have reported hypercapnia with blood-gas monitoring to be a reliable index of cerebral oxygenation, other investigators cast some doubt on the infallibility of this method in every case. Larson et al.[33] have demonstrated that patients may have levels of jugular venous oxygen saturation below the so-called critical level without exhibiting cerebral symptoms. Contrariwise, a number of patients have shown values in the "safe" zones only to awaken with neurologic deficits following carotid surgery. This method is obviously a good one and estimates accurately *total* cerebral oxygenation, but it may not reflect inadequacies in *regional* blood flow. Because of this consideration, hypocapnia rather than hypercapnia has been advocated by Ehrenfeld et al.[22] and Wylie and Ehrenfeld,[61] who suggest that cerebral perfusion into ischemic areas may be increased by obviating any intracerebral steal, thus improving regional blood flow where it is most needed.

While this matter is still controversial, it does appear that hypercapnia is unsuitable for augmenting cerebral blood flow during carotid clamping. Probably the use of normocapnia with normal or slightly elevated blood pressure is the safest course to follow in the operating room.

The use of a temporary inlying bypass shunt is a simple and reliable method of cerebral support.[50, 52, 54a] When one becomes familiar with its use complications are few and it may be employed in any operating room without the necessity of other complicated apparatus. Recent discussion has centered around the necessity for its routine use.

The effectiveness of any method of cerebral monitoring or cerebral protection during carotid endarterectomy must be demonstrated in patients with transient ischemia and asymptomatic bruits since they are without neurologic deficits prior to operation. Several series in the literature are available for comparison, using the parameters of operative mortality, incidence of transient neurologic deficits, and incidence of permanent deficits.

When no special protection other than general anesthesia and maintenance of normal or slightly hypertensive blood pressure is used, operative mortality has been reported as 3 per cent, the incidence of transient weakness as 13 per cent, and of permanent deficits as 7 per cent.[18] With hypercapnic general anesthesia without a shunt, operative mortality has been 4.4 per cent, and permanent neurologic worsening 2.9 per cent.[62] In the Joint Study Project, with various methods of cerebral protection, operative mortality was 3.5 per cent, transient deficits 1.8 per cent, and permanent deficits 7.7 per cent.[24] Using internal carotid stump pressure of 50 mm. Hg or more as the deciding factor as to whether or not to employ a shunt, Hays et al. reported operative mortality as zero, the incidence of permanent deficits as 1 per cent, and that of transient deficits as 2.5 per cent.[30a]

Table 11–2 shows the data in the author's series employing a shunt, all operations being performed by a single surgeon. The operative mortality has been 0.3 per cent and the incidence of neurologic deficts 1.9 per cent. There were no deaths due to stroke.

Table 11–2. Operation-Related Neurologic Deficits in Patients with Transient Cerebral Ischemia and Asymptomatic Bruits Using a Temporary Inlying Shunt*

| | No. of Patients | No. of Operations | Operative Mortality | | | | Operative and Postoperative Deficits | | | |
| | | | Deaths | Patient Mortality | Procedure Mortality | Death from Strokes | Transient | Permanent | | Total Deficits |
								Mild	Severe	
Transient cerebral ischemia	199	264	1	0.5%	0.4%	0	2 – 0.76%	2 – 0.76%	2 – 0.76%	6 – 2.3%
Asymptomatic bruits	39	54	0	0	0	0	0	0	0	0
Total	238	318	1	0.4%	0.3%	0	2 – 0.63%	2 – 0.63%	2 – 0.63%	6 – 1.9%

*Number of Patients – 238. Number of Operations – 318.

An additional strenuous test for any method of cerebral protection is its efficacy in the patient with ipsilateral carotid stenosis and contralateral total carotid occlusion, when the former is being operated upon. In a series of 92 such patients, Bloodwell et al.,[10] using only general anesthesia and hypercapnia, reported an operative mortality due to stroke of 7.6 per cent and neurologic worsening of 5.4 per cent. In a series of 86 carotid operations on 64 patients with unilateral stenosis and contralateral occlusion, in which a shunt was used routinely, there was no operative death and no instance of aggravation of neurologic deficits.[52]

Granted, a shunt may not be necessary in every case but, in the absence of precise knowledge as to which patient needs it, the writer advocates its routine use for all partially occlusive lesions. It adds very little to the operating time but does add a great deal of security. Combined with general anesthesia, normal blood pressure, and gentleness during dissection, it is the simplest and most reliable method of temporary cerebral support for keeping the complications of carotid surgery at a minimal and acceptable level. Results with its use are generally superior to those reported with other methods of cerebral protection.

TOTAL CAROTID OCCLUSIONS AND ACUTE STROKES

When atherosclerotic plaques are partially occlusive and the distal internal carotid artery is patent on the arteriogram, restoration of cerebral blood flow by surgical reconstruction is almost uniformly successful. This is not the case, however, if the internal carotid is totally occluded. Table 11–3 shows the data on totally occluded carotid arteries treated by carotid endarterectomy.[52] Thus, 40 per cent of the arteries may be rendered patent by operation while in 60 per cent flow

Table 11–3. Data on Totally Occluded Carotid Arteries Treated by Endarterectomy

Number of patients operated upon	112
Number of operations for total occlusion	118
Number of operations for partial occlusion	31
Total number of operations	149
Number of operative deaths	7
Patient mortality	6.2%
Operative procedure mortality	4.7%
Number of totally occluded arteries with flow restored	48 — 40.7%
Number of totally occluded arteries with flow *not* restored	70 — 59.3%

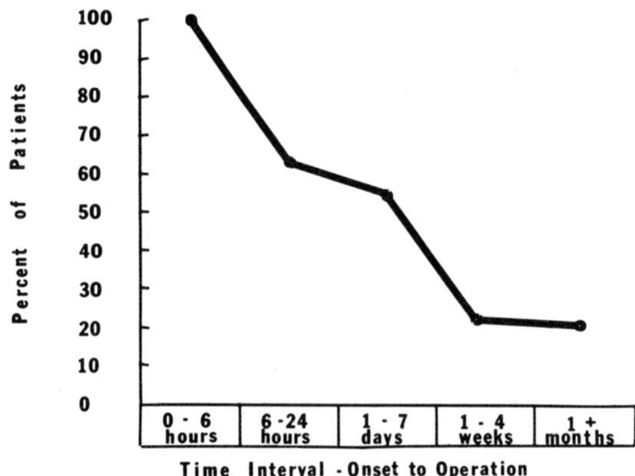

Figure 11–12.   Graph showing relationship between time of onset of occlusion and successful restoration of blood flow in totally occluded internal carotid arteries.

cannot be restored. A considerable difference of opinion has existed regarding the advisability of operation on the totally occluded carotid.[49]

Several factors are responsible for successful restoration of blood flow. Probably most important is the time interval from onset of occlusion to operation. The earlier patients are operated upon the greater likelihood of success (Fig. 11–12). It is surprising to find that even after several weeks of occlusion it is still possible to restore flow in a few instances.

At times the arteriograms are helpful in predicting a successful outcome. Films may show filling of the ophthalmic artery, the siphon, or distal internal carotid on the occluded side via collaterals from the ipsilateral external carotid or vertebral or from contralateral vessels through the circle of Willis. Patients taking anticoagulants at the time total occlusion occurs appear to have a better chance for restoration of flow than those not on the drugs. The Fogarty balloon catheter has been helpful in removing fresh thrombi from the distal internal carotid in a few instances. One must exercise caution in any attempts to remove old thrombi from the distal internal carotid as too-vigorous manipulation can perforate the artery and result in the formation of a carotid–cavernous sinus fistula, a very troublesome complication.[5]

Other unknown factors must exist to explain successful restoration of flow in some cases. In occasional patients a vessel has been noted, probably the ascending pharyngeal, leaving the carotid bifurcation more distal than usual, on the internal carotid side. It is possible that such an abnormally situated vessel distal to the total block has been responsible for keeping the internal carotid patent, since there are no other branches leaving this artery in the neck.

The nature of the stroke itself in the individual patient is probably the most important factor determining surgical intervention, since a large proportion of acute frank strokes are caused by total carotid occlusions.

Mortality rates up to 60 per cent have been reported following operation for acute strokes in the early course of the disease, whereas if arteriography and operation are delayed at least two weeks or more following onset of the stroke, mortality and morbidity rates are significantly less.[8, 10, 18, 27, 60] Pathologic studies have shown that it requires more than eight days for an area of cerebral infarction or softening to become sufficiently stabilized that intracranial hemorrhage will not occur when an increased flow of blood under pressure is restored to the area by carotid endarterectomy.

One should not perform emergency operations on patients with acute profound stroke, rapidly progressing stroke, or rapidly improving stroke, but allow them to stabilize for two to six weeks and then consider them for studies and possible operation. Rarely, if a patient is in the hospital when an acute stroke occurs, and operation can be done within six hours of onset, emergency endarterectomy may be justifiable.

There are several reasons for considering surgery in these patients at a *delayed* time, however, after the neurologic status has apparently stabilized. In the first place, restoration of cerebral blood flow may result in more rapid clinical improvement. A number of patients whose deficits appeared irreversible have made remarkable improvement following surgical restoration of cerebral blood flow.[51] Secondly, a patient may continue to have recurrent disabling transient ischemic attacks which may be relieved by removal of an occlusive plaque. Finally, removal of a lesion from either carotid will increase cerebral blood flow and may prevent the occurrence of another stroke on one or both sides.

On the basis of these considerations the patient with a totally occluded carotid artery should not be routinely operated upon nor should he be categorically rejected for operation. Judicious consideration of the following factors will aid in the selection of patients for operation and the appropriate timing of the procedures. If seen within six to 12 hours of onset of occlusion the patient may be operated upon with a reasonable expectation of restoration of cerebral blood flow. Thereafter, the success rate progressively declines so that after a week or two chances of restoring flow drop to 20 per cent (Fig. 11–12). Clinical considerations of the stroke itself are the most important factors determining operability. Patients with acute profound strokes of 12 hours' duration or more should not be operated upon as an emergency but be allowed to stabilize for at least two weeks.

By avoiding operation on acute strokes and by using a shunt rou-

Table 11–4.   Operative Mortality Following Carotid
Endarterectomy

ERA I — 1957–1963 — INCLUSIVE

Clinical Category	No. of Patients	No. of Operations	No. of Deaths	Patient Mortality	Procedure Mortality
Frank stroke	105	126	11	10.5%	8.7%
Transient cerebral ischemia	87	117	2	2.3%	1.7%
Chronic cerebral ischemia	10	12	0	0	0
Asymptomatic bruit	14	17	0	0	0
Total	216	272	13	6%	4.8%

ERA II — 1964–1970 — INCLUSIVE

Clinical Category	No. of Patients	No. of Operations	No. of Deaths	Patient Mortality	Procedure Mortality
Frank stroke	121	147	6	5%	4.1%
Transient cerebral ischemia	245	310	2	0.8%	0.6%
Chronic cerebral ischemia	7	9	0	0	0
Asymptomatic bruit	59	81	0	0	0
Total	432	547	8	1.8%	1.5%

tinely for all partially occlusive lesions, one can lower the operative
mortality associated with carotid endarterectomy. Table 11–4 summarizes the data which are the basis for this statement. In the last seven
years mortality for transient ischemia patients has been 0.6 per cent
and overall procedure mortality 1.5 per cent.[52]

RESULTS OF CAROTID ENDARTERECTOMY

Successful anatomic restoration of blood flow by operation may
be accomplished in more than 98 per cent of patients with partially
occluded arteries. Several studies have demonstrated that arteries
reconstructed by endarterectomy remain patent for many years without evidence of constriction[7, 21, 52, 61] (Fig. 11–13). The incidence of
reoperation for recurrent carotid stenosis at the site of previous endarterectomy, with or without a patch graft, is extremely low, being less
than 0.2 per cent.

The highly successful restoration of cerebral blood flow in partially occluded arteries is not the case, however, when the internal carotid is totally occluded. In the latter case, restoration of patency is at most 40 per cent.

Operative mortality following carotid endarterectomy is shown in Table 11–4. A total experience of 14 years has been divided into two eras of seven years each to show the improvement with increasing experience.[52] Mortality in patients with frank strokes is highest, being 4 per cent in the recent era, while in patients with transient cerebral ischemia it is 0.6 per cent. There were no operative deaths in patients with chronic ischemia and asymptomatic bruits. Of the 21 deaths, 15 were due to cerebral causes, five to myocardial infarction, and one to pulmonary embolism. Most of them occurred in the frank stroke group (17 of 21).

In a later analysis (1973) of 1013 carotid operations, results are similar, with recent mortality for frank strokes being 4.4 per cent and that for transient ischemia being 0.46 per cent.[54a]

In a follow-up study of patients subjected to carotid endarterectomy it was found that 52.3 per cent of the long-term deaths were from cardiac causes, while only 13.4 per cent of the deaths were due to strokes. These deaths represented 3.9 per cent of the entire series

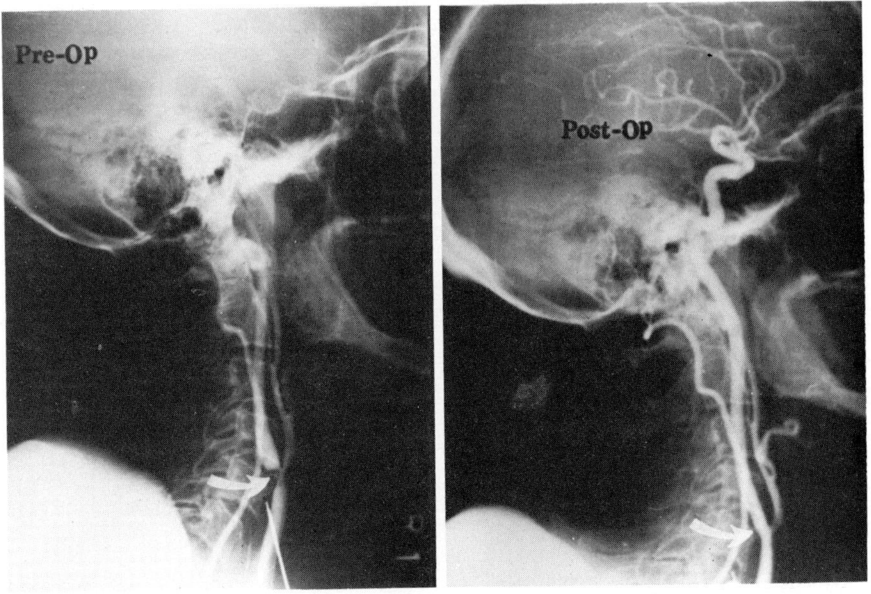

Figure 11–13. A, Preoperative carotid arteriogram of patient with tight stenosis in right internal carotid artery. B, Postoperative arteriogram of same patient three years following endarterectomy showing normal caliber of arterial lumen after simple closure of arteriotomy without a patch graft. These endarterectomized vessels remain patent for many years without evidence of recurrent stenosis.

Table 11–5. Long-Term Functional Results After Carotid Endarterectomy in Surviving Patients

CLINICAL CATEGORY	NO. OF PATIENTS	NO. OF DEATHS		NO. OF SURVIVORS	LONG TERM NEUROLOGIC STATUS					TOTAL IMPROVED
		Opera-tive	Long Term		Normal	Improved	Same	Worse	Normal or improved then worsened	
Frank stroke	217	16	75	126	38 (30.2%)	74 (58.7%)	6 (4.7%)	3 (2.4%)	5 (4.0%)	112 (88.9%)
Transient cerebral ischemia	293	4	79	210	170 (81%)	33 (15.7%)	0	4 (1.9%)	3 (1.4%)	203 (96.7%)
Chronic cerebral ischemia	17	0	8	9	3 (33.3%)	2 (22.2%)	1 (11.1%)	0	3 (33.3%)	5 (55.5%)
Asymptomatic bruit	65	0	10	55	51 (92.7%)	0	1 (1.8%)	2 (3.6%)	1 (1.8%)	51 (92.7%)
Total	592	20	172	400	262 (65.5%)	109 (27.3%)	8 (2%)	9 (2.2%)	12 (3%)	371 (92.8%)

operated upon, a figure considerably lower than the expected mortality from stroke in patients with cerebrovascular insufficiency treated by nonsurgical methods.[52]

The long-term functional results after carotid endarterectomy in 400 surviving patients are given in Table 11–5.[52] The goals of therapy should be kept in mind in every patient with cerebrovascular insufficiency. One is concerned almost as much with morbidity as with mortality; that is to say, the quality of survival is important. The disability in a patient who cannot talk, write, walk, or care for himself is entirely different from that seen in patients with severe intermittent claudication or heart disease, for example.

Frank Strokes

The functional results of any method of treatment for frank strokes are difficult to assess since the clinical course is so variable and the natural history of improvement so well known. A patient who survives an initial stroke usually improves, at least for a time and to some degree. Likewise, as the years pass, patients with cerebrovascular insufficiency who were previously normal or improved following operation, in some instances may deteriorate and worsen functionally.

It is difficult to judge the efficacy of carotid surgery for frank strokes because of the lack of adequate control studies. Several reports bear on this matter, however. Table 11–6 shows a comparison between a medically treated group of patients followed up to 42 months and a surgically treated group followed up to 96 months after operation.[6, 48] In another study of functional results following operation for frank strokes in patients with totally occluded carotid arteries, it was concluded that in patients in whom blood flow was restored recovery was more rapid and to a greater degree than occurred in the course of the natural history of recovery from a stroke.[49]

A group of frank-stroke patients operated upon early in the course of their disease was analyzed in an effort to determine which patients exhibited marked improvement following operation. It was found that

Table 11–6.   Functional Results in Medically and Surgically Treated Patients with Frank Strokes

Author	Method of Therapy	Length of Follow Up	Number of Patients	Normal or Improved	Unchanged	Worse	Deaths
Bauer et al.	Medical	Up to 42 mos.	73	37%	28.8%	9.6%	24.6%
Thompson et al.	Surgical	Up to 96 mos.	135	61.5%	4.4%	1.5%	°32.6%

°Of 44 deaths, 12 were operative and 32 long-term.

those patients with mild preoperative deficits, such as monoparesis or dysphasia, who were improving, were those most likely to return to a normal or near-normal status. Only rarely did a patient with a profound frank stroke with flaccid hemiplegia, severe mental obtundity, aphasia, or coma make any dramatic improvement when subjected to operation in the acute phase, and many did not survive operation.[51]

In summary, it appears that in patients with *frank strokes* endarterectomy has decreased the mortality from subsequent stroke, has lowered the incidence of recurrent strokes, and probably has been responsible for improvement in neurologic status beyond that expected from the natural course of the disease. Further control studies are needed.

Transient Cerebral Ischemia

Patients with transient cerebral ischemia are ideal candidates for surgical therapy since disabling symptoms can be relieved and frank strokes prevented. Our data indicate that these goals have been accomplished[52] (Table 11–5). A number of reports testify to the beneficial effects of carotid endarterectomy in reducing the occurrence of transient ischemic attacks and lowering significantly the incidence of subsequent strokes. At the same time operative mortality and morbidity have become acceptable for this elderly group of atherosclerotic patients.[8, 10, 17, 18, 18a, 21, 24, 52, 54a, 61, 62]

Chronic Cerebral Ischemia

In patients with chronic cerebral ischemia mental improvement has been limited. No patient has had a stroke during the follow-up period but cerebral deterioration has been common. The principal result of operation appears to be the prevention of strokes by removal of occlusive carotid plaques. Indications for operation in this category are obviously narrow.

Results of operation upon patients with asymptomatic carotid bruits will be considered in detail in the section that follows.

CAROTID ARTERY BRUITS

Auscultation of the neck for the presence of carotid bruits is an important examination in patients with cerebrovascular insufficiency syndromes. In fact, this should be done in every routine physical examination, especially in patients over the age of forty and in those with evidence of atherosclerosis elsewhere in the body. Recently developed sophisticated stethoscopes for the heart are inadequate for the head and neck. The standard 3 cm. bell stethoscope remains most satisfactory for cervical auscultation.

The word "bruit" is derived from the Latin *rugire*, which means "to roar." It is used here synonymously with the word "murmur." A bruit is the auditory manifestation of "uniformly oriented vortical eddies produced when a rapidly moving fluid stream encounters an obstacle."[3] The physical characteristics of murmurs in the head and neck have been described by Allen,[3] and by Allen and Mustian.[4]

The differential diagnosis of cervical murmurs includes physiological murmurs of no significance; venous hum; arteriovenous fistula; angiomatous malformations; intracranial neoplasms; Paget's disease of the skull; fever; anemia; thyrotoxicosis; atherosclerosis of the innominate, subclavian, vertebral, and carotid arteries; loops, kinks, and fibromuscular hyperplasia of the carotid arteries; and transmitted cardiac murmurs.

The incidence and significance of cervical bruits in the young and in the elderly, with and without cerebrovascular disease, has been the subject of several reports.[26, 37] In children and young adults these murmurs are of little significance, are usually heard at the base of the neck, and are of rapidly decreasing incidence with increasing age. Over the age of 40, however, cervical murmurs are much more significant, the carotid bruits being those most commonly encountered, with a reported incidence of about 10 per cent.

The most important cervical bruit is the mid-carotid one, heard over the carotid bifurcation near the angle of the jaw. It is usually highly localized and disappears quickly as one listens inferiorly.

Carotid bruits vary in intensity from soft to very harsh and may be graded from zero to four-plus on a quantitative basis. They appear when stenosis is 50 per cent or greater and may actually disappear at 85 to 90 per cent stenosis.[48] They vary in timing from systolic to continuous.

The most frequent cause of a mid-carotid bruit is an atherosclerotic plaque at the bifurcation of the common carotid artery, which usually involves the origin and first few centimeters of the internal carotid but occasionally is limited to the external carotid. Rarely a bruit is present in the absence of any radiographically demonstrable carotid pathology. This has been attributed to a hemodynamic phenomenon which may result from total occlusion of the opposite carotid.[4]

Several studies have been done on patients with overt cerebrovascular insufficiency, correlating stenotic lesions demonstrated on arteriograms with carotid bruits. The degree of correlation is very high when bruits are audible, ranging from 75 to 85 per cent.[37] Ninety per cent of audible bruits arise from internal carotid plaques, the remainder coming from the external carotid or other uncommon lesions.

Overall correlation between demonstrable carotid disease and bruits is about 60 per cent, since lesions may be present on the arteriogram when no bruit is audible. These include stenoses of less than 50 per cent, severe stenoses with a lumen diameter of one mm. or less, and total occlusions of the internal carotid.[51] A carotid bruit, when present, thus constitutes a significant finding in patients with cerebrovascular insufficiency.

Considerable controversy exists concerning the advisability of recommending arteriography and endarterectomy for patients with asymptomatic carotid bruits. The following data bear on this question.

Over a 13-year period Thompson et al.[52,53,54a,54b] performed 87 elective carotid endarterectomies on 65 patients with asymptomatic carotid bruits. General anesthesia was used, together with a temporary inlying bypass shunt for cerebral protection. There was no operative mortality. One patient had a mild transient weakness, and a second has a mild permanent deficit related to operation. During long-term follow-up, no patient has died of a stroke; one patient had a mild stroke with full recovery, while a second had a severe stroke one year after operation.

For a control series to compare with the surgical series, 59 patients with asymptomatic carotid bruits who were not operated upon when the bruit was first detected, were followed. There were various reasons for not operating upon these patients at the time they were first seen. In the early days of the study it was unclear as to whether they should be operated upon at all. In some patients the bruit was unilateral and very soft. In some cases the patient did not wish to have arteriography or surgery considered, while in others the patient's referring physician did not wish to have anything done. Occasionally, the treatment of other diseases took precedence over management of the bruit. In a few cases the patients did not return for regular follow-up after being instructed to do so.

These individuals were followed up to eight years after detection of the bruit, with an average follow-up of about 24 months. During this time 30 of the 59 patients (51 per cent) have remained asymptomatic. Fifteen (25 per cent) developed transient cerebral ischemia and were operated upon. Four of these had disappearance of the bruit with total occlusion of the internal carotid artery prior to operation. Fourteen patients (24 per cent) had frank strokes without transient ischemic attacks, from two days to four years following detection of the bruit. Eleven of these had total carotid occlusions with disappearance of the bruit associated with onset of stroke. Thus 29 of the 59 patients (49 per cent) developed transient ischemia or frank strokes during the follow-up period. When a stenotic carotid artery becomes totally occluded, there is a significant incidence of acute hemiplegic stroke with its attendant mortality and morbidity.

The long-term clinical consequences of asymptomatic carotid bruits may be listed thusly: (1) nothing may happen; (2) transient cerebral ischemic attacks may supervene; (3) frank strokes may occur without intervening episodes of transient ischemia; (4) total occlusion of the artery may occur without symptoms; and (5) total occlusion may occur resulting in either a transient ischemic episode or a frank stroke. The hazard depends directly upon the lesion giving rise to the bruit and upon the status of all vessels supplying the brain, both primary and collateral. Thus, little hazard is posed by bruits arising from stenosis of the external carotid or from loops, kinks, or fibromuscular hyperplasia. On the other hand, bruits coming from atherosclerotic plaques involving the internal carotid become symptomatic, in most instances, if followed long enough.[54b]

Javid et al.[31] have studied the natural history of carotid atheromas. On follow-up arteriograms they noted no change in size of the atheromas in 38 per cent of the lesions studied, and an increase in size in 62 per cent of the lesions. Thirty-four per cent increased at a rate greater than 25 per cent a year.

In another report these same authors[32] cite their experience with endarterectomy for asymptomatic bruits in 50 patients. One patient died after operation (2 per cent) and two patients suffered postoperative strokes (4 per cent). During long-term follow-up two patients developed non-fatal strokes (4 per cent). Because of the high long-term mortality from causes other than strokes, they believe that endarterectomy for asymptomatic bruits is inadvisable in hypertensive patients over the age of 65 with a history of myocardial infarction. In younger patients without several risk factors, however, they recommend endarterectomy for severe internal carotid stenosis.

In the final analysis, arteriography is the definitive diagnostic maneuver necessary to establish the etiology of a carotid bruit and to determine its significance as a stroke hazard.

As cerebral arteriography has become increasingly safer, it should probably be recommended more often for studying patients with asymptomatic carotid bruits of grade two intensity or greater. The overall general status of each patient should be considered very carefully, however, before recommending this procedure. It should not be done if there already exists some contraindication to endarterectomy.

If the arteriograms show that the bruit arises from a lesion which poses no stroke hazard, operation need not be considered. If a significant atherosclerotic stenosis is found in the internal carotid, endarterectomy may be recommended. Specific indications include (1) bilateral stenoses, (2) unilateral stenosis with contralateral occlusion, (3) stenosis in the artery to the dominant hemisphere, (4) known progressive atherosclerotic lesions elsewhere in the peripheral vasculature,

Table 11–7.   Indications for Carotid Endarterectomy in
Cerebrovascular Insufficiency

A. Indications
  1. Transient cerebral ischemia
  2. Stable strokes — selected
  3. Asymptomatic bruits — selected
  4. Chronic cerebral ischemia — selected

B. Contraindications
  1. Acute profound strokes
  2. Progressing strokes
  3. Severe intracranial disease
  4. Other severe generalized disorders (e.g., cancer)

---

and (5) contemplated major surgery of another sort where a hypotensive episode might well result in a stroke.

Since no unnecessary risks should be taken, appropriate measures for cerebral protection such as a temporary inlying shunt must be employed during carotid endarterectomy to avoid producing neurologic deficits. Operative mortality should be below one per cent and complications less than two per cent.

In summary, asymptomatic carotid bruits may originate in the internal carotid artery from atherosclerotic plaques which predispose to strokes in certain individuals over the age of 40. Arteriography is necessary at present to determine the significance of these bruits. If hazardous lesions are demonstrated, carotid endarterectomy may be performed to prevent the occurrence of ischemic cerebral episodes. Further studies of the natural history of asymptomatic carotid bruits are needed, as are non-invasive screening techniques to delineate the anatomic location and configuration of bruit-producing lesions and their hemodynamic significance prior to arteriography.

INDICATIONS FOR AND TIMING OF CAROTID ENDARTERECTOMY

Clinical considerations in each of the four categories of patients determine the indications and contraindications for carotid endarterectomy. Table 11–7 is a summary of indications for operation. The principal indication is transient cerebral ischemia, since strokes can be prevented, troublesome episodes of ischemia are largely abolished, and long-term survival rates are improved. Indications for operation in the other three categories are limited, and candidates for operation must be selected very carefully.

Table 11–8 summarizes the appropriate timing of operation for the various clinical categories. The procedure may be carried out at a time of election, delayed from several days to several weeks, or done as an emergency. Although *delayed* operation is an important principle in stroke surgery, *emergency* operation is not often necessary and probably has done more harm than good during the period of development of this field of surgery.

Occasionally, one finds patients in whom occlusive lesions are located in the carotid artery on the paradoxical side relative to the neurologic signs and symptoms. A number of patients having such lesions removed surgically have responded as would have been expected had the lesions been located on the appropriate side. This observation is in keeping with the concept of total cerebral blood flow on the basis of collateral circulation, which gives one a sound basis for recommending endarterectomy of inappropriate lesions.

Operation is contraindicated for cervical occlusions in the presence of severe intracranial disease. Mild intracranial disease, however, is an indication rather than a contraindication for operation. Age itself is not necessarily a contraindication to operation when the patient's general condition otherwise does not pose any undue hazard.

Patients with significant bilateral occlusions should have bilateral endarterectomies, but in separate stages at least one week apart. A number of strokes have occurred in patients with previous unilateral operations whose asymptomatic lesions in the unoperated artery were simply being followed.[48] Bilateral operation in a single stage is inadvisable because of the complications which may ensue. These include

Table 11–8. Timing of Carotid Endarterectomy for Cerebrovascular Insufficiency

A. Elective operation
   1. Stable stroke, recent or old
   2. Transient cerebral ischemia
   3. Asymptomatic bruit
   4. Chronic cerebral ischemia (rare)

B. Delayed operation (days to weeks)
   1. Acute stroke
   2. Fluctuating stroke

C. Emergency operation (rare)
   1. Frank stroke
      a. Disappearance of bruit
      b. Slowly worsening
      c. Fluctuating
   2. Transient cerebral ischemia
      a. Severe stenosis, especially if bilateral
      b. Disappearance of bruit
   3. Carotid thrombosis immediately following arteriography or endarterectomy

respiratory difficulties secondary to edema of the neck or transient hypoglossal paresis, postoperative hypertension from bilateral carotid sinus denervation, and aggravation of neurologic deficits from cerebral edema following the prolonged anesthesia and bilateral carotid blood flow interruption required for endarterectomy.

SURGERY OF INNOMINATE, COMMON CAROTID, SUBCLAVIAN AND VERTEBRAL ARTERIES

Occlusive lesions in the great vessels arising from the aortic arch and in the vertebral arteries may cause symptoms of cerebrovascular insufficiency. Such lesions are characteristically located at the origins of these vessels and are usually segmental in extent (Fig. 11–2). Even with total occlusion of the innominate, subclavian, and common carotid arteries, the distal vasculature is nearly always patent. By virtue of this fact, most occlusions of the great vessels can be successfully reconstructed by surgical means. Numerically speaking, these lesions comprise only a small proportion of the total extracranial occlusions responsible for cerebrovascular insufficiency since those at the common carotid bifurcations are by far the ones most frequently encountered. Multiple stenoses may occur in the great vessels, the carotids, and the vertebral arteries.

Symptomatology varies depending upon the location of the lesions. Thus one may find patterns of carotid insufficiency, of vertebral-basilar insufficiency, or combinations. When the subclavian artery is involved there may be symptoms of arterial insufficiency of the upper extremity in addition to or without cerebral manifestations.

Arteriographic verification of lesions of the great vessels must be done prior to operative intervention. Retrograde techniques employing either the femoral, axillary, or brachial arteries, depending upon the clinical situation, are most satisfactory for these studies.

Innominate and Common Carotid Arteries

When the innominate artery is stenotic or occluded there may be symptoms arising from the distribution of the right carotid, the right subclavian, or the right vertebral artery systems. Diagnostic features include differences in blood pressure and arterial pulsations in the two arms and a murmur heard over the innominate artery. Occasionally, with occlusive lesions in the innominate artery, when the distal subclavian, carotid, and vertebral arteries are patent, one encounters the syndrome known as the "innominate steal," with reversal of flow in both the right carotid and right vertebral arteries, giving symptoms of left hemiparesis and brain stem ischemia.[35]

Subclavian Arteries and "Subclavian Steal" Syndrome

Subclavian occlusive lesions may cause vertebral-basilar insufficiency, arterial insufficiency of the corresponding arm, or may give no symptoms whatsoever. Differences in blood pressure and arterial pulsations in the arms, and bruits in the supraclavicular areas are diagnostic features of these lesions.

An interesting syndrome known as the "subclavian steal" has recently been described.[14, 20, 44] In this situation the proximal subclavian artery, usually the left, is occluded while the ipsilateral vertebral artery is patent. There is reversal of flow in the vertebral artery with blood flowing *from* the brain into the arm distal to the subclavian occlusion *via* the patent vertebral vessel. With loss of blood from the brain stem and cerebellum one may have manifestations of vertebral-basilar insufficiency. Symptoms may be precipitated by exercise of the ipsilateral arm. Detailed serial arteriograms are necessary to establish the diagnosis of the subclavian steal syndrome. Unless symptomatic, patients with subclavian steal syndromes need not be subjected to surgical reconstruction.

Vertebral Arteries

Stenoses at the takeoff of the vertebral artery from the subclavian may cause symptoms of vertebral-basilar insufficiency. Anatomic variations in the origin of the vertebral artery are not uncommon. At times the artery is vestigial or even completely absent on one side. Ordinarily if one vertebral is widely patent, circulation in the vertebral-basilar system is adequate and symptoms are minimal or absent. The situation may vary, however, depending upon the presence of occlusive lesions in the carotid system and in the basilar artery itself. Total occlusion of the vertebral artery at its origin is usually accompanied by thrombosis throughout the entire cervical extent of the vessel and precludes surgical restoration of patency.

Many patients with the clinical syndrome of vertebral-basilar insufficiency have occlusive lesions in the carotid system as well as in the vertebral vessels. Experience has shown that endarterectomy of the carotid arteries may so favorably influence the vertebral symptoms that further surgery on the vertebral artery is not required.[35] Restoration of carotid circulation increases total cerebral blood flow, improves the collateral to the posterior system, and so relieves the manifestations of ischemia. The importance of detailed serial arteriographic studies of both the carotid and the vertebral-basilar systems under these circumstances is thus apparent.

As mentioned above, patients with a single vertebral occlusion may exhibit no symptoms, provided the opposite vertebral is patent. It

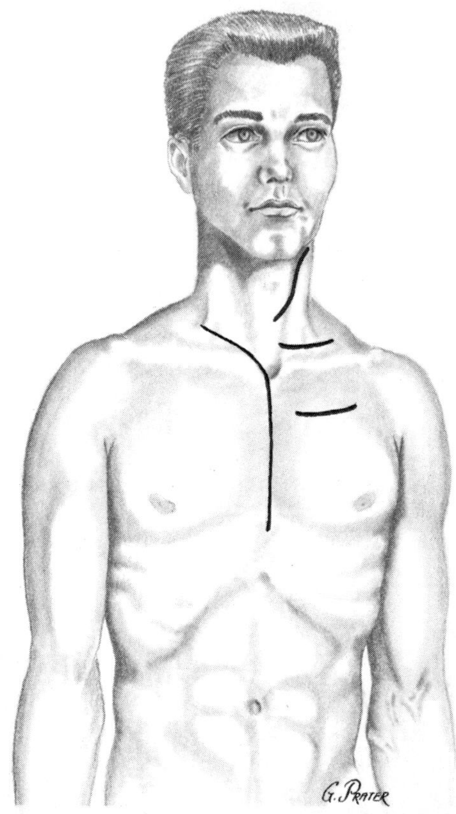

Figure 11–14. Locations of sternal-splitting, intercostal space, and cervical incisions used for operations upon the aortic arch, common carotid, subclavian, and vertebral vessels.

is also well known that total subclavian occlusion may occur without cerebral or extremity symptoms. In view of these observations and the fact that vertebral-basilar symptoms are frequently relieved by carotid surgery alone, it has become increasingly apparent that surgical reconstruction of the vertebral artery is infrequently indicated. Patients with bilateral vertebral stenoses or with stenosis of a single remaining artery are the principal candidates for operation. These are few indeed, comprising less than three per cent of the number of patients requiring carotid endarterectomy. When vertebral reconstruction is indicated, however, the results of operation are quite satisfactory.

Surgical Techniques

Revascularization procedures for occlusion of the great vessels and vertebral arteries must be highly individualized because of the many possible sites of the lesions. Technical procedures have changed considerably during the past decade. Figure 11–14 shows the locations of the various incisions which have been employed for these operations. These include intrathoracic approaches and extrathoracic cervical incisions. The former may be done through a sternal-splitting incision, anterior thoracic incisions via the second or third intercostal space, or a lateral thoracic approach through the fifth intercostal space.

In the past, stenoses of the innominate, common carotid, and subclavian arteries were treated by direct endarterectomy or with bypass grafts taking origin from the arch of the aorta. Figures 11–15 and 11–16 illustrate sites of arteriotomies and the type of bypass graft employed. Many variations are possible.

Although blood-flow restoration was quite satisfactory, it soon became obvious that mortality and morbidity for these procedures was quite high (20 per cent mortality).[16] Consequently, new methods were devised for treating these lesions, resulting in the use of extrathoracic approaches and cervical bypass procedures almost routinely. Figures 11–17, 11–18 and 11–19 illustrate the types of extrathoracic cervical bypass operations which may be employed. Either 8 mm. Dacron or saphenous vein may be used as the prosthesis. These operations are simpler to perform, carry a low mortality (2 to 3 per cent) and morbidity, and are quite satisfactory.

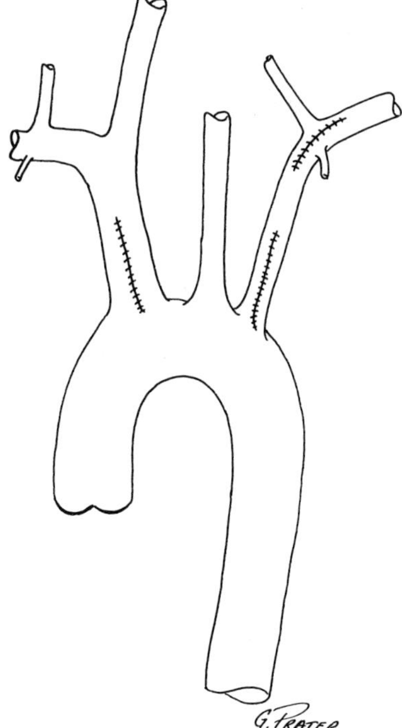

Figure 11–15. Diagram showing arteriotomies which may be used for endarterectomy of the innominate, subclavian, and vertebral arteries. (From Thompson, J. E.: *Surgery for Cerebrovascular Insufficiency (Stroke).* Courtesy of Charles C Thomas, Publisher, Springfield, Illinois, 1968.)

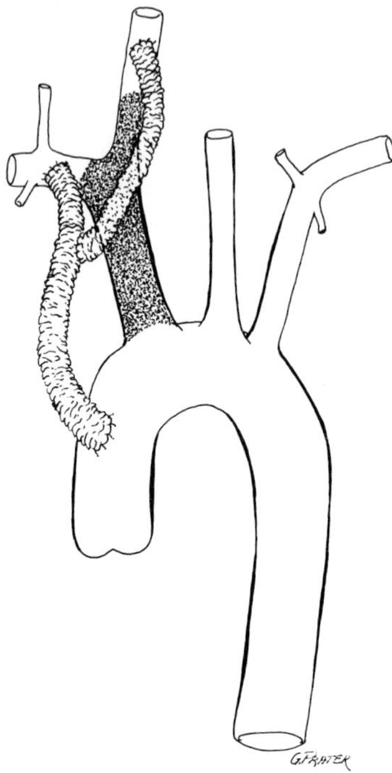

Figure 11-16. Illustration of the type of bypass graft which may be used for reconstruction of occlusive lesions of the aortic arch vessels. In this case the occluded innominate artery has been bypassed with 8 mm. Dacron from the aortic arch to the distal right subclavian and common carotid arteries. Many variations of this technique are possible.

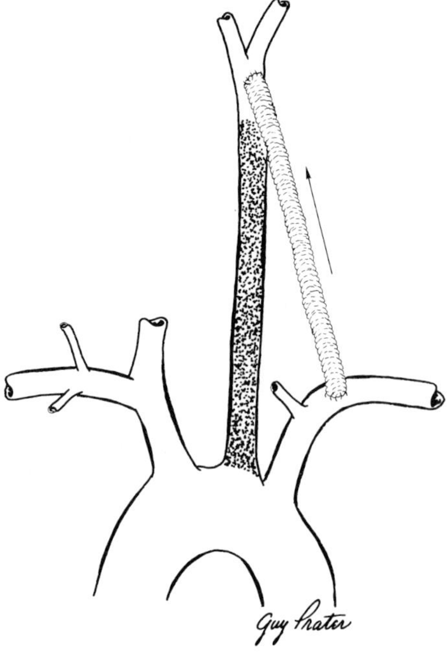

Figure 11-17. Drawing of a long extrathoracic cervical bypass graft from subclavian to carotid artery for reconstruction of left common carotid artery occlusion. This operation eliminates the necessity for an intrathoracic procedure.

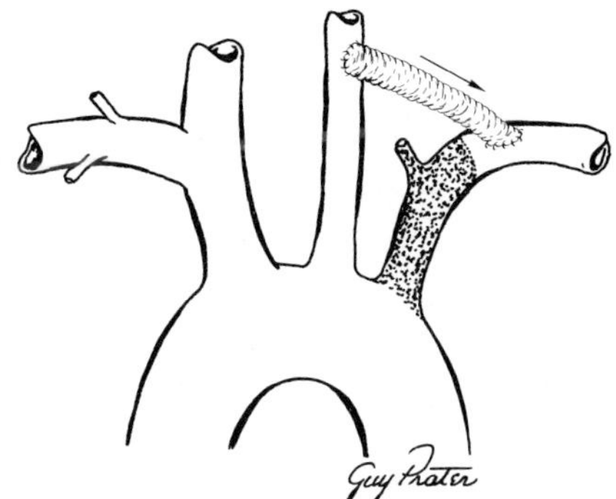

Figure 11–18. Extrathoracic cervical bypass from left common carotid to left subclavian artery for restoration of blood flow into an occluded left subclavian artery. This same maneuver restores flow into the vertebral artery when it is patent and only the proximal portion of the subclavian is occluded.

In a good-risk patient one may still elect to perform endarterectomy of the innominate artery using an intrathoracic approach, although cervical subclavian-to-subclavian bypass may be used for innominate occlusions (Fig. 11–20). Stenoses of the common carotid and proximal subclavian arteries are best handled by means of the simpler cervical bypass maneuvers. There are many variations in technique depending upon the location of the lesions.[16, 61]

Increasing experience has shown that construction of these bypasses does not produce symptomatic "steal" syndromes. Compensatory increase in blood flow sufficient to vascularize the various distal beds occurs in the parent artery.

In summary, extrathoracic cervical bypass operations are the procedures of choice for stenotic lesions of the great vessels, with the occasional exception of the innominate artery, which may be handled by direct endarterectomy. Because of the excellence of distal runoff in most cases, these operations carry a very high percentage of successful restoration of blood flow, both immediate and long-term, with consequent relief of symptoms.

Although many more vertebral arteries are being visualized in the study of patients with cerebrovascular insufficiency, fewer are being

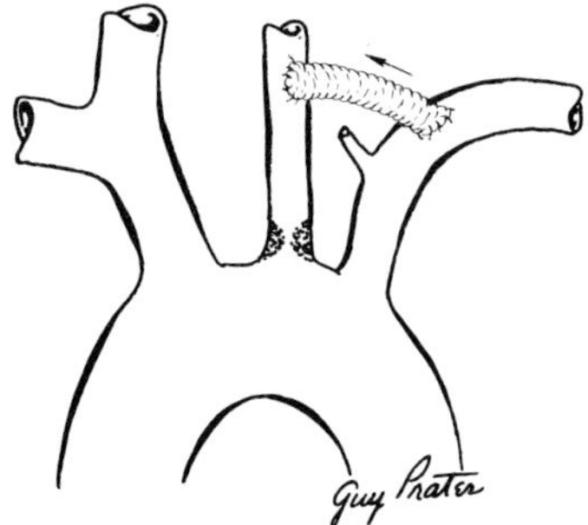

Figure 11–19. Diagram of extrathoracic cervical bypass graft from left subclavian to left common carotid artery for treatment of common carotid stenosis at its origin from the aortic arch. Either saphenous vein or 8 mm. Dacron tube may be utilized.

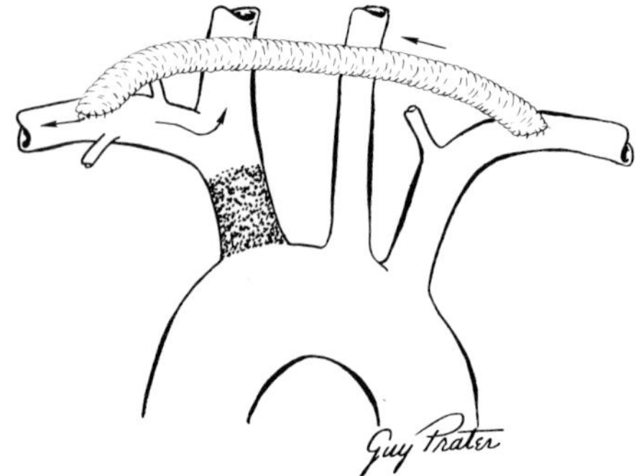

Figure 11–20. Extrathoracic cervical bypass procedure which may be used to reconstruct a totally occluded innominate artery. Here the bypass originates from the left subclavian artery, crosses the neck, and is attached to the right subclavian, revascularizing the subclavian, vertebral, and carotid arteries. A variation of this technique is the axillary-to-axillary bypass, with the graft passing subcutaneously in the anterior extrathoracic plane.

subjected to operative reconstruction. When reconstruction is required, a variety of techniques is available for restoration of vertebral blood flow. An isolated vertebral stenosis is best approached through a supraclavicular incision (Fig. 11–14). At times this operation is difficult because of the depth of the operative field. Simple endarterectomy of the vertebral origin is usually inadvisable because of the small size of the artery, and may be hazardous because of its friability. A patch graft of vein or Dacron is ordinarily used for reconstruction of the vertebral origin (Fig. 11–21). The artery may be ligated and divided at its takeoff and then reimplanted into the distal subclavian at a more convenient site. When the vertebral artery is tortuous, arterioplasty may be performed by suturing the vertebral to the subclavian artery, employing a side-to-side anastomosis (Fig. 11–22).

In the presence of subclavian plaques the orifice of the vertebral artery may be endarterectomized through the lumen of the subclavian artery (Fig. 11–15).

Bypass techniques are also useful for vertebral reconstruction. A bypass may be constructed from the distal subclavian to the distal vertebral. Depending upon the site of the lesions, bypass grafts may orig-

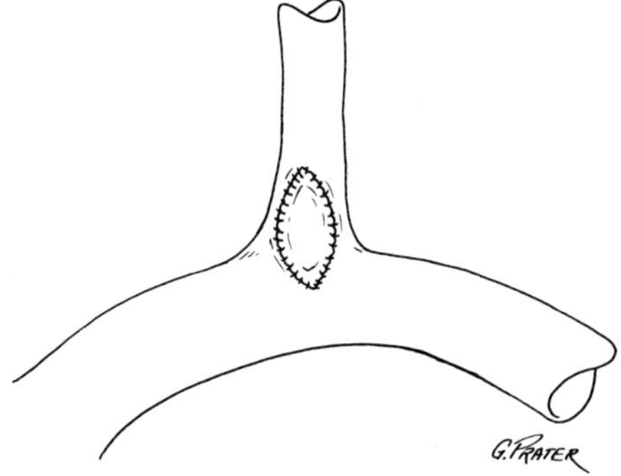

Figure 11–21. Vertebral artery reconstruction using a patch graft to enlarge the stenosed origin. (From Thompson, J. E.: *Surgery for Cerebrovascular Insufficiency (Stroke)*. Courtesy of Charles C Thomas, Publisher, Springfield, Illinois, 1968.)

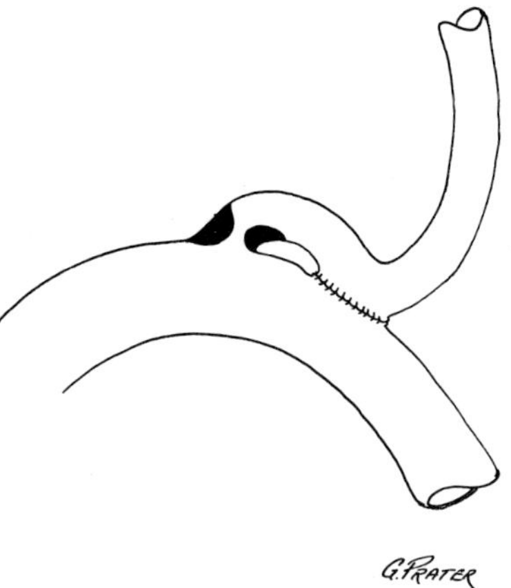

Figure 11–22. Vertebral arterioplasty of a tortuous artery with side-to-side anastomosis to the subclavian artery. (From Thompson, J. E.: *Surgery for Cerebrovascular Insufficiency (Stroke).* Courtesy of Charles C Thomas, Publisher, Springfield, Illinois, 1968.)

inate from the aortic arch or from the common carotid arteries and revascularize the vertebral-basilar system via the distal subclavian (Fig. 11–16).

Occasionally, in poor-risk patients who exhibit symptoms of a subclavian steal syndrome the simplest operation is ligation of the appropriate vertebral artery near its point of origin. This is obviously inferior to reconstruction but may be used in exceptional circumstances to abolish symptoms of vertebral-basilar ischemia.

Patients subjected to operation for occlusive lesions in the aortic arch branches and vertebral arteries become asymptomatic or are improved in 85 to 90 per cent of the cases reported.[16, 61]

REFERENCES

1. Adams, J. E., Smith, M. C., and Wylie, E. J.: Cerebral blood flow and hemodynamics in extracranial vascular disease: Effect of endarterectomy. Surgery 53:449, 1963.
2. Alexander, S. C., and Lassen, N. A.: Cerebral circulatory response to acute brain disease: Implications for anesthetic practice. Anesthesiology 32:60, 1970.
3. Allen, N.: The significance of vascular murmurs in the head and neck. Geriatrics 20:525, 1965.
4. Allen, N., and Mustian, V.: Origin and significance of vascular murmurs of the head and neck. Medicine 41:227, 1962.
5. Barker, W. F., Stern, W. E., Krayenbuhl, H., and Senning, A.: Carotid endarterectomy complicated by carotid cavernous sinus fistula. Ann. Surg. 167:568, 1968.
6. Bauer, R. B., Meyer, J. S., Gotham, J. E., and Gilroy, J.: A controlled study of surgical treatment of cerebrovascular disease—42 months' experience with 183 cases. In: *Cerebral Vascular Diseases.* Millikan, C. H., Siekert, R. G., and Whisnant, J. P. (Eds.). New York, Grune and Stratton, 1966.
7. Blaisdell, F. W., Lim, R., and Hall, A. D.: Technical result of carotid endarterectomy. Am. J. Surg. 114:239, 1967.
8. Blaisdell, F. W., Clauss, R. H., Galbraith, J. G., Imparato, A. M., and Wylie, E. J.:

Joint study of extracranial arterial occlusion. IV. A review of surgical considerations. J.A.M.A. *209*:1889, 1969.

9. Bland, J. E., Chapman, R. E., and Wylie, E. J.: Neurological complications of carotid artery surgery. Ann. Surg. *171*:459, 1970.

10. Bloodwell, R. D., Hallman, G. L., Keats, A. S., and Cooley, D. A.: Carotid endarterectomy without a shunt. Arch. Surg. *96*:644, 1968.

11. Borhani, N. D., and Meyer, J. S. (Eds.): *Medical Basis for Comprehensive Community Stroke Programs.* National Institutes of Health, 1968.

12. Brice, J. G., Dowsett, D. J., and Lowe, R. D.: Haemodynamic effects of carotid artery stenosis. Brit. Med. J. *2*:1363, 1964.

13. Carrea, R., Molins, M., and Murphy, G.: Surgical treatment of spontaneous thrombosis of the internal carotid artery in the neck. Carotid–carotideal anastomosis. Report of a case. Acta Neurol. Lat. Amer. *1*:71, 1955.

14. Contorni, L.: The vertebro-vertebral collateral circulation in obliteration of the subclavian artery at its origin. Minerva Chir. *15*:268, 1960.

15. Crawford, E. S., De Bakey, M. E., Blaisdell, F. W., Morris, G. C., Jr., and Fields, W. S.: Hemodynamic alterations in patients with cerebral arterial insufficiency before and after operation. Surgery *48*:76, 1960.

16. Crawford, E. S., De Bakey, M. E., Morris, G. C., Jr., and Howell, J. F.: Surgical treatment of occlusion of the innominate, common carotid, and subclavian arteries: A 10 year experience. Surgery *65*:17, 1969.

17. De Bakey, M. E., Crawford, E. S., Cooley, D. A., Morris, G. C., Jr., Garrett, H. E., and Fields, W. S.: Cerebral arterial insufficiency: one to 11-year results following arterial reconstructive operation. Ann. Surg. *161*:921, 1965.

18. De Weese, J. A., Rob, C. G., Satran, R., Norris, F. H., Lipchik, E. O., Zehl, D. N., and Long, J. M.: Surgical treatment for occlusive disease of the carotid artery. Ann. Surg. *168*:85, 1968.

18a. DeWeese, J. A., Rob, C. G., Satran, R., Marsh, D. O., Joynt, R. J., Summers, D., and Nicols, C.: Results of carotid endarterectomies for transient ischemic attacks—five years later. Ann. Surg. *178*:258, 1973.

19. Eastcott, H. H. G., Pickering, G. W., and Rob, C.: Reconstruction of internal carotid artery in a patient with intermittent attacks of hemiplegia. Lancet *2*:994, 1954.

20. Editorial: A new vascular syndrome— "The subclavian steal." New Eng. J. Med. *265*:912, 1961.

21. Edwards, W. S., Wilson, T. A. S., and Bennett, A.: The long-term effectiveness of carotid endarterectomy in prevention of strokes. Ann. Surg. *168*:765, 1968.

22. Ehrenfeld, W. K., Hamilton, F. N., Larson, C. P., Jr., Hickey, R. F., and Severinghaus, J. W.: Effect of CO_2 and systemic hypertension on downstream cerebral arterial pressure during carotid endarterectomy. Surgery *67*:87, 1970.

22a. Engell, H. C.: Studies in cerebral circulation. Bull. Amer. Coll. Surg. *58*:7, 1973.

23. Fields, W. S., Bruetman, M. E., and Weibel, J.: Collateral circulation of the brain. In: *Monographs in the Surgical Sciences.* Baltimore, The Williams & Wilkins Co., 1965.

24. Fields, W. S., Maslenikov, V., Meyer, J. S., Hass, W. K., Remington, R. D., and MacDonald, M.: Joint study of extracranial arterial occlusion: V. Progress report of prognosis following surgery or nonsurgical treatment for transient cerebral ischemic attacks and cervical carotid artery lesions. J.A.M.A. *211*:1993, 1970.

25. Fisher, C. M.: Clinical syndromes in cerebral arterial occlusion. In: *Pathogenesis and Treatment of Cerebrovascular Disease.* Fields, W. S. (Ed.). Springfield, Ill., Charles C Thomas, 1961.

26. Gilroy, J., and Meyer, J. S.: Auscultation of the neck in occlusive cerebrovascular disease. Circulation *25*:300, 1962.

27. Gonzalez, L. L., and Lewis, C. M.: Cerebral hemorrhage following successful endarterectomy of the internal carotid artery. Surg. Gynec. Obstet. *122*:773, 1966.

28. Hardesty, W. H., Roberts, B., Toole, J. F., and Royster, H. P.: Studies of carotid-artery blood flow in man. New Eng. J. Med. *263*:944, 1960.

29. Harris, E. J., Brown, W. H., Pavy, R. N., Anderson, W. W., and Stone, D. W.: Continuous electroencephalographic monitoring during carotid artery endarterectomy. Surgery *62*:441, 1967.

30. Hass, W. K., Fields, W. S., North, R. R., Kricheff, I. I., Chase, N. E., and Bauer, R. B.:

Joint study of extracranial arterial occlusion: II. Arteriography, techniques, sites, and complications. J.A.M.A. *203*:961, 1968.

30a. Hays, R. J., Levinson, S. A., and Wylie, E. J.: Intraoperative measurement of carotid back pressure as a guide to operative management for carotid endarterectomy. Surgery 72:953, 1972.

31. Javid, H., Ostermiller, W. E., Hengesh, J. W., Dye, W. S., Hunter, J. A., Najafi, H., and Julian, O. C.: Natural history of carotid bifurcation atheroma. Surgery *67*:80, 1970.

32. Javid, H., Ostermiller, W. E., Hengesh, J. W., Dye, W. S., Hunter, J. A., Najafi, H., and Julian, O. C.: Carotid endarterectomy for asymptomatic patients. Arch. Surg. *102*:389, 1971.

33. Larson, C. P., Jr., Ehrenfeld, W. K., Wade, J. G., and Wylie, E. J.: Jugular venous oxygen saturation as an index of adequacy of cerebral oxygenation. Surgery *62*:31, 1967.

34. Larson, C. P., Jr.: Anesthesia and control of the cerebral circulation. In: Wylie, E. J. and Ehrenfeld, W. K.: *Extracranial Occlusive Cerebrovascular Disease.* Philadelphia, W. B. Saunders Co., 1970.

35. Loeb, C., and Meyer, J. S.: *Strokes Due to Vertebro-Basilar Disease.* Springfield, Ill., Charles C Thomas, 1965.

36. Lyons, C., Clark, L. C., Jr., McDowell, H., and McArthur, K.: Cerebral venous oxygen content during carotid thrombintimectomy. Ann. Surg. *160*:561, 1964.

37. McDowell, F., Rennie, L., and Ejrup, B.: Arterial bruit in cerebrovascular disease. In: *Cerebral Vascular Diseases.* Millikan, C. H., Siekert, R. G., and Whisnant, J. P. (Eds.). New York, Grune and Stratton, 1966.

38. Meyer, J. S., Gotoh, F., Tomita, M., and Akiyama, M.: New technics for recording cerebral blood flow and metabolism in subjects with cerebrovascular disease. In: *Cerebral Vascular Diseases.* Millikan, C. H., Siekert, R. G., and Whisnant, J. P. (Eds.). New York, Grune and Stratton, 1966.

39. Millikan, C. H., Siekert, R. G., and Whisnant, J. P.: The clinical pattern in certain types of occlusive cerebrovascular disease. Circulation *22*:1002, 1960.

40. Millikan, C. H.: The pathogenesis of transient focal cerebral ischemia. Circulation *32*:438, 1965.

41. Moore, W. S., and Hall, A. D.: Carotid artery back pressure. A test of cerebral tolerance to temporary carotid occlusion. Arch. Surg. *99*:702, 1969.

42. Paulson, O. B.: Cerebral apoplexy (stroke): Pathogenesis, pathophysiology and therapy as illustrated by regional blood flow measurements in the brain. Stroke *2*:327, 1971.

43. Quinn, James L., III.: Brain scanning. In: *Cerebral Vascular Diseases.* Toole, J. F., Siekert, R. G., and Whisnant, J. P. (Eds.). New York, Grune and Stratton, 1968.

44. Reivich, M., Holling, H. E., Roberts, B., and Toole, J. F.: Reversal of blood flow through the vertebral artery and its effect on cerebral circulation. New Eng. J. Med. *265*:878, 1961.

45. Roberts, B., Hardesty, W. H., Holling, H. E., Reivich, M., and Toole, J. F.: Studies on extracranial cerebral blood flow. Surgery *56*:826, 1964.

46. Thompson, J. E., and Austin, D. J.: Surgical treatment of arteriosclerotic occlusions of the carotid artery in the neck. Surgery *51*:74, 1962.

47. Thompson, J. E., Kartchner, M. M., Austin, D. J., Wheeler, C. G., and Patman, R. D.: Clinical considerations in the surgical management of strokes. Circulation *33*:I-162, 1966.

48. Thompson, J. E., Kartchner, M. M., Austin, D. J., Wheeler, C. G., and Patman, R. D.: Carotid endarterectomy for cerebrovascular insufficiency (Stroke): Follow up of 359 cases. Ann. Surg. *163*:751, 1966.

49. Thompson, J. E., Austin, D. J., and Patman, R. D.: Endarterectomy of the totally occluded carotid artery for stroke: Results in 100 operations. Arch. Surg. *95*:791, 1967.

50. Thompson, J. E.: Cerebral protection during carotid endarterectomy. J.A.M.A. *202*:1046, 1967.

51. Thompson, J. E.: *Surgery for Cerebrovascular Insufficiency (Stroke).* Springfield, Ill., Charles C Thomas, 1968.

52. Thompson, J. E., Austin, D. J., and Patman, R. D.: Carotid endarterectomy for

cerebrovascular insufficiency: Long-term results in 592 patients followed up to thirteen years. Ann. Surg. *172*:663, 1970.

53. Thompson, J. E., and Patman, R. D.: Endarterectomy for asymptomatic carotid bruits. The Heart Bulletin: *19*:116, 1970.

54. Thompson, J. E.: Prevention of complications of cerebral arteriography and surgery. In: *Management of Arterial Occlusive Disease.* Dale, W. A. (Ed.). Chicago, Year Book Medical Publishers, Inc., 1971.

54a. Thompson, J. E.: The development of carotid artery surgery. Arch. Surg. *107*:643, 1973.

54b. Thompson, J. E.: The role of surgery in controlling cerebral ischemia. In: Ingelfinger, F. J., Ebert, R. V., Finland, M., and Relman, A. S. (Eds.) *Controversy in Internal Medicine II.* Philadelphia, W. B. Saunders Co., 1974.

55. Toole, J. F., and Patel, A. N.: *Cerebrovascular Disorders.* New York, McGraw-Hill Book Co., Inc. 1967.

56. Waltz, A. G.: Regional cerebral blood flow: Responses to changes in arterial blood pressure and CO_2 tension. In: *Cerebral Vascular Diseases.* Toole, J. F., Siekert, R. G., and Whisnant, J. P. (Eds.). New York, Grune and Stratton, 1968.

57. Weibel, J., and Fields, W. S.: *Atlas of Arteriography in Occlusive Cerebrovascular Disease.* Stuttgart, Georg Thieme Verlag, 1969.

58. Wells, B. A., Keats, A. S., and Cooley, D. A.: Increased tolerance to cerebral ischemia produced by general anesthesia during temporary carotid occlusion. Surgery *54*:216, 1963.

59. White, C. W., Jr., Allarde, R. R., and McDowell, H. A.: Anesthetic management for carotid artery surgery. J.A.M.A. *202*:1023, 1967.

60. Wylie, E. J., Hein, M. F., and Adams, J. E.: Intracranial hemorrhage following surgical revascularization for treatment of acute strokes. J. Neurosurg. *21*:212, 1964.

61. Wylie, E. J., and Ehrenfeld, W. K.: *Extracranial Occlusive Cerebrovascular Disease.* Philadelphia, W. B. Saunders Co., 1970.

62. Young, J. R., Humphries, A. W., Beven, E. G., and de Wolfe, V. G.: Carotid endarterectomy without a shunt. Arch. Surg. *99*:293, 1969.

Chapter Twelve

DISEASES OF THE RENAL VESSELS

JOSEPH J. KAUFMAN, M.D.

The incidence and character of diseases of the renal vessels have been fully appreciated only since the development of renal angiography during the past decade. The chief clinical problems are hypertension secondary to renal artery stenosis, renal artery aneurysms, arteriovenous fistulas, and renal vein thrombosis. In this chapter we discuss diagnostic methods and the indications and techniques of surgical correction of renovascular lesions.

RENAL ARTERY STENOSIS AND RENOVASCULAR HYPERTENSION

Goldblatt, in the 1930's, proved that experimental constriction of the renal artery resulted in a secondary form of hypertension caused by the release of a pressor substance or precursor from the kidney, but the clinical implications of his work have been appreciated only during the last 15 or 16 years. The diagnosis and surgical treatment of this important form of secondary hypertension have constituted major advances in medicine, radiology, and surgery. It is estimated that renovascular hypertension exists in approximately 5 per cent of persons with high blood pressure. Since there are at least 20 million hypertensive individuals in the United States alone, it follows that renovascular disease may be responsible for high blood pressure in as many as one million people. Although it was initially believed that atherosclerosis affecting the ostia of the renal arteries or proximal renal arteries was the most common form of renal artery stenosis, an increasing number of young hypertensive patients have been shown to have fibroplasias of the walls of the renal vessels.

Unfortunately, knowledge of the etiology of stenosing diseases of the renal vessels has not kept pace with advances in diagnosis and surgical treatment. The anatomical arrangement of the renal vessels undoubtedly exposes the ostia to kinetic influences which predispose to the formation of atherosclerotic plaques, often out of proportion to the existence of functionally critical atherosclerosis in other vessels.[46] Fibroplasias of the arterial walls have been classified pathologically so that distinct, but sometimes overlapping, involvements of the intima, media, or adventitia can be distinguished.[39] Although some types occur primarily in children (subintimal fibroplasia) and although a preponderance of medial fibroplasia occurs in young women, exceptions to these patterns are legion.

History of Renovascular Surgery

Approximately 45 years ago, Callahan and Schiltz[7] reported ligating the neck of a renal artery aneurysm. In 1948, Mathé[36] reported resection of an aneurysmal sac of a renal artery. The technique of thrombendarterectomy was described in 1949 by Dos Santos.[14] Ten years after these events, although awareness of hypertension secondary to renal disease was increasing, there still was little interest in diseases of the renal vessels.

Despite recognition of the relationship of kidney disease to hypertension, it was not until the work of Goldblatt and associates in 1934[19] that a cause and effect relationship was established between renal artery stenosis and hypertension. The first documented cure of hypertension by nephrectomy was reported by Bulter in 1937.[6] Additional evidence of the curability of hypertension caused by renovascular disease was reported by Leadbetter and Burkland in 1938[32] and subsequently by Barker and Walters,[2] Boyd and Lewis,[5] and Freeman and Hartley.[17]

Freeman and his associates[18] described the first case of hypertension cured by corrective renovascular surgery in 1954. Their operation consisted of thrombendarterectomy from above the renal arteries to the bifurcation of the common iliac arteries. Following Freeman's milestone, a number of surgeons began to report the correction of hypertension by operation on the renal arteries. The pioneers in the field were Ellis et al.,[15] who implanted the renal artery into the aorta (1955), Hurwitt et al.,[24] who performed the first splenorenal anastomosis (1956), and DeCamp et al.,[11, 12] who performed a splenorenal anastomosis on a solitary kidney of a ten-year-old girl in 1955 and an excision and end-to-end anastomosis of the renal artery in 1956. Poutasse,[45] in 1956, did the first successful bilateral renal artery homograft. In 1958, bilateral simultaneous renal endarterectomy was done by Starzl and Trippel.[57] One of the largest experiences in the treatment of renovascular hypertension was reported by Morris et al.,[42] who popularized the use of the bypass graft. Stoney and Wylie[58] introduced the free hypogastric autograft. Autotransplantation for renal artery stenosis was successfully used by Marshall et al.,[35] Serrallach-Mila et al.,[52] and Kaufman et al.[25]

Diagnosis

Clinical clues as to the possible existence of renal artery stenosis include an absence of family history of high blood pressure, onset of hypertension below the age of 35 years or over the age of 50, accelerated hypertension, a bruit over the upper abdomen, restlessness and anxiety, and a frequent finding of secondary hyperaldosteronism. However, none of these clinical features is pathognomonic, and there is a generous overlap among the clinical features of essential and renal hypertension. Therefore, special diagnostic tests have been used and are particularly indicated in young patients.

The radioactive renogram with iodohippurate I^{131} was more popular several years ago than it is today. Its value has been questioned by investigators because of the high incidence (19 per cent) of false positive studies and the lack of specificity of the changes seen in the secretory and excretory phases of the renogram.[38]

Renal scanning using iodohippurate I^{131} and the Anger camera scintiphotographic techniques are subject to the same criticisms in that they are relatively nonspecific. However, in our hands, this test has had its greatest value as a simple means of determining functional adequacy after renovascular repair.

The intravenous urogram is the simplest and the most frequently used test. When multiple criteria are analyzed, a positive correlation between the intravenous urogram and the angiographic and surgical findings is possible in 93 per cent of patients.[37] False positive tests occur but are rare, and false negative studies usually are associated with segmental lesions, bilateral disease, or marginal unilateral renal artery stenosis. Even in the case of bilateral lesions, there is often asymmetrical functional impact on the kidneys, and the urogram frequently will be positive for the more seriously affected side. The radiographic parameters to be considered are kidney size, early nephrogram, pyelocalyceal appearance time and differential pyelocalyceal concentration with dehydration, hydration, or drug-induced diuresis. Hence, the intravenous urogram appears to be the most practical and useful diagnostic test for hypertensive patients with suspected renal artery stenosis, provided that rapid sequence studies are done and films are taken at one-minute intervals after injection of a bolus of the contrast agent. A stenosing lesion of the renal artery is highly suspect when there is a disparity in kidney size of 1 cm. or more, a delay in appearance time of the contrast medium in the calyces, a relative hyperconcentration of contrast medium on the involved side, and a delay in washout of contrast medium from the ischemic kidney[31] (Fig. 12–1). Although all criteria may exist, it is not uncommon to find only one or two radiographic indications of unilateral renal ischemia in the intravenous urogram.

RENAL ARTERIOGRAM AND THE ANATOMICAL LESIONS

Improvements in the techniques of aortography and renal arteriography have been made possible since the Seldinger catheteri-

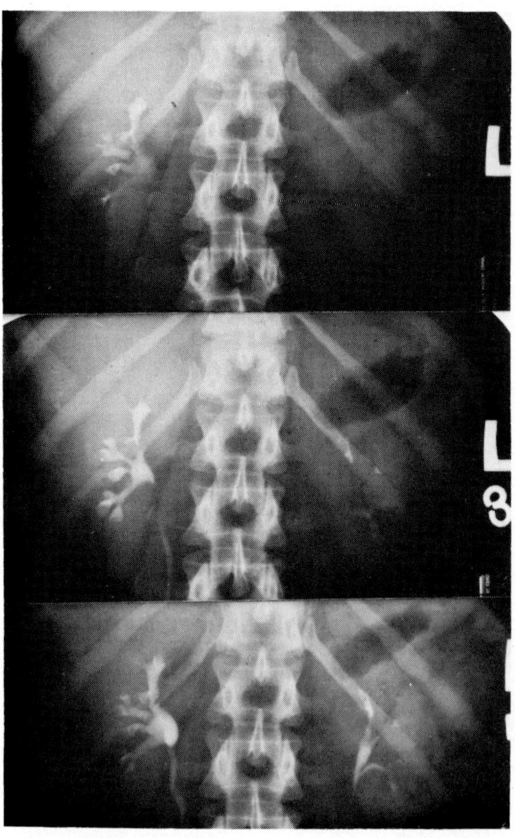

Figure 12–1. Rapid sequence IVP showing small left kidney and delay in pyelocalyceal opacification in a patient with functionally significant left renal artery stenosis. Note first filling of left renal calyces at three minutes and the small volume of the pyelocalyceal contents in the five-minute film.

zation method was devised and image intensifiers were perfected. In experienced hands, the test need not be unduly uncomfortable or hazardous. Midstream aortic flush is important to determine the number of renal arteries and to demonstrate stenosing lesions at the aortic take-off of the vessels (Fig. 12–2). Upright aortography was described in 1962,[27] and although it is not widely practiced today, it was useful in showing the relationship of nephroptosis to renal artery stenosis. Selective catheterization of the renal arteries has become routine in the study of patients with suspected renovascular lesions since it provides the best definition of the fine details of the renal vasculature. New techniques employing magnification demonstrate detailed architecture of the vessels, making possible visualization of small aneurysms (periarteritis nodosa), small areas of infarction and scarring, and minute arteriovenous shunts.

The distinction of mural dysplasias from atheromatous lesions usually is not difficult because of the predilection of these lesions for different areas of the renal vessels and because of their characteristic radiographic appearances. Atherosclerotic plaques often occur in the proximal one-third of the renal artery or at its orifice, and they tend

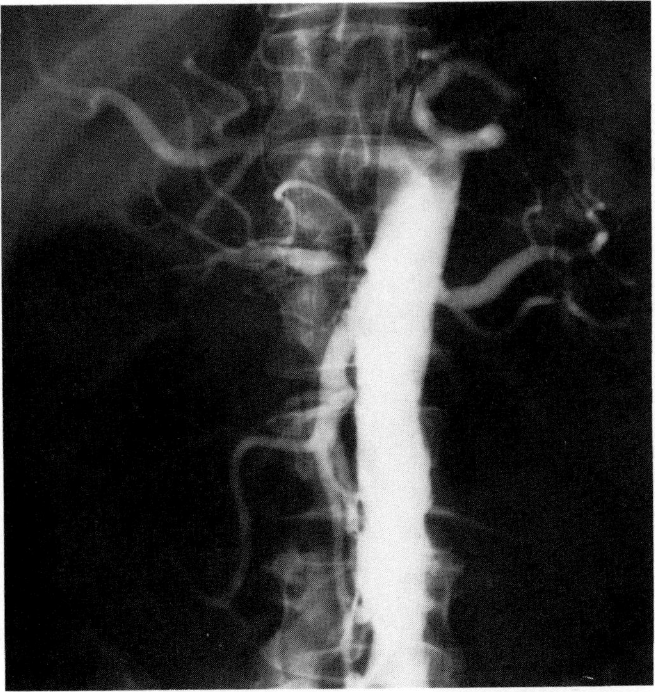

Figure 12–2. Aortogram of 54-year-old patient showing atherosclerotic plaque of right renal artery.

to be eccentric (Fig. 12–3). Coexistent atherosclerosis of the aorta and iliac vessels is commonly seen.

Atherosclerotic lesions usually occur in men over the age of 50, whereas fibroplasias occur in younger patients from infancy[21] to middle age and predominantly in women.

Most of the fibroplasias affecting the wall of the renal vessels occur in the middle or distal thirds of the main renal artery and some extend into branches (Fig. 12–4). McCormack et al.[39] have classified mural lesions into *intimal fibroplasia, medial fibroplasia,* and *subadventitial fibroplasia.* Intimal fibroplasia often appears as a smooth, often focal, stenosis involving the distal portion of the renal artery or its branches (Fig. 12–5). Dissecting aneurysms may occur.

Medial fibroplasia is the most common mural dysplasia, accounting for 70 to 75 per cent of cases. It often involves both arteries (30 to 35 per cent), occurs chiefly in women between the ages of 25 and 45, and is frequently associated with renal ptosis. It produces a characteristic beading effect on arteriography, with a series of fibrous rings alternating with aneurysmal dilatations of varying sizes (Fig. 12–6). Microscopically, the internal elastic membrane may be thinned, lost, or reduplicated, and the media is thickened with collagenous tissue (Fig. 12–7). The lesion is often extensive and frequently involves the

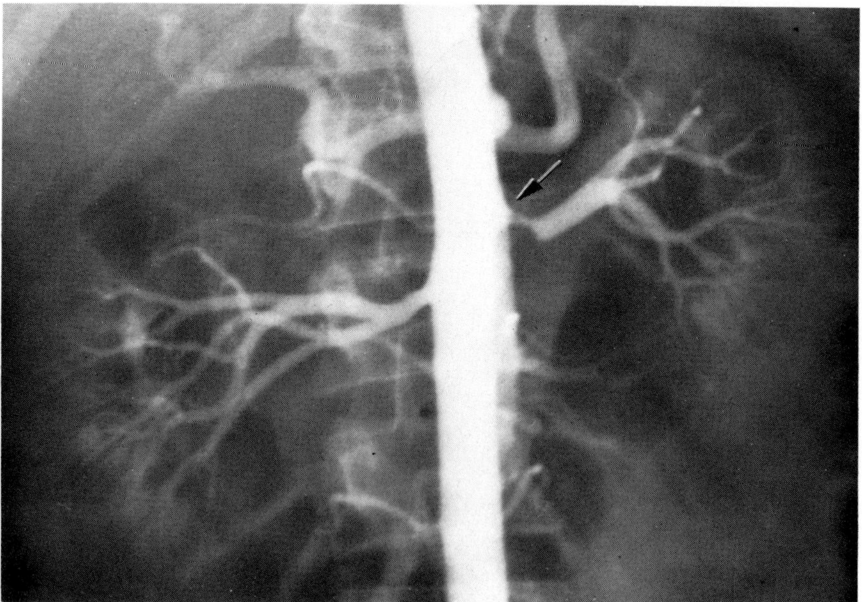

Figure 12–3.   Arteriogram showing atherosclerotic plaque of an eccentric type in the first portion of the left renal artery.

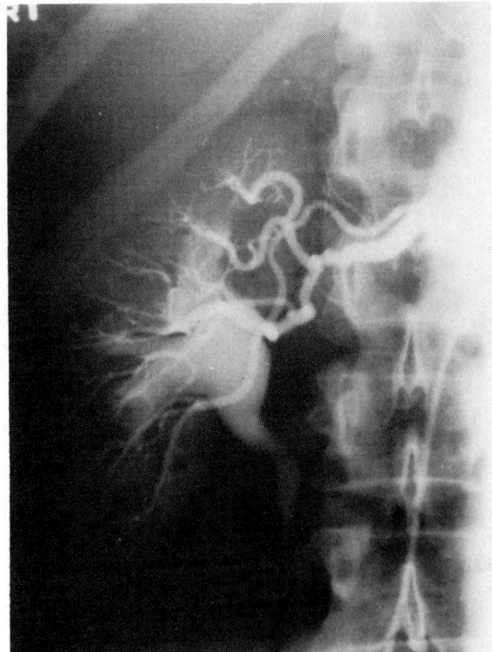

Figure 12–4. Selective right arteriogram showing medial fibroplasia of the distal third of the vessel extending into the proximal portion of the primary branches.

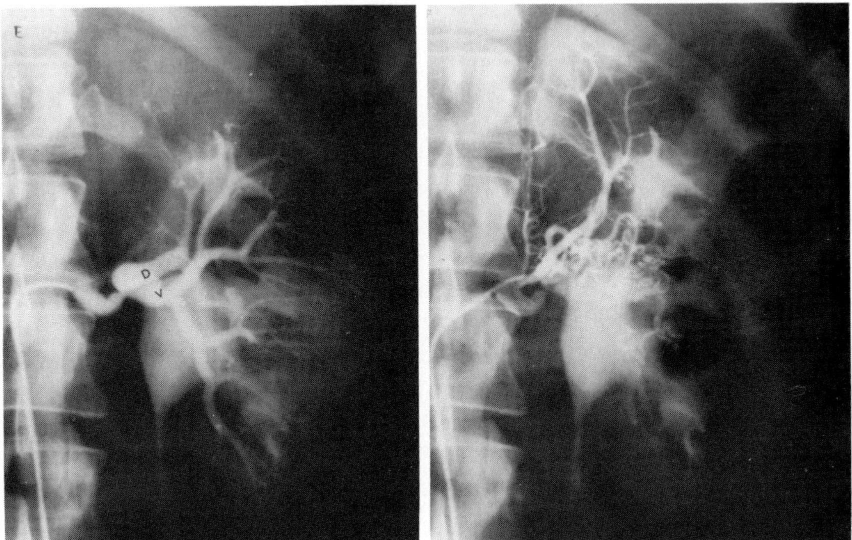

Figure 12–5. Selective left arteriogram showing severe stenosis of the subintimal type affecting the distal third of the vessel. Note the abundant collateral blood supply to the kidney, illustrated by injecting a superior branch proximal to the area of stenosis.

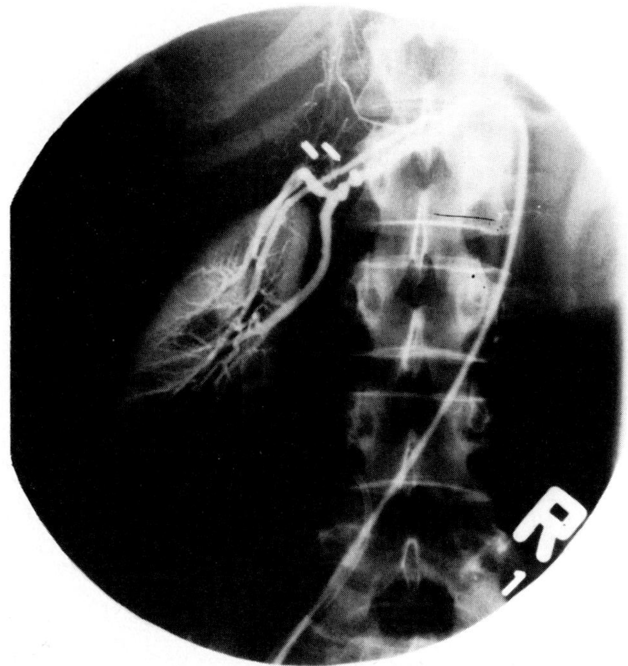

Figure 12–6. Aortogram showing medial fibroplasia of the distal third of the right renal artery.

distal two-thirds of the renal artery and may extend into the primary branches.

Fibromuscular hyperplasia differs from medial fibroplasia in that there is unorganized smooth muscle and fibrous tissue condensation within the media. Dissecting aneurysms occur more frequently in this form of dysplasia, probably as a result of disruption of the internal elastica.

Subadventitial fibroplasia produces stenoses of variable lengths. It often occurs in the proximal portion of the renal artery and is seen at times in children. Because of the frequent association of medial fibroplasia and a history of pregnancies or contraceptive steroid drug therapy, it is tempting to implicate a hormonal cause for the condition occurring in women. It is impossible to accurately diagnose these fibroplastic lesions angiographically since there may be components of each of the processes in several layers of the artery.

It is appropriate to discuss *renal artery aneurysms* together with stenosing lesions of the renal vessels since the two conditions coexist or may be causally related. Aneurysmal dilatation of the arterial wall associated with medial fibroplasia is a frequent finding. These may occur as small swellings or saccular formations (Fig. 12–8). Dissect-

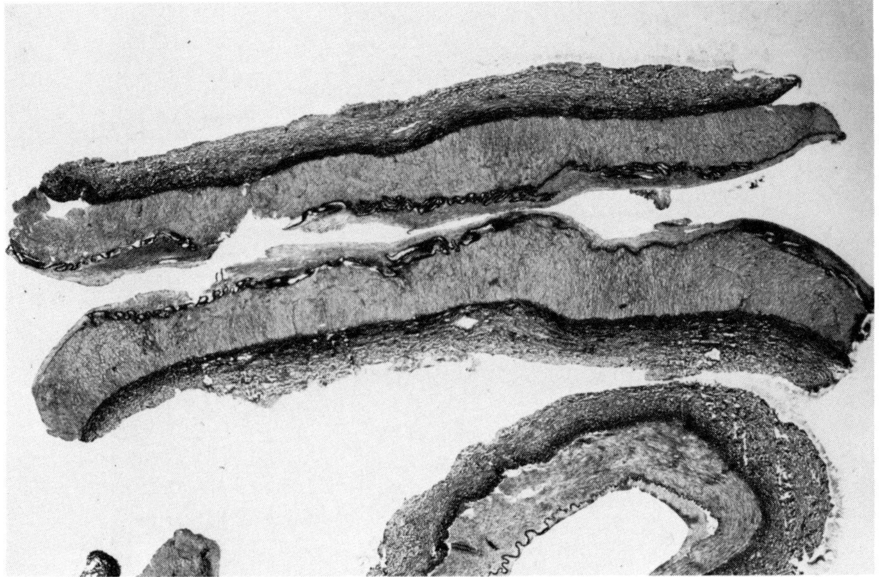

Figure 12-7. Photomicrograph showing longitudinal section of renal artery which displays medial fibroplasia, duplication, and fragmentation of the internal elastica.

ing aneurysms are similarly encountered in the variant forms of mural dysplasia and probably are caused by disruption of the internal elastica (Fig. 12-9). True aneurysms occur in the main renal artery or in its primary branches (Fig. 12-10). False aneurysms occur

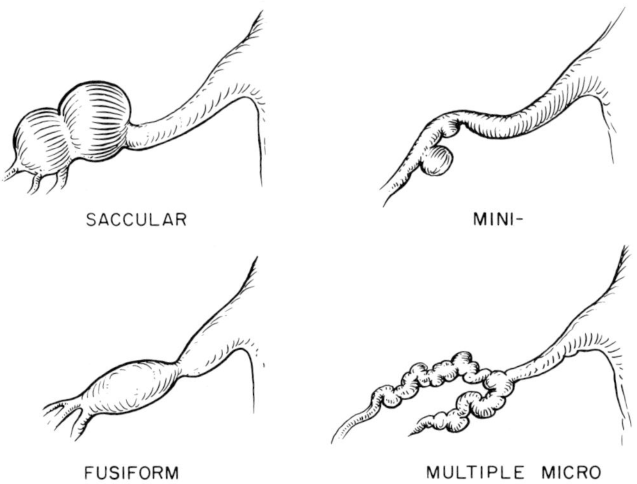

Figure 12-8. Variant forms of renal artery aneurysms.

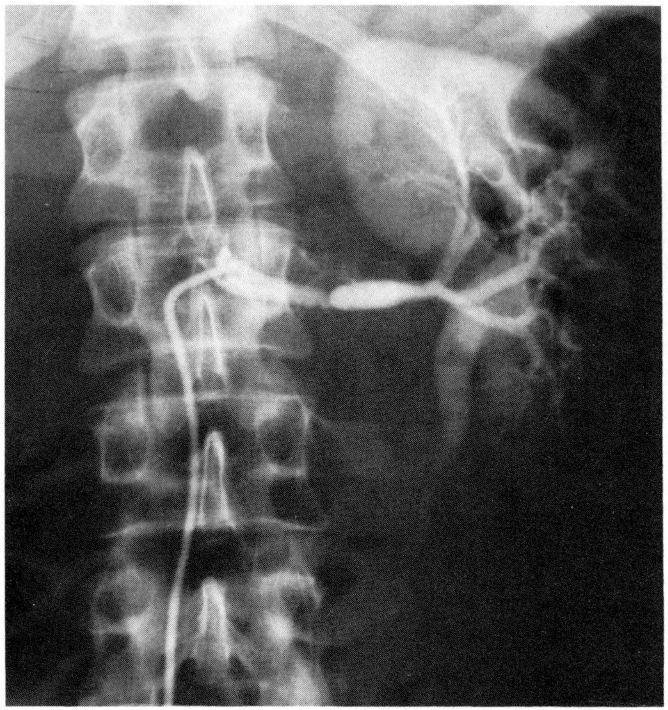

Figure 12-9. Patient with intimal fibroplasia showing early dissection of the arterial wall.

as a result of spontaneous or traumatic rupture of a portion of the renal artery wall. There is a propensity for calcification within the walls of aneurysms undoubtedly related to traumatic turbulence.

The relation of renal artery aneurysms to hypertension is unclear, and relatively few studies have been done to correlate excess renin elaboration and renal artery aneurysms.[10] It is our impression that such aneurysms rarely produce hypertension unless infarction has resulted from clotting within the aneurysmal sac. Arteriovenous shunts, acquired or congenital, may produce hypertension, but this probably is related to high cardiac output sequelae and not to the release of vasoactive substances. Arteriovenous fistulas of the congenital type usually have a cirsoid appearance (Fig. 12–11), whereas acquired types generally occur as single communications following a penetrating wound or iatrogenic trauma such as needle biopsy or nephrolithotomy.

MEASUREMENT OF PRESSOR SUBSTANCES

The measurement of pressor substances by bioassay and, more recently, by immunoassay methods has been a major advance in the

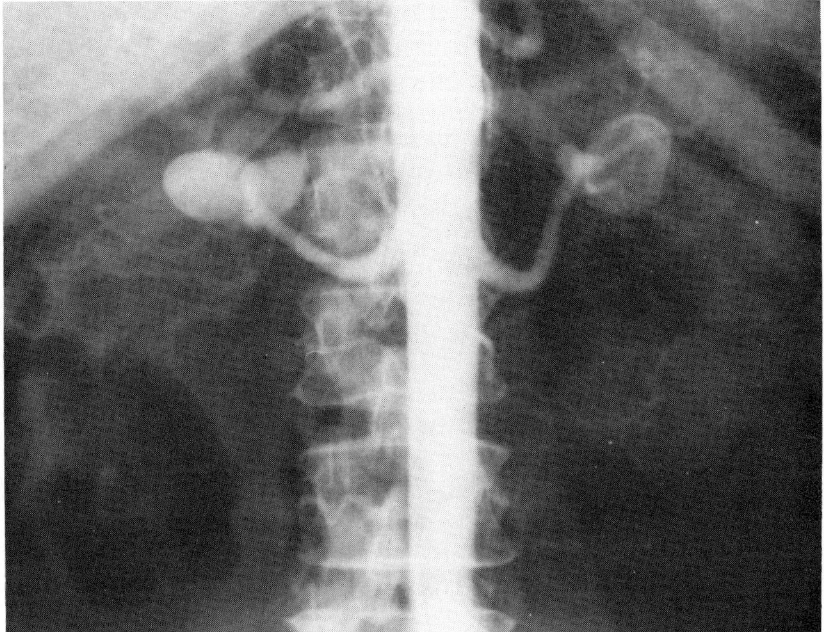

Figure 12-10. Patient with bilateral large renal artery aneurysms.

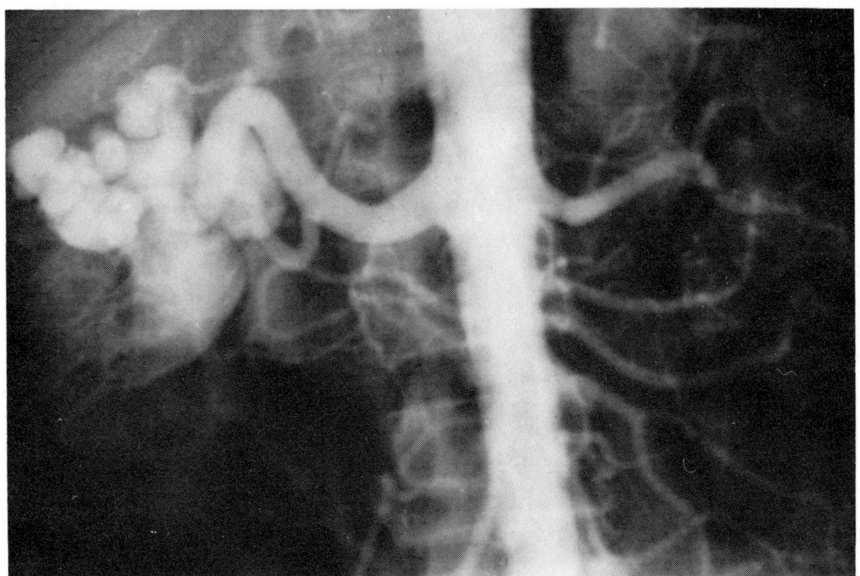

Figure 12-11. Congenital aneurysm of cirsoid type showing massive dilatation of the arteries and arteriovenous shunts.

diagnosis of renovascular hypertension, and a high correlation of the differential renal vein plasma renin assay and curability by nephrectomy or angioplasty has been established.[29, 60] The sampling of renal vein effluent by retrograde catheterization of the femoral vein is a relatively easy procedure without major risks. We have found in laboratory experiments that renin activity increases abruptly and predictably shortly after renal artery constriction, but that absolute levels of renin activity tend to decrease as chronicity of the hypertension ensues.[29] There seems to be little controversy in regard to the advantage of divided renal vein renin assay over peripheral renin assay in the diagnosis of renovascular hypertension. Peripheral renin assay determinations are subject to considerable variation depending upon volume states, and do not serve as a satisfactory screening test because of multiple entities affecting renin release in hypertensive individuals. While we and others have considered that a high degree of correlation, in the range of 90 per cent, is obtainable between the divided renal vein renin assay and the results of surgical treatment of renovascular hypertension, there is still a small group of skeptics who believe that the value of divided renal vein renin assay has been overstated. It is generally conceded that a correlation of 1.5 to 1 between the affected and the opposite renal vein venous effluent is a valid indication of functionally significant renal artery stenosis found on arteriography (and particularly when correlated with a positive intravenous urogram). Foster and Dean, and Stamey feel that there are many false positive or negative renin assays, and that the divided kidney function test is still an important part of the preoperative workup on these patients.[16, 56]

A recent discovery of an angiotensin II blockade has opened new vistas of possibilities for the diagnosis and possibly the treatment of renovascular hypertension. Brunner, Gavras, Laragh and Keenan have found that SAR[1]-ALA[8]-angiotensin II is an octapeptide competitive inhibitor of angiotensin II. The sarcosine and alanine amino acids replace two other amino acids of the octapeptide, changing the pressor activity of angiotensin II to a non-pressor agent. The high specificity of the compound has made it possible to investigate the role of angiotensin II in the pathogenesis of high blood pressure and has offered the possibility of treating patients with angiotensin mediated hypertension. The drug action correlated with the levels of plasma renin activity and had no biological action other than to block angiotensin II and reduce the blood pressures in high renin patients. They postulate that this competitive angiotensin II blockade will be useful for the identification of angiotensin II-dependent disorders, of particular value in screening patients with surgically curable renal hypertension. In a small series of patients with unilateral renal artery stenosis, angiotensin II blockade made it possible to determine within one to two hours that the increased blood pressure was due to an excess of circulating angiotensin II and thereby to predict accurately that the hypertensive disorder could be cured by surgical vascular repair.

DIFFERENTIAL KIDNEY FUNCTION TESTS

Differential kidney function tests deserve mention even though they have not been widely practiced since the emergence of the divided renal vein plasma renin assay. They are of great historical and physiological interest, however. Following partial occlusion of the renal artery (50 per cent), there is a reduction of glomerular filtration rate and a lowered filtered load of sodium, resulting in a decreased secretion of sodium and water. Increased fractional reabsorption of sodium and water leads to a higher osmolality in the final urine and to a hyperconcentration of those solutes that are poorly reabsorbed, viz., PAH, inulin, and creatinine.

Although divided kidney function tests are not universally employed because they are cumbersome and associated with greater morbidity than other commonly used tests, they may be useful when other tests are equivocal. In a comparative study in which both divided kidney function tests and divided plasma renin activity determinations were done in 25 patients with arteriographically demonstrated lesions, we found three subjects with negative or equivocal divided kidney function tests who had positive plasma renin ratios for ischemia.[29] Contrariwise, one cured patient with a negative plasma renin ratio had a positive divided kidney function test. Furthermore, the divided kidney function test provides the most accurate data regarding the contribution of each kidney to total renal economy.

Determination of Pressure Gradients and Renal Blood Flow

The validity of pressure gradient determinations at the time of surgical intervention for renal artery stenosis has recently come under some doubt as a result of reports indicating that intrarenal hemodynamics may produce spurious values.[59] Animal experiments have shown that increased intrarenal resistance produced pharmacologically may minimize or obliterate a gradient as renal blood flow is being significantly reduced.[33] By and large, however, a pressure differential of 25 mm. Hg or more has correlated well with a functionally significant lesion curable by nephrectomy or vascular repair.

A useful adjunct is the determination of renal blood flow. Electromagnetic flowmeters are now widely available, and their use is easy and practical.[41]

Intraoperative renal blood flow is readily and accurately measured with long-handled probes and a square-wave electromagnetic flowmeter. It is important that the probes be calibrated in the laboratory prior to their use. Customarily, we employ 4, 5 or 6 mm. probes. The determination of renal arterial blood flow is particularly indicated when there are bilateral lesions, and before and after repair of lesions. In our hands, when coupled with strain gauge manometry, the best index of functional stenosis and operative repair is provided.

RENAL BIOPSY

The pathological findings in renal vascular hypertension are inconstant. Hypercellularity and hypergranulation of the juxtaglomerular apparatus (JGA), thought to be pathognomonic a few years ago, are no longer considered constant features of the condition. This confirms the impression that the JGA may trigger secondary hypertension, but it is not necessarily a factor in sustaining the hypertensive state. Ischemic tubular atrophy, interstitial scarring, hyalinosis of arterioles, and round cell infiltration are also features of severe vascular insufficiency, but these, too, are difficult to correlate with surgical curability. Nevertheless, tubular atrophy has some prognostic value in that it indicates a severity of the condition frequently associated with irreversibility and may indicate need for nephrectomy rather than arterioplasty.[1] Bilateral percutaneous "preoperative" renal biopsy is not recommended since its value has not been established.

SURGICAL TREATMENT OF RENAL ARTERY STENOSIS AND RENAL ARTERY ANEURYSMS: INDICATIONS FOR SURGICAL TREATMENT

Indications for surgical treatment of stenosing disease and aneurysms of the renal artery are being crystallized as a result of cumulative experience with these conditions. Frequently, hypertension secondary to renal artery stenosis is resistant to antihypertensive drug therapy. In addition, medical therapy will not halt the progression of this disease, whereas vascular reconstruction, in selected cases, appears to provide successful long-term beneficial results and may actually arrest the fibrosing stenotic process.

Follow-up of patients with renal artery stenosis treated conservatively and by surgical vascular repair during the last 15 years has provided an insight regarding the natural history of stenosing diseases of the renal vessels. While firm predictions of the progression or stability of the disease cannot be made, certain trends in the evolution of such processes are evident. There is both experimental and clinical evidence to suggest that a reduced flow to the renal artery in the presence of a constricting disease process may predispose to further reductions in the caliber of the vessels. In addition, we have observed that after reconstructive procedures, there is often an apparent reversal in the progression of the disease secondary to restoration of hemodynamic dilatation.

Atherosclerosis of the renal vessels, which predominantly affects men in the fifth, sixth, and seventh decades, appears to progress at variable rates, but in at least one-third of such patients treated conservatively, advancement of the stenosis and deterioration of renal function will occur over periods of one to eight years (Fig. 12–12). We have witnessed several cases of renal infarction resulting from progression of the stenosis culminating in thrombosis. In addition, even though 60 per cent of patients with atherosclerosis can be cured or dramatically improved by nephrectomy or repair, about 10 per cent will die of cardiovascular complications within a few years, irrespective of treatment. Shapiro et al.[54] observed that 33 per cent of patients with atherosclerotic renal artery stenosis treated surgically were dead within one to six years postoperatively, and they compared this to 40 per cent mortality over an equal period in 72 unoperated patients. Operative intervention, therefore, is advised in such patients, provided they are good surgical risks, the hypertension cannot be controlled by medical management, or renal function is deteriorating.

The mortality from progressive arterial disease in younger patients with fibrous mural dysplasias is considerably less than that in the atherosclerotic group. However, even in patients with mural dysplasias, the frequency of bilateral involvement and the technical difficulties in repairing disease extending to branches prevents an overoptimistic longterm view.

The best prognosis is probably in patients with medial fibroplasias, fortunately the type of mural dysplasia most frequently encountered.[40] The stenosing process appears to be slowly progressive; it may cause dissection but rarely results in thrombosis, and, hence, the outlook is more favorable. When the diseased artery can be successfully bypassed progression of the disease to distal branches seems to be significantly retarded.

Subadventitial fibroplasia tends to be more rapidly progressive than other forms of fibrous stenosing disease, and our experience with serial arteriography has shown a progressive obstruction of the renal artery from one year to the next, making vascular repair imperative (Fig. 12–13).

Because of its propensity to develop dissections, intimal fibro-

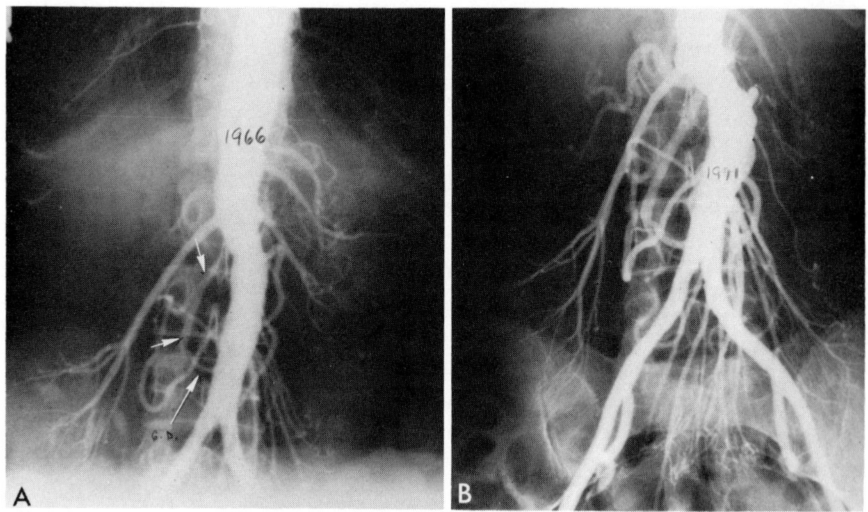

Figure 12–12. *A,* Postoperative aortogram 6 days following endarterectomy showing good patency of both renal arteries compared to preoperative appearance. *B,* Aortographic appearance five years later (1971) showing virtually complete occlusion of left renal artery and progression of aortic atherosclerosis.

plasia, which occurs primarily in children and young adults, requires surgical repair whenever possible.

In our experience with 293 cases, the operative mortality has been 2.5 per cent. Of 507 patients treated surgically for renal vascu-

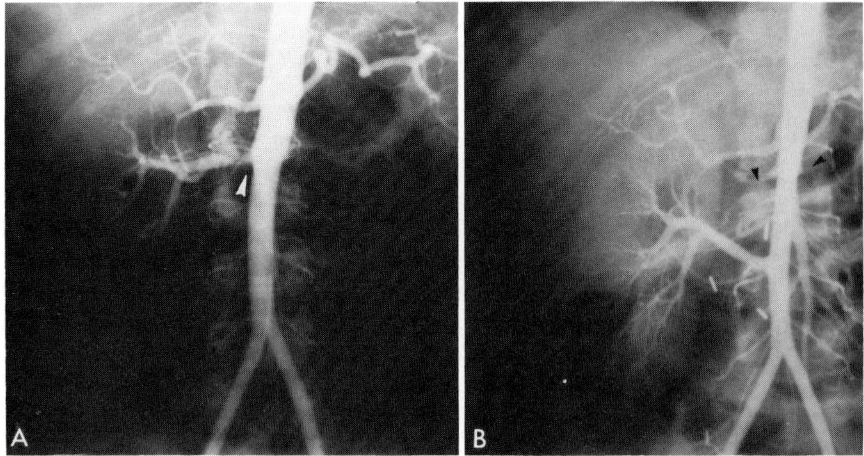

Figure 12–13. Seven-year-old boy with severe subadventitial fibrosis of the right renal artery. When this child underwent a left nephrectomy for stenosing disease of the left renal artery at the age of four, only minimal involvement of the right renal artery was seen *(A).* However, within two years, a high degree of stenosis had developed, and subsequently a hypogastric artery interposition graft was used to repair the solitary renal artery *(B).*

lar disease in the Cooperative Study of Renal Vascular Hypertension,[59] there were 35 deaths (6.9 per cent). Of interest is a mortality rate of 7 per cent for 172 primary nephrectomies as compared to a rate of only 4.1 per cent in 218 patients undergoing unilateral vascular reconstruction (indicating, perhaps, that nephrectomy was selected for the more seriously ill or poorer risk patients). A mortality rate of 8.4 per cent in 36 patients undergoing bilateral reconstructive procedures increased to 22.2 per cent in patients undergoing unilateral arterial reconstruction with contralateral nephrectomy as a single procedure.

Renal Artery Aneurysms

Surgical treatment of renal artery aneurysms is clearly indicated when the lesion is greater than 2 cm. and the patient is a good surgical risk. Likewise, when renal vascular hypertension is confirmed by the finding of elevated plasma renin activity on the affected side, surgical intervention is justified. Less well-defined indications are aneurysms of smaller size with or without hypertension and particularly without laboratory confirmation of disparate renin elaboration.

Rupture of renal artery aneurysms is rare, and the danger has probably been exaggerated. It occurs primarily in patients whose lesions are greater than 2 cm. in diameter and are not calcified. Pregnancy is, unquestionably, a predisposing factor to rupture.[22] In general, then, uncalcified aneurysms greater than 2 cm. in size in young women should be treated surgically, and aneurysms associated with hypertension (and rarely with pain or hematuria) should also have the benefit of vascular repair or nephrectomy.

ARTERIOVENOUS FISTULAS

Arteriovenous fistulas may be congenital or acquired. The congenital type usually has an angiomatous or cirsoid appearance (Fig. 12–11), whereas the acquired types (unless they are in association with renal carcinoma) generally occur as single communications following penetrating wounds or iatrogenic trauma such as needle biopsy, partial nephrectomy, or nephrolithotomy. Characteristically, and when functionally significant, arteriovenous fistulas cause arterial hypertension (widened pulse pressure), cardiac enlargement, and congestive heart failure. The majority, however, produce no other functional disorder and are detected by the finding of an abdominal machinery-like bruit and the characteristic appearance on arteriography.

PREPARATION OF THE PATIENT
UNDERGOING RENOVASCULAR SURGERY

Although in the past operation on patients receiving certain antihypertensive drug therapy was contraindicated because of difficulty controlling blood pressure in the presence of catecholamine depletion, modern anesthetics and techniques have virtually eliminated blood pressure problems during operation.

Potassium is repleted preoperatively in patients with hypokalemia (secondary hyperaldosteronism) to circumvent myocardial irritability. An intravenous infusion is administered the night before the operation, and, where difficulty is anticipated because of the serious nature of the problem or high risk of the patients, a central venous catheter is desirable and should be placed in position before the operation. A catheter is placed in the bladder before the operation and an infusion of 10 per cent mannitol in a 0.5 per cent normal saline is started at the beginning of the procedure. Approximately 500 ml. is allowed to run in before renal artery clamping. When vascular repair is planned, systemic heparin (50 to 75 units/kg. of body weight) is given intravenously approximately five minutes before renal artery clamping. Heparin effect is allowed to wear off, but in occasional cases where bleeding is excessive, protamine (0.75 mg. to 1.0 mg./kg. of body weight) is administered intravenously to counteract the heparin effect.

Recent evidence indicates that furosemide and ethacrynic acid have a protective action on the ischemic kidney.[43] These agents may be given on the morning of the operation. Postoperatively, if oliguria occurs following unilateral or bilateral procedures, furosemide (80 to 1000 mg.), administered intravenously, intramuscularly, or orally, is useful in promoting diuresis.

Postoperatively, blood pressure is carefully monitored, and marked elevations or depressions are treated with parenteral vasopressor (norepinephrine, angiotensin) or vasodepressor agents (nitroprusside, diazoxide, hydralazine, Aldomet, or reserpine), respectively.

OPERATIVE PROCEDURES FOR RENOVASCULAR
HYPERTENSION

Surgery for renovascular hypertension may be ablative or reconstructive. Before the indications and techniques for vascular reconstruction were appreciated, the majority of patients with renal artery stenosis and hypertension were treated by nephrectomy. Since, in the vast majority of cases, the kidney distal to the stenosis is anatomically sound and minor pathological changes are reversible after the correction of hypertension, the indications and desirability for attempted vascular reconstruction became obvious. In addition, the frequent occurrence of bilateral stenosis and the progressive nature of the diseases have strengthened the movement for arterioplasty in order to conserve tissue. Among 383 patients collated from the literature[26] prior to 1962, the ratio of nephrectomy to arterioplasty was approximately 2 to 1. In our personal series there were 72 primary nephrectomies, 12 partial nephrectomies, and 168 angioplasties. Twenty-two secondary nephrectomies were required after unsuccessful arterioplasty.

In 16 of our patients, bilateral reconstructive procedures were done at one stage, and 8 were performed at separate stages some months or years apart. In other cases of bilateral disease, the stenosis on the unoperated side was not considered of significant magnitude to justify intervention.

SURGERY OF RENAL ARTERY ANEURYSMS

Simple aneurysms of the renal artery are of two types: *arteriosclerotic* and *mural dysplastic*. Aneurysms may also be classified as *true* and *false;* these have been described earlier in this chapter. Miscellaneous classifications include the congenital, mycotic, and traumatic aneurysms. They may be soft and thin-walled or calcified, and they may be single or multiple. Commonly, arteriosclerotic aneurysms and aneurysms associated with fibromuscular arterial dysplasias occur at the branching of the renal artery where there is weakness of the vessel wall. However, true congenital aneurysms may occur anywhere in the renal arterial tree (Fig. 12–10).

Intrarenal aneurysms of large size (e.g., congenital or vascular malformations) usually necessitate nephrectomy or, less frequently, partial nephrectomy. When a large aneurysm is calcified and a major portion of the kidney has undergone infarction, nephrectomy is often the only possible treatment (Fig. 12–14). The treatment of extrarenal single or double aneurysms is excision of the aneurysm and primary arteriorrhaphy. Occasionally, it may be necessary to insert a patch of vein or synthetic material at the area of excision (Fig. 12–15). In some cases it may be necessary to excise an aneurysm and to perform one or more anastomoses of the afferent and efferent vessels. Figure 12–16 illustrates two types of surgical correction of aneurysms in a patient with bilateral large aneurysms without hypertension. The af-

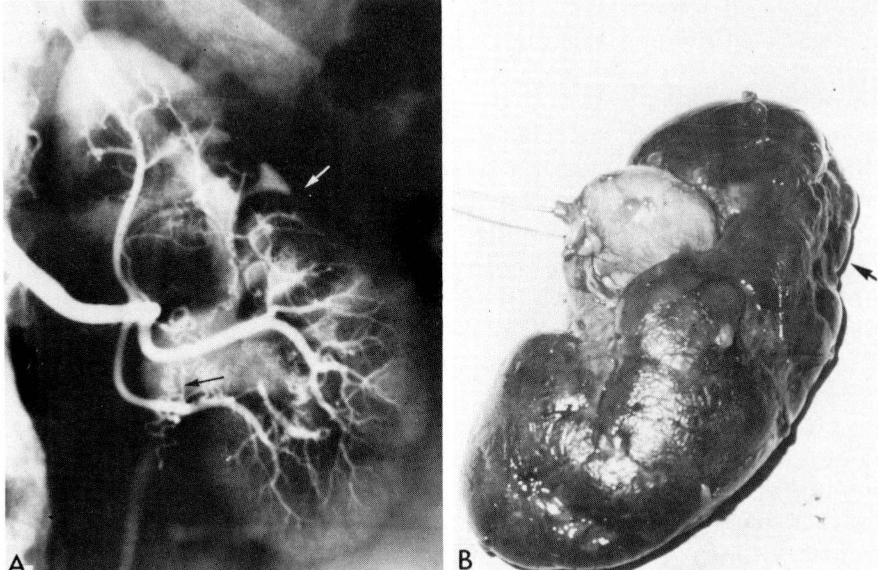

Figure 12–14. A, Left selective arteriogram showing clotted aneurysm represented by filling defect distal to the branching of the main renal artery, segmental atrophy of the renal cortex, and abundant collateral circulation to the ischemic renal segment. B, Surgical specimen showing aneurysm and atrophic cortex of the kidney.

ferent and efferent vessels entered and left the aneurysmal sac of the right kidney at its base, allowing excision of the aneurysm and arteriorrhaphy. On the left side, because the vessels entered and left the midportion of the aneurysm, and because the aneurysm was calcified, primary aneurysmorrhaphy was not possible; therefore, the aneurysm was resected, and both an end-to-end anastomosis and an end-to-side anastomosis were done. The preoperative arteriogram is shown in Figure 12–10; the postoperative arteriogram is seen in Figure 12–16C.

Modern preservation techniques have allowed ex-situ repair of renal arterial branches in association with correction of renal artery aneurysms. Microsurgical or magnification techniques are practical and following repair the kidney is transplanted heterotopically to the ipsilateral iliac fossa or the contralateral iliac fossa, according to the usual arterial transplantation techniques. The ureter need not be divided and the "bench" surgery can be done on towels spread on the patient's abdomen provided that kidney preservation is done by initial perfusion and cooling.[47, 48, 49]

Small arteriovenous communications often require no treatment, but if there is major shunting resulting in systemic cardiovascular effects, correction of the fistula is indicated. This may be done by

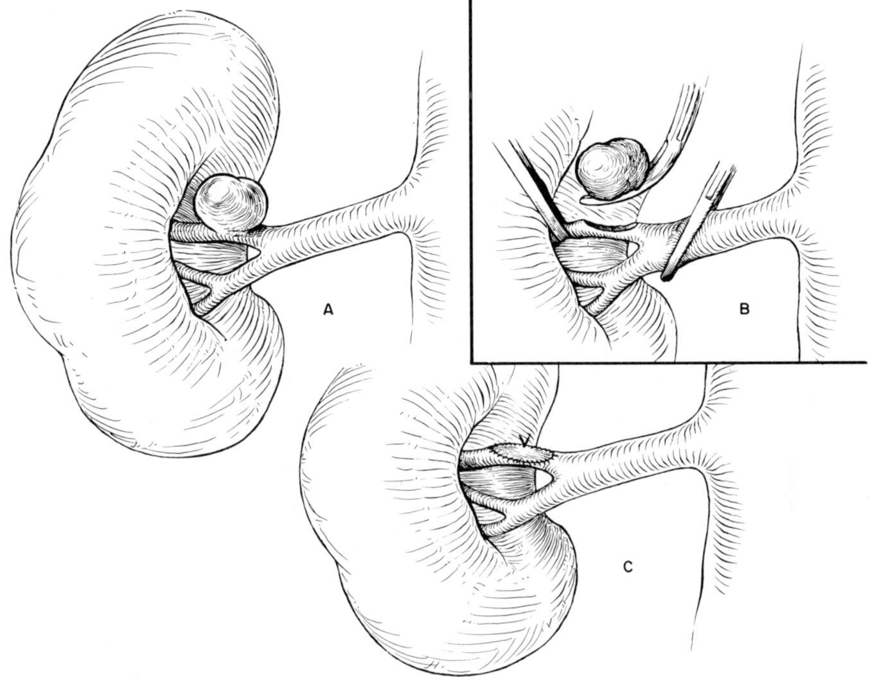

Figure 12–15. Method of excising renal artery aneurysm with placement of a gusset of vein or synthetic material.

ligating the afferent artery to the aneurysm and excising that portion of the kidney containing the fistula. Large arteriovenous communications, or those associated with renal cell carcinoma, are customarily handled by nephrectomy.

Formerly, when mass ligatures were placed about the renal pedicle in the performance of nephrectomy, major arteriovenous fistulas were not uncommon. The treatment of this condition usually required separating the two vessels and performing individual ligation of the artery and vein.

Surgical Exposure of the Renal Vessels

The customary approach to the renal vessels is through an anterior abdominal incision, and, although we have employed extraperitoneal approaches, the transperitoneal access is favored. With the patient in the supine position, the abdomen is opened either by a midline paramedian incision extending from the xiphoid to the midlower abdomen, or by a transverse incision in the upper abdomen, cutting both rectus muscles and the external and internal oblique

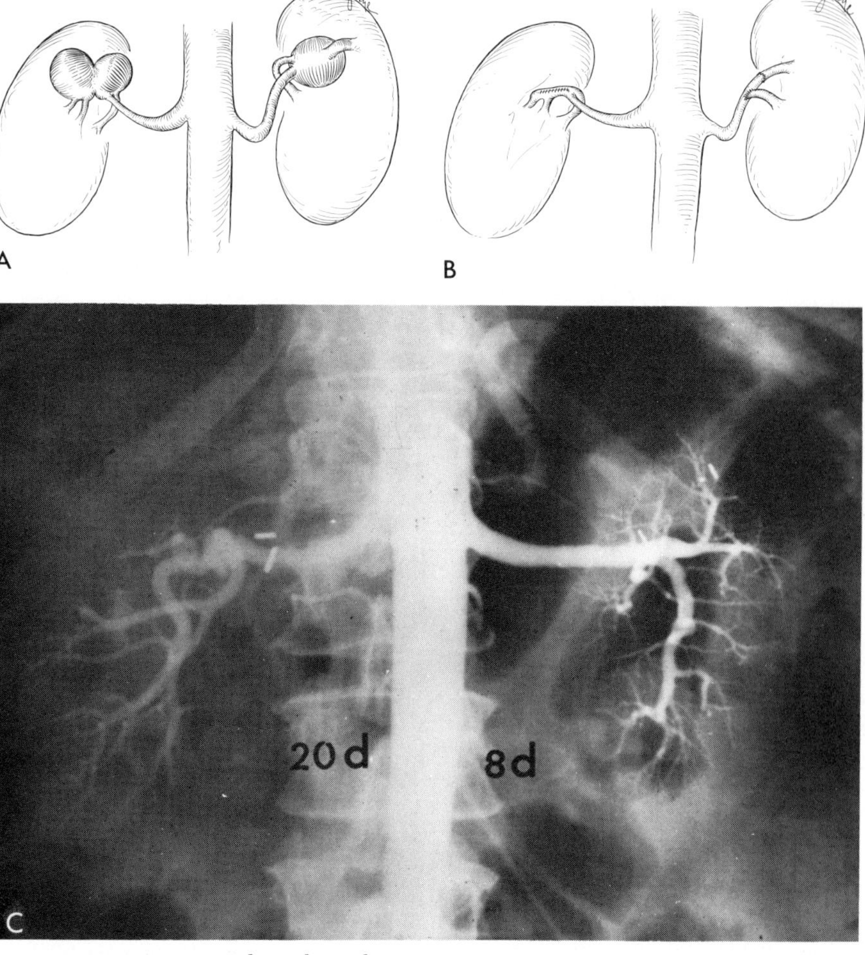

Figure 12–16.   *A,* Bilateral renal artery aneurysms seen in Figure 12–10 (arteriogram). *B,* Methods of treating aneurysm by excision and aneurysmorrhaphy (right) and excision and reanastomosis of the branches (left). *C,* Postoperative arteriogram showing excision of aneurysms and repair.

muscles on the side of the intended repair. For obese or muscular patients, the thoracoabdominal approach provides the best exposure. There are two good approaches to the renal vessels, either by reflection of the right or left colon and hepatic or splenic flexures, respectively, or by duodenal mobilization. In the first method the peritoneum is incised along the paracolic reflection. On the right side, the incision is continued through the hepatocolic ligaments, and the duodenum is mobilized by Kocher's maneuver after incising the peritoneum along the lateral border of the duodenum. If the cecum is not sufficiently free to be retracted, it is also mobilized. The right colon is retracted, together with the duodenum, to the left, thus exposing the vena cava. Usually, the right gonadal vein is ligated and divided at its entry into the vena cava. On the left side, the splenic flexure is mobilized by incising the lienocolic ligament. Occasionally, it may be necessary to enter the avascular space behind the spleen. Another approach to the left renal vessels is provided by making an incision in the left mesocolon and by retracting the inferior mesenteric vein laterally or by dividing the inferior mesenteric vein.

The most direct approach to the aorta, vena cava, and proximal portions of the renal vessels is afforded by mobilizing the duodenum upward, as shown in Figure 12–17. The small bowel is eviscerated or packed in a Lahey bag, and the transverse colon is lifted upward. The peritoneal reflection along the inferior border of the ascending portion of the duodenum is incised, and the duodenum is rotated upward. This will open the retroperitoneal area and give direct exposure to the great vessels.

The key structures in gaining access to the right renal artery are the vena cava and the left renal vein crossing over the aorta and lying anterior to the right and left renal arteries. The vena cava

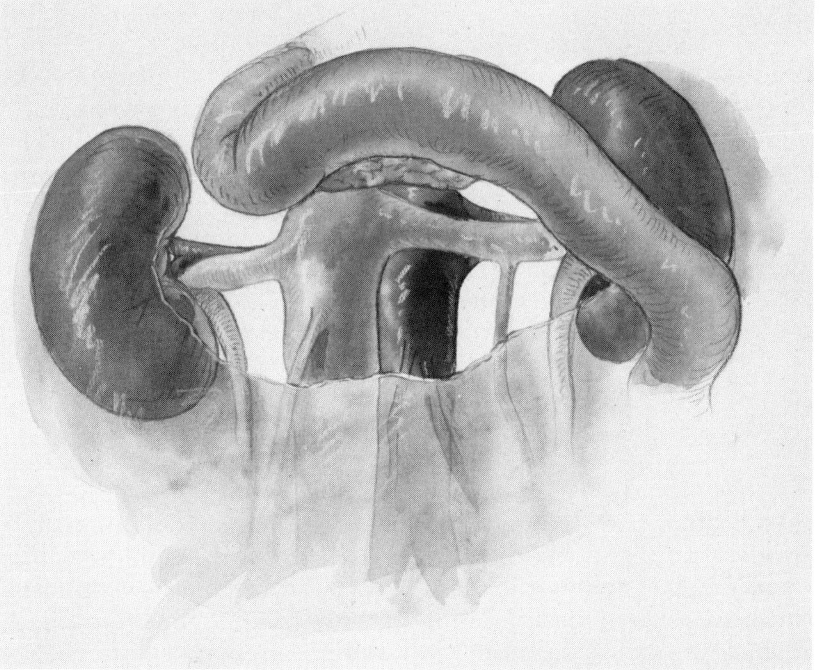

Figure 12–17. Mobilization of the ascending portion of the duodenum to provide exposure to the aorta, vena cava, and renal vessels.

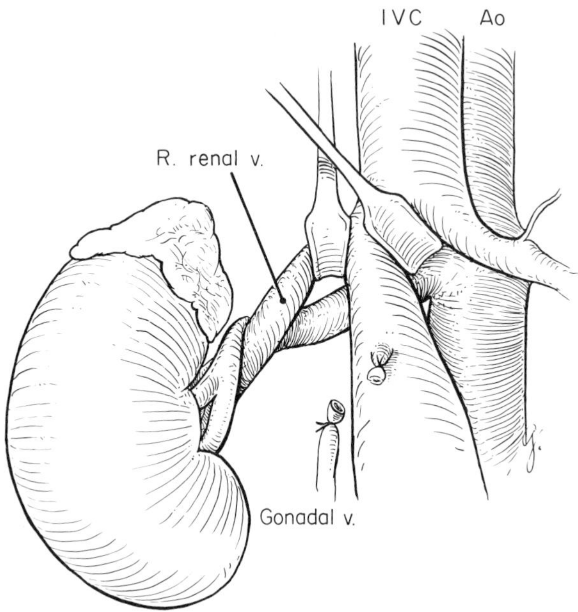

Figure 12–18. Exposure of the right renal artery after dividing the right gonadal vein, mobilizing the vena cava and left renal vein, and retracting the vena cava and right renal vein.

should be mobilized, and it is particularly useful to place a vein retractor at the angle between the left renal vein and the vena cava and to elevate this juncture superiorly and to the right (Fig. 12–18). On the left side, it is important to divide the gonadal vein and adrenal veins. This will allow upward or downward mobilization and retraction of the left renal vein and permit exposure of the proximal portions of the renal arteries (Fig. 12–19). The renal vessels are encircled with plastic tapes which are non-abrasive and which aid in subsequent dissection and in the performance of flow and pressure studies.

NEPHRECTOMY

Indications for nephrectomy are: 1. unilateral renal infarction or nonfunction, 2. multiple branch lesions, 3. severe unilateral parenchymal disease, with or without associated renal artery stenosis, 4. unsuccessful previous arterioplasty or partial nephrectomy, and 5. poor flow through a repaired vessel after vascular repair. The technique of nephrectomy is found in standard textbooks.

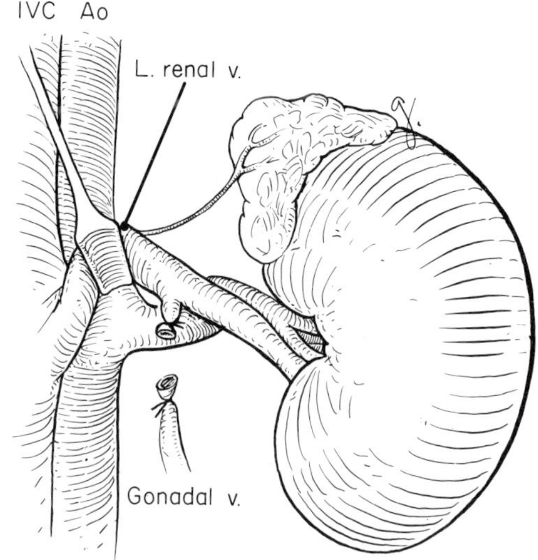

Figure 12–19. Exposure of the left renal artery after division of the left gonadal vein and upward retraction of the left renal vein.

PARTIAL NEPHRECTOMY

The indications for partial nephrectomy are relatively uncommon. Patients with branch lesions producing segmental ischemia may be treated either with arteriotomy and dilatation or by partial nephrectomy. The removal of the lower pole of the kidney is perhaps the most commonly indicated type of partial nephrectomy, but mid-segmental renal resection is also possible and is certainly indicated wherever the branch lesion is well defined. In most series the results of partial nephrectomy in curing hypertension are not as good as are the results from arterioplasty or nephrectomy. Since the diagnostic and predictive tests are less reliable when only a small segment of the kidney is ischemic, the cause and effect relationship between the segmental lesion and the hypertension is less clear than in other cases. In addition, incomplete removal of all ischemic tissue is difficult to achieve. Injection of the branch with indigo carmine or methylene blue is useful to define the zone of ischemia. When the branch is occluded or too small to inject, the main renal artery can be injected, and the zone that is *not* discolored may be resected. The kidney generally has fairly well-defined segmental arterial distributions (Fig. 12–20). These are the upper middle segment and lower middle segment, the lower pole, the upper pole, and the posterior mid-segment. There is usually a major branch to the posterior surface of the kidney arising just proximal, at, or just distal to the two major branches supplying the anterior half of the kidney.

The technique of partial nephrectomy is as follows: the renal ar-

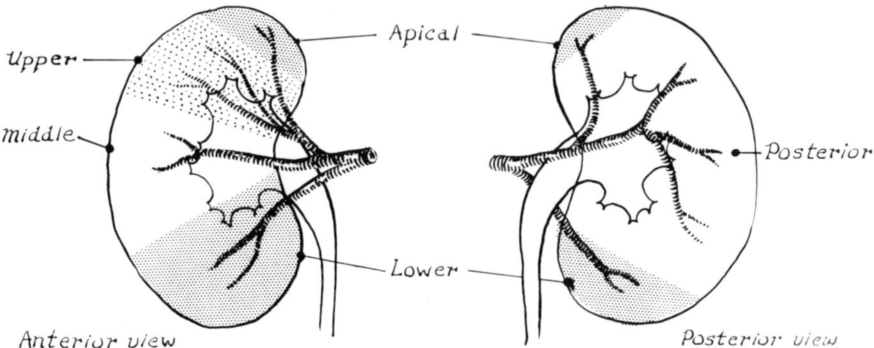

Figure 12–20.   Segmental renal blood supply.

tery is dissected and a tape is placed about it. Tapes then are placed about the successive branches until the involved branch is identified. After injection of indigo, the branch is ligated, which further defines the zone of ischemia by rendering that portion of the kidney soft. The main renal artery is then temporarily occluded with an arterial clamp, Rumel tourniquet, or Schwartz clip. The capsule over the involved segment is incised and peeled back, and the ischemic portion of the kidney is sharply excised. The excision will often include several pyramids. Transected calyces and infundibula are closed with continuous 5–0 chromic catgut sutures. Transected arteries and veins are secured with mattress or figure-8 sutures of 4–0 chromic catgut. Nonabsorabable suture material is not used in the kidney because, if extruded or accidentally exposed to urine, urinary calculi will form on it. After excision of the involved segment, the clamp of the main artery is released and additional sutures are taken as needed to complete hemostasis. The capsule is then folded back over the area and closed with continuous 4–0 chromic catgut suture.

ENDARTERECTOMY

Thrombendarterectomy is applicable in patients with localized atheromatous stenosis of the renal artery. In most series, 55 to 65 per cent of stenosing lesions are caused by atheromatous plaques. Since these usually are located at the ostia or in the proximal portions of the renal arteries, they may be approached by renal, aortic, or aortorenal arteriotomy. Care must be exercised in the dissection to remove the plaque entirely, since residual roughened portions may invite subsequent dissection. Caution should also be taken to prevent the escape of particles of atheromatous material, which can cause atheroembolism and segmental renal infarcts.

The method that has been commonly employed consists of placing an exclusion clamp about the aortorenal juncture (Fig. 12–21) and making a longitudinal arteriotomy on the anterior wall of the renal artery, extending into the aorta if necessary. An ear curet or Cannon dissector is used to separate the plaque from the wall, after which the artery is thoroughly irrigated with a weak solution of heparinized saline (50 mg/500 ml). The arteriotomy is closed with continuous 5–0 or 6–0 sutures of silk or Teflon-coated Dacron, but when the lumen appears inadequate, or when there is a tendency for

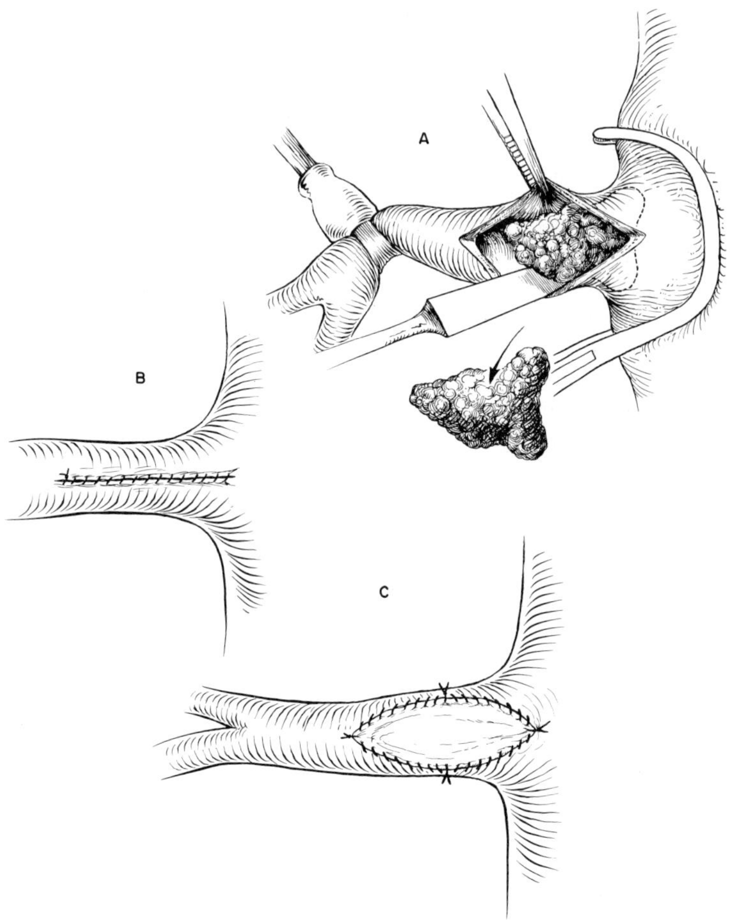

Figure 12–21. Technique of right renal endarterectomy with primary closure *(B)* or with patch *(C)*.

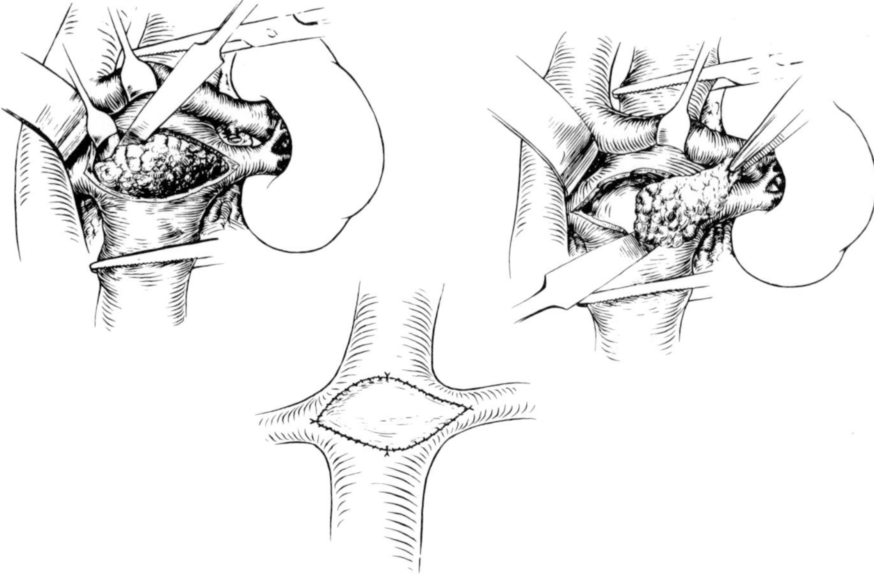

Figure 12–22. Technique of bilateral aortorenal endarterectomy through a transverse aortotomy.

the thin-walled vessel to buckle, a gusset of vein, anterior rectus sheath, or Dacron is used.

Bilateral endarterectomy is indicated when there is significant stenosis of both renal arteries. This requires aortic cross clamping above and below the renal arteries, hence it is somewhat more difficult than unilateral endarterectomy. A transverse or longitudinal aortotomy is made, and atheromas are removed from within the aorta by circumcising the orifice and dissecting the plaques distalward. The other method commonly employed is a transverse aortotomy, extending the incision into the renal arteries and performing a renal endarterectomy together with removal of the aortic plaques (Fig. 12–22). The vessels may be sutured primarily, or a gusset of Dacron, fascia or saphenous vein may be used.

Endarterectomy is, of course, easier in young patients who have good residual vessel walls. When cross-clamping the aorta, the usual precautions should be taken by giving the patient mannitol, administering systemic heparin, and releasing the aortic clamps slowly.

RESECTION AND REANASTOMOSIS

Resection of the diseased portion of the renal artery with reanastomosis is ideal for selected cases in which the disease is well defined. However, the arteriogram frequently fails to indicate the true extent of the disease, and longer segments than may be seen are often involved. In such cases reanastomosis may be difficult and sometimes predisposes to the redevelopment of stenosis at the area of anastomosis. Where resection of the diseased vessel requires an insertion graft, it is often easier to perform an aortorenal bypass, since the proximal anastomosis can be done at a lower level on the aorta, where exposure is better.

BYPASS GRAFTS

The bypass graft is the most popular reconstructive operation because it is technically the simplest and because extensive involvements of the renal artery frequently can best be handled in this way. Autologous vein grafts are popular among vascular surgeons because of their experience with long-term patency in other areas. However, certain features of aortorenal bypasses are unique. A successful bypass has an excellent chance of remaining patent because of the short length of the graft, its fixation, and high flow rates, conditions that generally do not apply to other areas in which the bypass is employed.

Enthusiasm for the use of synthetic grafts has waned among vascular surgeons because of thrombotic closures over intermediate and long-range observations. However, in our view, the Dacron microweave graft has been extremely successful, and we have witnessed no early or even late occlusions in the absence of obvious technical fault or poor case selection. Their ready availability in a variety of sizes and lengths, their ease of handling, and the high patency rates in our hands have been impressive.[28] Reported occlusions with Dacron grafts have largely been based on experience in replacement of peripheral vessels where long distances have been bridged.

Formerly, we employed 6-mm. tubes of microweave Dacron, but currently we employ the external veloured Dacron grafts exclusively. Observations regarding the fate of Dacron grafts used elsewhere in the arterial tree have demonstrated, however, that the early graft lining is in fact thrombogenic and the ultimate graft lining is composed of compacted fibrin rather than endothelium.[4] Recent evidence has accumulated which advocates the "trellis" concept of synthetic graft construction.[50] This concept evolved when it was noted that if the external surface of a porous synthetic graft is filamentous rather than smooth, the graft becomes firmly encapsulated and the lining is ultimately cellular. This cellular lining purportedly occurs via mesenchymal penetration through the interstices of the graft or "fallout seeding" from the blood stream.[51]

The principle of the "veloured" graft construction asserts that when the interstices of a porous graft are webbed by synthetic filaments (velour), mesenchymal ingrowth may occur rapidly and completely.[50] This concept is based upon the observation that fibroblasts will migrate along synthetic filaments in tissue culture.[34] Thus, it is conceivable that cellular penetration of a porous graft occurs when the interstices are bridged by a three-dimensional "trellis" of such synthetic monofilaments. This is undoubtedly the mechanism of encapsulation of the graft. The origin of the cellular lining of the velour graft is considerably more obscure. Sauvage suggests that the "organization of thrombus deposit on the inner wall was facilitated by the ingrowth."[51]

Pre-clotting of the grafts is not necessary, and synthetic suture material such as Teflon-coated Dacron should be used to anastomose synthetic grafts to obviate deterioration. Figure 12–23 illustrates the technique of placement of bypass grafts of Dacron. Customarily, we place the graft on the renal side, using continuous or interrupted

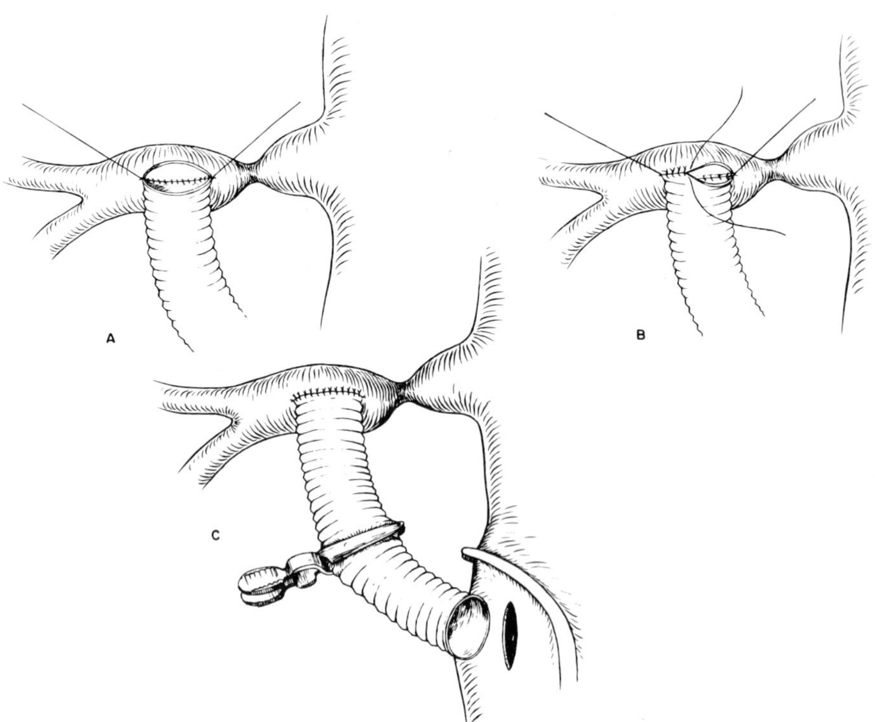

Figure 12–23.   Technique of placement of the aortorenal bypass graft (Dacron).

sutures of 5–0 or 6–0 synthetic material. The renal artery is then allowed to perfuse after removing the clamp on the proximal part of the vessel. Subsequently, the graft is anastomosed to the side of the aorta between the renal artery take-off and the inferior mesenteric artery. In general, we prefer end-to-side anastomosis of the graft to the renal artery, since this tends to fix the graft in position and prevents kinking.

One of the chief advantages of use of synthetic tubes over autologous vessel grafts is that fibroplasias apparently do not affect the synthetic prosthesis, but may extend into the autologous vessel graft and cause restenosis (Fig. 12–24. 4–0 suture material and K-type needles with cutting point facilitate the suturing of Dacron grafts. Although we have advocated retrocaval placement of right-sided grafts, this probably is not necessary. The following principles apply to the use of synthetic grafts and are recommended: 1) use only Dacron (preferably of external velour type); 2) avoid excessive lengths and kinking; 3) avoid septum formation at anastomotic areas by careful suturing; 4) use a graft the diameter of which is between 1½ and 2 times that of the renal artery for end-to-side anastomosis; and 5) use anticoagulants intraoperatively and antibiotics prophylactically during the postoperative period.

Since 1967 we have employed the hypogastric artery as a free bypass autograft in 35 patients. The hypogastric artery was too short to bridge the distance in an additional patient in whom a synthetic graft was then used. The hypogastric artery should be normal if it is being considered as an autologous bypass; thus, preoperative aortograms should include the iliac vessels. When normal, the hypogastric artery is ideally suited to serve as a bypass, since it is one of the large arteries that can be sacrificed with little risk. Most patients requiring bypass grafts are young individuals with fibroplasia, and the coexistence of the disease in the hypogastric arteries in such patients appears to be infrequent. The viscoelastic properties of the hypogastric artery duplicate those of the normal renal artery, and constrictions at anastomotic sites might be expected to be infrequent.[30] It is appealing to substitute an artery for an artery, and all of the patients in whom we have employed the hypogastric artery as a bypass have had excellent clinical and technical results, with the exception of the one (cited above) in whom the graft was placed into a diseased segment of the renal artery, with subsequent stenosis at the site of anastomosis.

The long-term fate of autologous hypogastric artery grafts is not known, but we now have six- and seven-year arteriograms showing maintenance of patency. We prefer to use the hypogastric artery as an aortorenal insertion graft with an end-to-end anastomosis to the renal artery. We advise the use of interrupted sutures of 5–0 or 6–0

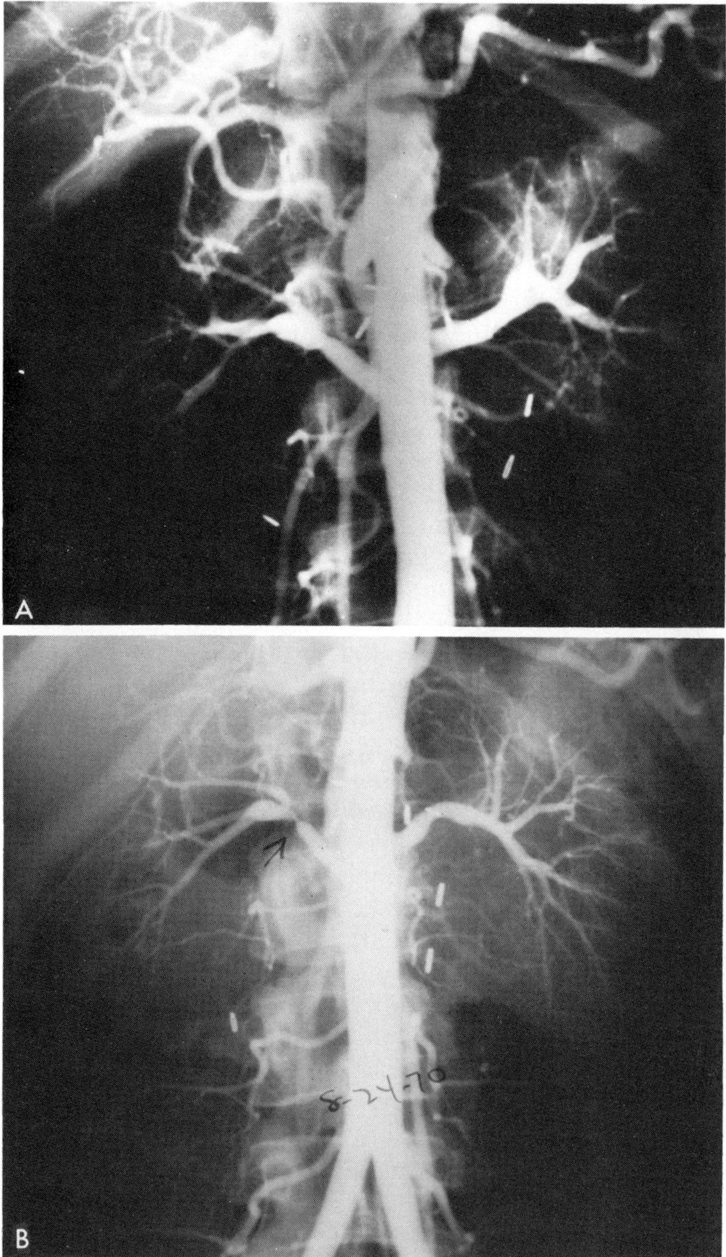

Figure 12-24. *A,* Early postoperative aortogram showing bilateral hypogastric artery interposition grafts. *B,* Aortogram of same patient six months later showing restenosis of the hypogastric artery bypass to the right renal artery, where the graft was sutured to the diseased renal artery. Patient underwent a subsequent revision.

polypropylene or silk, and frequently place all the sutures before tying them in order to allow for accurate placement and good visualization of both vessels during the performance of the anastomosis. Similar technique is used for suturing autologous saphenous veins. Interrupted suture technique is also used for the aortic anastomosis. In one case, in which the disease had extended into the proximal portion of the two primary branches, we employed the hypogastric artery with its anterior and posterior branches to provide an insertion graft from the aorta into the primary renal artery branches (Fig. 12–25). The chief disadvantage of the hypogastric artery bypass is the short length of the vessel; however, we have found that even a 1½ cm. segment serving as an interposition graft is better than direct renoaortic anastomosis.

There are still questions as to the comparative long-term patency rates among autologous vein, autologous artery, and synthetic grafts, and at least 10 additional years of observation will be necessary to allow a valid judgment of their respective values. Some recent evidence would seem to indicate that atherogenesis may occur more commonly in autologous vein grafts than in Dacron or autologous arterial grafts.[52]

SPLENORENAL ANASTOMOSIS

Use of the splenic artery as a bypass is one of the original operations devised to correct renal artery stenosis.[12] Unfortunately, the operation is more difficult than the free aortorenal bypass, and in addition, diseases of the right renal artery outnumber those of the left by at least four to one in our experience. In older patients, in whom left renal artery stenosis is somewhat more common, splenic artery disease is also more commonly encountered. Hence, the opportunities to borrow the splenic artery for renal revascularization are relatively few.

Customarily, the splenic artery is isolated by mobilizing the duodenum (Kocher's maneuver), dividing the inferior mesenteric vein, and following it cephalad to its entry into the splenic vein. The splenic artery is in juxtaposition to the splenic vein. There are numerous small branches of the splenic artery as it runs behind the pancreas, and these must be carefully ligated and divided. It is best to free the portion of the splenic artery that lies behind the pancreas and to avoid dissection too far laterally where branches to the spleen arise. Similarly, it is not necessary to dissect the splenic artery close to the aorta, and a segment only of 4 to 5 cm. need be freed to reach the left renal artery. The distal end of the splenic artery is ligated,

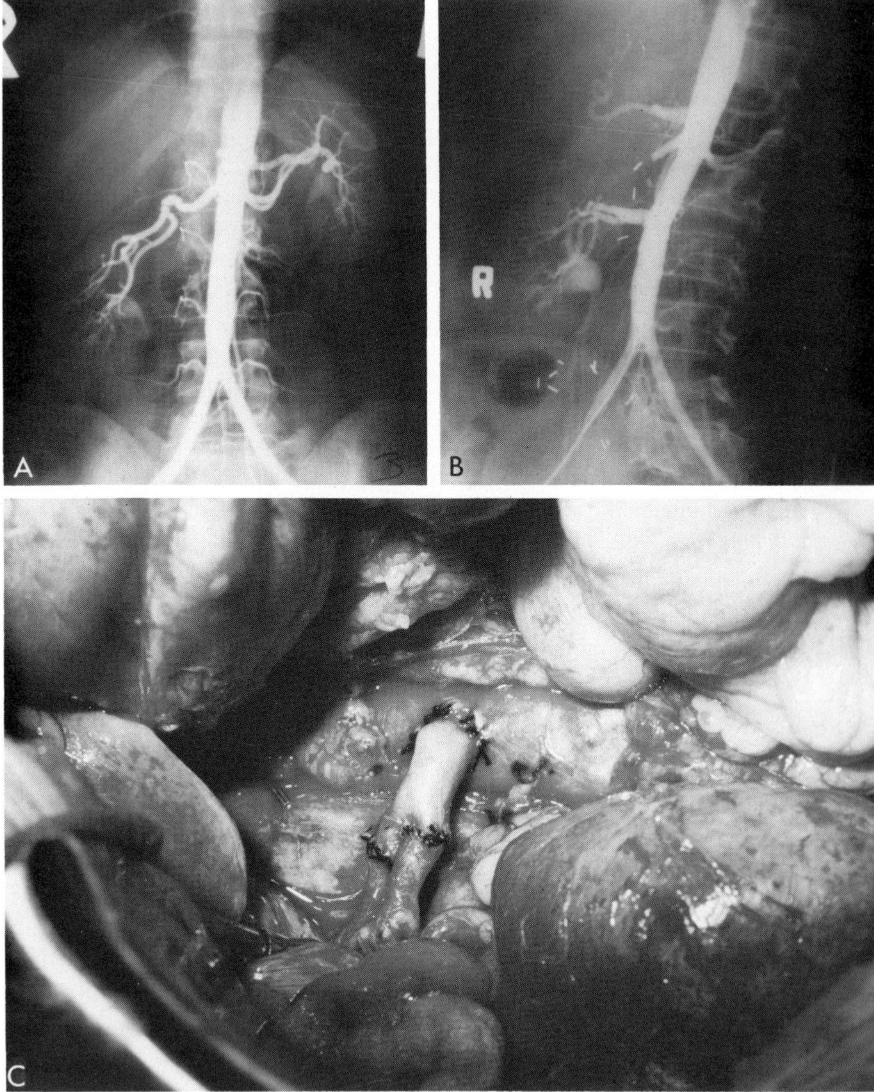

Figure 12–25. *A,* Aortogram showing fibroplasia of right renal artery extending into the primary branches. *B,* Aortogram one week following hypogastric interposition graft in which both major branches of the hypogastric artery were used to replace the two primary branches of the renal artery. *C,* Photograph of aortorenal bypass using hypogastric artery in pantaloon fashion.

and the proximal end is temporarily occluded. Following this, an end-to-end or elliptical end-to-side anastomosis is done (Fig. 12–26). The spleen need not be removed, since it received adequate blood supply from the short gastric vessels. Excellent access to the splenic and renal artery is possible through a left thoracoabdominal incision

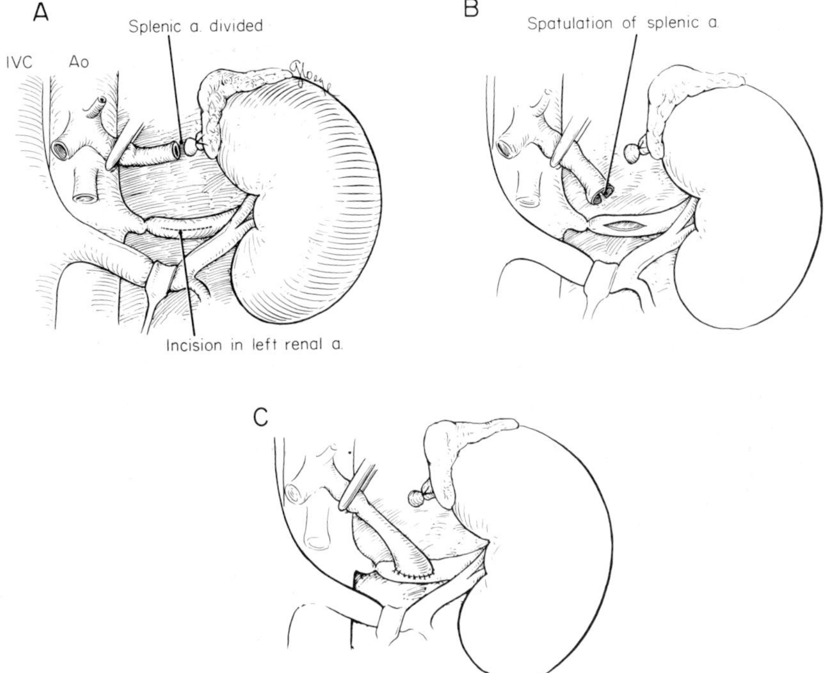

Figure 12–26. Technique of splenorenal end-to-side bypass.

in muscular or obese patients. In general, we have been pleased with the results of the splenorenal bypass, particularly in male patients. We are not as enthusiastic regarding splenorenal bypass in women and children since early thrombotic occlusion is more frequently encountered in these groups. Pancreatic injury, the chief danger of the procedure, must be carefully avoided. Figure 12–27 shows the postoperative appearance of a splenorenal anastomosis in a young man with subintimal fibroplasia of the left renal artery.

MISCELLANEOUS ARTERIOPLASTY

Endarterectomy, aortorenal bypass, splenorenal bypass, and resection of diseased segments with end-to-end reanastomosis are the more common types of repair in use for renal artery stenosis. Other procedures such as arterioplasty with a patch using fascia, vein wall, arterial wall, or Dacron have not proved to be of consistent value. Reimplantation of the renal artery into the aorta is not a popular procedure, for it is difficult to obtain a perfect anatomical result.

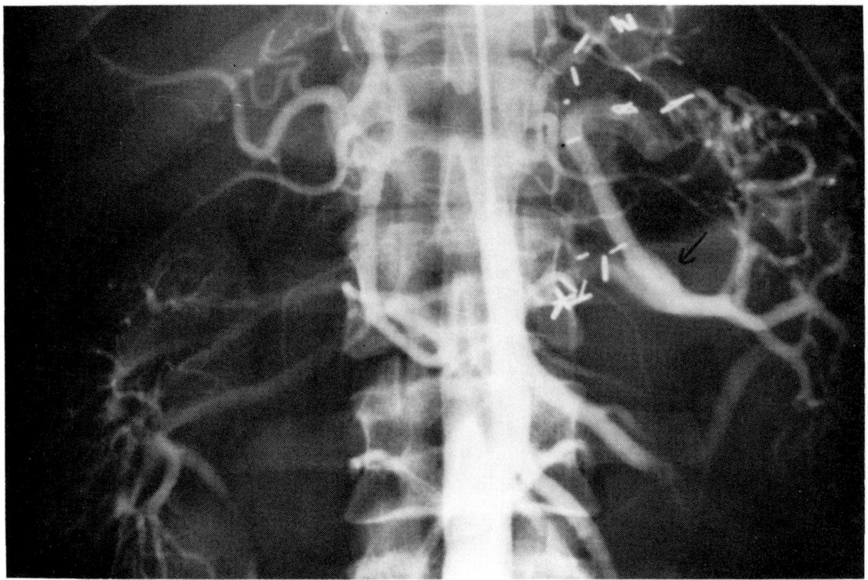

Figure 12–27.   Postoperative arteriogram showing end-to-side splenorenal anastomosis (arrow).

Renal autotransplantation has gained popularity since a number of reports have indicated good results.[25, 48] The chief advantage of autotransplantation is that the kidney can be moved to the iliac fossa, where anastomosis to the iliac vessels or hypogastric artery affords better exposure than with in situ repair of the vessels. Therefore, the operation is indicated when access to the upper abdominal aorta and proximal renal arteries is unusually difficult or when ex situ repair of the renal vessels or branches is necessary. In the latter case, the kidney can be lifted out of the wound after the renal artery and renal vein are divided, repair of branch disease can be done with initial perfusion and cooling of the kidney, according to the technique we have discussed,[44, 47] and the kidney can be placed in the iliac fossa on the ipsilateral side. No revision of the ureter is necessary, because the ureter can be left at its original length; the resulting redundancy does not constitute a urinary drainage problem (Fig. 12–28). We have performed autotransplantation in 11 patients, four of whom had solitary kidneys. In one patient a functional failure occurred because of poor perfusion of small vessels that were being fed entirely by collateral channels in the presence of total occlusion of the main renal artery.

Results of our experience in treatment of renal artery stenosis are shown in Table 12–1.

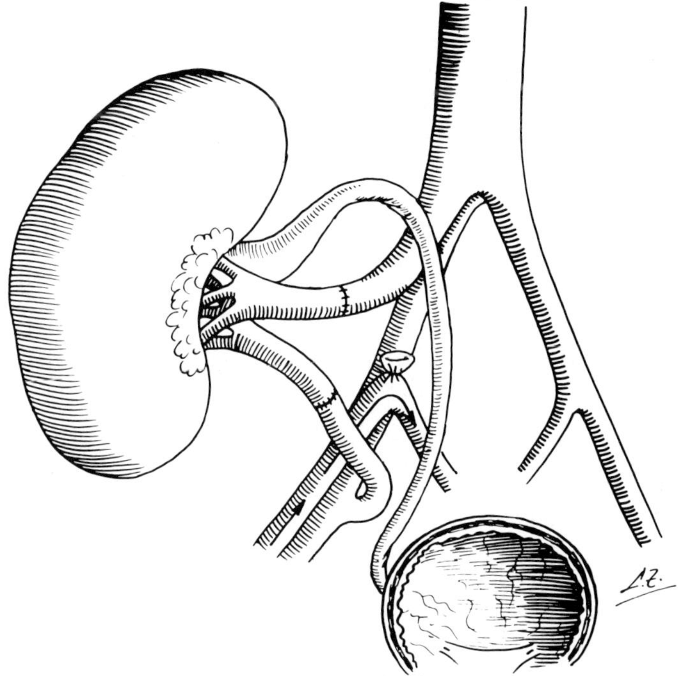

Figure 12–28.   Technique of renal autotransplantation for repair of renal artery stenosis.

RENAL ARTERY EMBOLISM

Renal artery embolism is not as common as other forms of major arterial disease, but Hoxie and Coggin[23] found 205 cases among 14,411 autopsies. Most patients with renal artery embolism have a history of rheumatic heart disease. The majority are a result of thrombi dislodged from a fibrillating atrium or from a valvular site. Renal artery embolism should be suspected when a patient with heart disease complains of flank pain, hematuria and or oliguria. Presumptive diagnosis is made by excretory urographic examination showing nonfunction, and a retrograde pyelogram showing normal pyelocalyceal architecture; definitive diagnosis is made by renal arteriogram.

Most of the cases of renal infarction reported in the literature have been treated by nephrectomy, but more aggressive approaches toward this condition are evidenced by the number of case reports of renal artery embolectomy appearing in the literature. Evidence is mounting to suggest that many cases of renal artery embolism can be treated expectantly with results that compare favorably to those obtained after embolectomy; i.e., the same number of kidneys will be functioning or functionless. This, however, is still a moot issue and will probably not be crystallized for another 10 years.

Surgical removal of renal artery emboli depends on the site of the infarct and, to some extent, on the duration. Emboli lodged in the main renal artery or in the primary branches may be satisfactorily removed, whereas emboli in small branches often may not. Although there are rare examples of successful late embolectomies, it is generally accepted that early intervention is mandatory; when unilateral anuria or oliguria have existed for longer than 48 hours, it is ex-

Table 12–1.   Surgical Results in Renovascular Hypertension Unilateral Procedures

	Procedures 293		Patients 273	
(106)	*Primary Nephrectomy* 72	*Secondary Nephrectomy* 22	*Partial Nephrectomy* 12	*Average %*
Cured	45 (62%)	12 (55%)	6 (50%)	(56%)
Improved	23 (32%)	8 (36%)	3 (25%)	(31%)
Failed	4 (6%)	2 (9%)	3 (25%)	(13%)
		Bypass Procedures		
(108)	Synthetic 54	Vein 19	Hypogastric artery 35	
Cured	33 (61%)	8 (42%)	33 (94%)	
Improved	11 (20%)	4 (21%)	1 (3%)	
Failed	10 (19%) (4 deaths)	7 (37%)	1 (3%)	
Graft closure (Partial or complete)	6 (of the 10 failures) 4* 1**	4 (3)*	1*	
(47)	Endarterectomy 23	Resection and Anastomosis 10	Splenorenal Anastomosis 14	
Cured	9 (39%)	5 (50%)	7 (50%)	
Improved	6 (26%)	4 (40%)	5 (36%)	
Failed	8 (35%)	1 (10%)	2 (14%)	
Thrombosis	1 (of the 8 failures)	2	2	
		Miscellaneous		
(32)	Arteriolysis 5	Reimplantations 2	Patch-plasty 3	Autotransplantation 9/11 cured · Aneurysmorrhaphy 11

*Nephrectomy performed after unsuccessful repair.
**Secondary repair.

tremely unlikely to obtain late good functional recovery. Systemic anticoagulant therapy is advisable with or without operation to prevent subsequent formation of emboli. Other conservative measures, such as selective catheterization of the renal artery with infusion of heparin or fibrinolysin, are of questionable value at this time.

RENAL ARTERY THROMBOSIS FOLLOWING BLUNT TRAUMA

Renal artery thrombosis following blunt trauma is a rare condition, and only approximately 15 cases have been reported.[20] However, its true incidence is probably greater than indicated from collated reports, since many patients are seen with atrophic kidneys which probably represent old unrecognized renal artery injury and thrombosis caused by blunt abdominal trauma sustained in previous years.

The mechanism of injury in renal artery thrombosis following blunt trauma has been postulated by Collins and Jacobs.[9] They believe that a sudden force may set the mobile kidney into motion and stretch its vascular pedicle. This ruptures the arterial intima, the least elastic component of the artery, and allows subintimal dissection and hematoma formation. Subintimal hematomas may cause partial or total occlusion of the artery. Prompt recognition is important if repair is to be done before onset of ischemic injury to the kidney. Partial occlusion must not be mistaken for spasm on arteriogram, for delay in diagnosis decreases the chances of success following arterial reconstruction. Repair is feasible even with total occlusion of the renal artery, as the distal renal artery is usually patent.

In all cases, exploration should be performed through a transabdominal approach in an effort to restore vascular continuity and preserve renal function. Because of the sensitivity of the kidney to anoxia, immediate operation is imperative. When hematoma formation is extensive, a bypass graft from aorta to distal renal artery may be possible. When the arterial injury is localized, thrombectomy and angioplasty may be possible.[55] If the renal parenchyma is necrotic, or if vascular reconstruction is impossible, a nephrectomy should be performed, provided the other kidney is normal.

CONCLUSION

The current status of diagnosis and treatment of renovascular hypertension and related renal vascular problems has been described. Despite great strides that have been made in management of these clinical problems, there are many areas left to be explored and clarified. Of real urgency is the need for knowledge of the evolution of stenosing diseases and of methods to prevent the occurrence and progression of renovascular lesions. A gratifying degree of diagnostic and therapeutic expertise has been achieved as a result of the combined efforts of internists, physiologists, urologists, and vascular surgeons.

REFERENCES

1. Barajas, L., Lupu, A., Kaufman, J. J., Latta, H., and Maxwell, M. H.: The prognostic value of the renal biopsy in unilateral renovascular hypertension. Nephron 4:231, 1967.
2. Barker, N. W., and Walters, W.: Hypertension associated with unilateral atrophic pyelonephritis: Treatment by nephrectomy. Proc. Mayo Clin. 13:118, 1938.
3. Belzer, F. O., Keaveny, T. V., Reed, T. W., and Pryor, J. P.: A new method of renal artery reconstruction. Surgery 68:619, 1970.
4. Berger, K. E., Sauvage, L. R., Rao, A. M., and Wood, S. J.: Healing of arterial prosthesis in man: Its incompleteness. Ann. Surg. 175:118, 1972.
5. Boyd, C. H., and Lewis, L. G.: Nephrectomy for arterial hypertension. J. Urol. 39:627, 1938.
6. Butler, A. M.: Chronic pyelonephritis and arterial hypertension. J. Clin. Invest. 16:889, 1937.
7. Callahan, W. P., and Schiltz, F. H.: Aneurysm of the renal artery. Surg. Gynec. Obstet. 43:724, 1926.
8. Chapman, W. H., O'Brien, D. J., McRoberts, J. W., and Ansell, J. S.: Renin assays in hypertension: Use of peripheral renin as screening test. J. Urol. 104:362, 1970.
9. Collins, H. A., and Jacobs, J. K.: Acute arterial injuries due to blunt trauma. J. Bone Joint Surg. 43-A:195, 1961.
10. Cummings, K. B., Lecky, J. W., and Kaufman, J. J.: Renal artery aneurysms and hypertension. J. Urol. 109:144–148, Feb. 1973.
11. DeCamp, P. T., and Birchall, R.: Recognition and treatment of renal arterial stenosis associated with hypertension. Surgery 43:134, 1958.
12. DeCamp, P. T., Snyder, C. H., and Bost, R. B.: Severe hypertension due to congenital stenosis of artery to solitary kidney: Correction by splenorenal anastomosis. Arch. Surg. 75:1023, 1957.
13. Del Greco, F., Simon, N. N., Goodman, S., and Roguska, J.: Plasma renin activity in primary and secondary hypertension. Medicine 46:475, 1967.
14. Dos Santos, J. S.: Note sur la desobuction des anciennes thromboses artérielles. Presse Méd. 57:544, 1949.
15. Ellis, F. M., Helden, R. A., and Hines, E. A.: Aneurysm of the abdominal aorta involving the right renal artery. Ann. Surg. 142:992, 1955.
16. Foster, J. H., and Dean, R. H.: Criteria for the diagnosis of renovascular hypertension. Surgery 74:926, 1973.
17. Freeman, G., and Hartely, G.: Hypertension in a patient with solitary ischemic kidney. J.A.M.A. 111:1159, 1938.
18. Freeman, N. E., Leeds, F. H., Elliott, W. G., and Roland, S. I.: Thrombendarterectomy for hypertension due to renal artery occlusion. J.A.M.A. 156:1077, 1954.
19. Goldblatt, H., Lynch, J., Hanzal, R. F., and Sommerville, W. W.: Studies on experimental hypertension. J. Exp. Med. 59:347, 1934.
20. Grablowsky, O. M., Weichert, R. F. III, Goff, J. B., and Schlegel, J. U.: Renal artery thrombosis following blunt trauma: Report of four cases. Surgery 67:895, 1970.

21. Harrison, E. G., Jr., and McCormack, L. J.: Pathologic classification of renal arterial disease in renovascular hypertension. Proc. Mayo Clin. 46:161, 1971.

22. Harrow, B. R., and Sloane, J. A.: Aneurysm of renal artery: Report of five cases. J. Urol. 81:35, 1959.

23. Hoxie, H. J., and Coggin, C. B.: Renal infarction: Statistical studies of 205 cases and detailed report of an unusual case. Arch. Intern. Med. 65:587, 1940.

24. Hurwitt, E. S., Seidenberg, B., Haimovici, H., and Abelson, D. S.: Splenorenal arterial anastomosis. Circulation 4:532, 1956.

25. Kaufman, J. J., Alferez, C., and Vela-Navarette, R.: Autotransplantation of a solitary functioning kidney for renovascular hypertension. J. Urol. 102:146, 1969.

26. Kaufman, J. J., Lupu, A. N., and Maxwell, M. H.: Renovascular hypertension: Clinical characteristics, diagnosis and treatment. Cardiovasc. Clin. 1:79, 1969.

27. Kaufman, J. J., and Hughes, D. L.: Upright aortography: An aid to the study of renal artery stenosis. Radiology 79:1017, 1962.

28. Kaufman, J. J., and Moloney, P. J.: Results of synthetic bypass grafts in the treatment of renal artery stenosis. J. Urol. 98:140, 1967.

29. Kaufman, J. J., Lupu, A. N., Franklin, S., and Maxwell, M. H.: Diagnostic and predictive value of renal vein renin activity in renovascular hypertension. J. Urol. 103:702, 1970.

30. Kaufman, J. J., and Lupu, A. N.: Treatment of renal artery stenosis using hypogastric artery autografts. J. Urol. 106:9, 1971.

31. Kaufman, J. J., Schanche, A. F., and Maxwell, M. H.: Excretory urography in the diagnosis of renovascular hypertension: Methods of enhancing its value. J. Urol. 89:498, 1963.

32. Leadbetter, W. F., and Burkland, C. E.: Hypertension in unilateral renal disease. J. Urol. 39:611, 1938.

33. Lupu, A., Kaufman, J. J., and Maxwell, M. H.: Renal artery constriction: Physiological determinants of pressure gradients. Ann. Surg. 167:246, 1968.

34. Mansfield, P. B.: Tissue culture endothelium for vascular prostheses. Presented at a Meeting of the American College of Chest Physicians, Chicago, Illinois, October, 1969.

35. Marshall, V. F., Whitesell, J., McGovern, J. H., and Miscall, B. G.: The practicality of renal autotransplantation in humans. J.A.M.A. 196:1154, 1966.

36. Mathe, C. P.: Aneurysm of the renal artery: Report of five cases, one treated by resection of aneurysmal sac without sacrificing the kidney. J. Urol. 60:543, 1948.

37. Maxwell, M. H., and Lupu, A. N.: Excretory urography in renal arterial hypertension. J. Urol. 100:395, 1968.

38. Maxwell, M. H. Lupu, A. N., and Taplin, G. V.: Radioisotope renogram in renal arterial hypertension. J. Urol. 100:376, 1968.

39. McCormack, L. J., Poutasse, E. F., Meaney, T. F., et al.: A pathologic-arteriographic correlation of renal arterial disease. Am. Heart J. 72:188, 1966.

40. Meaney, T. F., Dustan, H. P., and McCormack, L. J.: Natural history of renal arterial disease. Radiology 91:881, 1968.

41. Moran, J. M.: Blood flowmeters. New Eng. J. Med. 276:225, 1967.

42. Morris, G. C., Jr., DeBakey, M. E., Crawford, E. S., Cooley, D. E., and Zanger, L. C. C.: Late results of surgical treatment for renovascular hypertension. Surg. Gynec. Obstet. 122:1255, 1966.

43. Nanninga, J. B., Deam, M., Holland, J. M., and Grayhack, J. T.: Adjuncts to renal preservation. Surg. Forum 21:527, 1970.

44. Petritsch, P. H. Sacks, S. A., Newell, M. E., and Kaufman, J. J.: Ex-vivo renal surgery: Further use of a new perfusate. Am. J. Surg. 128:408–414, 1974.

45. Poutasse, E. F.: Surgical treatment of renal hypertension: Result in patients with occlusive lesions of renal arteries. J. Urol. 82:403, 1959.

46. Rogers, W. H., Rukskul, A., Camishion, R. C., and Padula, R. T.: In-vivo cinephotographic analysis of aortic and major arterial flow patterns. Arch. Surg. 103:93, 1971.

47. Sacks, S. A., Petritsch, P. H., and Kaufman, J. J.: Canine kidney preservation using a new perfusate. Lancet 1:1024–1028, May 12, 1973.

48. Sacks, S. A., Petritsch, P. H., Linder, R., and Kaufman, J. J.: Renal autotransplantation: Further use of a new perfusate. Am. J. Surg. 128:402–407, 1974.

49. Sacks, S. A., Petritsch, P. H., and Kaufman, J. J.: Simplified in-situ and ex-situ renal preservation. Preliminary Observations: International Research Communications System, March 1973. (73–3) 20–11–1 for reprint requests.
50. Sauvage, L. R., Berger, K. E., Wood, S. J., Nakagawa, Y., and Mansfield, P. B.: An external velour surface for porous arterial prostheses. Surgery 70:940, 1971.
51. Sauvage, L. R., Berger, K. E., Mansfield, P. B., Wood, S. J., Smith, J. C., and Overton, J. B.: Future directions in the development of arterial prostheses for small- and medium-caliber arteries. Surg. Clin. North Am. 54:213, 1974.
52. Scott, H. W., Jr., Morgan, C. V., Bolasny, B. L., Lanier, V. C., Younger, R. K., and Butts, W.: Experimental atherosclerosis in autogenous venous grafts. Arch. Surg. 101:677, 1970.
53. Serrallach-Mila, N., Paravisini, J., Alberti, J., Mayol-Valls, P., Casellas, A., Torner-Soler, M., and Nolla-Panades, J.: Nuevo metodo de revascularizacion en la cirugia de la hipertensión renovascular el autotransplante renal. Angiologia 18:93, 1966.
54. Shapiro, A. P., Perez-Stable, E., Scheibe, E. T., et al.: Renal artery stenosis and hypertension. Am. J. Med. 47:175, 1969.
55. Skinner, D. G.: Blunt traumatic renal artery thrombosis: A successful thrombectomy and revascularization. Ann. Surg. 177:264–267, 1973.
56. Stamey, T.: Personal communications.
57. Starzl, T., and Trippel, O.: Reno-mesenteric-aortoiliac thrombendarterectomy in patients with malignant hypertension. Surgery 46:556, 1959.
58. Stoney, R. J., and Wylie, E. J.: Arterial autografts. Surgery 67:18, 1970.
59. Thomas, C. S., Brockman, S. K., and Foster, J. H.: Variability of the pressure gradient in renal artery stenosis. Surg. Gynec. Obstet. 126:339, 1968.
60. Winer, B. M., Lubbe, W. F., Simon, M., and Williams, J. A.: Renin in the diagnosis of renovascular hypertension. Activity in renal and peripheral vein plasma. J.A.M.A. 202:121, 1967.
61. Young, J. D., Palmer, J. M., Cerny, J., and Franklin, S. S.: Operative mortality in renovascular hypertension. To be published in Reports of Cooperative Study of Renal Hypertension. Morton H. Maxwell, Coordinator, 1971. To be published, J.A.M.A.

Chapter Thirteen

MESENTERIC VASCULAR DISEASE

FRANK C. SPARKS, M.D.

INTRODUCTION

Several clinically definable syndromes produce vascular insufficiency or infarction of the intestine. Only in the past two decades have vascular surgeons been able to repair successfully stenosis and occlusion of the mesenteric vessels. Improved arteriographic techniques have helped to define newer syndromes such as external compression of the celiac artery, and have made possible earlier and more accurate diagnoses. New drugs have been shown to increase mesenteric flow, and may prove to be important in the treatment of non-occlusive mesenteric vascular disease.

Thus, it is important that surgeons become familiar with each of the syndromes in order to recognize the underlying disease process, make the correct diagnosis, and institute proper treatment. In this chapter the historical background, etiology, pathophysiology, symptoms, diagnostic studies, and treatment of each of the major syndromes will be discussed separately.

CHRONIC ISCHEMIA SECONDARY TO STENOSIS OF THE CELIAC AND MESENTERIC ARTERIES

History

In the early 1900's, Schnitzler[103] and Warburg[128] described mesenteric angina. Then, in 1921, Kline[66] pointed out the effects of cardiac decompensation on partial occlusion of this artery. His was the first paper in the English literature to describe the relationship between stenosis of the superior mesenteric artery and visceral angina. In 1936, Dunphy[40] emphasized the relationship between intestinal angina and fatal mesenteric artery occlusion, reporting that seven of 12 patients with fatal mesenteric infarction had a history of previous intestinal angina.

Two advances were reported in 1957: first, Mikkelsen[85] suggested that chronic intestinal ischemia be treated with bypass grafting or reimplantation of the superior mesenteric artery; second, Shaw[106] reported a patient with chronic intestinal ischemia and malabsorption who, while hospitalized, developed acute mesenteric occlusion that was treated successfully by thromboendarterectomy of the superior mesenteric artery. A year later, Mikkelsen[84] reported the first case of intestinal angina diagnosed preoperatively and treated by elective thromboendarterectomy. Morris[88] reported the first elective bypass revascularization to the superior mesenteric artery in 1959.

Pathology

Arteriosclerosis obliterans is the most common cause of stenosis of the celiac and mesenteric arteries,[100] and usually involves the proximal 2 cm. (Fig. 13–1) of the superior mesenteric and celiac arteries.[19, 47, 66] Thromboangiitis obliterans (Buerger's disease), atherosclerotic aneurysms, dissecting aneurysms, periarteritis, fibromuscular hyperplasia, and external compression of the vessels by tumors are less frequent causes.

The extent of injury caused by acute vessel occlusion is dependent upon the size and location of the vessel, the duration of occlusion, the efficiency of collateral circulation, and the presence or absence of bacteria within the lumen of the bowel.[74] Should the length of intestine involved prove to be greater than collateral and intramural vessels can supply, mucosal necrosis, sloughing, and then death will follow.[92] If blood supply is sufficient to prevent gangrene but insufficient for repair of the damaged mucosa, a combination of necrosis and bacterial invasion takes place and results in muscular atrophy or hypertrophy, fibrosis, and stenosis.[89, 96, 98] With short segment involvement and adequate collateral circulation, transient ischemia is followed by vasodilatation and complete healing, with no permanent lesions.[9]

Collateral circulation may be a significant factor in maintaining intestinal viability. In 1869, Chiene[22] wrote about a patient with thrombosis of the celiac, superior mesenteric, and inferior mesenteric arteries who had adequate blood supply to the abdominal vis-

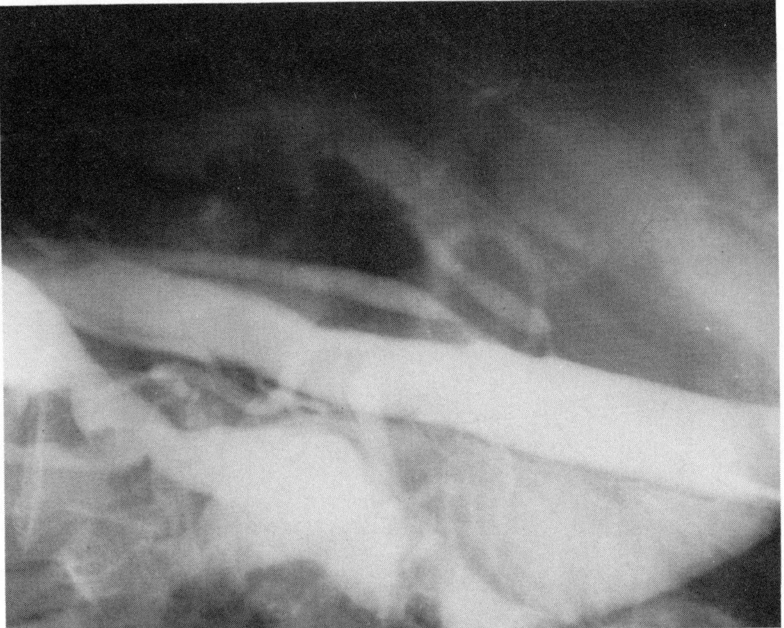

Figure 13–1. Lateral projection of arteriogram showing marked atherosclerotic narrowing of the proximal celiac and superior mesenteric arteries.

cera from parietal branches of the aorta. The arteriogram of a similar patient is seen in Figure 13–2. This patient complained of claudication in both legs. There were no abdominal symptoms. Arteriogram showed complete occlusion of the celiac, superior mesenteric, and inferior mesenteric arteries.

Signs and Symptoms

Postprandial pain in the middle and upper abdomen is the first symptom of intestinal ischemia. This occurs 20 minutes to two hours after a meal, is initially crampy, and becomes steady as disease progresses. Marked weight loss secondary to anorexia and malabsorption is a constant feature.[27] Initial constipation and bloating may be followed by diarrhea and fatty stools as malabsorption occurs. Except for signs of generalized arteriosclerosis, an upper abdominal bruit may be the only significant physical finding. The disease occurs most often in males at an age of 55 to 60 years.

Laboratory Studies

Although necessary to exclude other causes of pain, complete barium examination of the gastrointestinal tract is uniformly unre-

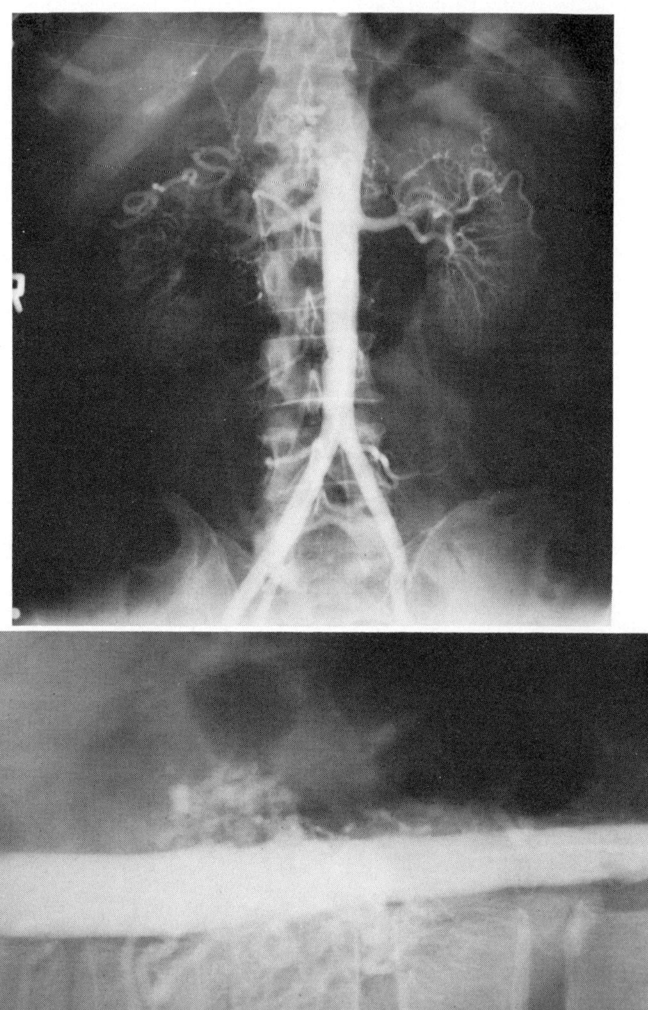

Figure 13–2. Arteriograms in a patient without abdominal symptoms. The celiac, superior mesenteric, and inferior mesenteric arteries are all occluded.

warding. Stool examination and absorption studies show malabsorption late in the course of the disease. Increased fecal fat and nitrogen, decreased d-xylose excretion, and decreased serum carotene levels become evident in this stage of the disease. Triolein [131]iodine and oleic acid [131]iodine absorption also may be depressed.

Definitive diagnosis depends upon arteriographic examination of the mesenteric vessels in both the anterior and lateral projections. The demonstration of collateral circulation, such as a tortuous, dilated, "meandering" inferior mesenteric artery (Fig. 13–3), is helpful in confirming the diagnosis. Angiography will delineate stenosis of the distal mesenteric vessels in those patients who are not amenable to vascular reconstruction.[47]

Treatment

Vascular reconstruction is indicated both to relieve symptoms and to prevent intestinal infarction with its high mortality rate. Since it is believed that stenosis of two of the three arteries is necessary to cause symptoms,[35, 37, 47, 85, 88, 100] the only patients who are advised against revascularization are patients with single vessel stenosis or

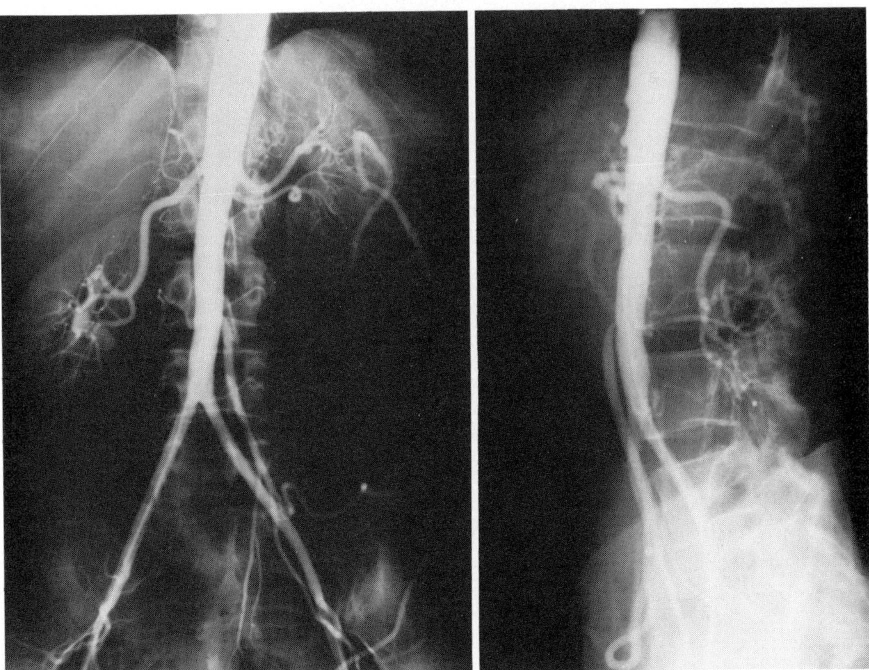

Figure 13–3. Arteriograms in a patient with intestinal angina. The celiac and superior mesenteric arteries are occluded. Note the dilated, tortuous, "meandering" inferior mesenteric artery with 90 per cent stenosis at its orifice.

occlusion and patients with a high risk of not surviving a major abdominal operation. At operation, thorough exploration of the abdomen is done to rule out other causes of the patient's symptoms.

Despite early success with thromboendarterectomy,[15, 47, 107, 114] a bypass is preferred because of difficulty in operative exposure, the tendency of rethrombosis, and the generally poor results reported.[5, 48, 80, 86, 94, 100] Morris[88] points out that measurement of pressure gradients between the aorta and the mesenteric vessels is helpful in determining whether one or two bypass grafts are necessary. In his series of 31 cases, single artery bypass was sufficient in 14 patients and double artery bypass was necessary in 17 patients to reduce the gradient in all vessels.

Since Mikkelsen[85] first proposed aortomesenteric bypass, numerous modifications have been devised to accommodate individual anatomic and physiologic problems. These include thoracic aorta-to-mesenteric artery bypass,[87] splenomesenteric bypass, aorta-to-iliocolic bypass,[97] implantation of the superior mesenteric artery into the aorta[64] and the common iliac artery,[125] sidearm bypass from aortofemoral bypass,[88] and common iliac to mesenteric bypass.[80] Axillomesenteric bypass has been performed when there was thrombosis of the aorta below the renal arteries.[113]

Rob[100] states that splenic artery to superior mesenteric artery bypass rarely is indicated because the orifices of both vessels are almost invariably involved by arteriosclerosis. Either knitted Dacron prostheses or saphenous vein allografts are suitable for the bypass. For elective revascularization, Rob[101] has found a Dacron prosthesis preferable to autogenous vein and suggests that the short distance from the aorta to the mesenteric artery accounts for this success.

CELIAC AXIS SYNDROME

History

This syndrome, also known as the median arcuate ligament syndrome, is controversial.[42] Those who question its validity as an entity contend that (1) the symptoms are vague and subjective, (2) patients with the identical angiographic findings often are asymptomatic,[37, 43, 81] and (3) symptoms secondary to isolated stenosis are contrary to the widely held view that stenosis of two of three mesenteric vessels must be involved.[35, 37, 47, 85, 88, 100] All of these may merely have delayed the recognition of the celiac artery compression syndrome as a specific clinical entity.[21]

Lipshutz[69] described external compression of the celiac axis in

1917. Michels[82] confirmed this observation in 1955. Marable[71] and Dunbar[38] from the United States and Harjola[55] from Finland were the first to describe symptoms due to this condition. Marable,[71] Carey,[17] Lord,[70] and Stoney[116] believe that the median arcuate ligament causes the external compression of the celiac artery as a result of the abnormally high origin of the celiac artery in relation to the aortic hiatus in the diaphragm. However, Caldwell[20] and George[51] both found this to be a normal variation in approximately 20 per cent of patients.

Snyder[111] thought that the compression was caused by surrounding fibrous and neural tissue of the celiac ganglion. He pointed out that division of the median arcuate ligament invariably involves section of the fibers of the celiac ganglion, and suggested that this is the necessary surgical maneuver. In support of this, Carey[17] demonstrated that celiac neuronectomy in animals resulted in a 30 per cent increase in flow of an experimentally induced stenotic celiac vessel.

Harjola[56] reported that the operative findings showed the stenosis to be caused by a fibrotic celiac ganglion in seven patients, a fibrotic band of hiatus (median arcuate ligament) in three patients, and a combination of both in one patient. In these patients, there was a good correlation between the gross operative findings and the microscopic picture of the tissue causing the constriction.

Lindner[68] studied 75 fresh cadavers and found marked variation of the median arcuate ligament and the celiac plexus, and of their anatomic relationship to the celiac artery. These findings suggest that the celiac plexus alone, or with the median arcuate ligament, may be the cause of the stenosis.

Drapanas[37] stated that 13 per cent of all abdominal arteriograms will show this entity. In 17 patients that he studied, six were asymptomatic, six had other conditions responsible for the abdominal symptoms, and two of the remaining five patients had no relief of symptoms from corrective vascular procedures. Meaney[81] found external compression of the celiac artery in 18 of 109 arteriograms. Critical histories of patients with more than 50 per cent stenosis of the celiac artery were analyzed in detail and compared with those of a control group without celiac artery disease or with minimal occlusive changes. There was no difference in symptoms in these two groups.

Edwards[43] urged caution in attributing a causal relationship between celiac artery compression and pain. Because only two of five patients responded to operation, Edwards examined 200 randomly selected normal volunteer hospital personnel between the ages of 17 and 30. Thirteen had epigastric bruits, although only one complained of dyspepsia. Twenty-four others admitted dyspepsia without a bruit. These figures provide no evidence that the incidence of bruit is higher in young persons with dyspepsia than in those without, and give no support to a causal relationship between bruit and dyspepsia.

Signs and Symptoms

The most common symptom is postprandial epigastric pain unrelated to the type of food ingested. Abdominal distention, nausea, vomiting, and diarrhea are less commonly reported. All patients demonstrate a systolic epigastric bruit that is not transmitted into the aorta or the femoral vessels. A typical patient who has received good results postoperatively is a young woman who has had long-standing epigastric pain of the type described, with concomitant systolic bruit and characteristic roentgenographic findings.[71]

Angiography in the lateral projection demonstrates a significant degree of stenosis of the proximal portion of the celiac axis (see Fig. 13–1). The superior and inferior mesenteric arteries are normal in appearance. The patients are in an age group in which atherosclerotic changes of the visceral arteries are uncommon. All of Marable's[72] patients had normal gastrointestinal x-ray examinations, D-xylose tolerance, and triolein uptake studies.

Operative Therapy

After careful exploration of the abdomen to eliminate other sources of abdominal pain, the celiac axis is exposed by dividing the gastrohepatic ligament. Arterial pressures are measured in the aorta and celiac axis to determine whether a gradient exists. If so, dissection is carried down the anterior surface of the celiac artery, dividing the lymphatic and neural structures insofar as necessary. The median arcuate ligament, that portion of the aortic hiatus overlying the celiac artery, and the ganglionic tissue are divided in the midline for a distance sufficient to expose the origin of the celiac axis. Pressure measurements are again taken from the aorta and celiac axis. If a gradient persists, reimplantation of the celiac artery, bypass, or vein patch angioplasty is done.

Results

Despite the many questions raised regarding the validity of this syndrome, excellent results have been obtained in a carefully selected patient group. Edwards[43] collected reports of 61 patients from five centers. Fifty-nine had adequate followup, 47 (79 per cent) were asymptomatic, 8 (14 per cent) were improved, and 4 (7 per cent) were unimproved. In Marable's series of 30 patients, there was no operative mortality and the only morbidity was postoperative diarrhea in one patient.[72]

ACUTE OCCLUSION OF THE SUPERIOR MESENTERIC ARTERY

History

Superior mesenteric artery occlusion with gangrene was recognized in 1843[120] and treated successfully by resection in 1894.[44] Klass[65] was the first to attempt direct operation on the superior mesenteric artery, reporting two cases of embolectomy in 1951. Stewart[115] reported the first successful embolectomy on this artery. DeBakey resected a superior mesenteric artery aneurysm in 1953,[29] and a thoracoabdominal aneurysm involving the celiac mesenteric and renal arteries in 1956.[30] Shaw accomplished the first embolectomy without bowel resection,[106] and then did the first two successful thromboendarterectomies for acute occlusion in 1958.[107]

Etiology

Jackson[58] collected 1500 cases of mesenteric infarction and found 62 per cent to be due to arterial occlusion, 33 per cent to venous occlusion and 5 per cent mixed. Arteriosclerosis accounted for 39 per cent of arterial occlusion and emboli for 42 per cent; in the remaining 19 per cent no organic obstruction was found. With arteriosclerotic occlusion, 67 per cent were within 2.5 cm. of the ostium of the artery, and 33 per cent were in small branches. Acute thrombosis of the superior mesenteric artery usually occurs after the vessel is already partially occluded by atherosclerosis.[53] Thromboangiitis and other inflammatory vascular diseases usually affect the smaller, more distal mesenteric arteries, with resultant short segment intestinal infarction.

Emboli usually originate from mural thrombi associated with a myocardial infarction, or from an auricular thrombus associated with atrial fibrillation.[10, 26, 39] Less commonly, the emboli originate from valvular prostheses or from vegetations from acute and subacute bacterial endocarditis. In 12 per cent of the cases reported by Jackson,[58] emboli orginated from a rheumatic heart in sinus rhythm. Intestinal ischemia secondary to emboli of atheromatous plaques occurring spontaneously[90, 117] or following angiography has been reported. Decreased cardiac output often is the precipitating event in both arteriosclerotic and nonorganic mesenteric infarction, as was first pointed out by Trotter.[123] Previous operation, dehydration, hypovolemic shock, vasopressors, and arrhythmias are among the many factors associated with mesenteric infarction.

In 1926, Cokkinis[25] observed that acute occlusion of the orifice of the superior mesenteric artery produced gangrene from the ligament of Treitz to the mid ascending colon. Occlusion of a proximal jejunal or ilial arcade does not lead to ischemia, but occlusion of a terminal arcade may produce intestinal infarction if 5 to 10 cm. of bowel is devascularized.

Acute occlusion of superior mesenteric artery produces hemorrhagic infarction in about 90 per cent of cases and anemic infarction in the remainder.[58] Initially intense vasospasm of the intramural vessels produces a pale, firm, contracted bowel with mucosal ulceration. As the initial vasospasm subsides, three to four hours later, the musculature relaxes and the capillaries become engorged with blood, producing bowel with splotchy bluish-red areas of discoloration. The intestine then becomes dark blue and blood soaked as full thickness gangrene progresses to perforation in 12 to 24 hours. At this stage the peritoneal cavity contains serosanguineous fluid from the bowel wall, and the intestinal lumen contains blood from necrosis of the mucosa. The length of the segment involved and the adequacy of collateral circulation determine the speed and extent of infarction that occurs.

Signs and Symptoms

The clinical picture of acute mesenteric infarction depends upon whether the ischemia is caused by thrombosis or an embolus. Thrombosis usually occurs in an arterial bed which has had stimulus for collateral circulation due to stenosis or occlusion of more than one of the three visceral arteries supplying the bowel. Consequently, severe ischemia develops slowly. The onset of pain is less abrupt when ischemia is caused by thrombosis than when it is caused by an embolus. Vomiting occurs later. Progression to frank infarction of the bowel may occur because of the insidious nature of the process. Many patients give a history of previous intestinal ischemia with postprandial pain, weight loss, and malabsorption.

Emboli often cause occlusion of mesenteric arteries with little collateral blood supply. Therefore, the onset of pain is abrupt and severe, and is accompanied by marked upper and lower gastrointestinal emptying as a result of the muscular spasm in the bowel wall. Consequently, the catastrophic nature of the process is recognized early, and embolectomy may be done promptly with an expectation of total success.[127, 137] About one half of the patients with mesenteric emboli have had previous peripheral emboli associated with atrial fibrillation.

The pain of ischemic bowel infarction varies in location, depending upon the length of bowel involved. It is at first colicky, but then becomes steady as the bowel loses its ability to contract. Initially, the pain is out of proportion to the physical findings. Generally, some tenderness is present, but signs of peritonitis are absent until late in the course of the disease when infarction has progressed completely through the bowel wall from mucosa to serosa. Although the vomitus or stools may contain blood, Dunphy[41] stressed that gastrointestinal bleeding is not a necessary consequence of acute intestinal ischemia. Bowel sounds are absent after the initial phase. Temperature and pulse may go up only as infarction progresses to frank gangrene.

Mavor[80] has emphasized that neither embolus nor thrombus precipitates sudden peritonitis and shock as was previously taught. Cardiovascular collapse occurs only late in the disease with full thickness gangrene, peritonitis, sepsis, and large fluid shifts into the peritoneum.

Laboratory Studies

Serial white blood counts show an early progressive leukocytosis with left shift. Serum amylase and transaminase levels may be elevated, but there are no studies documenting the value of enzyme elevations in leading to an earlier diagnosis.[133] Paracentesis has been advocated for establishing an early diagnosis,[52] and will reveal large numbers of polymorphonuclear leukocytes in the fluid.

Plain films of the abdomen show probable or definite infarction in 46 per cent of cases secondary to arterial emboli and in only 12 per cent of cases secondary to thrombosis.[121] Specific changes include (1) abnormal separation of bowel loops which, in the absence of ascites, indicates bowel wall thickening; and (2) interstitial bowel-wall gas or gas in the portal venous system. Nonspecific findings include (1) small-bowel dilatation or "pseudo-obstruction," although initially there may be an absence of gas due to spasm; (2) colonic dilatation, especially of the transverse colon; (3) air fluid levels in the small bowel and colon; and (4) decreased fecal volume in the colon. Barium studies of the intestine should be done after arteriography and may show irregular mucosal thickening progressing to an enteritis-like pattern with stenosis.[105]

Arteriography should be done preoperatively in all patients in whom bowel ischemia is suspected, based upon the history and physical examination.[134] It can be done rapidly while the patient is being prepared for surgery and need not delay operative intervention. Arteriography done in both the frontal and lateral projections helps to delineate the cause of ischemia and the operative procedure to be done. If arteriography suggests nonocclusive mesenteric ischemia, operation may be delayed while attempts are made to increase mesenteric flow. If, on the other hand, arteriography shows occlusive disease, immediate operation and embolectomy or bypass is indicated.

Treatment

Klass[65] postulated, 20 years ago, that the surgical treatment of mesenteric occlusion should be directed toward revascularization of the mesenteric artery rather than toward resection. Resection is applicable only in short segment infarction secondary to small peripheral emboli or occlusion of the peripheral vasa recta arteries, usually from arteritis. Hopefully, diagnosis of the cause of the infarction has been made from the preoperative arteriogram. If not, the mesenteric vessels should be explored below the pancreas and examined for evidence of an embolus or a thrombus, and for pulses. Palpation of mesenteric pulses can be deceptive. If there is doubt as to the strength of the arterial pulse, pressure should be measured in the aorta and the superior mesenteric artery. If a reproducible gradient exists, revascularization should be attempted. Distal and proximal control of the superior mesenteric artery can be obtained at the base of the mesentery. A Fogarty catheter is passed distally to remove any propagated thrombus, and then proximally to clear an embolus. If the catheter meets resistance proximally and cannot pass into the aorta, or if the resultant pulse is inadequate, stenosis of the origin of the artery should be suspected and a bypass constructed.

Despite early success with thromboendarterectomy,[15, 47, 107, 114] this procedure is now considered second best to a bypass because of the difficulty in exposure in a critically ill patient, the tendency to rethrombose, and the poor results obtained.[5, 48, 78, 80, 86, 94, 100]

Many different bypass procedures have been done and are discussed under chronic occlusion of the superior mesenteric artery. In these desperately ill patients, the simplest, quickest, and most expedient bypass should be selected. This usually will be an aortomesenteric bypass.

The material used is important: autogenous saphenous vein is preferable in acute occlusion with contamination due to gangrenous bowel.[100] If the vein is too small, a composite graft of saphenous vein can be quickly constructed, or cephalic vein can be utilized. An appealing alternative is the use of homograft bank veins or arterial heterografts.[119] However, heterograft or homograft tissue is extremely hazardous when infection is present.[3]

An operative arteriogram should be obtained if there is any doubt as to the adequacy of the revascularization or removal of distal propagated thrombus.

Welsh[130] was the first to note that apparently gangrenous bowel might actually be viable. Shaw[107] has advocated a "second-look technique," leaving in all bowel which is questionably viable and re-exploring the patient 24 hours after revascularization. The principle of re-exploration is now well established,[133, 134] as it is not possible to predict limits of viability of the bowel at the time of either embolectomy or bypass. Rob[101] goes so far as to advocate resecting only those segments of intestine that have actually perforated, re-exploring the abdomen a few hours to a few days later.

Results

The overall mortality rate of acute mesenteric infarction has remained relatively unchanged at nearly 90 per cent despite an increased awareness of the disease and attempts at revascularization.[4, 48, 60, 94] This may be the result of many factors, including delay in diagnosis, etiology of occlusion, length of bowel involved, and degree of associated cardiac disease. Failure to reach an early diagnosis has resulted in patients coming to operation desperately ill with massive midgut necrosis and peritonitis. Early diagnosis lowers the mortality rate by 15 to 20 per cent.[60, 94]

Mesenteric embolic occlusion, mesenteric venous thrombosis, and short segment infarction all carry a significantly lower mortality than do mesenteric artery thrombosis and non-occlusive infarctions, both of which have a mortality greater than 95 per cent.[4, 94] Acidosis, hyperkalemia, histamine, serotonin, absorption of toxic intestinal substances, cardiac failure, blood volume depletion, vasoactive substances, and upper gastrointestinal bleeding have all been postulated as contributing to death after intestinal revascularization.[4, 12, 24, 73, 102] Williams[132] found evidence for a "negative inotropic factor" causing early decreased cardiac output which would be potentiated by hyperkalemia, acidosis, hypovolemia and sepsis.

NON-OCCLUSIVE MESENTERIC INFARCTION

Despite an obviously severe reduction in intestinal blood flow, 20 to 50 per cent of patients with mesenteric infarction have no demonstrable occlusion of the arterial or venous systems.[60, 94] These patients often have a prolonged decrease in cardiac output secondary to myocardial infarction, arrhythmia, aortic insufficiency, congestive heart failure, or septic or hypovolemic shock.[61]

In a series of 18 patients with non-occlusive mesenteric infarction reported by Fogarty,[46] four factors seem to set these patients apart from those with occlusive gangrene: increased age (average 74 years), severe congestive failure, increased red cell mass or viscosity, and digitalis intoxication. Digitalis is known to have a selective vasoconstrictive action in the mesenteric vasculature.[45] Concomitant stenosis of the mesenteric arteries has been found in one third of the patients with non-thrombotic intestinal infarction.[57] These factors plus compensatory shunting of blood, preferentially to the heart, kidneys and brain lead to intestinal hypoxia that in itself precipitates secondary muscle spasm and further reduces effective intestinal blood supply. Often these patients are on vasopressors, which also contribute to the vasoconstriction and ischemia. Hemorrhagic necrosis occurs, with segmental cyanosis and mottling of the entire length of the intestine.

It is important to remember that abdominal complaints in these patients usually occur secondary to the decreased cardiac output. The severity of the complaints depends upon the degree and length of hypotension, the use of vasopressor drugs, and the presence of any concomitant mesenteric atherosclerosis. Abdominal findings are similar to those in other patients with intestinal ischemia.

Arteriography, while showing no pathognomonic findings in non-occlusive mesenteric ischemia, often demonstrates spasm and unequal flow in the superior mesenteric arterial bed.[134] The smaller arterial branches may show short segmental constrictions and reduced filling.[1] Arteriography is important because it demonstrates that there most often is no anatomically correctable lesion in the superior mesenteric artery in these patients.

Treatment

Therapy should be directed initially toward increasing the cardiac output in an effort to prevent ischemic bowel from progressing to frank gangrene. Digitalis should be withheld and potassium administered in digitalis toxicity.

Glucagon is an attractive potential drug for the treatment of intestinal ischemia, since it has been shown in dogs to increase the splanchnic blood flow[118] and to reverse the vasoconstrictive effect of digoxin.[26, 45] Glucagon has positive inotropic and chronotropic effects on the myocardium and a vasodilating effect on the coronary arteries.

Blood volume deficits should be replaced. When the hematocrit is elevated, phlebotomy is useful, with replacement by crystalloid or colloid solutions. Dextran and heparin have been used in a further effort to decrease viscosity.

Epidural block has been shown by Liang[67] to increase survival in experimental mesenteric artery occlusion. Jackson[59] reported five patients with acute postoperative intestinal ischemia who responded to serial epidural blockade. The advantages of epidural block are ease of administration and usefulness in both the preoperative and postoperative periods. Direct splanchnic block has been used to decrease the vascular resistance but unless a catheter is left in the retroperitoneal space splanchnic block cannot be sustained.[14]

Phenoxybenzamine has been shown to be useful in the laboratory to decrease the mesenteric resistance and increase the mesenteric artery flow,[14] but, unfortunately, this drug is not available for widespread use.

Surgical intervention to remove dead bowel is often necessary but will most likely be successful only in those patients whose decreased cardiac output can be improved. Because involvement frequently is widespread from the stomach to the colon, resection often is not feasible. With smaller areas of necrosis, the bowel should be resected. Because of frequent extension of gangrene in the postoperative period, anastomosis is best avoided in these patients and, instead, the bowel should be exteriorized.

The mortality rate with this disease runs from 88 to 100 per cent.[14, 94] Improvement in these figures can be expected to come only with earlier recognition, improvement in cardiac output and mesenteric blood flow, and expedient operation when indicated.

MESENTERIC VENOUS THROMBOSIS

History

Mesenteric venous thrombosis was first reported as a separate entity in 1935.[36, 129] Warren, at that time, was able to collect 70 cases from the literature and add two of his own.[129] He listed the following predisposing factors: (1) infection from appendicitis, pelvic abscesses, peritonitis and general sepsis; (2) hypercoagulable states such as polycythemia vera, splenic anemias, and carcinomatosis; (3) trauma, including iatrogenic injuries; and (4) mechanical causes resulting from congestion or stasis, such as from cirrhosis with portal hypertension, or from external pressure from tumors, adhesions, or congenital bands. Berry[7] reported 13 cases of primary mesenteric venous thrombosis without predisposing factors. It was estimated that 25 to 55 per cent of all occlusions of the mesenteric veins are of this primary type.[91] Although venous stasis, intimal damage, and hypercoagulability of the blood have not been implicated in these cases of primary mesenteric venous thrombosis, 14 of 31 patients reported by

Naitove[91] had a previous history of thrombophlebitis, suggesting that this disease may represent a visceral form of the more common peripheral thrombophlebitis.

Pathology

The bowel wall is markedly thickened, edematous, and cyanotic. The moderately dilated lumen is filled with dark, bloody fluid.[79] The mesentery is also thickened and discolored. Early in the disease the arteries can be seen to be pulsating, but later with advanced necrosis they will also thrombose. The diagnosis can be made by careful dissection of the involved mesentery.[124] Thrombi can be seen to extrude from the mesenteric veins, whereas the arteries are patent. These thrombi often extend into normal-appearing mesentery and, in fact, may extend up to the liver in advanced disease. Less frequently, they also extend into the inferior mesenteric vein. Necrosis and gangrene begin at the mucosal surface and extend outward. Bacterial invasion begins early and leads to peritonitis and perforation. The microscopic picture is that of hemorrhagic infarction.

In primates and in man, the portal vein may be ligated in most instances without fear of extensive thrombosis in the venous circulation.[23] When occlusion of the proximal superior mesenteric vein occurs slowly, there also may be no ill effects, owing to the extensive collateral supply. Only when the thrombotic process begins in the smaller tributaries or extends to them does hemorrhagic infarction begin.

Signs and Symptoms

A prodromal period, especially in primary mesenteric venous thrombosis, may last for a few days or even weeks. It often occurs with vague abdominal pain associated with anorexia and a change of bowel habit. The pain may be steady or cramping, and may increase in severity as the stage of the disease progresses to either diarrhea or constipation. Hematemesis and melena are uncommon. Here again, the pain is out of proportion to the physical findings. Moderate dehydration and low grade fever often are present. Examination of the abdomen shows distention, some tenderness with guarding, and hypoactive bowel sounds. Rebound tenderness and ridigity occur only late, with perforation. Rectal examination is unrevealing except for guaiac-positive stool. Often peripheral thrombophlebitis is noted. A marked leukocytosis and elevated hematocrit are characteristic. X-ray findings include a thickened bowel wall with either a dilated or narrowed lumen, and are suggestive of infarction in 30 per cent of cases.[121] Serosanguineous peritoneal fluid usually can be found on abdominal paracentesis.

Treatment

Operation should be performed as soon as the diagnosis is suspected. The patient is prepared for surgery by correcting the hypovolemia with balanced salt solution and blood. In cases of polycythemia, phlebotomy and myelosuppressive agents are indicated.[93] All necrotic intestine is resected. Grossly normal-appearing mesentery may contain thrombi. Therefore, resection should include adjacent normal bowel and mesentery until all grossly thrombosed veins are removed. Failure to do so will lead to recurrent infarction. A primary end-to-end anastomosis is usually successful. However, Trinkel[122] advised exteriorization of the bowel because four of five patients on whom he reported had disruption of a primary anastomosis. A second-look operation may be advisable when primary anastomosis is done, since the recurrence rate in this disease is 25 per cent.[91]

Anticoagulation therapy with heparin should be started no later than 12 to 24 hours after operation, and then continued with Coumadin for six to 10 weeks. Although there is not universal agreement on the value of anticoagulants,[16] Naitove[91] reported no deaths in patients with primary mesenteric venous thrombosis in whom anticoagulants were administered, in contrast to a 50 per cent mortality in the group in which the drugs were not used.

Further therapy consists, when applicable, in treating polycythemia, draining abscesses, correcting mechanical obstruction, and discontinuing oral contraceptives.[13]

COLONIC ISCHEMIA

History

Iatrogenic colonic ischemia secondary to inferior mesenteric artery ligation during resection of the colon for carcinoma,[108] aortoiliac reconstruction, and aneurysmectomy[8, 95, 99, 110, 136] has been appreciated for the past two decades. Spontaneous and reversible colonic ischemia was first reported by Boley in 1963.[9] The relationship of colonic ischemia to ulcerative colitis has been further elaborated by Schwartz[104] and by Kilpatrick.[62]

Pathology

Etiologic factors other than iatrogenic include arterial occlusion secondary to emboli[18] or arteriosclerosis obliterans,[75, 126] periarteritis nodosa, rhematoid arthritis, diabetes,[2] decreased cardiac output with concomitant arteriosclerosis obliterans,[76, 98] and oral contraceptives.[63] Colonic ischemia without major vascular occlusion has also been reported.[75]

Colonic ischemia produces a spectrum of pathologic, clinical, and radiologic manifestations, all of which have been reproducible in the experimental laboratory.[10, 34, 49, 77]

Mild colonic ischemia with adequate collateral circulation involving a short segment of the colon produces only submucosal edema and hemorrhage which may go on to mucosal ulceration. However, the mucosa ultimately heals and leaves no radiographic or clinical evidence. Moderate colonic ischemia with sufficient blood to prevent necrosis of the intestine but insufficient for the repair of the damage to the mucosa leads to persistent ischemic colitis or stricture. Marked colonic ischemia leads to full-thickness gangrene and perforation.[75]

The histologic picture depends upon the stage of the disease. Mucosal infarction and ulceration, submucosal and muscularis mucosae inflammatory changes, muscular atrophy, and hypertrophy are all seen. These changes are distinctive and should not be confused with atypical ulcerative colitis or Crohn's disease. Colonic ischemia may affect any portion of the colon but is more frequent at the splenic flexure and descending colon.

Predisposing factors common only to the colon and not to the rest of the intestine are (a) colonic bacterial flora, (b) low normal colonic blood flow relative to the rest of the intestine,[49] (c) decrease in colonic blood flow secondary to functional motor activity,[50] (d) a more pronounced decrease in colonic blood flow secondary to increased intraluminal pressure,[54] and (e) a relatively greater response to autonomic nervous system stimulation.[31, 131] In addition, the collateral blood supply to the colon has been found to be absent or inadequate in a significant number of cases.[32, 83, 112] All these factors would suggest that the colon is more susceptible to ischemia than is the remainder of the bowel.

Signs and Symptoms

The great majority of patients with colonic ischemia are above 60 years of age and have signs of both cardiovascular and peripheral vascular disease. There is usually an acute onset of lower abdominal cramping, which may become constant and localized over the site of colonic ischemia as progressive ischemia occurs. Vomiting and bloody diarrhea are common. The amount of blood is less than that seen with diverticular bleedings. The temperature is slightly elevated. There is abdominal tenderness over the area of the involved colon. Although some degree of peritoneal irritation has been noted in reversible colonic ischemia, its presence should suggest full-thickness gangrene and perforation. Rectal examination will show guaiac-positive stool. Sigmoidoscopy will show blood-stained mucous. If the lesion is low enough to be visualized directly, submucosal hemorrhages are seen early, followed by non-specific mucosal ulceration later in the course of the disease. The leukocyte count is elevated early in this disease.

Boley[19] has emphasized that the diagnosis of reversible colonic ischemia can be only suspected on the initial examination, and that early and serial barium enema studies are the keys to making this diagnosis.

Radiographic Aspects

The radiographic features of ischemic colitis have been well documented[75, 105] and include (1) thumbprinting or "psuedo-tumors" which represent submucosal hemorrhage and are therefore present only in the early stages; (2) mucosal irregularity secondary to ulceration and similar to ulcerative colitis but lacking the fissures seen in Crohn's disease; (3) stenosis localized to one segment of the bowel and differentiated from carcinoma by the absence of "half-shadowing"; and (4) sacculation which is diagnostic and occurs in the antimesenteric border of the bowel.

Serial barium enemas will show a progression of the disease from the "thumbprints" to the shallow ulcers of segmental colitis, then either progression to complete healing or to segmental colitis with stricture. Persistence of the filling defects excludes the diagnosis of colonic ischemia.

Arteriography. Marston[75] states that most cases of spontaneous ischemic colitis occur without proximal obstruction of the inferior mesenteric artery. In these cases, angiography usually gives either negative results or films which are difficult to interpret. However, Dunbar[39] demonstrated embolic occlusion of the iliocolic and right colic arteries in a case of reversible cecal infarction.

Treatment

In the absence of physical findings suggestive of intestinal gangrene or perforation, and of confirmatory evidence from a barium enema that ischemic colitis is in fact present, treatment is nonoperative. This consists of systemic antibiotics, IV fluids, nasogastric suction, colonic decompression and careful saline irrigations with a rectal tube, antispasmodics, and analgesics. Close monitoring of the patient to ensure that the disease has not progressed to full-thickness gangrene and peritonitis is most important. If the disease is stable after the first few days, it is unusual for reversible ischemic colitis to progress to full-thickness gangrene.

If the patient presents with signs of peritoneal irritation suggesting gangrene, if the clinical course deteriorates, or if the diarrhea, bleeding, or both, persist for more than a week, irreversible changes have occured, and surgical intervention is indicated. Should operation be performed during the acute stages of the disease, the colon should be resected back to viable mucosa and no anastomosis performed. Should operation be performed during the chronic obstructive phase for stenosis, the bowel may be resected and a primary anastomosis performed after the usual bowel preparation. If any reconstructive vascular procedure is to be performed, however, it should be done prior to the resection of the bowel.

Boley[11] stresses that "the treatment of colonic ischemia consists of early identification and continued surveillance, an ultra-conservative approach where reversibility is probable and a very aggressive surgical approach where permanent ischemic damage is suggested."

REFERENCES

1. Aakhus, T., and Braband, G.: Angiography in acute superior mesenteric insufficiency. Acta Radiol. 6:1, 1967.
2. Ambruoso, V. N., and Peraru, F.: Massive gangrene of the colon due to distal obstruction. Surgery 61:228, 1967.
3. Barker, W. F.: Personal communication.
4. Bergan, J. J., Haid, S. P., and Conn, J. J., Jr.: Systemic effects of intestinal revascularization. Am. J. Surg. 117:235, 1969.
5. Bergan, J. J.: Recognition and treatment of intestinal ischemia. Surg. Clin. N. Amer. 47:109, 1967.
6. Berger, R. L., and Byrne, J. J.: Intestinal gangrene associated with heart disease. Surg. Gynec. Obstet. 112:529, 1961.
7. Berry, F. B., and Boughs, J. A.: Agnogenic venous mesenteric thrombosis. Ann. Surg. 32:450, 1950.
8. Birnbaum, W., Rudy, L., and Wylie, E. J.: Colonic and rectal ischemia following abdominal aneurysmectomy. Dis. Colon Rectum. 7:293, 1964.
9. Boley, S. J., Schwartz, S. S., Lash, J., and Sternhill, V.: Reversible vascular occlusions of the colon. Surg. Gynec. Obstet. 116:53, 1963.
10. Boley, S. J., Kraiger, H., Schultz, L., Robinson, K., Siew, F. P., Allen, A. C. and Schwartz, S.: Experimental aspects of peripheral vascular occlusion of the intestine. Surg. Gynec. Obstet. 121:789, 1965.
11. Boley, S. J., and Schwartz, S. S.: Colonic ischemia: Reversible ischemic lesions. In *Vascular Disorders of the Intestine.* New York, Appleton-Century Crofts, 1971.
12. Boley, S. J., Cohen, M. I., Winslow, P. R., Becker, N. H., Treiber, W., McNamara, H., Bleith, F. J., and Gliedman, M. L.: Mesenteric ischemia: A cause of increased gastric blood flow, hyperacidity, and acute gastric ulceration. Surgery 68:222, 1970.
13. Brennan, M. F., Clarke, A. M., and MacBeth, W. A.: Infarction of the midgut associated with oral contraceptives. Report of two cases. N. Eng. J. Med. 279:1213, 1968.
14. Britt, L. G., and Cheek, R. C.: Non-occlusive mesenteric vascular disease. Ann. Surg. 169:704, 1969.

15. Brittain, R. S., and Earley, T. K.: Emergency thrombo-endarterectomy of the superior mesenteric artery. Ann. Surg. *158*:138, 1963.
16. Campbell, S. J., and Mears, T. W.: Mesenteric thrombosis. Am. Surg. *23*:543, 1957.
17. Carey, J. P., Stemmer, E. A., and Connolly, J. E.: Median arcuate ligament syndrome. Arch. Surg. *99*:441, 1969.
18. Carnevale, N. J., and Delany, H. M.: Cholesterol embolization to the cecum with bowel infarction. Arch. Surg. *106*:94, 1973.
19. Carucci, J. J.: Mesenteric vascular occlusion. Am. J. Surg. *85*:47, 1953.
20. Cauldwell, E. W., and Anson, B. J.: The visceral branches of the abdominal aorta: topographical relationships. Am. J. Anat. *13*:27, 1943.
21. Charrette, E. P., Iyengar, S. R. K., Lynn, R. B., Paloschi, G. G., and West, R. O.: Abdominal pain associated with celiac artery compression. Surg. Gynec. Obstet. *132*:1009, 1971.
22. Chiene, J.: Complete obliteration of coeliac and mesenteric arteries. J. Anat. Physiol. *3*:65, 1869.
23. Child, C. G., III, Holswade, G. R., McClure, R. D., Jr., Gore, A. L., Neal, E. D., et al.: Pancreaticoduodenectomy with resection of portal vein in macaca mulatta monkey and in man. Surg. Gynec. Obstet. *94*:31, 1952.
24. Chiu, C. J., Scott, H. J., and Guard, F. N.: Volume deficit versus toxic absorption: A study of canine shock after mesenteric arterial occlusion. Ann. Surg. *175*:479, 1972.
25. Cokkinis, A.: *Mesenteric Vascular Occlusion.* London, Bailliere, Tindall and Cox, 1926.
26. Danford, R. O.: The splanchnic vasoconstrictive effect of digoxin and its reversal by Glucagon. In *Vascular Disorders of the Intestine.* Boley, S. J., Schwartz, S. S., and Williams, L. F. London, Butterworths, 1971.
27. Dardik, H., Seidenberg, B., Parker, J., and Hurwitt, E. S.: Intestinal angina with malabsorption treated by elective revascularization. J.A.M.A. *194*:1206, 1965.
28. Davis, J. E.: Reversible vascular occlusion of the colon. Ann. Surg. *171*:789, 1970.
29. DeBakey, M. E., and Cooley, D. A.: Successful resection of mycotic aneurysm of superior mesenteric artery: Case report and review of literature. Am. Surg. *19*:202, 1953.
30. DeBakey, M. E., Creech, O., and Morris, G. C., Jr.: Aneurysm of thoracoabdominal aorta involving the celiac, superior mesenteric and renal arteries. Report of four cases treated by resection and homograft replacement. Ann. Surg. *144*:549, 1956.
31. Delaney, J. P., and Leonard, A. S.: Hypothalamic influence on gastrointestinal blood flow in the awake cat. Fed. Proc. *29*:260, 1970.
32. Demos, N. J., Bahuth, J. J., and Urnes, P. D.: Comparative study of arteriosclerosis in the inferior and superior mesenteric arteries. Ann. Surg. *155*:599, 1961.
33. Derrick, J. R., Pollard, H. S., and Moore, R. M.: The pattern of arteriosclerotic narrowing of the celiac and superior mesenteric arteries. Ann. Surg. *149*:684, 1959.
34. DeVilliers, D. R.: Ischemia of the colon: An experimental study. Brit. J. Surg. *53*:497, 1966.
35. Dick, A. P., Groff, R., Gregg, D., Peters, N., and Sarner, M.: An arteriographic study of mesenteric arterial disease. Gut 8:206, 1967.
36. Donaldson, J. K., and Stout, B. F.: Mesenteric thrombosis. Am. J. Surg. *29*:208, 1935.
37. Drapanas, T., and Bron, K. M.: Stenosis of the celiac artery (editorial). Ann. Surg. *164*:1085, 1966.
38. Dunbar, J. D., Molnar, W., Beman, F. F., and Marable, S. A.: Compression of the celiac trunk and abdominal angina. Am. J. Roentgen. 95:731, 1965.
39. Dunbar, J. D.: Reversible cecal infarction. Am. J. Surg. *112*:447, 1966.
40. Dunphy, J. E.: Abdominal pain of vascular origin. Am. J. Med. Sc. *192*:109, 1936.
41. Dunphy, J. E., and Zollinger, R. M.: Mesenteric vascular occlusion. New Eng. J. Med. *211*:708, 1934.

42. Editorial. Compression of coeliac axis. Br. Med. J. *1*:317, 1970.
43. Edwards, A. J., Hamilton, J. D., Nichol, W. D., Taylor, G. W., and Dawson, A. M.: Experience with coeliac axis compression syndrome. Br. Med. J. *1*:342, 1970.
44. Elliot, J. W.: The operative relief of gangrene of the intestine due to occlusion of the mesenteric vessels. Am. Surg. *21*:9, 1895.
45. Ferrer, M. I., Bradley, S. E., Wheeler, H. O., Enson, Y., Preisig, R., and Harvey, R. M.: The effect of digoxin in the splanchnic circulation in ventricular failure. Circulation *32*:524, 1965.
46. Fogarty, T. J., and Fletcher, W. S.: Genesis of non-occlusive mesenteric ischemia. Am. J. Surg. *111*:130, 1966.
47. Fry, W. J., and Kraft, R. O.: Visceral angina. Surg. Gynec. Obstet. *117*:417, 1963.
48. Galloway, J. M. D., Walker, P. A., and Mavor, G. E.: Mesenteric arterial occlusion as a vascular emergency. Br. J. Surg. *56*:431, 1969.
49. Geber, W. F.: Quantitative measurement of blood flow in various areas of small and large intestine. Am. J. Physiol. *198*:985, 1960.
50. Geber, W. F.: Functional hemodynamics of the colon. Angiology *15*:366, 1964.
51. George, R.: Topography of the unpaired visceral branches of the abdominal aorta. J. Anat. *69*:196, 1934.
52. Ghanem, M., Goodale, R. L., Spanos, P., Tsung, M. S., and Wangensteen, O. H.: Value of leukocyte counts in the recognition of mesenteric infarction and strangulation of shorter intestinal length: An experimental study. Surgery *68*:635, 1970.
53. Glotzer, D. J., and Shaw, R. S.: Massive bowel infarction: An autopsy assessing the potentialities of reconstructive vascular surgery. New Eng. J. Med. *260*:162, 1959.
54. Halpern, A., Selman, D., Shaftel, N., Shaftel, H. E., Kuhn, P. H., Samuels, S. S., and Birch, H. G.: The peripheral vascular dynamics of bowel function. Angiology *11*:460, 1960.
55. Harjola, P. T.: A rare obstruction of the coeliac artery. Ann. Chir. et Cynaec. Fenniae *52*:547, 1963.
56. Harjola, P. T., and Lahtiharju, A.: Celiac syndrome. Am. J. Surg. *115*:864, 1968.
57. Heer, F. W., Silon, W., and French, S. W.: Intestinal gangrene without apparent vascular occlusion. Am. J. Surg. *110*:231, 1965.
58. Jackson, B. B.: *Occlusion of the Superior Mesenteric Artery.* Springfield, Ill., Charles C Thomas, 1963.
59. Jackson, B. B., and Lykins, R.: Serial epidural analgesia in mesenteric arterial failure. Arch. Surg. *90*:177, 1965.
60. Jensen, C. B., and Smith, G. A.: A clinical study of 51 cases of mesenteric infarction. Surgery *40*:930, 1956.
61. Jordan, T. H., Boulafendis, D., and Guinn, G. A.: Factors other than major vascular occlusion that contribute to intestinal infarction. Ann. Surg. *181*:189, 1970.
62. Kilpatrick, Z. M., Farman, J., Yesner, R., and Spiro, H. M.: Ischemic proctitis. J.A.M.A. *205*:74, 1968.
63. Kilpatrick, Z. M., Silverman, J. F., Betancourt, E., Farman, J., and Lawson, J. P.: Vascular occlusion of the colon and oral contraceptives. New Eng. J. Med. *278*:438, 1968.
64. Kiser, J. L., and Utley, J. R.: Visceral artery reconstruction. Am. J. Surg. *116*:720, 1968.
65. Klass, A. A.: Embolectomy in acute mesenteric occlusion. Ann. Surg. *134*:913, 1951.
66. Klein, E.: Embolism and thrombosis of the superior mesenteric artery. Surg. Gynec. Obstet. *33*:385, 1921.
67. Liang, H., Bernard, H. R., and Dodd, R. B.: The effect of epidural block upon experimental mesenteric occlusion. Arch. Surg. *83*:407, 1961.
68. Lindner, H. H., and Kemprud, E.: A clinicoanatomical study of the arcuate ligament of the diaphragm. Arch. Surg. *103*:600, 1971.
69. Lipshutz, B.: A composite study of the coeliac axis artery. Ann. Surg. *65*:159, 1917.

70. Lord, R. S. A., Stoney, R. J., and Wylie, E. J.: Coeliac-axis compression. Lancet 2:795, 1968.
71. Marable, S. A., Molnar, E., and Beman, F. J.: Abdominal pains secondary to celiac axis compression. Am. J. Surg. 111:493, 1966.
72. Marable, S. A., Kaplan, M. F., Beman, F. J., and Molnar, W.: Celiac compression syndrome. Am. J. Surg. 115:97, 1968.
73. Marston, A.: Causes of death in mesenteric arterial occlusion. Ann. Surg. 158:952, 960, 1963.
74. Marston, A.: Mesenteric arterial disease; the present position. Gut 8:203, 1967.
75. Marston, A., Pheils, M. T., Thomas, M. L., and Morson, B. C.: Ischemic colitis. Gut 7:1, 1966.
76. Marston, A.: The bowel in shock. Lancet 3:365, 1962.
77. Marston, A., Marcuson, R. W., Chapman, M., and Arthur, J. F.: Experimental study of devascularization of the colon. Gut 10:121, 1969.
78. Marston, A.: Diagnosis and management of intestinal ischemia. Ann. Roy. Coll. Surg. Engl. 50:29, 1972.
79. Mathews, J. E., and White, R. R.: Primary mesenteric venous occlusive disease. Am. J. Surg. 122:579, 1971.
80. Mavor, G. E., Lyall, A. D., Chrystal, K. M., and Tsapogas, M.: Mesenteric infarction as a vascular emergency. Br. J. Surg. 50:219, 1962.
81. Meaney, T. F., and Kistner, R. L.: Evaluation of intra-abdominal disease of obscure cause. Arch. Surg. 94:811, 1967.
82. Michels, N. A.: Blood Supply and Anatomy of the Upper Abdominal Organs. Philadelphia, J. B. Lippincott Co., 1955, p. 141.
83. Michels, N. A., Siddharth, P., Kornblith, P. L., and Parke, W. W.: The variant blood supply to the descending colon, retrosigmoid and rectum based on 400 dissections. Dis. Col. Rec. 8:251, 1965.
84. Mikkelsen, W. P., and Zaro, J. A.: Intestinal angina. New Eng. J. Med. 260:912, 1959.
85. Mikkelsen, W. P.: Intestinal angina. Am. J. Surg. 94:262, 1957.
86. Morris, G. C., Jr., DeBakey, M. E., and Bernhard, V.: Abdominal angina. Surg. Clin. N. Amer. 46:919, 1966.
87. Morris, G. C., Jr., and DeBakey, M. E.: Abdominal angina—diagnosis and surgical treatment. J.A.M.A. 176:89, 1961.
88. Morris, G. C., Jr., Crawford, E. S., Cooley, D. A., and DeBakey, M. E.: Revascularization of the celiac and superior mesenteric arteries. Arch. Surg. 84:95, 1962.
89. Mozes, M., Adar, R., Tsur, N., David, R., and Deutsh, V.: Intestinal obstruction due to mesenteric vascular occlusion. Surg. Gynec. Obstet. 133:583, 1971.
90. Mulliken, J. B., and Bartlett, M. D.: Small bowel obstruction secondary to atheromatous embolism. Ann. Surg. 174:145, 1971.
91. Naitove, A., and Weismann, R. E.: Primary mesenteric venous thrombosis. Ann. Surg. 161:516, 1965.
92. Niederstein, K.: Die Zirkulationstorungen im Mesenterialgebiet. Deutsch. Z. Chir. 85:710, 1906.
93. Ostermiller, W., Jr., and Carter, R.: Mesenteric venous thrombosis secondary to polycythemia vera. Am. Surg. 35:338, 1969.
94. Ottinger, L. W., and Austen, W. S.: A study of 136 patients with mesenteric infarction. Surg. Gynec. Obstet. 125:251, 1967.
95. Ottinger, L. W., Darling, C., Nathan, M. D., and Linton, R. R.: Left colon ischemia complicating aorta-iliac reconstruction. Causes, diagnosis, management, and prevention. Arch. Surg. 105:841, 1972.
96. Pope, C. H., and O'Neil, R. M.: Incomplete infarction of the ileum simulating regional enteritis. J.A.M.A. 161:963, 1956.
97. Ranger, I., and Spence, M. P.: Superior mesenteric artery occlusion treated by ileocolic aortic anastomosis. Br. Med. J. 2:95, 1962.
98. Reeves, J. D., and Wang, C. C.: The stages of mesenteric artery disease. South. Med. J. 54:541, 1961.
99. Rob, C. G., and Snyder, M.: Chronic intestinal ischemia: A complication of surgery of the abdominal aorta. Surgery 60:1141, 1966.

100. Rob, C. G.: Surgical diseases of the celiac and mesenteric arteries. Arch. Surg. 93:21, 1966.
101. Rob, C. G.: Stenosis and thrombosis of the celiac and mesenteric arteries. Am. J. Surg. 114:363, 1967.
102. Rush, B. F., Jr., Host, W. R., Fewel, J., and Hsieh, J.: Intestinal ischemia and some organic substances in serum and abdominal fluid. Arch. Surg. 105:151, 1972.
103. Schnitzler, F.: Zur Zymptomatik des Darmarterien-verschlusses. Wien. Med. Wchnschr. 11/12:506, 1901.
104. Schwartz, S. S., Boley, S. J., Lash, J., and Sternhill, V.: Roentgenologic aspects of reversible vascular occlusion of the colon in its relationship to ulcerative colitis. Radiology 80:625, 1963.
105. Schwartz, S. S., Boley, S., Robinson, K., Krieger, H., Schultz, L., and Allen, A. C.: Roentgenologic features of vascular disorders of the intestine. Radiol. Clin. N. Amer. 2:71, 1964.
106. Shaw, R. S., and Rutledge, R.: Superior-mesenteric-artery embolectomy in treatment of massive mesenteric infarction. New Eng. J. Med. 257:595, 1957.
107. Shaw, R. S., and Maynard, E. P.: Acute and chronic thrombosis of the mesenteric arteries associated with malabsorption. New Eng. J. Med. 258:874, 1958.
108. Shaw, R. S., and Green, T. H.: Massive mesenteric infarction following inferior mesenteric artery ligation in resection of the colon for carcinoma. New Eng. J. Med. 248:890, 1953.
109. Slater, H., and Elliott, D. W.: Primary mesenteric infarction. Am. J. Surg. 123:309, 1972.
110. Smith, R. F., and Szilagyi, D. E.: Ischemia of the colon as a complication in the surgery of the abdominal aorta. Arch. Surg. 80:806, 1960.
111. Snyder, M. A., Mahoney, E. B., and Rob, C. G.: Symptomatic celiac artery stenosis due to constriction by the neurofibrous tissue of the celiac ganglia. Surgery 61:372, 1967.
112. Sonneland, J., Anson, B. J., and Beaton, L. E.: Surgical anatomy of the arterial supply to the colon from the superior mesenteric artery based upon a study of 600 specimens. Surg. Gynec. Obstet. 106:385, 1958.
113. Sparks, F. C., Ramp, J. M., and Imparato, A. I.: Axillo-mesenteric bypass for acute mesenteric infarction. Vascular Surgery 8:90, 1974.
114. Starzl, T. E., and Trippel, O. H.: Reno-mesenteric-aortoiliac thromboendarterectomy in patient with malignant hypertension. Surgery 46:556, 1959.
115. Stewart, G. D., Sweetman, W. R., Westphal, K., and Wise, R. A.: Superior mesenteric artery embolectomy. Ann. Surg. 151:274, 1960.
116. Stoney, R. J., and Wylie, E. J.: Recognition and surgical management of visceral ischemic syndromes. Ann. Surg. 164:714, 1966.
117. Taylor, N. S., Gueft, B., and Lebowich, R. J.: Atheromatous embolization: A cause of gastric ulcers and small bowel necrosis. Gastroenterology 47:97, 1964.
118. Tibblin, S., Kock, N. G., and Schenk, W. G.: Response of mesenteric blood flow to Glucagon. Arch. Surg. 102:65, 1971.
119. Tice, D. A., and Santoni, E.: Use of saphenous vein homografts for arterial reconstruction: A preliminary report. Surgery 67:493, 1970.
120. Tiedeman, F.: Von der verengung und schliessung der pulsadern in Rraukheiten. xiv + 316 pp., 3 pl. Heidelberg u Leipzig, K. Groos, 1843.
121. Tomchik, F. S., Wittenberg, J., and Ottinger, L. W.: The roentgenographic spectrum of bowel infarction. Radiology 96:249, 1970.
122. Trinkle, K.: The operative management of idiopathic mesenteric venothrombosis with intestinal infarction. Am. Surg. 35:338, 1969.
123. Trotter, L. B. C.: *Embolism and Thrombosis of the Mesenteric Vessels.* New York, Cambridge University Press, 1913.
124. Van Way, C. W., Brockman, S. K., and Rosenfeld, L.: Spontaneous thrombosis of the mesenteric veins. Ann. Surg. 173:561, 1971.
125. Van Zyl, J. J. W., and DuToit, F. D.: Superior mesenteric artery occlusion treated by common iliac-ileocolic anastomosis. Br. J. Surg. 53:522, 1966.

126. Wald, M.: Gangrene of the distal two thirds of the transverse colon, left colon, rectum and anal canal due to superior mesenteric vascular insufficiency. Dis. Col. Rect. 7:303, 1964.
127. Wangensteen, S. L., Golden, G. F., and Stapleton, S. L.: Successful superior mesenteric artery embolectomy. Am. J. Surg. 123:601, 1972.
128. Warburg, E.: Über dyspragia intermittens angiosclerotical intestinalis. München med Wchnschr. 52:1174, 1905.
129. Warren, S., and Eberhardt, T.: Mesenteric venous thrombosis. Surg. Gynec. Obstet. 61:102, 1935.
130. Welch, W. H.: Collected papers, Vol. I., 1920 (cited by Dumont, A. E., Tice, D. A., and Mulholland, J. H.: Arteriosclerotic occlusion of the superior mesenteric artery. Ann. Surg. 154:833, 1961).
131. Welsh, J. D.: Blood flow. Am. J. Dig. Dis. 8:614, 1963.
132. Williams, L. F., Jr., Goldberg, A. H., Polansky, B. J., and Byrne, J. J.: Myocardial effects of acute intestinal ischemia. Surgery 138:1969, 1966.
133. Williams, L. F.: Vascular insufficiency of the intestines. Progr. Gastro. 61:757, 1971.
134. Williams, L. F., Athanasoulis, C. A., and Wittenberg, J.: Ischemic bowel disease. Postgrad. Med. 53:136, 1973.
135. Wittenberg, J., Athanasoulis, C. A., Shapiro, J. H., and Williams, L. F., Jr.: Mesenteric angiography. New Eng. J. Med. 285:1539, 1971.
136. Young, J. R., Humphries, A. W., DeWolfe, V. G., and Lefevre, F. A.: Complications of abdominal aortic surgery. II: Intestinal ischemia. Arch. Surg. (Chicago) 86:51, 1963.
137. Zuidema, G. D., Reed, D., Turcotte, J. E., and Fry, W. J.: Superior mesenteric artery embolectomy. Ann. Surg. 159:548, 1964.

ARTERIAL TRAUMA

Many outstanding surgeons of the past years have considered repair of injured vessels to be a special challenge. It is unfortunate but true that in a world of wars, high-speed travel, and civilian violence, the repair of major injuries to the vascular system has become an important part of the surgeon's work.

Prior to the conflict in Korea, successful repairs of arterial injuries were only sporadic, and the major emphasis was directed to the choice of the optimal site of ligation. Gangrene and amputation followed ligation in a predictable percentage of instances.[20] In Korea, however, newly acquired techniques of vascular surgery, effective antibiotic support, and successful treatment of shock combined to allow Hughes,[17] Jahnke and Seeley,[17] and Spencer and Grewe[35] to initiate the modern era of treatment of vascular injuries so ably carried on by many surgeons in Vietnam and in civilian life.

This chapter will deal with arterial wounds but will also touch upon the problems of associated injuries and the niceties of judgment necessary to the best treatment of the whole patient.

TYPES OF ARTERIAL INJURIES

The agents responsible for injuries can be categorized as in Table 14–1.

From the surgeon's point of view, it is important to distinguish certain aspects of these injuries. The possibility of contamination exists in all penetrating wounds, whereas most other wounds are clean.

A considerable degree of local arterial injury may be present

Table 14-1.   Classification of Injuring Agents

Penetrating wounds
  Missiles
    High velocity gunshot wounds
    Low velocity gunshot wounds, shrapnel
  Edged instruments
    Knives, glass splinters, and other sharp penetrating agents
    Bone fragments (compound wounds)
  Injections into arteries
    Diagnostic studies
    Therapeutic errors
    Illicit drugs
Non-penetrating or blunt injuries
  Dislocations, divulsions
  Blunt agents
  Bone fragments (non-compounded fractures)

beyond the actual discontinuity in high-velocity gunshot wounds[39] and in the stretching injuries associated with dislocations and divulsion injuries. Such an injury requires at least some debridement of the artery, although excision back to normal-appearing artery is now all that is recommended in the treatment of high-velocity gunshot wounds.[32] It should be understood, however, that the wounding power of high-velocity missiles is such that even without disruption, a considerable length of artery may be grossly injured and thrombosed.

Trauma that does not penetrate the artery may, nonetheless, produce intimal fracture and thrombosis (Fig. 14–1).[15]

Inadvertent injection of toxic drugs may result in extensive arterial damage and thrombosis defying repair.[13, 27]

DIAGNOSIS

There are many clues to the recognition that arterial injury has occurred. A large hematoma, a history of copious blood loss, and shock are nonspecific signs. The observation of pulsatile or arterial blood in the wound or a pulsating hematoma are more positive signs. A penetrating wound associated with major nerve injury (as in the brachial plexus, one of the "crowded" areas) in a site where vessels and nerves are so intimately arranged, or even a wound the course of which suggests injury of a major artery, may demand exploration. A murmur heard downstream from an injury also suggests arterial involvement.

Loss of distal pulses or signs of peripheral vascular insufficiency

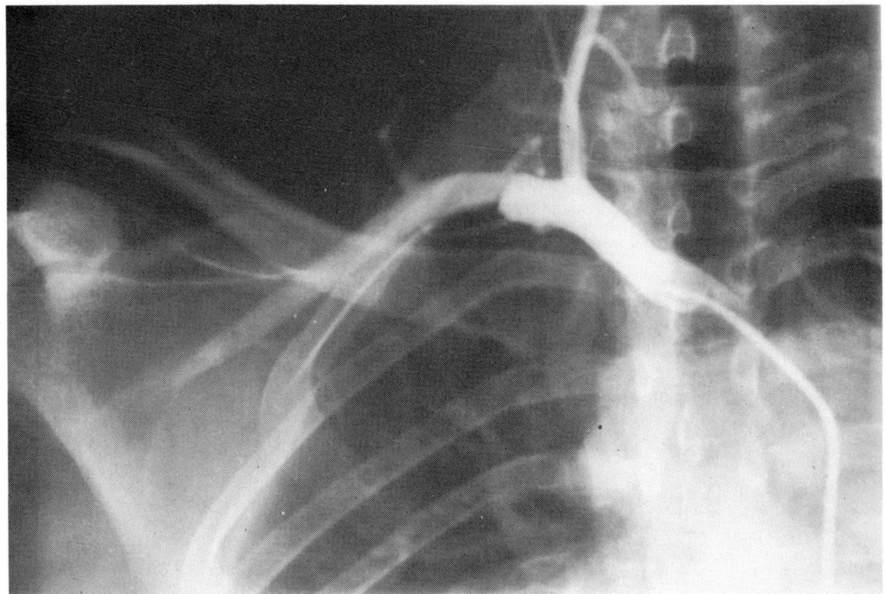

Figure 14–1. Arteriogram of an injury of the subclavian artery in which a dislocation of the intimal flap produced nearly complete obstruction. (From Hare, R. R., and Gaspar, M. R.: The intimal flap. Arch. Surg. *102*:552, 1071. By permission of American Medical Association Archives of Surgery and the authors).

in the absence of other suspicious signs demand exploration; as for example, a cold, hypesthetic, pale, and pulseless leg after a femoral fracture. Femoral fractures, closed or open, should always be approached with suspicion that there may be an associated arterial injury.

Where shock or loss of consciousness exists, more objective signs of injury are needed than simple palpation of pulses. The use of quick, noninvasive techniques such as measurement and comparison of arterial pressures at symmetrical sites or segmental plethysmography, should precede and define the need for arteriography.

If one suspects intra-abdominal arterial injuries, arteriography as an initial step may be helpful, provided the patient can tolerate the delay. At times, an intravenous pyelogram performed when arterial hemorrhage is not suspected may point to renal arterial injury such as an intimal fracture in the renal artery or an intrarenal arteriovenous shunt.[12] The finding of a nonfunctioning kidney on excretory urogram almost demands an arteriographic demonstration of the lesion.

Open carotid injuries or carotid injuries with major hematomas are easily recognized, and the decision to repair or not to repair the artery may be made by some surgeons on the absence or presence of

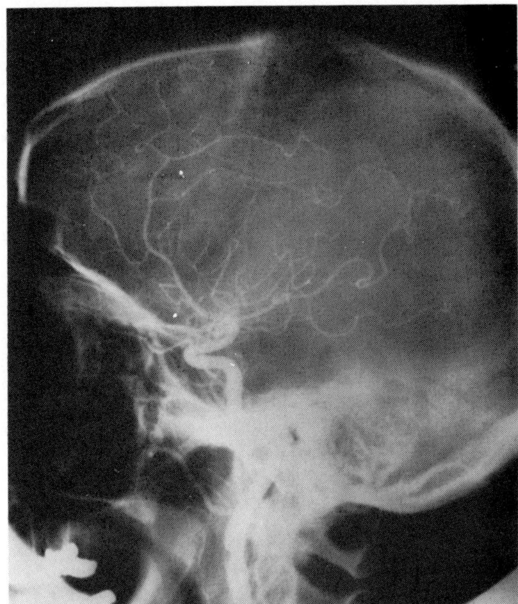

Figure 14–2. Blunt (hyperextension) trauma to the internal carotid artery resulting in intimal fracture and false aneurysm.

a neurological deficit.[8, 31] Closed carotid injuries with tears of the intima present a characteristic acute (Fig. 14–2) and chronic (Fig. 14–3) lesion. This lesion often shows slow progression to complete occlusion over 12 to 48 hours. Its early identification by a positive supraor-

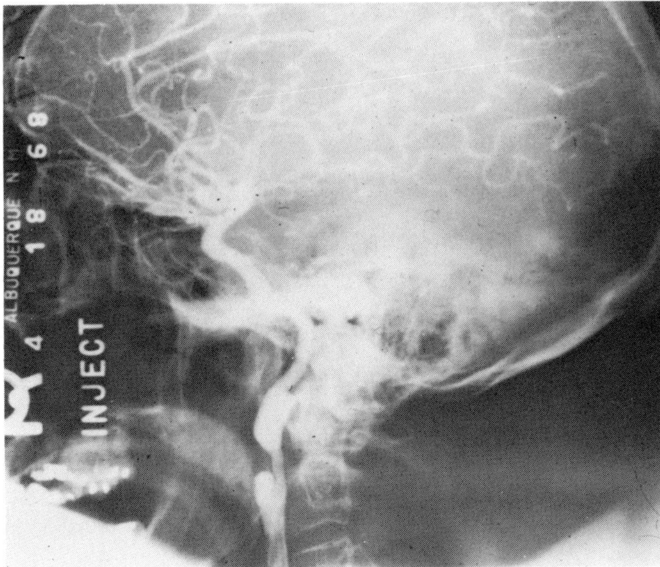

Figure 14–3. Late false aneurysm of the high extracranial internal carotid artery resulting from prior closed blunt trauma.

bital Doppler test may allow early repair before real neurological damage occurs.[24, 25]

Arteriography emerges as the most positive and accurate means of identifying arterial injury, although it is not perfect. Arteriographic diagnosis is based on arrest, or irregularity, of a column of contrast material, or extravasation locally or into adjacent veins.[23] In Figure 14–4 is shown an arteriographic study in which almost no clinical signs of injury existed, yet a clear injury was present. Furthermore, arteriography may identify the presence, if not the exact anatomy, of an arteriovenous fistula. The presence of an arteriovenous fistula in a vascular viscus such as the liver, spleen, or, especially, the kidney may be identified without other major signs of injury by the unusually rapid filling of the major veins.[12]

DISTRIBUTION OF INJURIES

The distribution of major arterial injuries from both military and civilian sources is shown in Table 14–2. Apparent differences may be reconciled by recognizing that civilian figures tabulate all injuries, of which perhaps only one half were repaired; the military figures represent only major injuries that were repaired.

RESULTS OF INJURY

The overall mortality rate in civilian injuries is between 10 and 11 per cent. Roughly three fourths of the injuries are suitable for direct suture or resection and suture, and one sixth are treated by venous grafts. Only rarely is it necessary to use a prosthetic graft. Injuries to the aorta and its intrathoracic branches account for three fourths of the deaths in most series of arterial injury.[9, 30]

The majority of civilian wounds are the result of low-velocity missiles, knives, blunt trauma, or fracture fragments, whereas the majority of military wounds are caused by high-velocity missiles or shrapnel fragments.

MANAGEMENT OF ARTERIAL INJURIES

General Aspects

Most arterial wounds are associated with multiple injuries, and the overall care of the patient plays an important part in the manage-

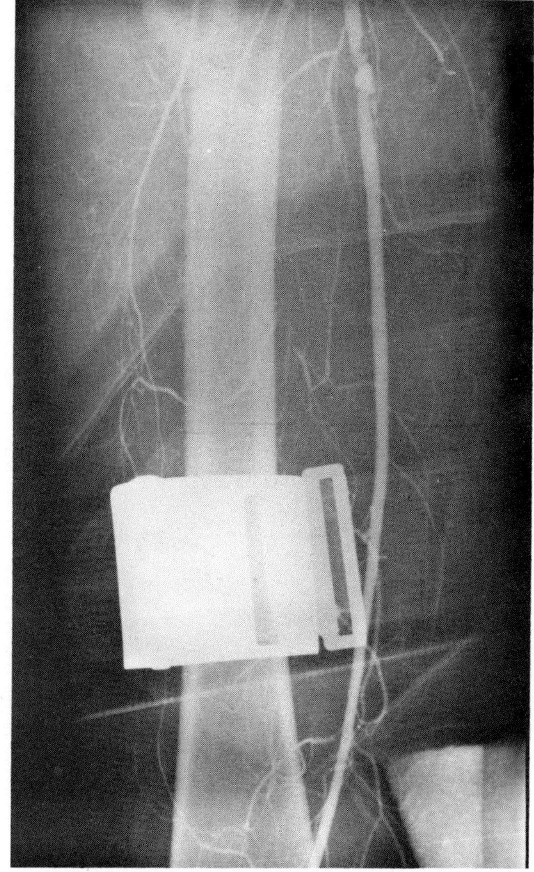

Figure 14–4. Arteriographic demonstration of femoral artery injury at site of femoral fracture. Lesion was suspected because of pulsating hematoma in presence of distal pulses.

ment. Prompt attention to full diagnosis, restoration of blood volume, assurance of continued ventilatory adequacy, splinting of wounds, and evaluation of the metabolic status of the patient are all important. The prompt establishment of therapeutic antibiotic levels is of special importance in the face of possible vascular reconstruction, especially in a contaminated field.

Certainly one of the highest priorities in the care of the injured patient is control of hemorrhage directed to the preservation of life. Later in order follows preservation of the limb, and last in immediate order of urgency is the restoration of complete normalcy to the limb. In other words, if ligation of an artery saves a life, and despite ligation, the limb lives but becomes ischemic on exercise, one can later consider the reconstruction to restore normal arterial flow.

The trained vascular surgeon is often tempted to proceed with technically feasible reconstructions in situations that are inappropriate. These will be reemphasized in later pages, but in brief they

Table 14–2. Anatomical Distribution of Arterial Injuries and Repairs

	CIVILIAN INJURIES (Combined from Perry et al.[30] and Drapanas et al.[9])		MILITARY REPAIRS (Rich and Hughes[33])	
	Number	*Per Cent*	*Number*	*Per Cent*
Carotids				
Common	9	1.3	12	3.3
Internal	3	0.5	3	0.8
Innominate	1	0.2	–	–
Subclavian	39	5.8	1	0.3
Axillary	50	7.5	22	6.0
Brachial	117	17.5	103	28.2
Radial or ulnar	143	21.4	–	–
Aorta	49	7.3	3	0.8
Hepatic, Superior mesenteric	4	0.7	–	–
Renal	6	0.9	1	0.3
Iliac	47	7.0	3	0.8
Common femoral	18	2.7	24	6.6
Superficial femoral	132	19.8	116	31.8
Popliteals	31	4.6	77	21.1
Tibials	19	2.8	–	–
	668	100.0	365	100.0

are situations where immediate or even ultimate reconstruction is not truly necessary, where sepsis and the need for a prosthesis make repair unduly hazardous, and where extensive injuries to other soft tissues make vascular repair fruitless.[32, 38]

All classical rules concerning open wounds apply to the care of contaminated wounds involving major vessels: adequate and accurate debridement, coverage of vital nerves, tendons, and vessels, and delayed primary closure of the skin. Whenever the surgeon is faced with a damaged artery in such a potentially contaminated wound, he is also faced with the specter of sepsis in the vascular repair. The late breakdown of many arterial wounds led Brisbin and his associates[5] to recommend that primary repair of wounds involving the following structures *not* be done:

(1) brachial artery between the profunda brachialis and the collaterals at the elbow;

(2) radial or ulnar artery *alone* at any level;

(3) profunda femoris;

(4) superficial femoral artery proximal to the geniculars;

(5) posterior tibial, anterior tibial, or the peroneal artery alone at any level.

The arterial disruptions that resulted in the publication of their recommendations were, to be sure, associated with other technical errors, but the argument must be given some validity. If ligation alone can be performed in a vessel without remarkable immediate threat to limb salvage, then it is hard to condone the extra hazards attendant upon repair, especially when the vessels under consideration are of such a size that one might not anticipate a high rate of lasting success.

In this respect it might be worth comparing the presumed risks of gangrene following simple ligation at several levels (Table 14–3). The figures of Beebe and DeBakey[2] are probably representative of the more serious major arterial injuries that, because of quick transportation to surgical care and speedy resuscitation, survived but were subjected to amputation.

Lateral suture without patching or end-to-end anastomoses can be performed with a high rate of success in almost any wound, provided that the suture line is not under tension and that it can be covered with viable tissue. Monofilamentous, nonabsorbable suture is preferred for the repair. When direct repair cannot be performed, then one must choose between no repair and placement of some kind of a graft. Use of autologous vein or artery in a contaminated wound is possible but hazardous. It has been suggested that, in the face of extensive tissue destruction and inability to cover a vein graft, stored porcine skin grafts can be used safely as temporary biological cover.[22] This procedure should be used only under the most unusual circumstances. The placement of bovine carotid or plastic prostheses in such a wound should be done only to save a life, for the possible complications if infection supervenes can be life-threatening. In the presence of any significant gross contamination, it is advisable to use not only coverage with systemic antibiotics, but also local antibiotic therapy by way of catheter irrigations.

There are circumstances, however, when a defect in a vessel must be bridged to restore the limb to normalcy, when one may elect to defer definitive repair to a later date when the infection is under control.

Table 14–3.   Risk of Ligation of an Artery*

| | RISK PER AUTHOR | | | |
SITE OF LIGATION	*Wolff*	*Hendrich*	*Makins*	*Beebe and DeBakey[2]*
Subclavian	4.8	9.7	–	28.6
Axillary	15.0	9.0		43.2
Common brachial	4.0	3.1		55.7
Brachial				25.8
Common iliac	50	100		53.8
External iliac	11.2	13.4	16.6	46.7
Common femoral	25.0	21.8	25.9	81.1
Superficial femoral	12.7	10.4	14.1	54.8
Popliteal	14.9	37.2	37.5	72.5

*Modified After Key[20] and Beebe and DeBakey.[2] All figures in percentages.

Lavenson and associates[21] reported use of the Doppler sensor, and stated this principle: if a Doppler tone can be heard in an extremity in which no repair is being considered, the extremity probably will survive without reconstruction. Definitive repair can then follow at a more appropriate time. Conversely, if no Doppler tone can be heard, amputation will most likely be necessary.[21]

This same principle can be applied to the circumstances in which a primary repair has broken down. After ligation of a disrupted vessel, the presence of a Doppler tone suggests that the limb will survive; absence of a Doppler tone foretells amputation, or a more exotic form of reconstruction may be considered. Some form of an extra-anatomic bypass can be considered if it can be done through clean fields. Even a precarious and unlikely bypass that preserves an extremity until collaterals develop and/or healing of the primary infection occurs may allow a satisfactory later reconstruction. Repeated attempts to salvage an infected reconstruction in the same operative field are contraindicated.

Use of sympathectomy in primary wounds is controversial, although Williams and associates[40] have brought forward evidence to support its use. There may be more value in chemical sympathetic blockade in the presence of venous injury. It is presumed that secondary venous dilatation allows better venous decompression and development of venous collaterals.[41]

Exposure of an arterial injury is best obtained through the classical elective incisions, assuring thus that proximal and distal control of the vessel can be acquired, so as to work in a dry field. Tourniquets, if present, should be removed as soon as they are found, and pressure used to control the bleeding. During the early stages of dissection, temporary use of a pneumatic tourniquet can be helpful.

Once hemorrhage is under control, systemic (intravenous) heparinization can be performed; distal heparinization is at times useful, but anticoagulants should not be carried through the postoperative period. Use of a Fogarty catheter to remove clots from both the distal arterial and venous systems is advised. This is particularly true of the major injuries to the femoral and iliac regions commonly associated with significant morbidity from the reflux of stagnant venous blood. Stallone and associates[36] once advocated a thorough rinsing through of the arterial and venous circulation, and careful venous embolectomy before final restoration of the flow. Venous clots should be expected when there is an unusually long delay between injury and operation.

Diagnosis of an arteriovenous fistula requires prompt attention. Classical teachings that one should defer operation until a collateral circulation had developed are hazardous; such circulation may *never* develop, and irreversible ischemia may follow instead.[38]

Major venous injuries should be repaired.[14] In many anatomical circumstances lateral repair is sufficient, but in the popliteal area, replacement of the popliteal vein with vein from the saphenous system of the contralateral extremity is urgent.[32, 37]

CONSIDERATION OF SPECIAL AREAS

Neck

Most authors divide injuries of the neck into those above and those below a line drawn horizontally through the ramus of the mandible. Arteriography is most helpful in the upper lesions because of the difficulty in recognizing changes in distal pulses.[11] Most patients with penetrating wounds require operation because of a massive hematoma or exsanguination. In the series described by Reul and associates[31] of 81 arterial wounds the internal carotid artery was wounded in only 10 instances; three fourths of the wounds involved the common carotid artery. Injury to other structures in the neck was common.[31]

Ligation instead of repair was advocated by Cohen and his associates[8] if a significant neurologic deficit existed preoperatively in war wounds. Reul, however, on the basis of 72 civilian carotid injuries, recommended repair, either by lateral suture, patch, end-to-end anastomosis, or graft interposition. Only three of 42 surviving patients who were normal on admission developed neurologic deficits, whereas only two of 14 patients who had deficits on admission were relieved of their deficit. The mortality in this series was 22 per cent: seven patients died of irreversible neurologic damage that existed on admission, four exsanguinated, four died of associated injury, and only one patient died of a complicating postoperative hemorrhage.[31]

No benefit was seen from the use of an internal shunt. The extent of injury and the preoperative deficit seemed to be most important in determining the outcome.[31]

Blunt trauma or trauma brought about by sudden acute and extreme motion of the head or the shoulders may result in an intimal injury to the high internal carotid artery opposite the body of the second cervical vertebra (Figs. 14–2 and 14–3).[24]

The supraorbital Doppler test introduced by Brockenbaugh[6] may be very useful in defining an acute reduction of internal carotid flow, especially in blunt trauma.[24, 25] This test uses the presence of a signal in the supraorbital artery as a criterion of internal carotid flow. If pressure is made on the superficial temporal arteries, normal internal carotid arteries will supply an increased flow and an augmentation of the Doppler tone in the supraorbital branch. If, however, flow is seriously restricted by any lesion in the internal carotid system, pressure on the superficial temporal artery causes a reduction in the signal.

Ocular plethysmography[1] or ocular dynamography,[19] if available, may indicate an encroachment on the carotid arterial system.

A 35-year-old woman sustained a "minor" closed injury to her neck, experiencing momentary confusion, then headache, and subsequent progressive neurologic deterioration. The Doppler supraorbital test was positive, and an arteriogram showed the typical picture shown in Figure 14–2, in which stenosis and false aneurysm formation are present because of the injury to the intima at the level of the body of the second cervical vertebra.

Surgical approach to the high carotid may be facilitated slightly by detaching the sternocleidomastoid muscle from the mastoid process.

If the injury lies in the segment of the neck between the clavicles and the mandible, exploration is usually carried out without arteriography because of the importance of not overlooking injuries to the other critical soft tissue organs in the neck.[11, 31] A major hematoma often makes operation mandatory.

Subclavian and Innominate Artery

Below the clavicles, injuries to the great vessels are best diagnosed by clinical signs of hemorrhage or distortion of anatomy on x-ray films. Because of the difficulty in obtaining prompt and accurate arteriographic studies in this anatomical area, overall clinical signs as well as simple local signs on x-ray film, in addition to a very suspicious attitude, are helpful in choosing patients for exploration.[11, 31]

In Flint and associates'[11] review of 146 patients with 206 injuries to the base of the neck, 49 per cent had arterial injuries but only 32 per cent had significant signs. Liberal indications for exploration must be followed in order to avoid missing some life-threatening injuries.[11] The approach of Brawley and associates[3] is similar. With a wound in this anatomic area, the patient receives highest priority for care until a vascular lesion either is proved by exploration or by arteriography *and* exploration, or is disproved by arteriography.

Flint and his associates[11] presented a useful discussion of incisions to manage these wounds. Horizontal incisions at the level of the clavicle, with resection of its medial portion, allow control of most subclavian wounds and some injuries of the innominate artery. This incision is quickly and easily extended by a median sternotomy or even by a flap composed of the proximal three ribs on either side if more proximal exposure is needed. Furious and exsanguinating hemorrhage into the chest may require initial control via an initial anterolateral thoracotomy in the third or fourth interspace.[11]

Brawley's incisions are slightly different: a median sternotomy extended into the right supraclavicular area allows excellent exposure of the right-sided vessels. On either side exposure and control of intrapleural hemorrhage may be achieved by third intercostal space thoracotomy, with pressure applied until the injured artery is exposed. Bleeding from the left subclavian artery is controlled this way, but definitive exposure by the supraclavicular route without sternotomy may be more satisfactory for *distal* left subclavian lesions.[3]

Thoracic Aorta

These include deceleration injuries described in the chapter on aneurysms. Penetrating injuries of the thoracic aorta almost inevitably bleed freely into one or another pleural cavities, and thus are not restricted by any tamponade. For this reason, hemorrhage is usually massive, and only a few injuries reach the hands of the surgeon. Definitive repair of those injuries that do reach the surgeon may require crossclamping of the aorta and endangers distal viscera and spinal cord injury. Unless a partial-occlusion clamp can be used, some kind of a makeshift shunt should be arranged.

Abdominal Injuries

Such wounds are usually associated with other major visceral injuries, but the immediate problem is control of hemorrhage. The discussion by Buscaglia and associates[7] describes the most expeditious approach to such injuries. If there is an injury of the suprarenal aorta, left renal artery, superior mesenteric artery, or celiac axis, the area is exposed by mobilizing the splenic flexure and left colon, spleen, and tail of the pancreas, to the right. If, on the other hand, the injury is expected to be of the inferior vena cava, the renal veins, or the portal vein, the exposure is obtained by means of Kocher's maneuver, mobilizing the duodenum and hepatic flexure forward and to the left.

Injuries to the cava in the intrahepatic or immediate infrahepatic area are controversial. A hematoma in this area that is not pulsatile or expanding may often be left alone, with satisfactory healing. Opening the hematoma may require suture of the cava in areas most difficult to expose, and at times require excision of the caudate lobe. However, complete exposure of the retroperitoneal duodenum to ensure its freedom from injury may demand incising such a hematoma. Control of bleeding from such an inaccessible portion of the cava may be assisted by placement of an intracaval balloon or a catheter-shunt that can have ligatures above and below the liver to allow continued flow through the catheter and maintain venous return to the heart.

Injuries to the great vessels in the lower abdomen can be exposed, by the usual approach, via the incision at the root of the mesentery.

Upper Extremity Injuries

Injuries to the axillary and brachial arteries often are associated with very damaging nerve injuries. There has been criticism of attempts to repair the brachial artery between the profunda brachialis and the collaterals of the elbow, and certainly isolated injuries of the radial or ulnar vessels do not usually demand repair.[5]

Longitudinal incisions along the course of the vessel are excellent in the upper arm; however, it may be desirable to gain control of the subclavian above the clavicle in axillary injuries in order to have a clear field. Full axillary exposure should be obtained, even dividing and resuturing the attachment of the pectoralis major.[3]

The axillary and brachial arteries are the sites of serious iatrogenic injuries, acquired either during open left heart catheterization or percutaneous arterial puncture for the modified Seldinger arteriographic techniques.[4, 26, 28] These injuries may result in hemorrhage with extensive extravasation, false aneurysm, or thrombosis. Thrombosis may occur because of embolization from a fibrin cuff on the catheter, excessive trauma to the vessel (including formation of a distal intimal flap), or thrombosis from a stenosing repair. Blind percutaneous punctures often have associated injuries to adjacent nerves.[26]

Early and accurate repair of these injuries is urged. The loss of a peripheral pulse without other signs of serious ischemia should ordinarily be sufficient indication for repair, for many extremities become symptomatic with use, and late repair is more complicated. Loss of a pulse must be assumed to be due to thrombosis and not spasm.[26, 38]

The identification of "spasm" at operation is an indication for careful arteriotomy to be sure that there is no intimal flap obstructing flow. Hydraulic dilatation is then in order, and operative arteriography is a must if so-called spasm persists.[34] Local vasodilators (papaverine, Priscoline) may be useful.

Initial repair of open catheterizations should be with fine, everting, interrupted mattress sutures after careful use of the Fogarty catheter, both proximally and distally.

Lower Extremity Injuries

The key to repair of femoropopliteal injuries is the use of the optimal elective incisions for control and exposure of the artery before debridement is attempted.[32, 33, 35, 37] In the "crowded" areas of the groin and the popliteal space, associated major nerve and vein injuries are common.

The thigh is prone to major wounds with great loss of tissue and serious contamination. Careful debridement, without skimping to gain coverage, is essential, as is coverage of the vascular repair. Lateral repairs or even replacement of the femoral vein are advised; ligation is believed to reduce the femoral arterial flow during the acute stages of recovery.[41]

The popliteal artery is subjected to injury in dislocations of the knees. Popliteal artery injury still results in amputation in about 35 per cent of war wounds. This has been shown to be due, in part, to associated venous injuries, and for this reason, replacement of an injured popliteal vein which is not suitable for lateral repair is urged. Both the artery and vein should be repaired with saphenous vein from the *opposite extremity* or with a vein from the arm. Repair of the vein results in very little post-phlebitic complications, whereas ligation is followed by serious consequences.[32, 37] Even though the vein may undergo thrombosis in four or five days, collaterals will develop in that period of time but not rapidly enough to drain a leg subjected to acute vein interruption.

Isolated repair of either a posterior tibial or anterior tibial artery is not often necessary. It can be accomplished in a particularly clean wound.[16] Most injuries of sufficient gravity to have destroyed both arteries will often cause sufficient other associated damage to veins and to nervous and skeletal structures that repair instead of amputation under these circumstances must be seriously considered. Rich[32] and Whelan[38] have both cited cases of questionable repairs, with complications of sepsis and hemorrhage, leading to ultimate amputation and even death, that make caution in the technical exercises most urgent.

FASCIOTOMY

Prolonged ischemia of either extremity, but especially of the lower leg, may result in dramatic edema in myofascial compartments, sufficient, in fact, to obstruct arterial inflow and result in serious nerve and muscle necrosis. Early recognition and treatment by fasciotomy involving all three compartments of the lower leg is essential. Although simple fascial incision, done blindly through a small skin incision, is often advocated, such a limited procedure may needlessly injure vessels and nerves; furthermore, the release of the fascia alone may not be adequate. Full-length incisions through skin and fascia are indicated. When fasciotomy is performed early, it is sometimes possible to achieve delayed primary closure of the skin in three or four days.[29] In any event, the fasciotomy scars are a good bargain in return for freedom from irretrievable nerve and muscle injury. Twenty per cent of extremity wounds require fasciotomy and at least one half of popliteal injuries do so.

A rare but dramatic injury occurs when the femoral artery is mistaken for the varicose saphenous vein and is stripped from the leg. Prompt recognition may allow restoration of flow with composite grafts to the lower leg, since such a stripping can rarely be carried below the knee, but most of these injuries have in the past resulted in amputation.[10]

LATE RESULTS OF VASCULAR REPAIR

A certain number of acute arterial repairs will fail early. In civilian injuries the figure is reported at between 10 and 20 per cent, of which most can be reoperated upon successfully.[9, 30] A certain number of arterial injuries, either repaired or not repaired, will result in later complications: these will be either occlusion or aneurysm formation, either of which can be treated by techniques much as described for other lesions. At times an arteriovenous fistula will not be recognized until long after the initial injury.

Associated venous thrombosis with or without primary venous injury may yield chronic edema in the classical postphlebitic pattern. Treatment consists of elevation, elastic support, and occasional surgical intervention for the treatment of postphlebitic ulceration.

One of the most frustrating late results of vascular injury with or without nerve injury is the syndrome of causalgia. This is a disabling burning pain associated with extreme degrees of vasospasm. The extremity must be protected from drafts or touch. Patients if neglected often become addicted or suicidal.

Treatment consists of initial attempts at sympathetic denervation, and if this does not relieve the pain, further destructive neurosurgical procedures such as spinothalamic tractotomy are indicated.

DRUG INJURIES

Therapeutic injections of drugs or the injection of drugs by drug addicts often result in serious peripheral injuries when inadvertent injection into an artery occurs. The arteries are often of small caliber, and the degree of local injury and chemical thrombosis results in an arterial wound that cannot be salvaged. In addition, there often is extensive edema due to venous thrombosis, with circulatory stasis in the tissues of the digits. Severe pain is characteristic. Heparin and dextran may limit the propagation of thrombosis, and dexamethasone (Decadron) together with elevation and immobilization in the position of function may alleviate the edema. Fasciotomy should be considered but is rarely applicable, since the major lesions occur at such a peripheral level.[13, 27]

Maxwell and associates noted that the upper extremity tolerated the drug injections better than the lower. They also noted a high percentage of candidal infections in the form of endocarditis and mycotic abscesses.[27]

REFERENCES

1. Barker, W. F., in discussion of Thomas, G. I., Spencer, M. P., Edmark, K. W., Jones, T. W., and Stavney, L. S.: Non-invasive carotid bifurcation mapping: its relationship to carotid surgery. Am. J. Surg. *128*:168, 1974.
2. Beebe, G. W., and DeBakey, M. E.: *Battle Casualties.* Springfield, Charles C Thomas, 1952.
3. Brawley, R. K., Murray, G. F., Crisler, C., and Cameron, J. L.: Management of wounds of the innominate subclavian and axillary blood vessels. Surg. Gynec. Obstet. *131*:1130, 1970.
4. Brener, B. J., and Couch, N. P.: Peripheral arterial complications of left heart catheterization and their management. Am. J. Surg. *125*:521, 1973.
5. Brisbin, R. L., Geib, P. O., and Eiseman, B.: Secondary disruption of vascular repair following war wounds. Arch. Surg. 99:787, 1969.
6. Brockenbrough, E. C.: Screening for prevention of strokes: Use of a Doppler flowmeter. Beaverton, Oregon Parks Electronics, 1970.
7. Buscaglia, L. C., Blaisdell, F. W., and Lim, R. C.: Penetrating abdominal vascular injuries. Arch. Surg. 99:764, 1969.
8. Cohen, A., Brief, D., and Mathewson, C., Jr.: Carotid artery injuries. An analysis of eighty-five cases. Am. J. Surg. *120*:210, 1970.
9. Drapanas, T., Hewitt, R. L., Weichert, R. F. III, and Smith, A. D.: Civilian arterial injuries: A critical appraisal of three decades of management. Ann. Surg. *172*:351, 1970.
10. Eger, M., Golcmon, L., Torok, G., and Hirsch, M.: Inadvertent arterial stripping in the lower limb. Surgery 73:23, 1973.
11. Flint, L. M., Snyder, W. H., Perry, M. O., and Shires, G. T.: Management of major vascular injuries in the base of the neck. Arch. Surg. *106*:407, 1973.
12. Freeark, R.: Role of angiography in the management of multiple injuries. Surg. Gynec. Obstet. *128*:761, 1969.
13. Gaspar, M. R., and Hare, R. R.: Gangrene due to intra-arterial injection of drugs by drug addicts. Surgery 72:573, 1972.
14. Gaspar, M. R., and Treiman, R. L.: The management of injuries to major veins. Am. J. Surg. *100*:171, 1960.
15. Hare, R. R., and Gaspar, M. R.: The intimal flap. Arch. Surg. *102*:552, 1971.
16. Hartsuck, J. M., Moreland, H. J., and Williams, G. R.: Surgical management of vascular trauma distal to the popliteal artery. Arch. Surg. *105*:937, 1972.
17. Hughes, C. W.: Acute vascular trauma in Korean War casualties: An analysis of 180 cases. Surg. Gynec. Obstet. 99:91, 1954.

18. Jahnke, E. J., Jr., and Seeley, S. F.: Acute vascular injuries in the Korean War: An analysis of 77 consecutive cases. Ann. Surg. *138*:158, 1953.
19. Kartchner, M. M., McRae, L. P., and Morrison, F. D.: Noninvasive detection and evaluation of carotid occlusive disease. Arch. Surg. *106*:528, 1973.
20. Key, E.: Embolectomy on vessels of the extremities. Br. J. Surg. *24*:350, 1936.
21. Lavenson, G. S., Rich, N. M., and Strandness, D. E., Jr.: Ultrasonic flow detector value in combat vascular injuries. Arch. Surg. *103*:644, 1971.
22. Ledgerwood, A. M., and Lucas, C. E.: Massive thigh injuries with vascular disruption. Role of porcine skin grafting of exposed arterial vein grafts. Arch. Surg. *107*:201, 1973.
23. Lumpkin, M. B., Logan, W. D., Coures, C. M., and Howard, J. M.: Arteriography as an aid in the diagnosis and localization of acute arterial injuries. Ann. Surg. *147*:353, 1958.
24. Machleder, H. I., and Barker, W. F.: The stroke on the wrong side. Arch. Surg. *105*:943, 1972.
25. Machleder, H. I., Batzdorf, U., Benson, J., and Barker, W.: Abstracts of Papers, XI World Congress of the International Cardiovascular Society. Barcelona, Spain, p. 161, September 1973, "Closed Injury to the Cervical Carotid Artery."
26. Machleder, H. I., Sweeney, J. P., and Barker, W. F.: Pulseless arm after brachial-artery catheterization. Lancet *1*:407, 1972.
27. Maxwell, T. M., Olcott, C. IV, and Blaisdell, F. W.: Vascular complications of drug abuse. Arch. Surg. *105*:875, 1972.
28. Page, C. R., Hagood, C. O., Jr., and Kemmerer, W. T.: Management of postcatheterization: brachial artery thrombosis. Surgery 72:619, 1972.
29. Patman, R. D., and Thompson, J. E.: Fasciotomy in peripheral vascular surgery. Arch. Surg. *101*:663, 1970.
30. Perry, M. O., Thal, E. R., and Shires, G. I.: Management of arterial injuries. Ann. Surg. *173*:403, 1971.
31. Reul, G. J., Jr., Rubio, P. A., Beall, A. C., Jr., and Jordan, G. L., Jr.: Acute carotid artery injury: 25 years' experience. (In press.)
32. Rich, N. M.: Vascular Trauma. Presented as part of "Postgraduate Course in Vascular Surgery," Clinical Congress of the American College of Surgeons, Chicago, 1973.
33. Rich, N. M., and Hughes, C. W.: Vietnam vascular registry: A preliminary report. Surgery 65:218, 1969.
34. Spencer, F. C.: Vascular injury and arteriovenous fistula. *In* Sabiston, D. C. (ed.): *Cardiovascular Surgery.* New York, Harper and Row, 1972.
35. Spencer, F. C., and Grewe, R. B.: The management of arterial injuries in battle casualties. Ann. Surg. *141*:304, 1955.
36. Stallone, R. J., Blaisdell, F. W., Cafferata, H. T., and Levin, S. M.: Analysis of morbidity and mortality from arterial embolectomy. Surgery 65:207, 1969.
37. Sullivan, W. G., Thornton, F. H., Baker, L. H., LaPlante, E. S., and Cohen, A.: Early influence of popliteal vein repair in the treatment of popliteal vessel injuries. Am. J. Surg. *122*:528, 1971.
38. Whelan, T. C. Personal communication.
39. Williams, G. D.: Peripheral vascular trauma. Am. J. Surg. *116*:725, 1968.
40. Williams, G. D., Crumpler, J. B., and Campbell, G. S.: Effect of sympathectomy on the severely traumatized artery. Arch. Surg. *101*:704, 1970.
41. Wright, C. B., and Hobson, R. W.: Hemodynamic effects of femoral venous occlusion in the subhuman primate. Surgery 75:453, 1974.

Chapter Fifteen

EXTRINSIC ARTERIAL COMPRESSION SYNDROMES

J. H. GROLLMAN, Jr., M.D.
and WILEY F. BARKER, M.D.

Not all diseases involving the arterial system are caused by intrinsic disease. There is a broad range of extrinsic processes which can encroach on arteries and even cause primary arterial symptoms. In order to institute proper therapy it is important to recognize the varied presentations of the syndromes as well as their arteriographic appearances.

THORACIC OUTLET SYNDROME

The thoracic outlet syndrome comprises a broad group of syndromes involving compression of the neurovascular bed at various points of the thoracic outlet. The various subgroups in this syndrome complex include the scalenus anticus, costoclavicular, cervical rib, and pectoralis minor syndromes; the names are derived from the presumed cause of the obstruction (see Fig. 2–3). The differentiation of these syndromes can be very difficult in that the symptoms are quite similar. These symptoms are secondary to compression of the neurovascular bundle, resulting in paresthesias and claudication in the involved extremity, and are brought out by various positions which increase the compression, such as hyperabduction and hyperextension of the shoulder.

Neuromuscular symptoms may be present without vascular insufficiency, but the identification of encroachment on the neurovascular bundle by changes in peripheral pulses may lead to the diagnosis and treatment of the neurological entrapment.

Physical examination consists of the exhibition of diminished pulsations at the wrist by Adson's maneuver or other extreme postural changes.[1, 2, 31]

Adson's maneuver is performed with the patient upright, with his shoulders back and down, especially with the arm on the affected side pulled down.[1, 2] The patient inspires and holds a deep breath, turning his head toward the affected side, thus tightening the anterior scalene muscle and obliterating the pulse; turning the head away usually causes the pulse to return, although at times any sharp deviation from the neutral, straightforward position diminishes the pulsation.

A second maneuver consists in achieving pulse diminution by extreme "bracing" in the military posture. The artery and nerves

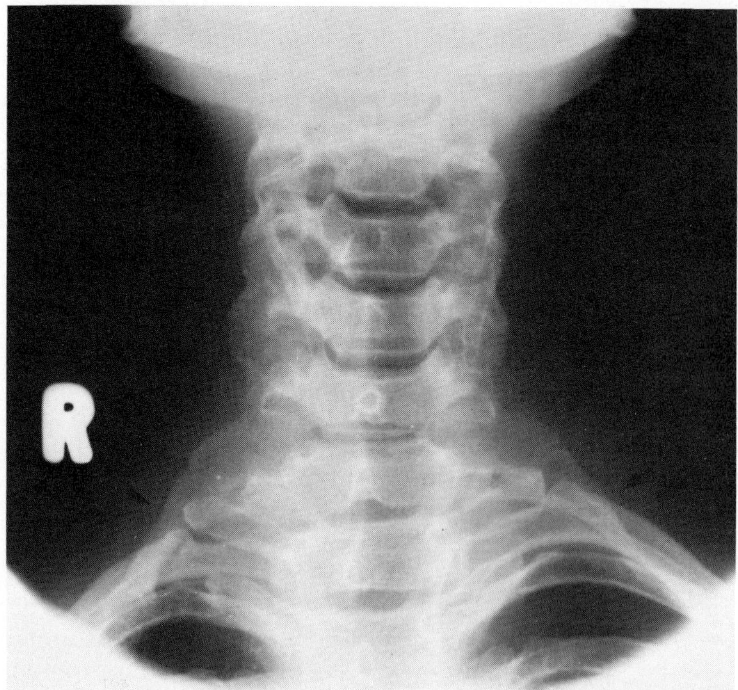

Figure 15–1. Bilateral cervical ribs (arrows). Thirty-eight-year-old female with bilateral thoracic outlet syndrome.

may be compressed by the scissors-like approximation of the clavicle and the first rib.[10]

A third series of maneuvers causes the neurovascular bundle to be stretched over the first rib under the coracoid process and tendon of the pectoralis minor, or stretched around the head of the sharply abducted humerus.[31] The arm is fully extended or abducted in the axis of the body (the Statue of Liberty position), and the pulse volume is evaluated. External rotation may exaggerate the changes. A variant of the postural encroachment may be identified with the arm directly outstretched away from the body, rotated externally and moved posteriorly—the same postural maneuver that causes anterior dislocation of the shoulder.

All these postural changes depend upon the identification of a change in pulse volume or the more gradual and less clear-cut onset of neurological symptoms. The use of a brachial segmental plethysmographic tracing in the several postures may identify pulse changes

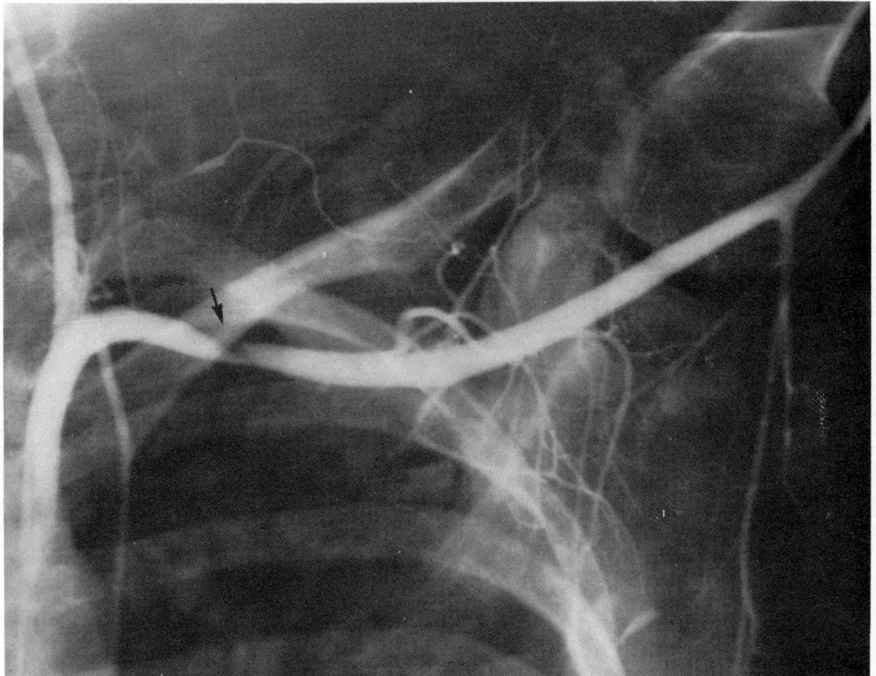

Figure 15–2. Extrinsic compression of left subclavian artery in region of costoclavicular space during hyperabduction of shoulder. Note the oblique defect coursing across the subclavian artery (arrow) typical of pressure by the scalenus anticus tendon. This 17-year-old female had symptoms of neurovascular compression on this side. Even though cervical ribs were present, surgical exploration revealed no relationship with the anomalous rib or a related cartilaginous band. The scalenus anticus and medius muscles were sectioned along with excision of the left first rib.

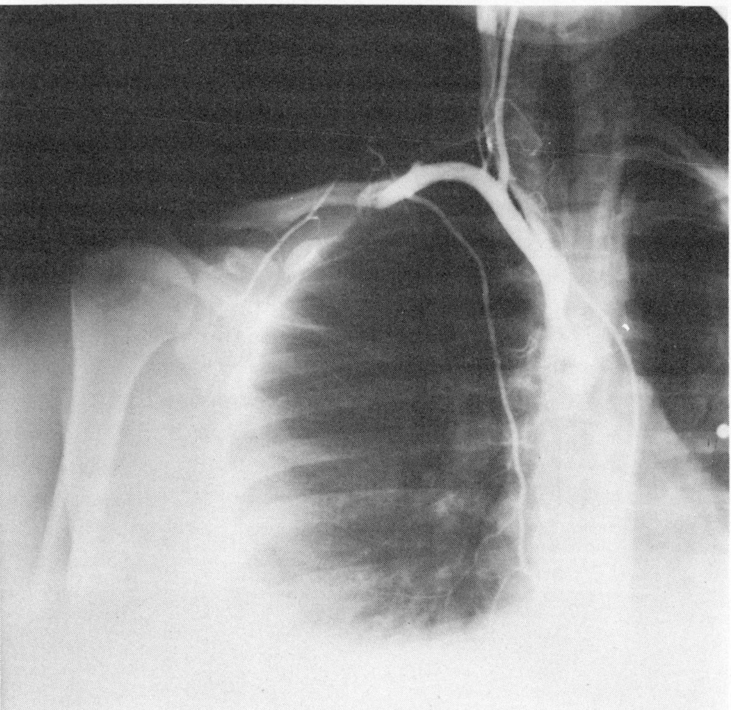

Figure 15–3. Occlusion of right subclavian artery in costoclavicular space with shoulders braced in a military position. The right subclavian artery presented a normal appearance in the neutral position. Twenty-six-year-old female with bilateral thoracic outlet syndrome. She subsequently underwent bilateral first rib resections and scalene muscle sections without relief of symptoms (see Fig. 15–4).

more exactly and more objectively, but radiologic studies provide exact anatomical localizations.

The diagnosis of the particular point of obstruction may best be made with radiographic studies in combination with the clinical examination.[19] Cervical spine and chest films should be examined for anomalous ribs (Fig. 15–1). Cervical spine views, especially obliques, are particularly advantageous in delineating small cervical ribs which may be completely overlooked on chest films.

Arteriography is best performed selectively, with a small catheter passed percutaneously by way of a femoral artery into the subclavian artery. Small amounts of contrast medium, in the range of 10 to 15 ml., should be injected both in the neutral position and in the position in which the radial pulse can be dampened. This may involve the performance of Adson's maneuver during the arteriogram or building the patient up on a roll of towels and hyperabducting the shoulders.

The characteristic radiologic findings of the scalenus anticus, costoclavicular, and cervical rib syndromes are narrowing or obstruction of the subclavial artery in the region of the intersection of the clavicle and the first rib anteriorly (Figs. 15–2 and 15–3). In the pectoralis minor syndrome the narrowing is seen as the subclavian artery passes under the tendon of the pectoralis minor muscle, near the coracoid process of the scapula (Fig. 15–4).

Several important points warrant emphasis. Asymptomatic patients may demonstrate stenosis in the region of the costoclavicular space (Fig. 15–5).[30] In addition, probably the most important aspect of the angiographic diagnosis is the demonstration of complicating factors such as aneurysm or thrombus formation with occlusion or peripheral embolism which in themselves are indications for surgical intervention (Fig. 15–6).[5, 19, 20] It should not be forgotten that occasionally tumors and clavicular fractures can simulate the syndrome.[6] Chest films and plain film evaluation of the cervical spine are imperative in distinguishing these possibilities.

Treatment of these extrinsic syndromes initially entails phy-

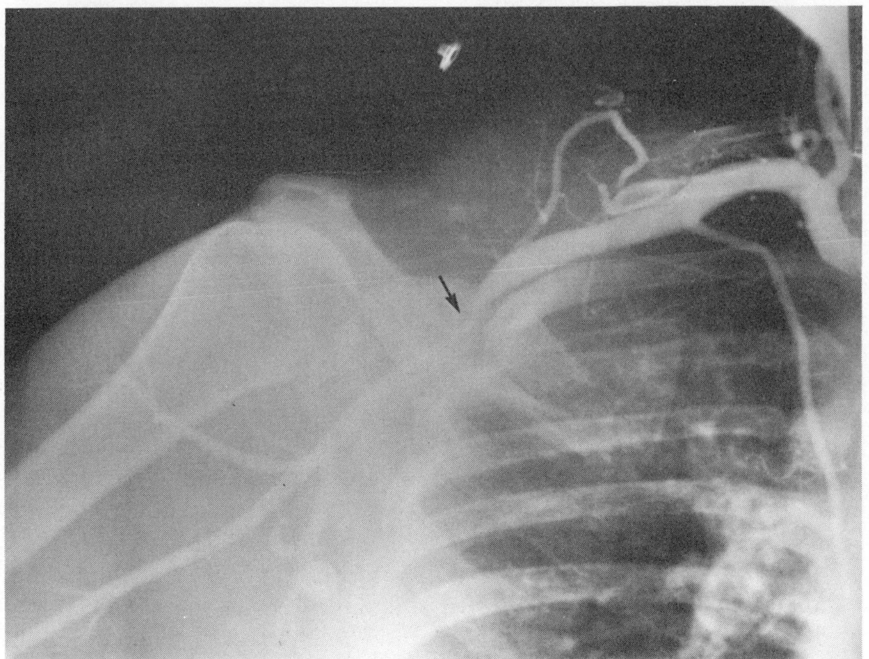

Figure 15–4. Same patient as in Figure 15–3. Postoperative arteriogram showing a stenosis (arrow) at the junction of the right subclavian and axillary arteries by the tendon of the pectoralis minor muscle brought out by abduction and bracing of the shoulder. This appearance was present bilaterally, with neutral arteriograms again showing no abnormalities. This abnormality was probably masked in prior studies by the proximal points of obstruction. Subsequent bilateral release of pectoralis minor tendon resulted in relief of symptoms.

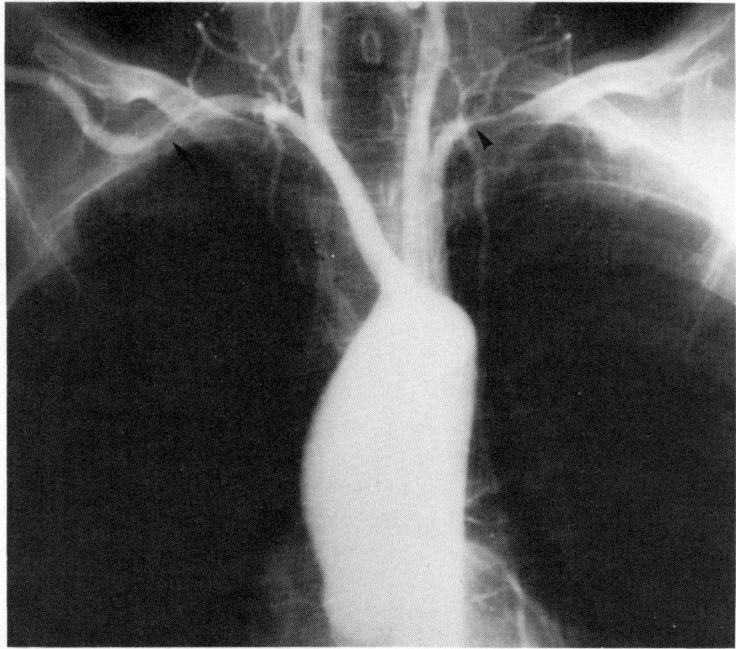

Figure 15–5. Incidental findings of a stenosis of the right subclavian and occlusion of the left subclavian artery (arrows) in the costoclavicular space during abduction of the shoulder during biplane thoracic aortography. The subclavian arteries had a normal appearance on a right posterior oblique aortogram with the arms along the patient's side. This 50-year-old female being studied for an aberrant right subclavian artery had no symptoms suggestive of a thoracic outlet syndrome.

siotherapy and postural improvement to relieve the abnormal encroachments.[9] If these simple measures are not successful, surgical intervention may be required. Initially, the surgical approach was a supraclavicular excision of the cervical rib. The importance of an abnormal scalenus anticus muscle even in the absence of the first of the cervical rib led to the introduction of simple scalenotomy. The surgical approach to scalenotomy is described in Chapter Six, where it is performed as part of the approach to the cervical sympathetic chain by the supraclavicular route. Although the cervical rib often need not be excised, it may be removed by this route with appropriate measures taken to protect the brachial plexus.

Clagett[4] and Roos[28] introduced the concept that the first rib is the offending structure common to all of the thoracic outlet syndromes. The removal of the first rib by the axillary route is made possible by the fact that a large number of these patients are asthenic.

With the patient in the lateral position and with the affected arm draped free, so that it can be retracted by an assistant who stands on a lift with a lock grip on the arm, a short incision is made just below

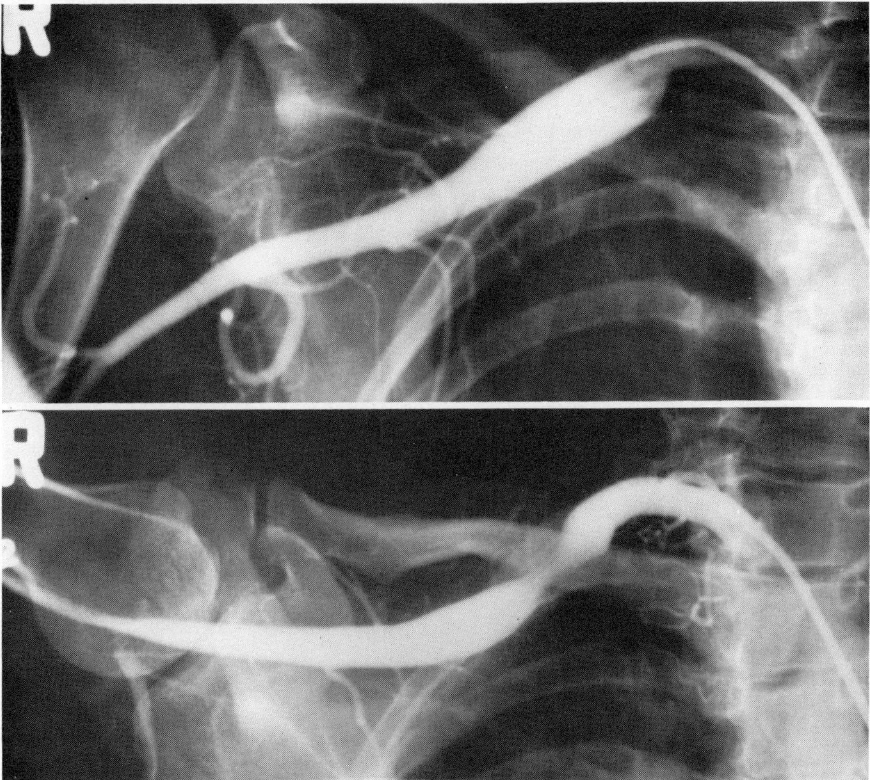

Figure 15–6. Fusiform dilatation of the right subclavian artery distal to compression at the thoracic outlet both in the neutral (top) and abducted (bottom) positions. In this 38-year-old female with symptoms of the thoracic outlet syndrome, a cervical rib was present which was found at surgery to be contributing to the compression. This rib was resected and the scalene muscles sectioned with relief of symptoms.

the axillary hairline between the pectoralis major and latissimus dorsi muscles. The dissection is carried down to the chest wall and then upward to the first rib. The neurovascular structures coursing over the rib are gently freed and retracted. If while working carefully above or below the rib one can begin to mobilize the pleura from under the rib, then by dissecting gently forward one can free the entire rib. If the first rib is divided anteriorly first, with traction outward and downward, the posterior portion can be divided with square-nosed shears or rongeurs at the very origin of the rib from the vertebral column. The axillary removal of the first rib, especially if it is necessary to combine it with removal of a cervical rib, is a far more difficult procedure in a heavily muscled individual than is the approach through the supraclavicular area.

Although the initial recommendations urged for the removal of the first rib by this route suggested a subperiosteal excision, the frequent recurrence of obstructive signs make it mandatory to remove the rib and its periosteum and muscular attachments. In unusual circumstances it may be necessary to remove the major portion of the second rib through this same approach. The key to this transaxillary approach is the vigorous upward and outward retraction of the arm by the assistant in whose charge the arm is given.

EXTRACRANIAL VERTEBRAL ARTERIAL COMPRESSION

Mechanical occlusion or narrowing of the vertebral artery resulting in symptoms of basilar artery insufficiency may be caused by impingement of cervical osteoarthritic spurs[12] (Fig. 15–7) and the

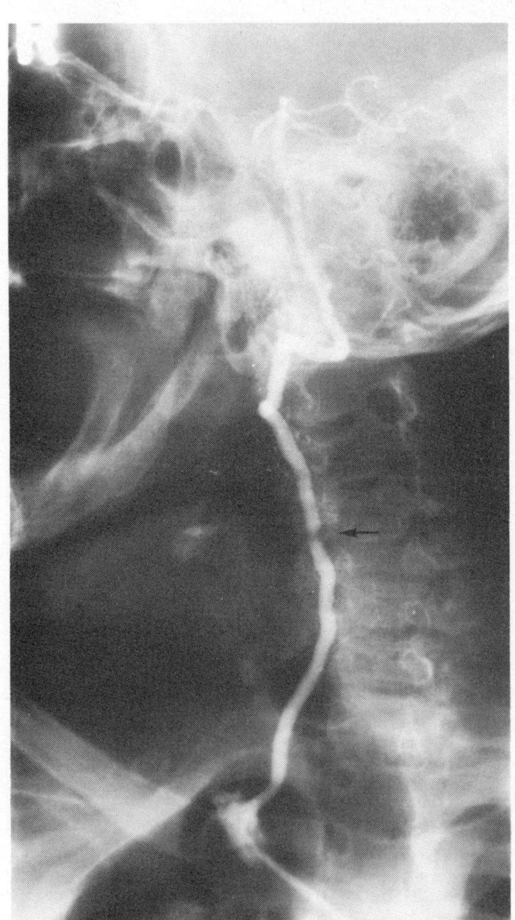

Figure 15–7. Osteoarthritic spur causing an extrinsic defect in the right vertebral artery at the C4–5 level (arrow). This patient noted dizziness and a feeling of faintness when turning his head sharply to the right. The aortic arch study demonstrated normal carotid origins and bifurcations but a hypoplastic left vertebral artery. The patient was advised not to turn his head to the right. (From Grollman, J. H., Jr., in *Selective Angiography*, W. Hanafee, Ed. Courtesy of Williams & Wilkins, Baltimore, Md.)

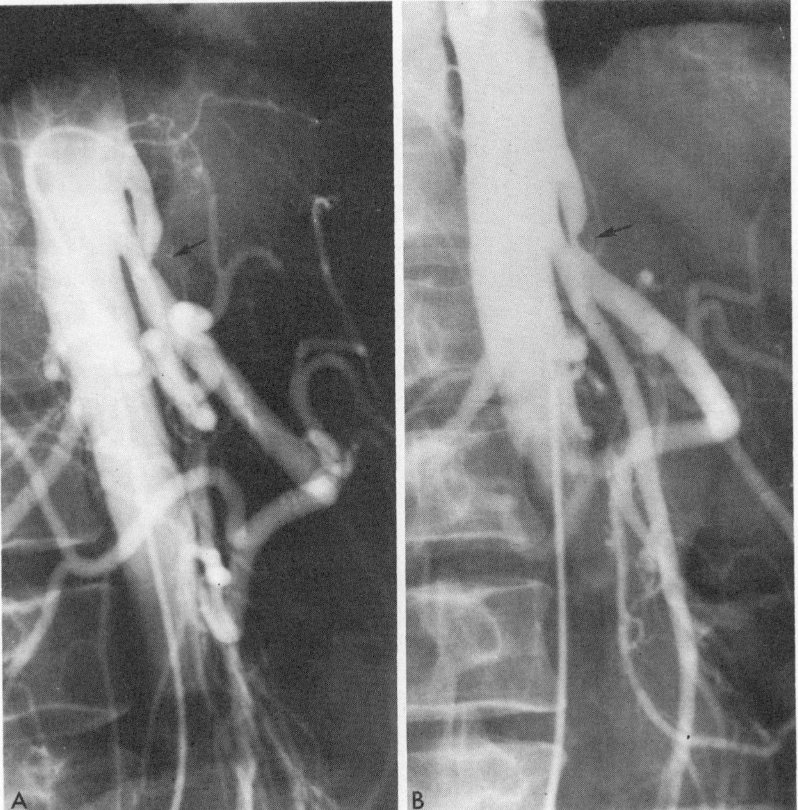

Figure 15–8.   Celiac axis compression by the median crural ligament of the diaphragm (arrows). This 49-year-old female complained of postprandial abdominal pain. *A,* Lateral aortogram. *B,* Steep left posterior oblique aortogram. Note that the latter projection really brings out the dorsal displacement of the celiac trunk to best advantage. Surgical therapy was refused by the patient.

compression action of certain adjacent cervical muscles, primarily the longus colli and scalene muscle groups, at the entrance of the vertebral artery into the sixth cervical transverse foramen.[15, 16] The diagnosis may be suggested when the symptoms are related to extreme positions of the head, particularly in the case of muscular compression, when turning the head to the contralateral side. Such maneuvers should be performed during angiography if symptoms of cerebral ischemia are considered to be related to head position.

Surgical approach to the intravertebral segment of the vertebral artery is not usually warranted without bilateral involvement: one adequate vertebral artery is usually sufficient to supply the basilar artery, especially if the carotid system and the circle of Willis are also adequate.

CELIAC AXIS COMPRESSION SYNDROME

Compression of the celiac trunk by the median arcuate ligament of the diaphragm may result in symptoms suggestive of intestinal angina. The etiology of the abdominal pain is unclear in that generally it is felt that two visceral arteries must be tightly stenosed in order to significantly compromise blood flow to the intestines.[7] There is, therefore, some doubt that the syndrome is due to stealing of blood from the mesenteric circulation by the celiac circulation. It has been suggested that symptoms are not due to ischemia but rather are on a neurogenic basis with compression of the celiac ganglion by the compressing ligament or associated fibrosis.[8, 13, 23]

The arteriographic diagnosis is best made on a lateral or a very steep left postero-oblique abdominal aortogram, with films exposed early during the injection because later the celiac trunk may be ob-

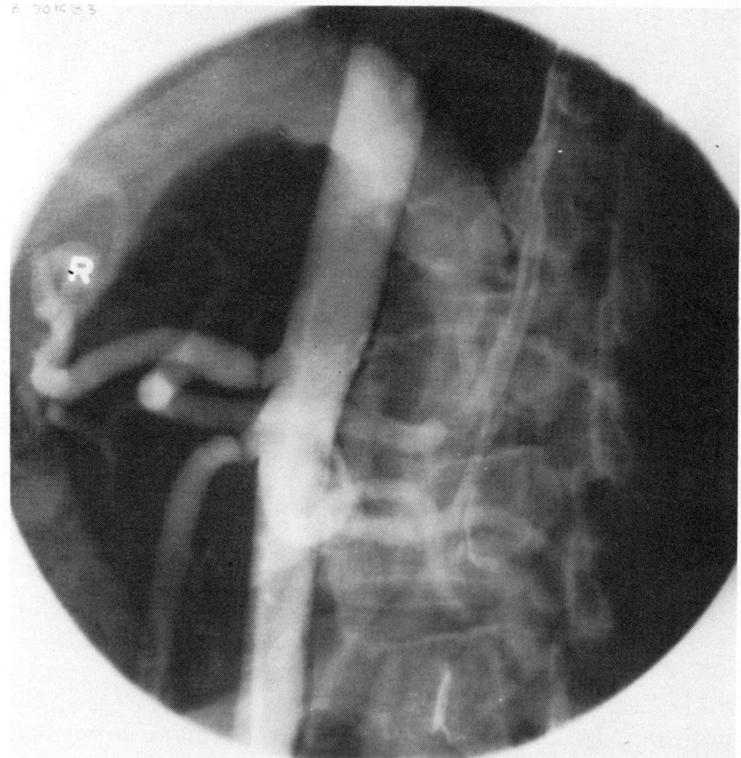

Figure 15–9.   Celiac axis and superior mesenteric artery compression by the median crural ligament in a patient with symptoms compatible with abdominal angina. In this case the compression is more prominent laterally than dorsally. (Courtesy of Robert Petersen, M.D.)

scured by overlapping branches. Dorsocaudal displacement of the celiac trunk with a smooth eccentric compression on its anterior wall will be seen (Fig. 15–8). Collateral flow to the celiac branches via enlarged pancreaticoduodenal, gastroduodenal and dorsal pancreatic arteries should be noted. The films should be obtained during expiration, as this will exaggerate the findings. A decrease in the degree of stenosis with inspiration has been described and is perhaps diagnostic of the abnormality.[26]

Rarely superior mesenteric (Fig. 15–9) and renal artery compression may be caused by extrinsic fibrotic bands from the diaphragm.[3, 21] In renal artery stenosis systemic hypertension may result.

Differential diagnosis includes arteriosclerosis, other primary arteriopathy and extrinsic neoplasm invading the arterial wall. Arteriosclerosis and fibromuscular dysplasia are usually circumferential, with no dorsal displacement of the vessel, however the latter is occasionally eccentric.[3] On the other hand, invasion of the wall by neoplasm may mimic this abnormality, but the involved area should not usually be limited to the celiac trunk but extend to other vessels as well. Inspiratory and expiratory lateral aortography may be very helpful in that a change in the degree of stenosis should not occur in these other possibilities (Fig. 15–10).

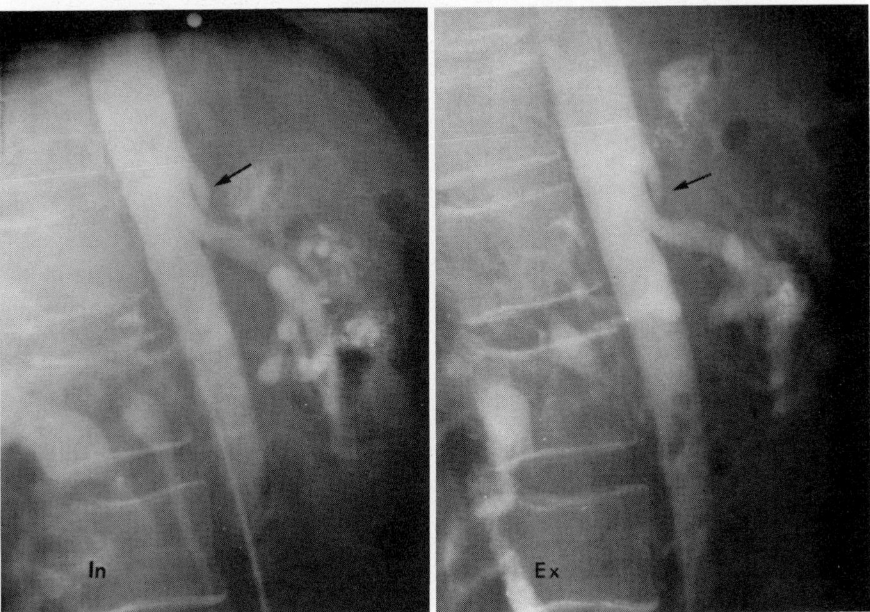

Figure 15–10. Occlusion of the celiac axis by pancreatic carcinoma with dorsal displacement resembling an extrinsic diaphragmatic band (arrows). The appearance did not change between inspiration (In) and expiration (Ex).

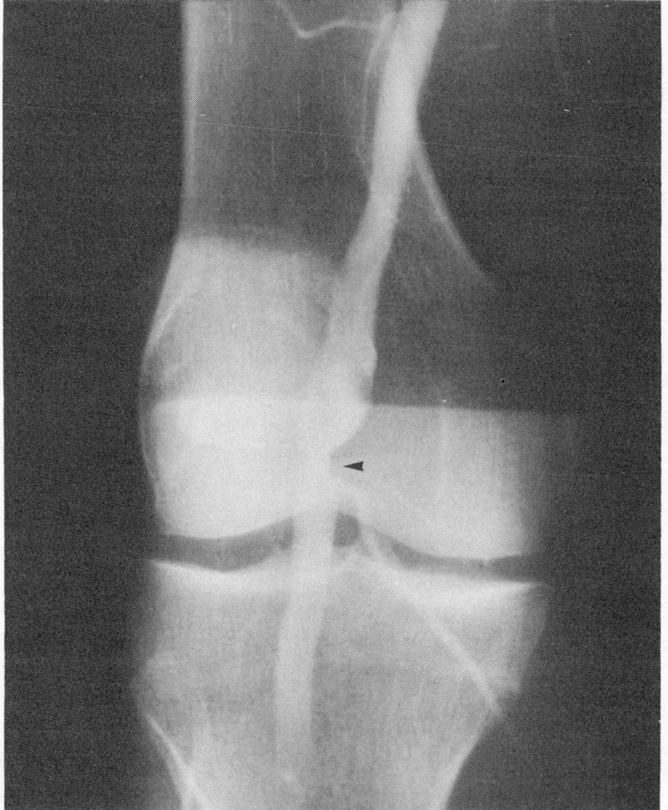

Figure 15–11. Popliteal artery entrapment by the medial head of the gastrocnemius muscle. The arrowhead indicates the point of compression. This patient complained of intermittent claudication of the right calf which was relieved by transection of compressing muscle bundle. (From Grollman, J. H., Jr., Lecky, J. W., and Rösch, J.: Miscellaneous diseases of arteries, or, all arterial lesions aren't fatty. Semin. Roentgen. 5:306, 1970.)

Surgical treatment of the occlusions and stenoses of the mesenteric vessels has been dealt with in the chapter on mesenteric vascular occlusions.

POPLITEAL ARTERY ENTRAPMENT SYNDROME

An unusual syndrome, occurring primarily but not solely in young male adults, consists of intermittent claudication due to entrapment of the popliteal artery by the medial head of the gastrocnemius muscle.[27]

The presence of an acute popliteal occlusion in a young patient who shows no other stigmata of primary vascular disease should suggest the diagnosis of extrinsic entrapment. Arteriographic examination of the contralateral extremity may show the same lesion and nearly assure the ipsilateral diagnosis. This abnormality can be recognized during arteriography by an unusual medial course of the popliteal artery or as an extrinsic band crossing obliquely (Fig. 15–11). Poststenotic dilatation and occlusion of the popliteal artery may occur.[22] Recognition of this anomaly is important, as surgical transsection of the medial head of the gastrocnemius muscle will be effective in relieving the symptoms and preventing subsequent thrombosis.[17, 29]

A variation of the syndrome was seen in a recent case in which the popliteal artery was encased by heavy fibrous fascia not related to a tendon (Fig. 15–12). In this patient, release of the popliteal artery resulted in complete remission of the symptoms.

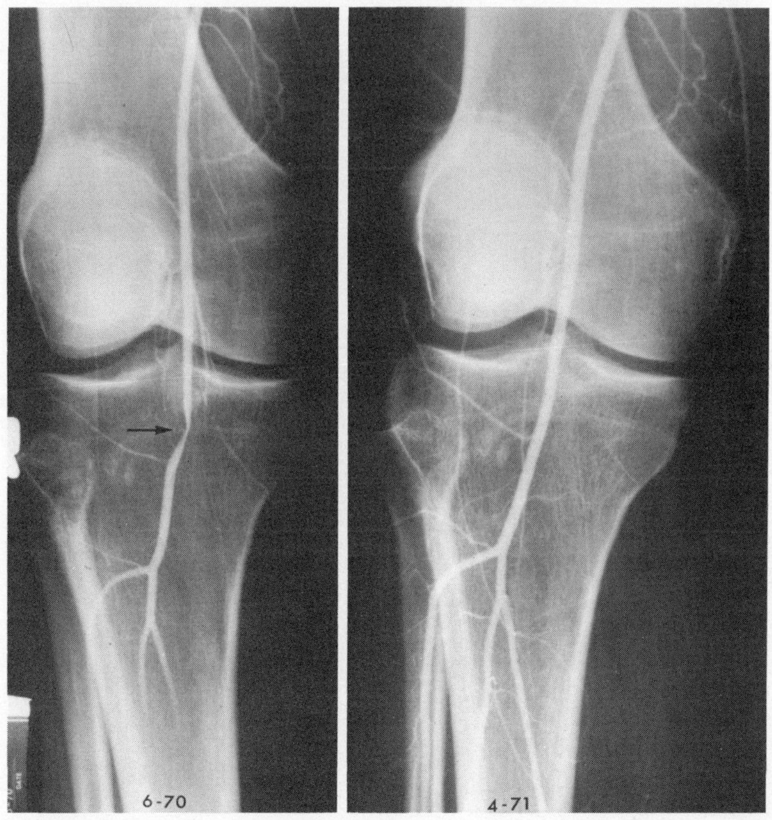

Figure 15–12. Popliteal artery entrapment by fibrous fascia. The medial defect (arrow) simulates entrapment by the medial head of the gastrocnemius muscle. Postoperatively, the symptoms of claudication were relieved and a femoral arteriogram was normal.

ANTERIOR TIBIAL COMPARTMENT SYNDROME

Swelling of the anterior tibial compartment muscles may cause ischemic symptoms and signs in the lower extremities. Trauma with acute hemorrhage in this region is the usual precipitating cause,[3, 24] but occasionally acute occlusion of the femoral or popliteal artery may lead to acute swelling in the anterior tibial compartment, resulting in a vicious circle of increasing ischemia.[14] Infrequently the syndrome may develop in patients without an acute precipitating cause, the basic problem seeming to be a tight anterior tibial compartment which, with heavy exercise, results in swelling and progressive arterial embarrassment.[18] Hughes et al. have reported a similar syndrome involving the personal (lateral) compartment,[14] and we have seen involvement of both the anterior and posterior peroneal compartments (Fig. 15–13).

The diagnosis is primarily clinical. Arteriography is necessary to

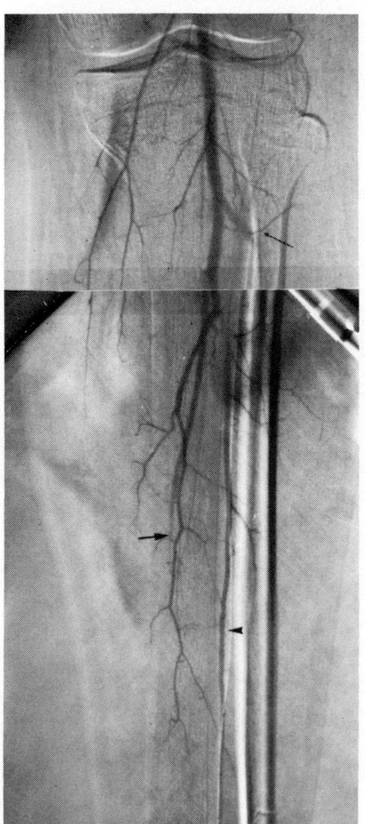

Figure 15–13. Anterior and posterior tibial compartment compression due to severe crush injury to the left leg. Serial filming over a 25-second interval demonstrated very slow flow in the anterior (small arrow) and posterior (large arrow) tibial arteries while the peroneal artery (arrowhead) fills normally. This patient's leg was edematous and pulseless. Emergency fasciotomy resulted in return of pulses.

show the site of occlusion, if existent, which generally will be at a more proximal level. In the absence of proximal occlusion, extreme slowing of the flow of contrast in the tibial and peroneal arteries will be noted (Fig. 15–13). Surgery is directed at treatment of the proximal obstruction and fasciotomy of the involved compartments.

MISCELLANEOUS COMPRESSION ARTERIOPATHIES

Trauma with hematoma formation, neoplasm, or inflammatory processes may secondarily compress arteries and result in ischemia at almost any place in the body. Usually the symptoms are secondary to the primary process, esepcially with neoplastic and inflammatory diseases. Therapy is, of course, generally directed to the primary process.

REFERENCES

1. Adson, A. W.: Surgical treatment for symptoms produced by cervical ribs and scalenus anticus muscle. Surg., Gynec. Obstet. 85:687, 1947.
2. Adson, A. W., and Coffey, J. R.: Cervical rib: method of anterior approach for relief of symptoms by division of scalenus anterior. Ann. Surg. 85:839, 1927.
3. Bron, K. M.: Splanchnic artery stenosis and occlusion: Incidence, arteriographic and clinical manifestations. Radiology 92:323, 1969.
4. Clagett, O. T.: Presidential address: Research and prosearch. J. Thor. Cardiov. Surg. 44:153, 1962.
5. DeVilliers, J. C.: A brachiocephalic vascular syndrome associated with cervical rib. Brit. Med. J. 2:140, 1966.
6. Dick, R.: Arteriography in neurovascular compression at the thoracic outlet, with special reference to embolic patterns. Am. J. Roentgenol. 110:141, 1970.
7. Drapanas, T., and Bron, K. M.: Stenosis of the celiac artery. Ann. Surg. 164:1085, 1966.
8. Dunbar, J. D., Molnar, W., Beman, F. F., and Marable, S. A.: Compression of the celiac trunk and abdominal angina. Amer. J. Roentgenol. 95:731, 1965.
9. Edwards, E. A.: Anatomic and clinical comments on shoulder girdle syndromes. In Barker, W. F.: Surgical Treatment of Peripheral Vascular Disease. New York, McGraw-Hill Book Co., 1962.
10. Falconer, M. A., and Weddell, G.: Costoclavicular compression of the subclavian artery and vein. Lancet 2:539, 1943.
11. Greenbaum, E. I., and O'Loughlin, B. J.: Value of delayed filming in the anterior tibial compartment syndrome secondary to trauma. Radiology 93:373, 1969.
12. Hardin, C. A.: Vertebral artery insufficiency produced by cervical osteoarthritic spurs. Arch. Surg. 90:629, 1965.
13. Harjola, P. T., and Lahtihara, A.: Celiac axis syndrome. Abdominal angina caused by external compression of the celiac artery. Am. J. Surg. 115:864, 1968.
14. Hughes, C. W., Lineberger, E. C., and Bowers, W. F.: Anterior tibial compartment syndrome: A plea for early surgical treatment. Milit. Med. 126:124, 1961.
15. Husni, E. A., Bell, H. S., and Storer, J.: Mechanical occlusion of the vertebral artery. J.A.M.A. 196:475, 1966.
16. Husni, E. A., and Storer, J.: Syndrome of mechanical occlusion of the vertebral artery. Angiology, 18:106, 1967.

17. Young, J. R., and Humphries, A. W.: Popliteal artery entrapment syndrome. Arch. Surg. *101*:771, 1970.
18. Kennelly, B. M., and Blumberg, L.: Bilateral anterior tibial claudication. Report of two cases in which the patients were cured by bilateral fasciotomy. J.A.M.A. *203*:487, 1968.
19. Lang, E. K.: Arteriographic diagnosis of the thoracic outlet syndrome. Radiology *84*:296, 1965.
20. Lang, E. K.: Neurovascular compression syndrome. Dis. Chest *50*:572, 1966.
21. Lecky, J.: Renal angiography. *Selective Angiography,* Waverly Press Inc., Baltimore, Maryland, 1972.
22. Love, J. W., and Whelan, T. J.: Popliteal artery entrapment syndrome. Am. J. Surg. *109*:620, 1965.
23. Marable, S. A., Molnar, W., and Beman, F. M.: Abdominal pain secondary to celiac axis compression. Am. J. Surg. *111*:493, 1966.
24. Moses, M., Ramon, Y., and Jahr, J.: The anterior tibial syndrome. J. Bone Joint Surg. *44A*:730, 1962.
25. Naffziger, H. C., and Grant, W. T.: Neuritis of the brachial plexus, mechanical origin; the scalenus syndrome. Surg. Gynec. Obstet. *67*:722, 1938.
26. Reuter, S. R.: Accentuation of celiac compression by median arcuate ligament of diaphragm during deep expiration. Radiology *98*:561, 1971.
27. Rich, N. M., and Hughes, C. W.: Popliteal artery and vein entrapment. Am. J. Surg. *113*:696, 1967.
28. Roos, D. V.: Transaxillary approach for first rib resection to relieve thoracic outlet syndrome. Ann. Surg. *163*:354, 1966.
29. Turner, G. R., Gosney, W. G., Ellingson, W., and Gaspar, M.: Popliteal artery entrapment syndrome. J.A.M.A. *208*:692, 1969.
30. Weibel, J., and Fields, W. S.: Arteriographic studies of thoracic outlet syndrome. Brit. J. Radiol. *40*:676, 1967.
31. Wright, I. S.: The neurovascular syndrome produced by hyperabduction of the arms. Am. Heart J. *29*:1, 1945.

Chapter Sixteen

ARTERIAL ANEURYSMS

The arterial aneurysm has been a challenge to the surgeon since at least the time of Antyllus who, in the second century, treated femoral aneurysms by proximal and distal ligation with evacuation of the clot. Loss of the leg from gangrene frequently followed this operation, however, leading John Hunter, in the eighteenth century, to ligate the femoral artery at a distance proximal to a popliteal aneurysm in order to try to preserve some collateral. Some aneurysms were cured, but some did thrombose. Sir Astley Cooper is credited with ligature of the abdominal aorta in 1817.

Matas[46] and Halsted[33] focused further attention on aneurysms. Colt, in 1903, recommended the introduction of wire in an attempt to achieve intraluminal thrombosis, according to Keen.[39] Blakemore and King advocated electrothermic wiring in 1938.[10] Bigger,[8] Elkin,[26] La Roque,[40] Matas,[47] and Vaughan[61] have described patients with aneurysms treated, with varying success, by ligation. No further significant advance in the management of major aneurysms occurred, however, until 1944, when Alexander and Byron[2] resected a thoracic aneurysm and oversewed the aorta. Gross,[32] in 1951, advocated arterial homografts in the treatment of coarctation, but Dubost et al.[21] introduced the modern treatment of aneurysms in 1952, when they resected an aneurysm and restored vascular continuity with arterial homografts. The vast experiences of surgeons such as Debakey et al.[18] and Szilagyi et al.[58] have since given important support to the development of the surgical treatment of aneurysms.

ETIOLOGIC CLASSIFICATION

In the current era, arteriosclerosis is the most common cause of aneurysm; trauma in its many forms is the next most common agent.

Sepsis as a primary cause is less frequent, although it may contribute to infection in the presence of injury. Syphilis, the great causative agent of ages past, rarely is seen as a responsible vector today. An unusual variant of the abdominal aortic aneurysm is the little understood inflammatory aneurysm described by Walker et al.[62]

Dissecting aneurysms as a result of cystic medial necrosis usually arise in the thoracic aorta but are seen in the classical infrarenal situation.

Pathogenesis

Two factors must be implicated in every aneurysm. The first is loss of structural integrity, whether it be due to trauma, atherosclerosis, sepsis, or iatrogenic mechanical pressure. Arterial hypertension is a common finding in many forms of aneurysmal disease, and controlled hypotension has been induced in the management of dissecting aneurysms.

Turbulence below an anatomical constriction has been implicated as a cause of aneurysm since Halsted's description.[33] Holman[34] was able to demonstrate the physical effects of turbulence with rubber tubing and prolonged flow past a subliminal constriction. The most common sites of arterial aneurysms are those below a minimal partial constriction: the preaortic fascia and aortic crus above the aortic aneurysm, the inguinal ligament above the femoral aneurysm, and the adductor hiatus above the popliteal aneurysm.

Undoubtedly, the basic size of the artery, as determined genetically, plays a role. Thomas[60] described the extreme of this variation. If one considers the effect of the law of LaPlace on the lateral tension of the artery, an artery one cm. in diameter, with a mean arterial pressure of 150 mm. Hg, has three times more tension on its wall than does an artery 0.5 cm. in diameter with a mean systolic pressure of 100 mm. Hg.

Eastcott suggested that aneurysmal dilatation may occur in spaces between nodes established by the patterns of resonance in the vibrating blood vessels, although these areas may also coincide with the areas between points of fixation by major branches.[22]

The multiplicity of aneurysms in a single patient speaks for a systemic factor in aneurysmal disease. Whychulis and associates[66] noted that 59 per cent of the patients in their series of popliteal aneurysms had a contralateral popliteal aneurysm. In our own experience, 18 patients who had an initial diagnosis of one peripheral aneurysm were found to have a total of 42 other aneurysms—aortic, popliteal, or femoral.[5]

Clinical Manifestations

The clinical manifestations are similar, but individual sites will show individual predilections. A pulsatile mass inevitably expands and finally either ruptures or undergoes intraluminal thrombosis, with subsequent distal embolism or thrombosis. During expansion, adjacent structures may be pressured, causing peripheral neuritic pains or venous occlusion and thrombosis. Expansion of the aneurysm may result in hemorrhage or dissection between structural layers. Atherosclerosis and hemorrhage may result in calcification, which is identifiable on radiologic examination (Fig. 16–1) but which is of little structural value in retaining the arterial pressure. Variations on these themes will be detailed in subsequent sections.

ARTERIOSCLEROTIC ABDOMINAL AORTIC ANEURYSM

Clinical Manifestations

The age at diagnosis of patients with aortic aneurysm is seen in Table 16–1. The percentage of patients suitable for operation proba-

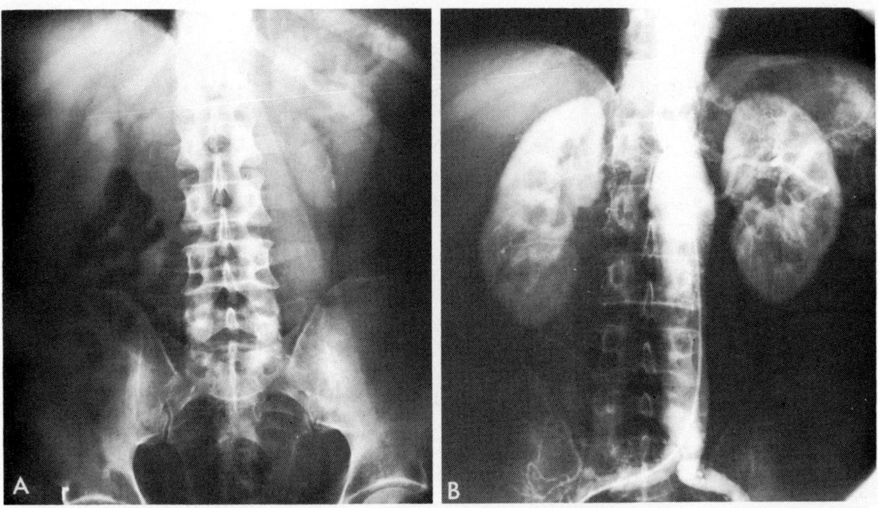

Figure 16–1. *A,* Plain film of patient with abdominal aneurysm. The calcification extends well to the left of the midline, a finding that might occur in tortuosity without dilatation. *B,* The arteriogram shows the true extent of the dilatation and the elongation.

Table 16–1. Age at Diagnosis of Patients
with Aortic Aneurysm

AGE AT DIAGNOSIS	PER CENT
Less than 50	3
51–60	23
61–70	48
71–80	24
81–	2

bly will be skewed toward a greater preponderance in the younger decades. Males are much more frequently involved than are females.

Patients who have aneurysmal disease are notorious for having involvement in many other systems. In Table 16–2 certain criteria from an earlier report of 100 patients from UCLA[12] are compared with more detailed criteria from a recent consecutive series of 99 patients.

These figures suggest that a larger percentage of our patients are being operated upon electively, but that this elective group is comprised of patients with greater risks as a consequence of their general status.

Diseases unrelated to the cardiovascular system are also encountered among these patients. Neoplasms in all sites, diverticulitis, gallbladder disease, and peptic ulcer all may be found, complicating the patient's course. Bouhoutsos and his colleagues[11] note the occurrence of peptic ulcer three to four times as frequently in aneurysmal disease as in stenotic arteriosclerosis.

Table 16–2. Aortic Aneurysm with other Systems Involved

	1955–1963	1970–1972
Total	100	99
Elective	66	73
Ruptured	34	26
Average age	65	67
Hypertension (>140 systolic or >90 diastolic)	37%	26%
MI (history)		25%*
MI (by EKG)		38%*
Congestive failure	10%	10%*
Angina pectoris		>10%*
Creatinine >2	not known	1%*
History of CVA		1%*
Claudication		8%*

*Percentages refer to the 73 unruptured patients only.

SYMPTOMS AND SIGNS

Most patients in the present series have had significant symptoms. To clarify the real risk of the ruptured aneurysm, the symptomatology has been classified as follows:

Asymptomatic: no pain or discomfort related to the aneurysm—45 patients

Symptomatic: acute or chronic pain believed due to the aneurysm but without true extravasation or rupture—28 patients

True extravasation or rupture—26 patients

The asymptomatic patients had either a palpable abdominal mass, a mass identified on x-ray studies, or an aneurysm found incidentally because of claudication. The increased risk of acute aortic thrombosis in the presence of claudication is described by Johnson and his associates.[36]

The diagnosis of an aortic aneurysm on physical examination alone depends upon the demonstration of a mass with pulsation demonstrable as distention. An elongated aorta without dilatation will manifest pulsation in only one direction. Pulsation felt in the midline well below the umbilicus is usually indicative of elongation concomitant with aneurysmal dilatation. A bruit may be heard, but this is not constant.

Concomitant occlusive disease of the common iliac system is present in approximately 10 per cent of patients. A much smaller number have occlusive disease of the renal or mesenteric system, but these lesions should be sought. Extra-abdominal lesions should also be considered. Stenosis of the carotid bifurcation is found in about five per cent. The femoral vessels frequently are atherosclerotic, but are often of large caliber and hence not obstructed. Femoral and/or popliteal aneurysms will be found in another five or 10 per cent of patients (Fig. 16–2).

The presence of the aneurysm may cause venous obstruction, especially on the left side. A left-sided or paired vena cava offers special surgical problems.[12] The intimate attachment of the duodenum may result in obstructive gastric symptoms of mild degree. Cayten and his associates[13] have described the problems of an associated horseshoe kidney.

LABORATORY DATA

Laboratory data are important in identifying the nature and extent of the lesion as well as associated disease.

Plain films of the abdomen and especially overexposed lateral views may show a rim of calcification (Fig. 16–1). If calcification is not easily seen, laminographic studies may help to identify an abdominal mass. Arteriography is useful, but the column of contrast

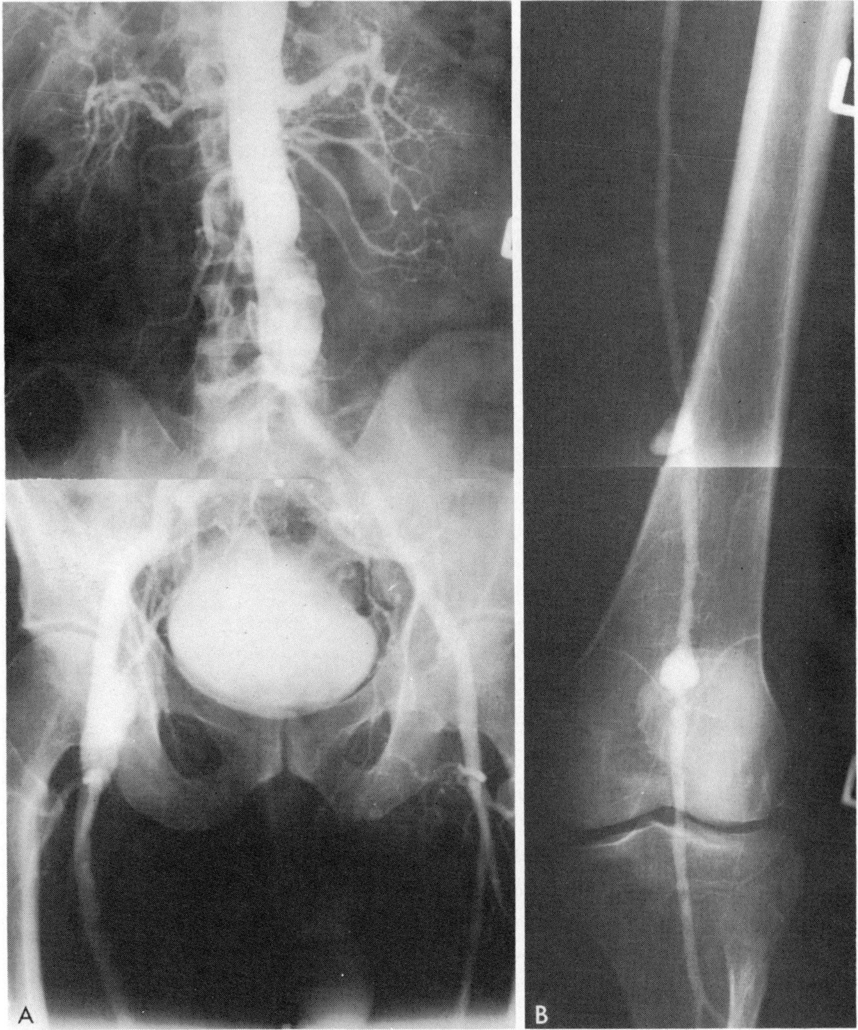

Figure 16-2. Arteriographic demonstration of one patient who has an aortic aneurysm, right femoral aneurysm and *B*, two separate popliteal aneurysms on the left. It is probable that he had experienced a thrombosis of his right popliteal aneurysm as well.

material often fills only the central channel. With this caveat then, that absence of dilatation means little, arteriography is often helpful, nonetheless, in defining the number of renal arteries, their involvement by the aneurysm, and possible stenosis. The status of the inferior and superior mesenteric vessels, of the common, internal, and external iliac arteries, and of the femoral vessels can be defined by arteriography as well.

If there is reason to suspect the progression of an aneurysm in a patient otherwise considered an unfavorable candidate for operation, repeated lateral films at appropriate intervals may be helpful. The introduction of echo-scanning has provided a useful tool, enabling an accurate anatomic diagnosis in the absence of calcification[41] (Fig. 16–3).

Operative Indications

The report of Estes,[28] focusing attention on the ominous prognosis for the patient with abdominal aortic aneurysms, was the justification for the rapid expansion of the field of surgery for aneurysm. Initially, the operation was attended with grave mortality risks, in the range of 15 per cent. Such mortality risk limited the application of operation in the earlier series to those patients who were at considerable risk of rupture. Bernstein and his associates[7] identified 7 cm. as the diameter above which rupture was common. Subsequently, improvement in operative and postoperative management led to the summation by Szilagyi et al.[58] that regardless of size, operation roughly doubled the survival expectancy; only in the presence of significant cardiovascular disease does the size become important. All aneurysms larger than 6 cm. constitute a serious risk to the patient, but in patients of less than 75 years of age, aneurysms of less than 6 cm. must be considered. The definition of "satisfactory risk" is not a matter of statistics but of individual experience, judgment, and conscience.[58] The experience of Esselstyn and his associates,[27] as well as that of Julian,[37] indicates that age alone is not a serious bar to operation.

We heartily agree with the principles stated in the preceding paragraph and urge that each surgeon consider *his own results* in selecting patients for operation. In our own hands, four deaths in 73 elective operations represents a figure similar to that now commonly reported. At one time, our hospital series ran to 89 consecutive aneurysmectomies without a death; hence, our indications for operation are now relatively liberal. It is impossible to state them exactly, but the following are our guidelines:

1. *Any* aneurysm in an otherwise intact patient whose cardiac, pulmonary, and renal status place him in an anesthetic risk of category three or less. Rarely will we elect operation past the age of 75 unless the patient has symptoms of pain, or unless clear enlargement can be demonstrated.
2. An aneurysm producing symptoms or showing signs of enlargement, even in a patient in anesthetic risk category four.
3. Substantially all aneurysms that are believed to be extravasating or rupturing.

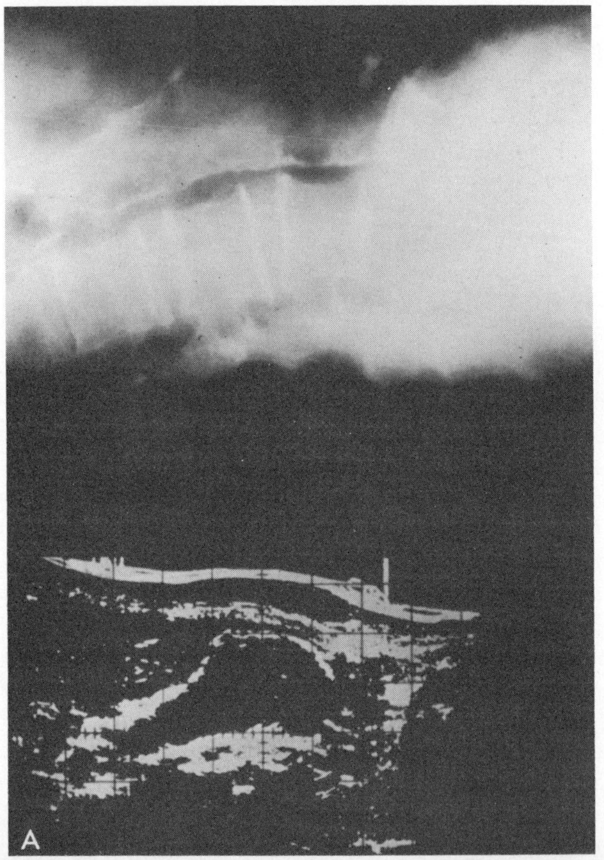

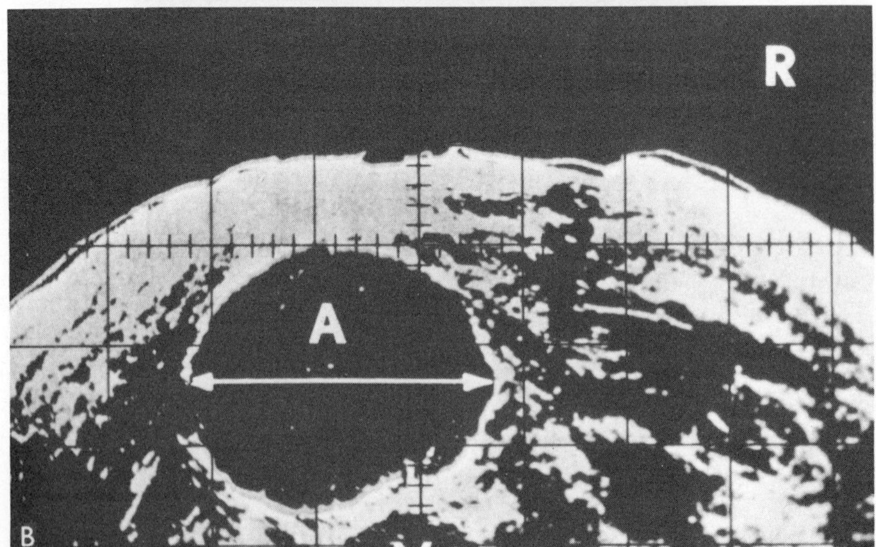

Figure 16–3. See legend on opposite page.

Size is not mentioned in these indications. During the period of this study there were as many deaths from small aneurysms in patients who died before operation as in the entire elective series.

In general, however, the younger the patient and the larger the aneurysm, the more urgently aneurysmectomy is indicated. The age to which a patient's parents lived may give some clues as to his possible life expectancy.

Cranley's[14] comments that only 25 per cent of patients with untreated aneurysm do die of rupture certainly lend weight to conservatism in those patients who are not good elective risks.

Preparation

It is essential that the patient come to operation fully hydrated and in the best metabolic balance possible. Some patients with marginal cardiac function should be digitalized. Serious pulmonary dysfunction may be treated best by elective tracheostomy to allow good respiratory control and toilette. Prolonged nasotracheal intubation postoperatively may also be useful but is often not so well tolerated for prolonged periods of time. When intermittent positive pressure respiratory therapy is to be utilized after operation, less respiratory gas is blown into the gastrointestinal tract when such intubation is used.

Smokers should stop smoking. Expectorants, postural drainage, and even specific antibiotic therapy should be used to prepare for operation any patient with significant productive cough.

Prophylactic antibiotics instituted in time to achieve good blood levels are now standard practice, but only two or three postoperative doses of such drugs are necessary, unless the antibiotics are being used to treat established urinary or respiratory infections. Our choice is Keflin 2 gm. and Cleocin 200 mg. at six-hour intervals by the intravenous route, beginning the night before operation.

With the patient in the supine position, the groins should be draped into the operative field. At times it is helpful to have the entire leg draped free, for examination, if not for surgical intervention. Straps or lateral supports should be used so that the patient may be tilted to the right in order to allow gravity to assist in retraction of the small bowel from the depths of the abdomen.

Figure 16–3. *A,* Comparison of lateral films of the abdomen demonstrating an unusually heavily calcified outline of the abdominal aortic aneurysm and a sagittal ultrasound study. *B,* Transverse ultrasound study shows a large abdominal aneurysm (A) which lies just anterior into the left of the vertebral column (V) which is only partly visible. The grid is 3 cm. (Figure *B* is reproduced with the permission of C. V. Mosby and Company).[14]

Anesthesia

Although conduction anesthesia has been used, the level must be so high that general anesthesia is generally preferred. The exact combination of agents is best left to the decision of a competent anesthesiologist. Adequate muscle relaxation is essential.

Monitoring techniques have become essential to best results. A large-bore catheter should be placed in the superior vena cava to monitor central venous pressure; it should not be used for routine fluid infusions, although it is available in an emergency. A Swann-Gans catheter can be used in the postoperative period, if necessary, to be certain of adequate left ventricular function but is usually not necessary during operation itself. Urinary output must be carefully followed by means of an indwelling urethral catheter. Continuous recording of arterial pressure by means of an indwelling radial artery line is of great value in avoiding prolonged periods of unrecognized hypotension and also allows frequent evaluation of blood gases. It is also helpful to be able to monitor flow in the extremities, either by monitoring digital pulse or by segmental plethysmography. These modalities, however, may interfere with preparation of the total extremity.

OPERATIVE TECHNIQUE

A long midline incision is the most common approach. After the usual abdominal exploration, the root of the small bowel mesentery is mobilized to expose the aneurysm. Little actual dissection of the aneurysm is done lest loose clot be spilled into the distal tree. Dissection is carried instead up to the level of the neck of the aneurysm. The left renal vein is identified and mobilized, and the left genital vein protected. The inferior mesenteric vein is also mobilized. Both the inferior mesenteric vein and the left renal vein may be divided, the latter as far to the right as possible without significant complications. Once the aneurysmal neck has been identified and it is established that an infrarenal anastomosis is possible, the size of the infrarenal aorta is estimated and the prosthesis chosen (Fig. 16–4).

The site of distal anastomosis is now selected, and any one of the several levels may be chosen (Fig. 16–5).

The Aortic Bifurcation

Although many surgeons use tube grafts between the proximal and distal infrarenal aortic segments, in the majority of instances serious occlusive disease is present at the level of the terminal aorta or proximal iliac arteries. Furthermore, dilatation of the common iliac artery may progress and result in needless late rupture.

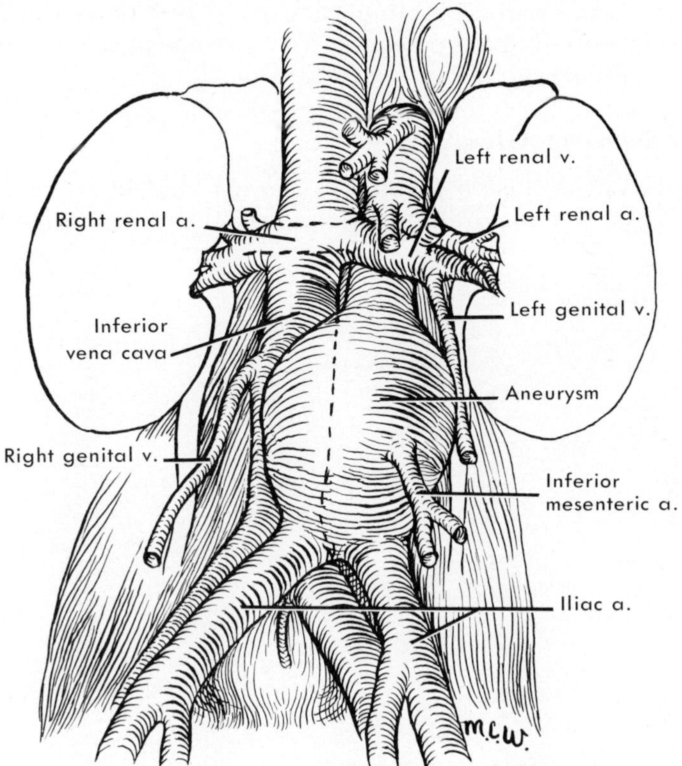

Figure 16–4. Anatomy of the classical aortic aneurysm.

Common Iliac Artery

If neither dilatation nor significant occlusive disease is present at this level, an end-to-end anastomosis is ideal.

External Iliac Artery

If there is troublesome aneurysmal, obstructive, or calcific disease in the common iliac artery, an end-to-side anastomosis to a soft spot in the mid-external iliac artery is useful. It preserves the possibility of retrograde flow into internal iliac system. A dilated or atherosclerotic common iliac artery is endarterectomized. A large (No. 14–18 French) catheter can be placed at this level through the external iliac system, to inject dilute heparin into the distal iliofemoral system to protect that system against clot from a proximal spillage and to serve as an intraluminal stent during the prosthesis-to-external iliac anastomosis (Fig. 16–5). Furthermore, this method allows one to keep the anastomosis out of the groin, especially if future femoropopliteal repair for a previously undissected groin may be a later advantage.[24] Szilagyi et al.[59] have implicated the groin as a critical area as far as infection is concerned.

On the other hand, Moore et al.[49] noted that the apprehensions of an earlier period about placement of a prosthesis across the fold of the groin are not warranted.

Common Femoral Artery

Significant occlusive disease in the external iliac system or an unusually small vessel in the area should indicate anastomosis to the

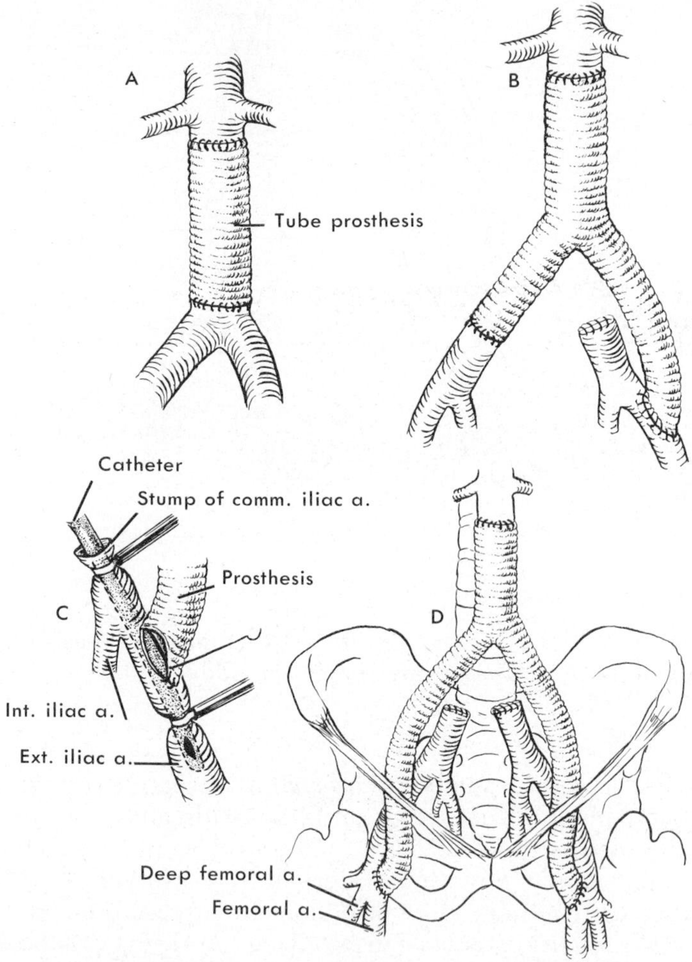

Figure 16–5.   Possible types of reconstruction. *A*, Tube graft. *B*, Bifurcation graft from aorta to right common iliac artery (end-to-end), and to left external iliac (end-to-side). Left common iliac stump is endarterectomized and oversewn; end-to-side anastomosis provides flow into both pelvic and femoral outflow tracts. *C*, If catheter is left in common iliac artery during distal anastomosis to external iliac artery, it may be used as a stent during repair. *D*, Bifurcation graft from aorta to both femoral arteries. It is attached end-to-side at the end of the common femoral artery facing the orifice of the superficial and profunda femoris branches. The common iliac stumps have been endarterectomized and oversewn.

distal end of the common femoral artery. This anastomosis is placed (Fig. 16–5) facing the orifice of the profunda femoris artery. A T-shaped arteriotomy is useful to achieve a satisfactory attachment of the prosthesis (as described in Chapter Eight).

If the distal anastomosis is to the area beyond the ureter, it is best to tunnel under the ureter on the right and under the combined ureter and sigmoid mesentery on the left.

Occasionally, the common iliac extends deeply into the pelvis, and the external iliac junction allows the ureter to lie so deeply in the pelvis that it is simpler to leave the ureter in place and to span the prosthesis over the ureter without causing any risk of ureteric obstruction.

DISSECTION OF THE ANEURYSM

Minimal dissection of the aneurysm itself is desirable. Once the sites of distal anastomosis are chosen, appropriate dissection to enable control of the common, internal, and external systems is achieved with tapes and tourniquets or light vascular clamps. Before occlusion of the aorta, however, blood is drawn for preclotting of the graft, and a dose of 3500 to 5000 units of heparin is given systemically. The aorta at the level of the renal arteries now may be cross-clamped. Circumferential control of the aorta is neither necessary nor particularly desirable, and a simple vertical placement of the clamp is satisfactory (Fig. 16–6).

Distal clamps are now placed, and, if desired, intra-arterial catheters are placed in the common iliac system. The aneurysmal wall is opened to the right of the orifice of the inferior mesenteric artery, and that artery is itself controlled with a small vascular clamp. The loose intraluminal debris and clot are removed, and an endarterectomy of the aneurysm itself is performed. This exposes the orifice of the lumbar and middle sacral vessels, which can easily be controlled with transfixing sutures. The external coats of the aneurysm are preserved. Care is taken to avoid dissection near the vena cava.

In males, it is desirable to try to preserve on at least one side the plexus of autonomic nerves that crosses the proximal common iliac artery.

At the upper limit of this incision in the aneurysm, the incision is carried laterally to include roughly the anterior 200 degrees of the circumference (Fig. 16–7). The chosen graft is now sutured in position at the upper limit of the aneurysm. Large sutures are placed across the posterior row and can include the retroaortic fascia. Care should be taken to identify and to avoid a retroaortic renal vein.

Walker has described an inflammatory aneurysm in which there

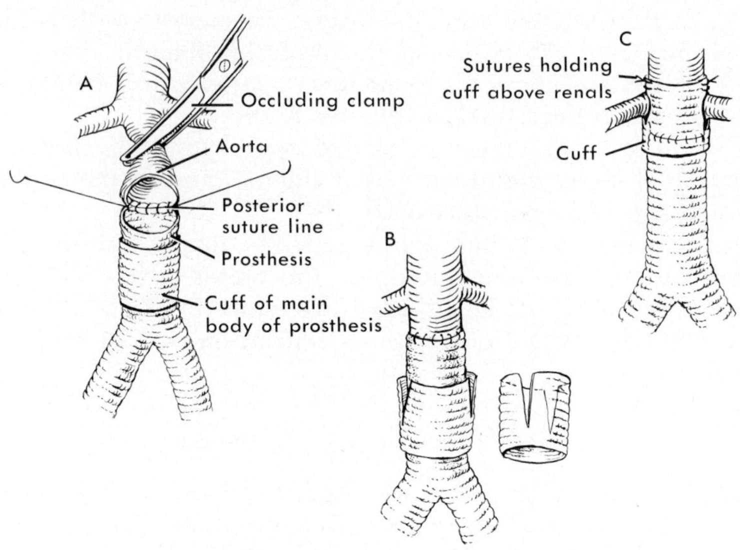

Figure 16–6.   Upper anastomosis in end-to-end repair. *A*, Suture line begun in posterior midline. *B*, Suture line completed. *C*, Suture line buttressed with bushing of prosthetic tube. In *B* the bushing is shown with a slit so that it can be drawn up over the level of the renal arteries and sutured in place as in *C*.

is intensive adherence of the duodenum to the thick white aneurysmal wall.[62] When this is encountered, it is useless and hazardous to try to dissect it free. Instead, the aorta must be cross-clamped and opened with an absolute minimum of dissection. The prosthesis is placed within the shell of the aneurysm, as described elsewhere. The inflammation has no specific cause yet identified and is restricted to the aorta.[62]

Although placement of the upper suture line near the renal arteries is both necessary and desirable, attention to the preservation of large proximal lumbar arteries is important. The arteria radicularis magna should come off at the level of the lower thoracic segments or at the level of the first or second lumbar segment, but it is occasionally derived from lower branches (see Chapter Two). There is no simple or safe way to identify this artery in the face of an aneurysm.[20, 31] Injury or even temporary occlusion for as little as seven minutes may result in paraplegia, according to the review by Zuber and his associates.[67] Suprarenal clamping and hypotension pose a particularly hazardous combination.

It is convenient to begin the suture line near the posterior midline (Fig. 16–6) with a relatively heavy suture (heavy for size, not for strength—3–0 or even 2–0). Mersilene coated with Teflon is the preferred suture, although polypropylene, which is smoother and less likely to cause a leaking suture hole, is also satisfactory.

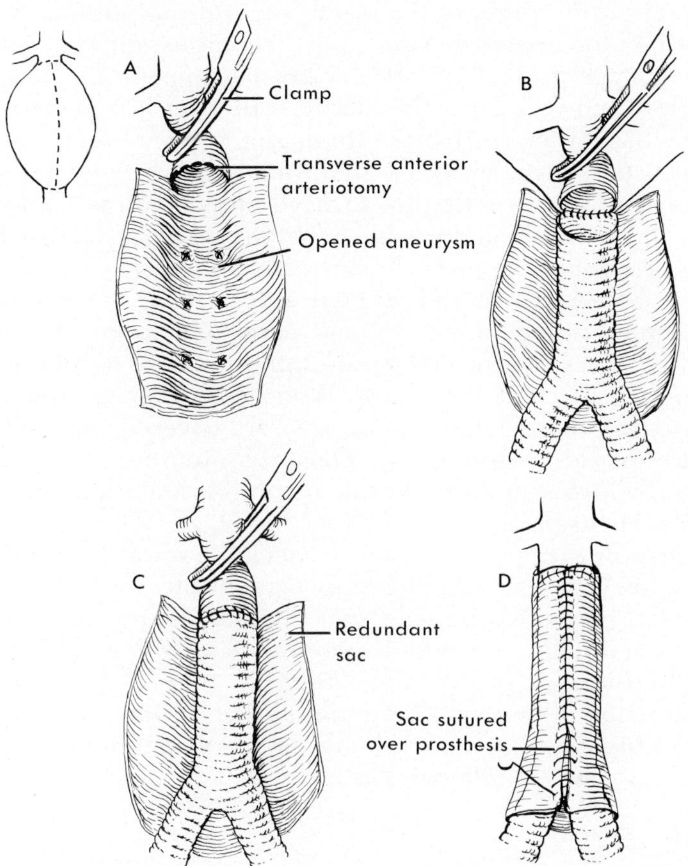

Figure 16-7. Upper anastomosis when prosthesis is placed in sac of aneurysm without resection (the preferred technique). *A,* T-shaped incision in aneurysmal sac. *B,* Posterior suture line to intact posterior wall. *C,* Prosthesis in place. *D,* Sac sutured loosely over the prosthesis.

The posterior portion of the suture line includes a bite in and out on the posterior aortic wall, then through the prosthesis. After the lateral incision is reached, a simple over-and-over, abutting suture continues the attachment of prosthesis to aorta (Fig. 16–7).

Once the suture line has been completed, an occluding clamp can be placed across the proximal prosthesis to test the competence of the anastomosis. Mattress sutures can be placed over any significant leaks, but these should be placed only after replacing the proximal aortic occluding clamp so as to reduce the chance of further tearing of the suture holes. Polypropylene sutures are excellent in this situation, and relatively finer suture material can be used here.

An alternative technique involves complete division of the aorta at the level of the origin of the aneurysm, with or without resection of the bulk of the aneurysm itself. This technique allows a cuff of the prosthetic material to be pulled over the anastomotic line (Fig. 16–6) to provide a bulwark for a thin aortic wall after a necessary endarterectomy has left only a paper-thin media.[12]

The distal anastomoses are performed with a twice-interrupted continuous suture. It is helpful to have either a large catheter or a probe (a Bâkes common duct dilator serves well) in the distal vessel to assure freedom from restriction.

Flow should be restored into one side as soon as the suture line is completed. Before doing so, the aorta and stagnant prosthesis should be blown free of clot by draining the flow through the opposite and unattached iliac limb. When cross-clamping any of the prosthetic materials, clamps whose jaws are covered with soft rubber or Silastic should be used on the Dacron to minimize the damage to the fabric, which can easily result in troublesome leaking through the prosthesis itself.

Declamping hypotension is a special hazard with prolonged occlusion. This can be minimized by expeditious restoration of flow, by early restoration to one side, and by fractional restoration of flow to the internal iliac and to the external iliac system separately, as advocated by Imparato et al.[35] (Fig. 16–8).

Restoration of flow into the internal iliac system first has the advantage of blowing any inadvertently overlooked intraluminal debris into the less critical outflow tract.

PROTECTION OF THE RENAL VASCULATURE

This consists of both gross anatomical and physiological protection. There is always a risk of dislocation of atheromatous and thrombotic debris into the renal arteries when a clamp is placed at the level of the renal arteries. It may be safer to use light clamps on the renal arteries for the few minutes of strict aortic occlusion, and even to place the clamp above the renal arteries to be sure there is not encroachment by clot or dislocated intima of the renal orifices. There are sufficient collaterals by way of adrenal branches, capsular anastomoses, and ureteric vessels to maintain renal viability for at least 20 to 30 minutes, but clamping for longer periods must be avoided.

In addition, however, adequate general hydration plus administration of mannitol and either ethacrynic acid (10–20 mg.) or furosemide (40 mg.) just before cross-clamping the aorta provides physiological protection by assuring an excellent glomerular filtration rate.[55]

Cayten et al.[13] have collected an experience with the manage-

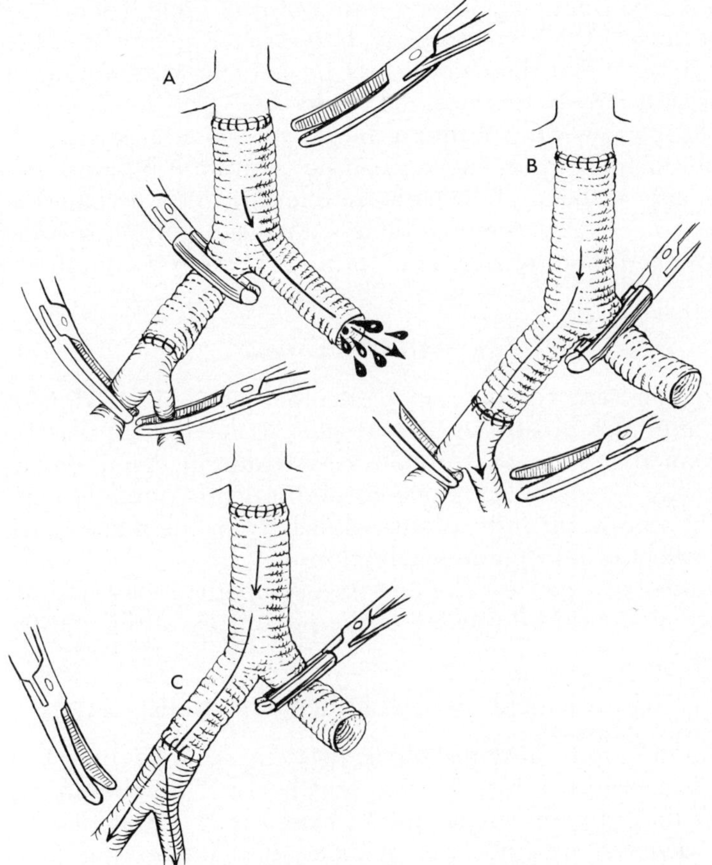

Figure 16–8. Restoration of flow. *A*, After the first iliac anastomosis has been completed, the aortic clamp is temporarily released, and intravascular debris is vented through the opposite iliac arm. *B*, The open iliac arm is cross-clamped with a silastic rubber shod clamp, and the clamp is removed from the right internal iliac artery first. *C*, After stable hemodynamic situation occurs, flow is restored to the external iliac system as well. A similar pattern is followed on the second side, opening flow into the internal iliac system first, then into the external iliac system (after Imparato).

ment of horseshoe kidneys in the presence of ruptured aneurysms, but their observations pertain as well to elective operations.[13]

CHOICE OF PROSTHESIS

Many excellent Dacron prostheses are available, and some of the criteria for choice of grafts have been discussed in previous chapters (Seven and Eight). The most effective prostheses are the externally velour-covered graft of Sauvage, not available in bifurcation units at the date of this publication, and the graft advocated by Wesolowski, which is excellent from a long-term point of view. Immediate blood loss because of a high porosity is a danger to the fragile patient. When it is crucial that blood loss be kept to a minimum, a tightly woven graft may be the optimal choice.

Unusual bleeding through the prosthesis or at a suture line that does not justify further sutures can be controlled by local Surgicel or by pledgets of Teflon felt. Heparin effects can be reversed with protamine if necessary. Some surgeons advocate routine reversal of the heparin effect before restoration of flow through the graft.

SYMPATHECTOMY

Concomitant lumbar sympathectomy can be performed more easily after the prosthesis is in place, if desired. Retraction of the aneurysm before reconstruction may result in distal embolization. There may be some reticence to perform this operation in the absence of significant indications, especially in the male in whom the sexual effect of retrograde ejaculation may occur.

Both sexes may experience post-sympathectomy neuralgia, and the patient should be warned of the possibility of this pain.

MANAGEMENT OF INFERIOR MESENTERIC ARTERY

Under certain circumstances, it is desirable to reimplant the inferior mesenteric artery in the prosthesis. This should always be done if there is any suggestion of cyanosis or pallor in the sigmoid colon after the prosthesis is in place and functioning. It is almost never necessary if there is pulsatile or vigorous back flow from the vessel by way of collaterals. On the other hand, restoration of a previously thrombosed vessel is rarely necessary. If, however, there is questionable reason to implant it, and if the internal iliac vessels are either thrombosed or excluded from the circulation because of the pattern of reconstruction, then reimplantation may be the wisest choice, to avoid colonic ischemia.

The technique of implantation may be that of a simple side-to-end attachment if the vessel is large. The technique is facilitated, however, by saving a 2 mm. rim of aortic wall and using it to allow more secure anastomosis to the prosthesis (Fig. 16–9). The prosthesis should be treated either by an only partially occluding clamp or by total occlusion and evacuation of all clot from the prosthesis before restoration of flow, so as to lessen the chance of spilling loose intraluminal clot into a distal arterial tree.

Accessory renal arteries of significant size should be similarly reimplanted in the prosthesis.

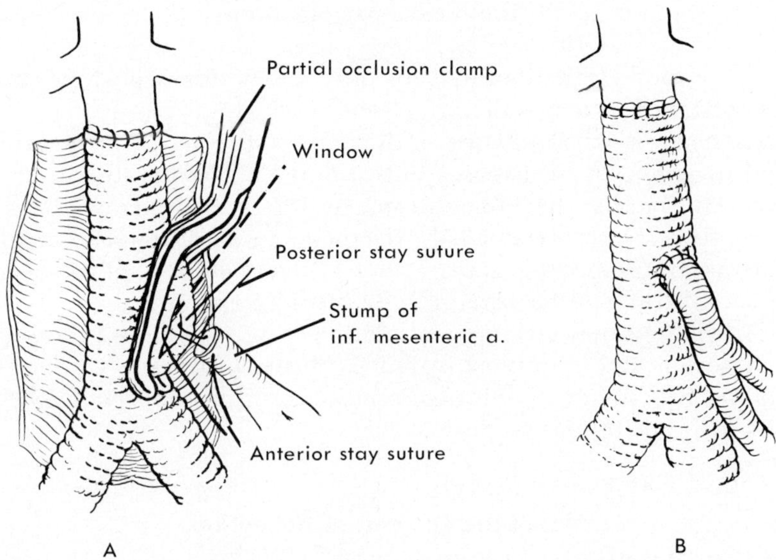

Figure 16–9.   Implantation of the inferior mesenteric artery. *A*, With bifurcation prosthesis in place, a partial occlusion clamp is applied and a small window is excised from the anterolateral aspect of the prosthesis. Anterior and posterior stay sutures are used to secure the cuff of the aortic wall and inferior mesenteric artery to the prosthesis: superior and inferior suture lines are thus defined which are easily placed. *B*, Shows the completed anastomosis. A similar technique can be used for replacement of any other critical mesenteric or renal branches.

CLOSURE

The shell of the aneurysm should be loosely wrapped around the prosthesis. A water-tight seal is unnecessary and could conceivably lead to periprosthetic hematoma and infection (Fig. 16–7).

The left renal vein may be reanastomosed if it has been divided, but it is probable that repair is unnecessary in most instances.

The peritoneal incision at the root of the small bowel mesentery and at the lateral margin of the sigmoid colon should be reapproximated loosely. If there is any unusual oozing of blood, drainage of the groin wound may be performed with a suction catheter lead under the inguinal ligament and along the course of the prosthesis. This suction drain should be removed *no later* than 48 hours after operation in most instances. Other abdominal drainage is not desirable.

Abdominal wound closure should follow the individual surgeon's routine. The usual closure employed by the author includes figure-of-eight mattress sutures of nonabsorbable material to the midline structures and support by retention sutures.

Especially in patients with pulmonary limitations, a tube gastrostomy is placed in the midportion of the greater curvature of the stomach, using a Witzel tunnel.

Postoperative Management

Antibiotics are maintained for only a few doses postoperatively unless directed at a specific infectious process.

Anticoagulants rarely are indicated in the early postoperative period in aneurysmal disease, but prolonged (six months to a year) Coumadin therapy has been used in those patients whose anti-prothrombin treatment is easily balanced in an attempt to ensure a better maturation of the graft. There is insufficient experience with antiplatelet drugs to be sure of their value in this role.

The patient may resume ambulation as soon as his cardiorespiratory system is stable in most instances. If the prosthesis extends into the groin, it is better to defer ambulation until fibroplasia has begun, on the fifth postoperative day.

Wrapping Instead of Resection

Robicsek et al.,[53] among others, have advocated wrapping an aneurysm if the risk of resection seems too great. This might well be applied to thoracoabdominal aneurysms and to aneurysms of the arch. Dacron cloth cut from tube grafts can be wound in a spiral about the vessels and sutured in place.

There is no doubt that this technique limits excessive expansion of the aneurysm. Sufficient manipulation to achieve adequate wrapping, however, may require such extensive dissection that resection may be simpler in most abdominal aneurysms. Furthermore, the actual manipulations may dislodge embolic fragments of intraluminal clot, which could be disastrous should they lodge in vital organs.

THE RUPTURED ANEURYSM

Once either intramural dissection, enclosed retroperitoneal dissection, or free intraperitoneal rupture has occurred, the mortality risk without operation is substantially 100 per cent. Thus, surgical intervention is indicated just as soon as this diagnosis is established. McKenzie[44] dramatized this with the suggestion that the first and most important thing for the surgeon to do once this diagnosis has been made is to start pushing the patient's bed to the operating room.

Delay for intravenous urography, electrocardiography, or resuscitation is hazardous. The only acceptable reason for delay is for the simplest blood typing. Indeed, surgical intervention with blood volume restoration using Ringer's solution and plasma may be even more important than a delay for cross-matching.

Diagnosis

The history of an aneurysm or the presence of a palpable pulsating mass together with acute pain and shock represent primary diagnostic criteria. At times, however, contained hemorrhage does not reflect itself in blood pressure changes. Pain is variable; it may be abdominal or it may be referred to the back or into the hip. If the diagnosis has not been suspected, abdominal calcification on abdominal roentgenograms consistent with an aneurysm, changes in the pattern of calcification from prior studies, or echo sound studies may provide the appropriate clue. Leopold et al.[41] have even shown one echo study in which the clinical diagnosis was made after the echogram showed a contained retroperitoneal hematoma. Ordinarily, however, the diagnosis of a ruptured aneurysm precludes further diagnostic evaluation.

Operative Technique

The only real difference between the operation for ruptured and unruptured aneurysm is the importance of the most rapid control of the proximal aorta.

One catastrophe that at times does occur during the hurried operation is the release of tamponaded pressure when free but contained intraperitoneal hemorrhage is released as the peritoneum is incised. A momentary pause before opening the peritoneal cavity should be taken to identify, by needle aspiration if necessary, the presence of free intraperitoneal blood. If such free hemorrhage is present, the further abdominal operation may be delayed until the chest has been opened and control of the aorta just above the diaphragm has been achieved. Indeed, some authors would advocate routine control of the aorta by means of this route during emergency operation.

If the thoracic route has not been used, three basic approaches may be utilized.

1. Direct. Quick finger exploration at the neck of the aneurysm, either below the colon or above the stomach via the gastrohepatic omentum will allow placement of a vertically oriented clamp albeit above the renal and mesenteric arteries.

2. Indirect. Pressure sufficient to compress the suprarenal aorta against the spine may be made with an assistant's fingers, a sponge stick, or an instrument like that devised by Nobis.[51] This is a Y-shaped instrument with a tough elastic closing the open Y, which, when thrust against the spine, is easily held in place to control proximal pressure.

3. Intraluminal. A large Foley catheter with a 30 ml. bag can be thrust upward into the lumen and distended to control the aorta. Similar intraluminal catheters can be used to control retrograde flow from the iliac arteries.

Acute Aorto-Caval Fistula

A special type of ruptured aneurysm is that which ruptures into the vena cava or one of the iliac veins. This should be recognized by the sudden increase in venous pressure, simulating pronounced cardiac failure. Peripheral edema may be massive. A murmur is usually heard, and a thrill is felt in the cava as soon as the abdomen is open. This occurrence does not require emergency operation, but urgent repair is desirable. Precautions must be taken to control the venous effluent and to prevent massive embolization of intraluminal debris during necessary dissection of the aorta.[4] Once the aorta has been controlled and opened, the venous defect can be repaired from within the aortic shell.

INTERNAL ILIAC ANEURYSMS

Internal iliac aneurysms are infrequent but troublesome. Martin et al.[45] have described a careful dissection from above downward lateral to the aneurysm until full control of the distal arterial supply is achieved. At times, however, the aneurysm extends so far into the gluteal branches that control is nearly impossible, and furious hemorrhage may follow attempts to cross-clamp the artery. Foley or Fogarty catheters placed into the distal vessels may achieve control long enough to place sutures in such a way as to allow closure, as in the technique of endoaneurysmorrhaphy. Careful dissection should avoid venous channels that may bleed copiously.

UPPER ABDOMINAL ANEURYSMS: THORACOABDOMINAL ANEURYSMS

Infrequently encountered are the aneurysms of the upper abdominal aorta that include the orifices of all the visceral arteries.

These are apt to be associated with pain and with visceral dysfunction. The first case reported with a successful outcome was that of Etheredge et al;[29] later reports by DeBakey et al.[18] and a discussion of the technical details by Stoney and Wylie[57] dealt with these problems.

Diagnosis presents a special problem in that the aneurysm may be difficult to feel. Arteriographic evaluation is essential.

The surgical approach described by Stoney and Wylie[57] is the preferred procedure (Fig. 16–10). A long, oblique incision from the right lower quadrant is carried at least as far as the posterior axillary line via the eighth intercostal space. The patient's left shoulder is now rotated forward through 45 degrees. The diaphragm is incised about 2 cm. from its peripheral posterior attachments, exposing the aorta. The spleen, tail of the pancreas, and left colon are mobilized forward. An initial occlusion of the upper aorta is necessary while either a side-to-end or end-to-end anastomosis to a graft is performed. Once the distal anastomosis is made to the distal aorta or iliac artery on one side in an end-to-side fashion, the upper limits of the aneurysm may be dissected, exposing and attaching to the prosthesis the several branches in order, the right renal artery being placed last.

If extensive collateralization to one stenotic vessel is present, one may take advantage of this fact, as illustrated by the following case of a 62-year-old woman admitted to the hospital with distal occlusive disease involving the right iliac and left superficial femoral arteries. She had had serious weight loss, and an arteriogram showed extensive collaterals through the right adrenal system to the celiac axis, which was totally occluded at its origin (Fig. 16–11). The vessels were treated successively as outlined above, but after reconstitution of the celiac artery, it was believed that the collateralization to the right renal artery could now serve to nourish the kidney during occlusion of the renal vessel for anastomosis.

The visceral branches may be attached directly to the graft with a cuff of aortic wall to facilitate suture, or they may be sewn end-to-end to previously prepared side arms sutured to the graft.

Dissecting Thoracoabdominal Aneurysms

An occasional dissecting thoracic aneurysm extends into the abdomen. Correction of the dissection at its source is ideal, but at times the false channel may present in the abdomen and require direct attack.

A 68-year-old man had had a resection and prosthetic replacement of the proximal part of his descending thoracic aorta six months before admission for dissection. He complained of pain and a rapidly distending abdominal

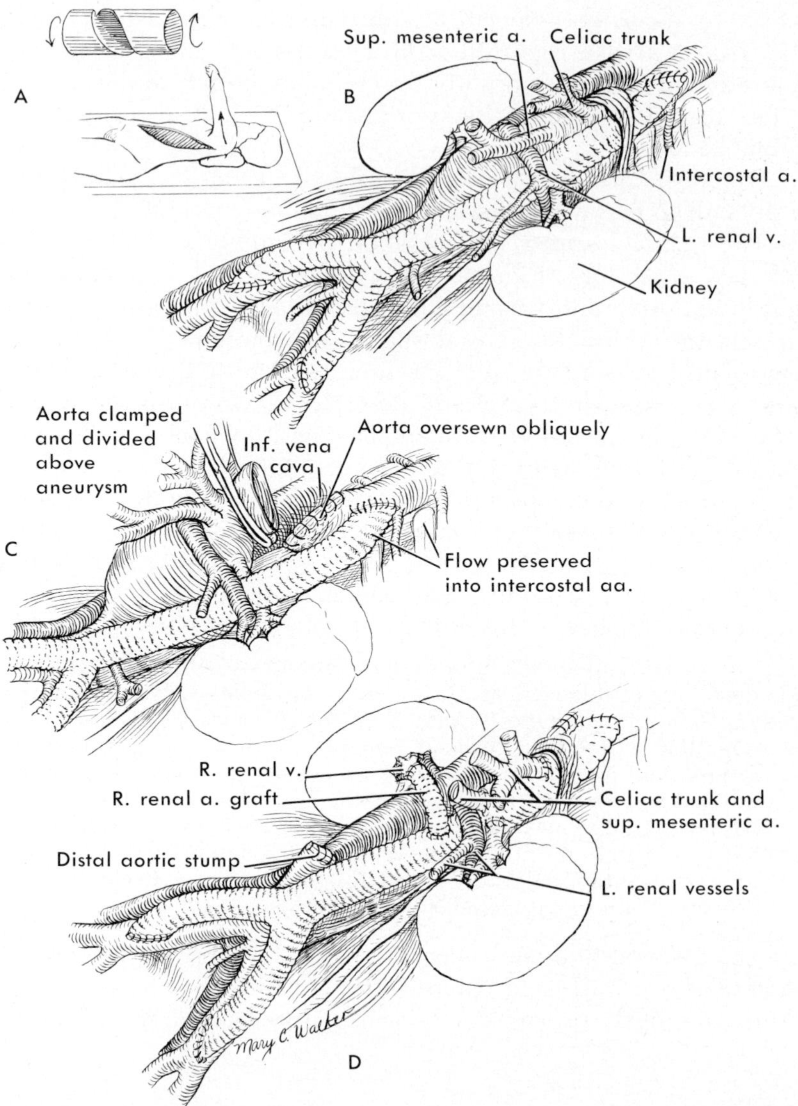

Figure 16–10.   Approach to the thoracoabdominal aneurysm. *A,* Thoracoabdominal incision after Stoney and Wylie.[57] (Redrawn with permission of the authors; the American Journal of Surgery, and the York Medical Group). A long, oblique abdominal incision is made from the right lower quadrant into the eighth interspace with the patient's hips flat on the table. When the incision has been made, the shoulders are rotated forward 45°, thus opening the incision like a cookie box. *B,* The bypass graft is placed from the proximal aorta to the distal aorta or the iliac arteries if necessary. *C,* Division of the thoracic aorta obliquely preserves the intercostals and upper lumbar arteries in an attempt to avoid paraplegia. *D,* Successive visceral branches are reattached to the graft. The most distal branches are perfused in a retrograde fashion through the bypass graft and the distal aorta and iliac arteries, as the more proximal branches are individually being attached to the bypass graft itself. The left renal vein may be divided at the level of the vena cava and reanastomosed. It may be left intact

(*Legend continued on opposite page.*)

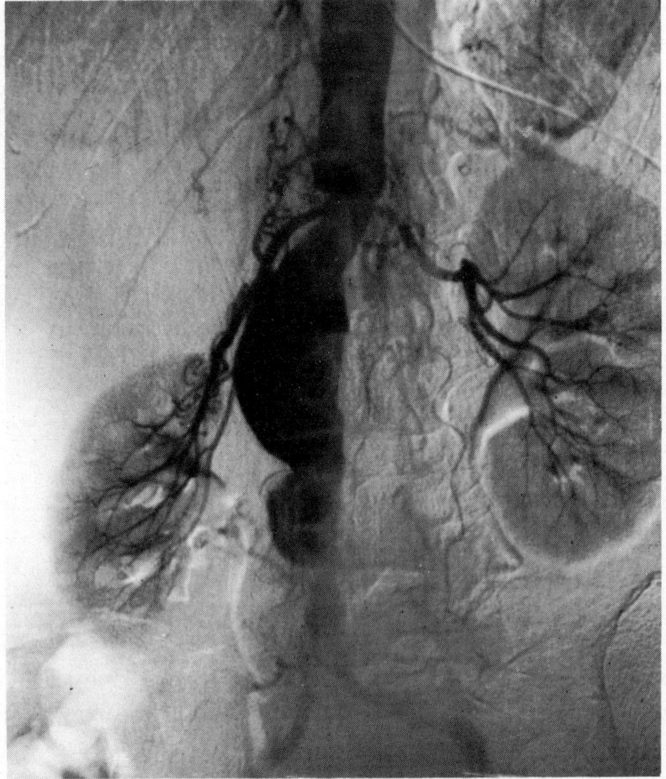

Figure 16–11. Arteriogram of a small upper abdominal aneurysm with stenosis of the left renal artery, total occlusion of both the celiac axis and superior mesenteric artery, stenosis of the right common iliac artery, and a stenosis of the inferior mesenteric artery.

mass. An arteriogram showed a true channel supplying one iliac artery and one kidney, whereas the false channel seemed to supply the other kidney, the superior mesenteric and celiac axis, and the other iliac artery. Echograms showed a narrow neck at the level of the infrarenal aorta. It was possible to cross-clamp the two channels at this level, fenestrate the common wall between the true and false channels, and attach a bifurcated prosthesis to the outer layer of aorta at its infrarenal level. The remainder of the infrarenal aneurysm was treated then as any other abdominal aneurysm.

Should any narrow spot be present, as is often the case at the level of the diaphragm (or the renal arteries as in this instance), the

---

posterior to the prosthesis; or the prosthesis may be passed behind it as shown here. In this sketch a short arm of Dacron tubing has been used to restore flow into the right renal artery, whereas the stumps of the left renal artery, superior mesenteric artery, and celiac axis are shown attached directly to the graft.

Table 16–3. Mortality in Treatment of Aortic Aneurysm
(Two Series)

	1963		1972	
	No. of Aneurysms	Mortality (Per cent)	No. of Aneurysms	Mortality (Per cent)
Elective asymptomatic	66	15	45	4
Elective, symptomatic, but unruptured	–	–	28	7
Ruptured	34	36	26	62

visceral branches can be reimplanted after establishing aorta-to-iliac shunts, just as with other upper abdominal aneurysms.

RESULTS

Elective Results

As a mechanism of understanding the philosophy that indicates repair of all aneurysms electively, it is worth comparing several aspects of our experience in the two series of aneurysms mentioned earlier (Table 16–3). The four deaths in patients who were operated upon electively are detailed in Table 16–4.

The complications encountered in the elective cases were many. On the other hand, in the 1972 series, 50 of the 73 patients had no complications whatsoever. The 23 patients who did have complications shared the complications shown in Table 16–5. The distal vascular occlusions listed could not be clearly identified as being purely embolic or purely thrombotic. Similarly, the three patients who had prolonged ileus may have had some degree of ischemic colitis as an origin, but no outright episodes of colonic ischemia were found.

Table 16–4. Mortality in Patients Operated on Electively
for Aortic Aneurysm

Status	Age	Cause of Death	Time of Death
Asymptomatic	69	CVA	3 weeks
	68	MI	10 days
Symptomatic	64	MI	2 days
	67*	Sepsis around graft	5 months

*This patient is included as a death, although there was no evidence of infection until shortly before death.

Table 16–5.   Complications in Elective Operations

	NO. OF PATIENTS
Pulmonary problems	
Infection (pneumonia)	3
Embolism*	3
Insufficiency	7
Myocardial infarction	1
Acute dysrhythmias	2
Congestive failure	1
Distal arterial occlusion	2
Venous thrombosis*	4
Protracted ileus	3
Dehiscence	1
Hepatitis	1
Splenic rupture	1
Prostatic obstruction	1
Ureteral fistula	1
Acute renal failure	1

*Although only one peripheral venous thrombosis was recognized, three others probably occurred as the source of the three pulmonary emboli.

It is likely that some of the patients with pulmonary insufficiency experienced some degree of aspiration as well.

Results of Operation for Ruptured Aneurysm.   The 18 patients who died during or after operation for ruptured aneurysms are detailed in Table 16–6.

Three patients listed as having acute cardiorespiratory failure manifested the lesion described by Blaisdell and associates,[9] a combination of cardiac insufficiency, pulmonary embolism, parenchymatous pulmonary changes, and possibly aspiration.

In Table 16–6 are mentioned six patients who died from the emergency operation more than 12 days after operation. Two of these died of acute renal failure, one of pulmonary sepsis, one of cardiorespiratory failure, and one of a combination of gastrointestinal bleeding, fulminant carcinoma, and aspiration. It is perhaps overstatement to ascribe this last mentioned death at 75 days to the operation, but it is included because the patient did not ever leave the hospital.

Inasmuch as the mortality rate from operation for the ruptured

Table 16–6.   Intraoperative and Postoperative Deaths
from Ruptured Aneurysms

Operative; hemorrhage and/or cardiac arrest	7
Coincidental extensive cancer	1
"Total" aneurysm	1
Cardiorespiratory failure, acute, in first 24 hours	3
Late deaths (13–75 days)	6

Table 16–7.   Improvement in Surgical Mortality of
Abdominal Aneurysms

		MORTALITY ASYMPTOMATIC EXCISION	RUPTURED
May et al.[48]	1961–70	10.4%	47.3%
Baker et al.[3]	1960–69	2.5%	—
Foster et al.[30]	1950–69	3%*	—
Stokes and Butcher[56]	1972	3.9%	—

*Small aneurysms.

aneurysm remains so high, it seemed worthwhile to consider whether, had operation been decided upon sooner, a successful conclusion might have resulted.

Results of Others

Many recent publications have attested to general improvement in the surgical mortality of abdominal aneurysms. A few selected examples are presented in Table 16–7.

Our operative indications have been based on the stable mortality risk of around 3 per cent for elective operations, whereas emergency resections are almost 20 times as hazardous. Especially disconcerting is the finding that such a large group of patients with ruptured aneurysms had had the diagnosis established or had indications for operation on the basis of claudication that would have led to elective treatment of the aneurysm (Table 16–8).

Two patients who died had had previous tube grafts for aneurysms: one ruptured above a short tube, and one ruptured an iliac aneurysm below the tube. Johnson and his associates[36] allude to the great risk of paraplegia and death in patients with abdominal aneurysms and distal occlusive disease who undergo acute thrombosis of the aneurysm.

This information suggests that the indications for operation previously described, namely the presence of an aneurysm of any size in an individual who is a reasonable operative risk, might have

Table 16–8.   Prior History of Patients with Ruptured Aneurysm

	NO. OF PATIENTS
Claudication—2 years or more	2
Diagnosis of aneurysm—1 week to 4 years	8
Pain—1 to 4 days	3
Pain—less than 12 hours	8

prevented death in perhaps six or eight of the patients operated upon only for rupture. Thus, the mortality might have been reduced to no more than 8 or 10 per cent for the overall series.

PERIPHERAL ARTERIAL ANEURYSMS

The most common aneurysms outside of the body cavities are the atherosclerotic lesions of the femoral and popliteal areas. Much more infrequent are aneurysms of the carotid or of the subclavian-axillary system due either to the cervical rib or to crutch trauma.

Femoral and Popliteal Aneurysms

Peripheral aneurysms that involve the limb vessels are about 5 per cent as common as aortic aneurysms. One third of these occur in the femoral area, and two thirds in the popliteal areas. About one third of these aneurysms are seen because of some surgical emergency.[16, 23] These figures are in agreement with our experience. Furthermore, most of these are atherosclerotic aneurysms and are associated with aneurysms in other sites. Whychulis and his associates[66] found that 59 per cent of their patients with popliteal aneurysms had contralateral popliteal aneurysms; in 45 per cent there was an aneurysm of the femoral artery or of the aorta. In our own experience, one group of 18 patients were found to have 42 aneurysms.[5]

FEMORAL ANEURYSMS

Cutler and Darling[16] described three types of femoral aneurysms. To these should be added a fourth and a fifth type (Table 16–9), although these two are quite rare. The proximal limit may be above the inguinal ligament; hence, some of these could properly be called iliofemoral aneurysms.

Approximately one third of femoral aneurysms cause either distal thrombosis, embolism, or both. Occasionally there is local hemorrhage and associated intense inflammatory reaction. The presence of a pulsatile mass is invariable. Because of the immediately adjacent femoral nerve and vein, neuritic pains or distal venous obstruction are also common. Iatrogenic injury, such as may be caused by ill-advised puncture of prominent pulsation, seemingly suitable for arteriography or for blood gas studies, may precipitate hemorrhage, extravasation, or even distal embolization.

Table 16–9.   Types of Femoral Aneurysms

Type I	Terminating proximal to the orifice of the superficial and deep femoral artery
Type II	Involving the superficial femoral and deep femoral arteries
Type III	A — Femoral aneurysm with chronic occlusion of the superficial femoral artery B — Femoral aneurysm with chronic occlusion of the deep femoral artery
Type IV	Aneurysms of the deep femoral artery
Type V	Aneurysms of superficial femoral artery

Diagnosis is ordinarily established by physical examination. Plain x-ray studies may show calcification. An arteriogram may show dilatation more commonly than in the popliteal system but is more helpful in identifying the status of the femoral branches. Echoscans may be useful in questionable cases.

Because of the frequency with which complications occur, and because of the obvious advantages of treating prophylactically rather than after the development of complications, resection of the aneurysm with reconstitution of arterial continuity is the treatment of choice. Total resection is not necessary, however, for isolation of the major branches allows a graft or prosthesis to be placed within the shell of the aneurysm, eliminating the hazard of injury to the vein or nerve. If the orifice of a patent profunda femoris artery can be attached to the side of the graft, it is well to do so. A cuff of the common femoral wall can facilitate the anastomosis. At times the vessels are so large that a small aortic bifurcation graft is suitable as a bifurcation prosthesis (Fig. 16–12A).

The preferred material for replacement is a piece of vein, especially in view of the slightly greater risk of sepsis in the groin; however, Dacron, especially the external velour prosthesis, or the bovine carotid heterograft is also satisfactory, when the available vein is too small.

POPLITEAL ANEURYSMS

The hazards of the popliteal aneurysm are even more significant than those of the femoral aneurysm. We have estimated, from our experience, that 10 per cent of acute femoropopliteal occlusions arise from popliteal aneurysmal complications. Furthermore, the infrequency with which successful reconstruction can be completed in the face of acute occlusion makes repair in the elective situation mandatory for all but the most unusual and debilitated patients.

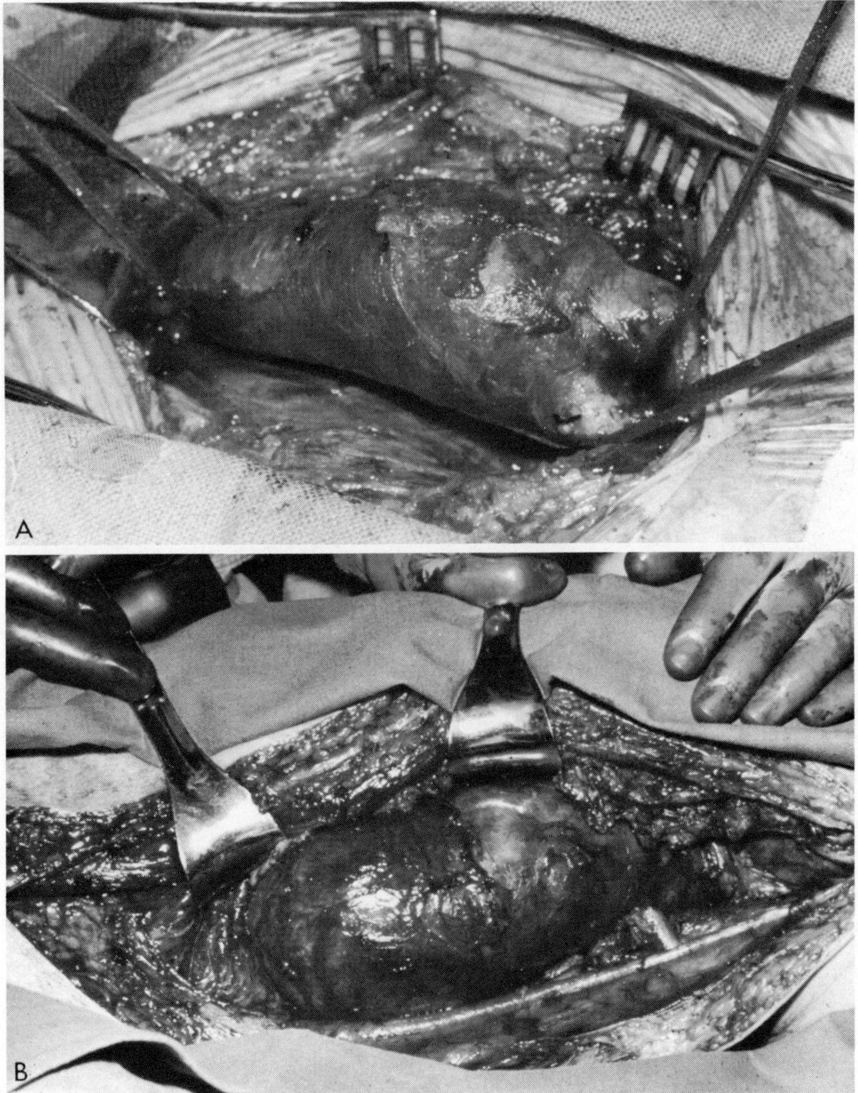

Figure 16–12. A, Photograph of a large femoral aneurysm (ultimately replaced by a bifurcation prosthesis). B, Popliteal aneurysm in the same patient shows the extensive elongation and kinking as well as the dilatation.

The presenting symptoms may be no more than those of a mass, pain from pressure on adjacent structures, venous thrombosis, or the previously mentioned acute occlusive symptoms. Spotty gangrene from peripheral embolization may lead to recognition of proximal aneurysms in either the femoral or popliteal area. Calcification outlining the aneurysm often does not seem to be reflected by the apparent, narrow channel seen on an arteriogram (Fig. 16–13 A and B).

From an historical point of view, the several levels of ligation mentioned in the introduction to this chapter are important, but there is little place for simple ligation today.

Both reconstructive and obliterative aneurysmorrhaphy played a part in the development of surgery, but their role was concerned more with correction of the aneurysm and less with restoration of normal, direct flow to the distal leg.

Linton[42] introduced the concept of preliminary sympathectomy and later resection of the aneurysm. Total resection of the aneurysm

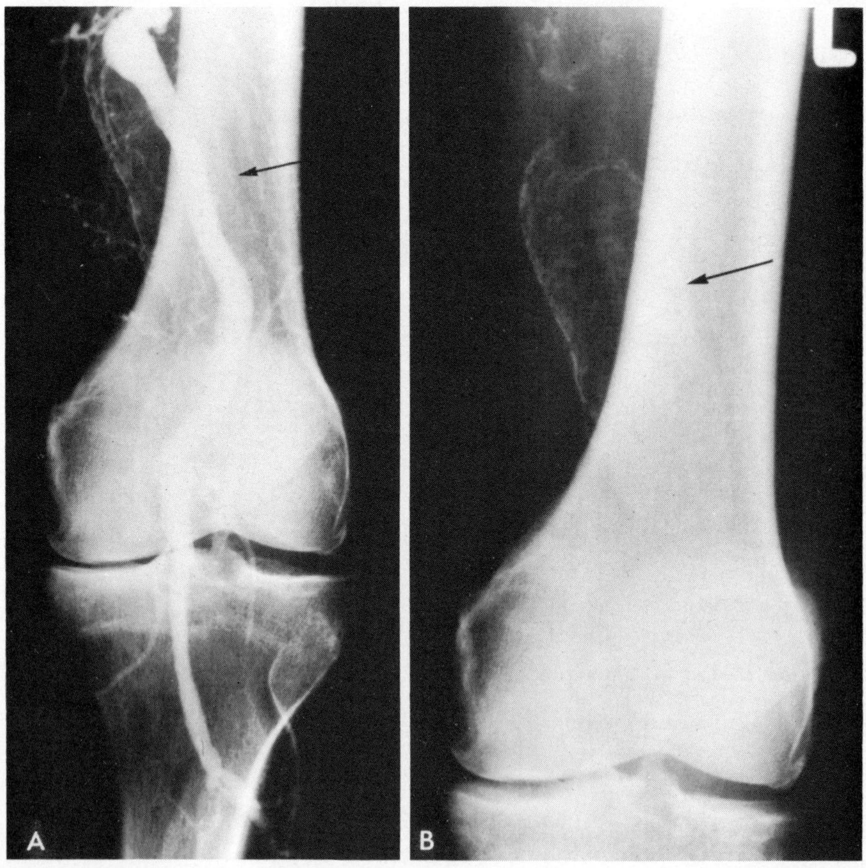

Figure 16–13. *A,* Arteriogram of popliteal aneurysm shows marked deviation of the channel within the lumen, but the caliber of the lumen appears as normal. *B,* Plain film shows the extent of the calcification in the aneurysm and indicates its true size. (Reproduced by permission of the Journal of Cardiovascular Surgery and Minerva Medicine).[5]

and restoration of flow by a graft or prosthesis was the next procedure in the evolutionary sequence of management.

Current techniques, just as with the femoral artery, recommend dissection within the shell of the aneurysm, provided reduction of the mass is necessary. Even simpler, however, is the technique of bypass and exclusion of the aneurysm[25] (Fig. 16–14).

The latter technique allows the surgeon to use either saphenous vein as the graft, even when there is a serious disparity in the size of host artery and vein. The same large size of the vessels in the aneurysmal patient at times requires use of the relatively large plastic prosthesis or bovine heterograft.

Elongation in peripheral aneurysms is even more dramatic than it is in abdominal aneurysms. Figure 16–12B indicates the degree to which elongation and kinking may occur. This kinking may be responsible for some of the symptoms of arterial insufficiency. In-

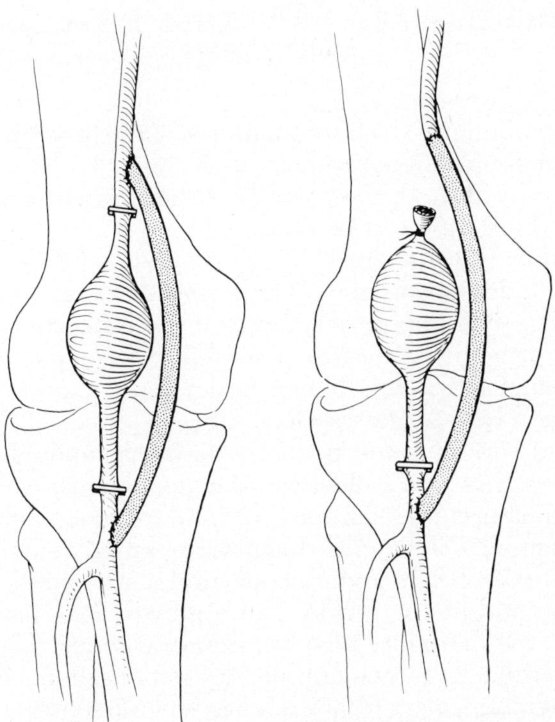

Figure 16–14. Sketches of technical management of the popliteal aneurysm by bypass without resection. On the left the aneurysm is excluded by clips or ligatures and a bypass graft placed side-to-end and end-to-side. On the right the graft is attached end-to-end proximally and end-to-side distally. (Reproduced from the Journal of Cardiovascular Surgery and Minerva Medicine).[5]

frequently, elongation is sufficient to allow end-to-end approximation without a prosthesis.

UPPER EXTREMITY ANEURYSMS

Aneurysmal disease of the upper extremity vessels is uncommon. In days past, *luetic aneurysms* in this area were a common and very serious problem. *Mycotic aneurysms* arising from emboli due to bacterial endocarditis have nearly disappeared with more effective antibacterial therapy. Poststenotic dilatation of the subclavian artery beyond a *cervical rib* may progress to true aneurysm formation. This occurrence may be treated by resection and replacement by prosthesis or vein. An increasing frequency of *axillary aneurysms* due to chronic trauma from the use of crutches is described by Abbott and Darling,[1] who recommended replacement of the aneurysm and the use of Canadian, as opposed to standard axillary crutches.

CONGENITAL ARTERIOVENOUS FISTULAS AND ANEURYSMS

This discouraging disease manifests itself in a variety of ways, ranging from simple hemangiomatous lesions, for which no therapy is necessarily indicated, to extensive lesions with serious systemic effects, for which little can be done.

The clinical presentation of a simple capillary hemangioma deserves little discussion here. The lesions may be resected for cosmetic reasons, with appropriate surgical reconstruction according to well-known principles, but it is essential to recognize any abnormal arterial or venous channels before undertaking a surgical procedure that might turn into a catastrophe.

A second variant is the patient who has a superficial hemangiomatous lesion that is a reflection of a deeper mass of vessels and possibly nonmature vascular networks. A third group appears as major venous dilatation. The venous channels are greatly enlarged and contain blood that is bright red, yet not under extensive pressure. No bruit will be audible as a rule. Limb growth may have been augmented, and the extremity may be slightly warmer. There is no evidence of cardiac enlargement or decompensation. Arteriography will show neither enlarged arteries nor visible shunts, but at a midphase of the arteriographic picture a flood of blood will suddenly appear in large venous channels; however, the exact point of anastomosis cannot be identified.

Resection of these lesions *in toto* is almost out of the question without destruction of bone, joints, muscles, and nerves. On rare occasions, a very isolated lesion is identified in a single muscle mass or even in part of a muscle mass, and it may be removed. Removal of large and superficial venous channels may be neccessary should ulceration develop near them and should there be a threat of hemorrhage. Resection of the veins should be performed by direct incision; blind stripping may result in catastrophic hemorrhage.

Intervention for even an apparently superficial lesion may be responsible for exsanguinating blood loss. A lesion that may seem on physical examination to be suitable for excision may extend directly through fascial and muscle planes so that bleeding is uncontrollable without massive ligatures that incorporate bolsters for pressure on the lesion. At times even the G-suit may be necessary to supplement maximal surgical efforts of hemostasis.

The fourth general category includes those lesions in which the arteries as well are truly involved and can be demonstrated to be enlarged and aneurysmal. This arterial change may come about because of either congenital abnormalities of the artery or continued long-term shunting of arterial blood through a myriad of shunts, or through the development of more significant arteriovenous fistulas secondary to minor trauma. The increased output through such arteriovenous shunts may result in cardiac decompensation which is refractory to digitalis and which may force some attempts at surgical treatment. Figure 16–15 shows such a congenital lesion in the left hand of a 15-year-old girl. There was a loud bruit over the distal radial artery and another in the superficial palmar arch. The radial artery "aneurysm," which was paper thin and alarmingly superficial, was resected in toto. Through a separate palmar incision under tourniquet control, all of the available hemangiomatous and dilated vascular tissue was removed, with at least early relief of the venous distention and disappearance of the bruits.

Figure 16–16 shows an arteriogram of a pelvic lesion in a 22-year-old man who presented with a tumor filling the pelvis, surrounding the base of the bladder and the pelvic colon, and extending into the walls of the pelvis. No bruits could be heard on physical examination, and there was no evidence of cardiac decompensation at this point. The arteriogram shows that both internal iliac systems are greatly enlarged, as is the inferior mesenteric system, and that they all contribute to the lesion. Surgical excision was deemed impossible short of hemicorporectomy. Operation was recommended and was to include the embolization of glass beads and ligation of multiple feeding arteries. The patient has declined the operation for the time being.

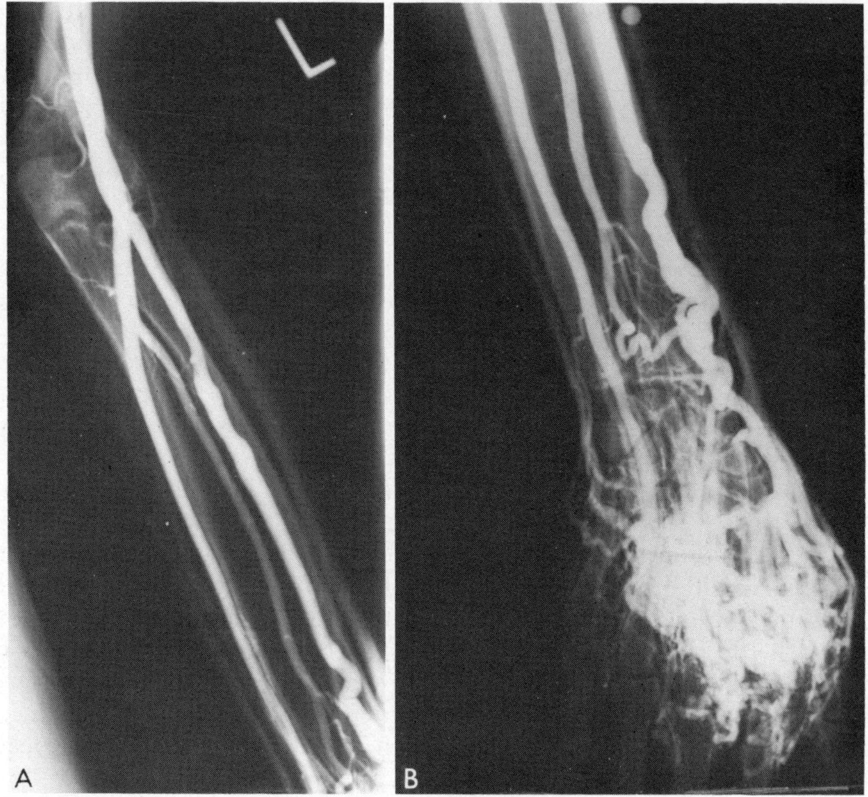

Figure 16–15.   Arteriograms of a young girl with *A*, aneurysmal dilatation of the radial artery and *B*, arteriovenous communications in the palm.

THORACIC ANEURYSMS

A discussion of the management of aneurysms of the thoracic aorta is beyond the scope of this book, since such lesions should be treated by the cardiothoracic surgeon experienced in various forms of extracorporeal bypass. A brief review of the more frequently seen lesions of the thoracic aorta is, nevertheless, included for the sake of completeness.

Since lesions arising in different portions of the thoracic aorta pose technical and hemodynamic changes unique to their location, the following discussion will be oriented primarily toward the anatomic, rather than pathologic, origin. The dissecting aneurysm, or hematoma, will be discussed separately, since its management, regardless of the site of origin, is a more complicated and potentially catastrophic problem.

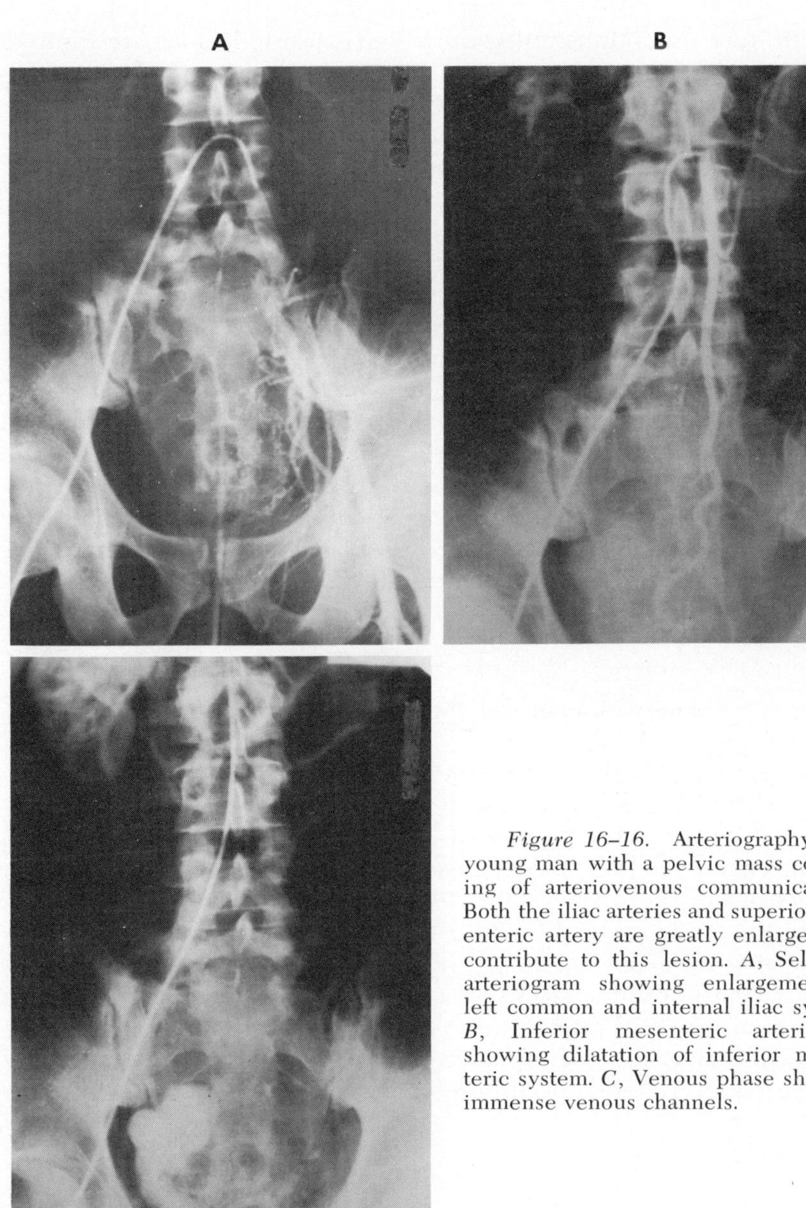

Figure 16–16. Arteriography of a young man with a pelvic mass consisting of arteriovenous communications. Both the iliac arteries and superior mesenteric artery are greatly enlarged and contribute to this lesion. *A*, Selective arteriogram showing enlargement of left common and internal iliac system. *B*, Inferior mesenteric arteriogram showing dilatation of inferior mesenteric system. *C*, Venous phase showing immense venous channels.

Aneurysms of the Ascending Aorta

With rare exceptions, these slowly expanding lesions are limited to the proximal ascending aorta and rarely involve the innominate artery or arch vessels. Not infrequently, however, with progressive enlargement of the aortic root, the otherwise normal aortic valve may become incompetent owing to annular dilatation.[63-65]

The most common causative factors are cystic medial necrosis, Marfan's syndrome, and arteriosclerosis. Although in the past syphilis was a common cause, this is now seldom seen.

The diagnosis is usually suspected when the prominent ascending aorta is noted on chest roentgenogram or by the appearance of aortic valvular insufficiency in the absence of any other obvious cause. Aortography confirms the diagnosis.

Such lesions are readily resected through a median sternotomy, and a tightly woven Dacron tube graft is inserted to bridge the defect. Myocardial protection is afforded by perfusion of both coronary arteries. In the presence of marked annular dilatation, the aortic valve must be replaced and a prosthetic aortic valve inserted. As with any other intracardiac procedure or those involving the ascending aorta, great care must be taken to avoid air embolization.

Aneurysms of the Transverse Aortic Arch

Aneurysms involving the transverse arch are, fortunately, uncommon. Whether of the saccular or fusiform variety, most commonly the cause is arteriosclerosis. Pressure on the trachea or recurrent laryngeal nerve may cause cough, stridor, or hoarseness. Rupture of the saccular variety poses a definite hazard, and compromise of the arch vessels by either thrombosis or embolic episodes is known to occur also.

Total cardiopulmonary bypass with partial or complete resection of the aneurysm and interposition of a fabric tube graft is the recommended treatment. A complicating feature in the technique is the need to supply adequate cerebral perfusion during the reconstruction.[15]

Aneurysms of the Descending Aorta

These aneurysms are second in frequency to the abdominal aortic aneurysms and are also most commonly caused by arteriosclerosis. They can also be caused by a severe deceleration injury (see Traumatic Thoracic Aneurysm). The diagnosis is most commonly suspected with the appearance of an abnormal shadow on the chest roentgenogram in the region of the aortic knob. Because of the symptoms of cough and pain, these lesions can frequently be misinterpreted as carcinoma of the lung. The presence of hypertension, together with serial chest x-ray films showing an expanding lesion, lend strong support to the diagnosis of an aneurysm. The most critical diagnostic study is a retrograde aortogram which, even in the presence of intraluminal clots, is extremely helpful in establishing the diagnosis.

Operation is performed through a left lateral thoracotomy with entrance into the pleural space through the bed of the resected fifth rib. Only partial bypass is necessary in the management of these lesions, and most commonly a left atrial to femoral artery technique is used. As the aorta is cross-clamped proximal and distal to the aneurysm, the pressure monitored in the upper and lower extremities is regulated by the amount of blood allowed to drain from the left atrium. An oxygenator, although not necessary in a left atrial to femoral artery bypass, is required if a femoral vein to femoral artery technique is used. The aneurysm is opened, the clot is evacuated, and the orifices of any patent intercostal artery are suture ligated for hemostasis; the posterior wall of the sac is not excised. This is an important maneuver, especially in lesions involving the aorta near the diaphragm, where jeopardy to the spinal artery is more likely. After fashioning of an adequate proximal and distal cuff of aortic wall, a woven Dacron graft (preclotted) is interposed.[19]

The use of an external shunt from the transverse arch to the descending aorta to avoid heparinization and a pump bypass system has been advocated by some.[38]

Traumatic Thoracic Aneurysms

Acute aortic disruption from a severe deceleration injury (e.g., automobile or airplane accident, fall from a great height) occurs in the vast majority of instances in the proximal ascending aorta and in the proximal descending aorta at the ligamentum arteriosum, two points of relative fixation of the aorta. Those occurring in the ascending aorta are virtually 100 per cent immediately fatal, whereas a surprising number of patients with partial or complete transection of their thoracic aorta in the region of the ligamentum arteriosum will survive for hours to days before exsanguinating. A few patients will recover from such an injury without the diagnosis having been made. Only subsequently, when an abnormal enlargement occurs in the region of the aortic knob and there is a history of deceleration injury, will the diagnosis of traumatic aneurysm be suspected. When such a patient is seen in the immediate post-injury period, the presence of mediastinal widening and/or blood in the left chest is diagnostic. Even so, confirmatory aortography should be carried out as preparations are made for immediate resection and grafting of the lesion. A technique similar to that used in treating the conventional descending thoracic aneurysm is employed.

When the patient is seen at a time remote from the injury, the differential diagnosis between carcinoma of the lung, neurogenic tumor, and traumatic aneurysm of the proximal descending aorta must be established. Again, the critical diagnostic study is an aortogram. Despite an interval of many years from injury to the appearance of the vascular lesion, recommendation for prompt operation is made because of the unpredictability of these aneurysms. Resection and restoration of aortic continuity by graft is performed by means of the previously described technique.[6, 50, 54]

Dissecting Aneurysms

A break in the integrity of the intima and inner layer of the media of the thoracic aorta with rapid intramural dissection of blood flow for varying distances distally is thought to be the precipitating event in such lesions and is perhaps more accurately termed dissecting hematoma.[52] Approximately one-half of such dissections initiate in the proximal ascending aorta just above the aortic valve. In most instances, they then rapidly dissect distally, frequently in a spiraling fashion, partially or completely occluding cerebral, visceral, or femoral arteries as they progress. If the site of the tear involves detachment of commissural support to the aortic valve, acute and flagrant aortic regurgitation occurs. The classical picture of tearing chest and back pain, sudden appearance of aortic valvular insufficiency, and possibly compromise or inequality of one or more of the peripheral pulses is diagnostic of acute dissection of the ascending aorta. Although aortography is almost invariably done, it probably is not essential. In a critically ill patient it might not be performed if the clinical picture is as classical as just described.

The differential diagnosis most commonly concerns acute myocardial infarction or perforation of the esophagus or stomach.

In the absence of irreversible organ damage, most patients with acute disruptions of the ascending aorta should be operated upon.[17] The approach is through a median sternotomy with total cardiopulmonary bypass. The proximal ascending aorta is transected to include the site of disruption. Integrity of aortic valve function can be restored by resuspension of the prolapsing intimal support of the valve commissure. Because of the friability of tissue in this region, such a repair should be carried out with a buttressing collar of Teflon felt. Once the site of the intimal disruption has been excised, the double-barrelled distal channel is reapproximated into a single lumen, and aortic continuity restored, usually by interposing a Dacron tube graft. Once intraluminal flow has been established the elevated intimal flap will drop back into its normal anatomic position.

When the dissection occurs in the descending aorta, the site of origin is invariably in the vicinity of the ligamentum arteriosum or in closer proximity to the orifice of the left subclavian artery. Rarely does the process dissect retrogradely toward the arch vessel. However, it may extend distally for varying distances and not uncommonly involve the renal and femoral arteries. Although the history and the clinical findings will be strongly suggestive of the diagnosis, aortography should be performed to be *certain* that the site of origin is not in an unusual location such as the transverse arch.

The technique of repair involves a left lateral thoracotomy through the bed of the resected fifth rib, control of the proximal and distal aorta, and institution of partial bypass as described under Descending Aneurysms. The essence of the technique involves excision of the site of disruption, with transection at some point distally which can be selected at a convenient level, hopefully where the distal aorta begins to resume a more normal size. As with the more typical aneurysms of the descending aorta, the anterior surface of the aortic wall is opened and the true lumen established. Again, intercostal vessels are ligated from within the aortic lumen. The distal, double-barreled aorta is converted into a single channel by a continuous whip stitch of Dacron suture. A preclotted graft is then interposed as previously described. Because of the friability of these tissues, great care must be exercised in obtaining a secure anastomosis, again relying on the use of buttressing pledgets of Teflon felt.

Because the risk of operation in these patients in the past was high, aggressive medical therapy attracted many advocates.[43, 52] Pharmacological control of the level of the arterial pressure by antihypertensive agents, and as a reduction in the force of left ventricular contraction with use of negative inotropic agents such as Indural, was an effective method to forestall progression of the process. It is still recommended by some as either a definitive modality of therapy or as a temporizing means to allow elective resection of the disease process. There is little question that if drug therapy cannot consistently maintain the blood pressure at the desired level, or if it fails to eliminate the pain associated with such a process, then operative intervention is mandatory.

REFERENCES

1. Abbot, W. M., and Darling, R. C.: Axillary artery aneurysm secondary to crutch trauma. Am. J. Surg. *125*:515, 1973.
2. Alexander, J., and Byron, F. X.: Aortectomy for thoracic aneurysm. J.A.M.A. *126*:1139, 1944.
3. Baker, A. G., Jr., Roberts, B., Berkowitz, H. D., and Barker, C. F.: Risk of excision of abdominal aortic aneurysms. Surgery 68:1129, 1970.
4. Baker, W. H., Sharzer, L. A., and Ehrenhaft, J. L.: Aortocaval fistula as a complication of abdominal aortic aneurysms. Surgery 72:933, 1972.
5. Barker, W. F.: Peripheral arterial aneurysms. J. Cardiovasc. Surg. (in press).
6. Beall, A. C., Jr., Arbegast, N. R., Ripepi, A. C., Bricker, D. L., Diethrich, E. B., Hollman, G. L., Cooley, D. A., and DeBakey, M. E.: Aortic laceration due to rapid deceleration. Surgical management. Arch. Surg. 98:595, 1969.
7. Bernstein, E. F., Fisher, J. C., and Varco, R. L.: Is excision the optimal treatment for all abdominal aortic aneurysms? Surgery *61*:83, 1967.
8. Bigger, I. A.: The surgical treatment of aneurysm of the abdominal aorta. Ann. Surg. *112*:879, 1940.
9. Blaisdell, F. W., Lim, R. C., Jr., and Stallone, R. J.: The mechanism of pulmonary damage following traumatic shock. Surg. Gynec. Obstet. *130*:15, 1970.
10. Blakemore, A. H., and King, B. G.: Electrothermic coagulation of aortic aneurysms. J.A.M.A. *111*:1821, 1938.
11. Bouhoutsos, J., Barabas, A. P., and Martin, P.: Arteriosclerosis amputation and peptic ulcer. Postgrad. Med. J. *48*:671, 1972.
12. Cannon, J. A., Van de Water, J., and Barker, W. F.: Experience with the surgical management of 100 consecutive cases of abdominal aortic aneurysm. Am. J. Surg. *106*:128, 1963.
13. Cayten, C. G., Davis, A. V., Berkowitz, H. D., and Roberts, B.: Ruptured abdominal aortic aneurysms in the presence of horseshoe kidneys. Surg. Gynec. Obstet. *135*:945, 1972.
14. Cranley, J. J.: *Vascular Surgery*, Vol. I. *Peripheral Arterial Diseases.* Hagerstown, Maryland. Harper and Row, Publishers, 1972.
15. Crisler, C., and Bahnson, H. T.: Aneurysms of the aorta. Curr. Probl. Surg. pp. 32–54, 1972.
16. Cutler, B. S., and Darling, R. C.: Surgical management of arteriosclerotic femoral aneurysms. Surgery 74:764, 1973.
17. Daily, P. O., Trueblood, H. W., Stinson, E. G., Wuerflein, R. D., and Shumway, N. E.: Management of acute aortic dissections. Ann. Thorac. Surg. *10*:237, 1970.
18. DeBakey, M. E., Crawford, E. S., Cooley, D. A., Morris, G. C., Jr., Royster, T. S., and Abbott, W. P.: Aneurysm of the abdominal aorta. Analysis of results of graft replacement therapy one to eleven years after operation. Ann. Surg. *160*:622, 1964.
19. Dillon, M. L., Young, W. G., and Sealy, W. C.: Aneurysms of the descending thoracic aorta. Ann. Thorac. Surg. 3:430, 1967.
20. Doppman, J. L., DiChiro, G., and Morton, D. L.: Arteriographic identification of spinal cord blood supply prior to aortic surgery. J.A.M.A. *204*:172, 1968.
21. Dubost, C., Allary, M., and Oeconomos, N.: Resection of an aneurysm of the abdominal aorta. Arch. Surg. *64*:405, 1952.
22. Eastcott, H. H. G.: *Arterial Surgery.* London, Sir Isaac Pitman and Sons, Ltd., 1969, p. 278.
23. Edmunds, L. H., Darling, R. C., and Linton, R. R.: Surgical management of popliteal aneurysms. Circulation 32:517, 1965.
24. Edwards, W. H., and Wright, R. S.: A technique for combined aorto-femoral-popliteal arterial reconstruction. Ann. Surg. *179*:572, 1974.
25. Edwards, W. S.: Exclusion and saphenous vein bypass of popliteal aneurysms. Surg. Gynec. Obstet. *128*:829, 1969.
26. Elkin, D. C.: Aneurysm of the abdominal aorta: treatment by ligation. Ann. Surg. *112*:895, 1940.

27. Esselstyn, C. B., Jr., Humphries, A. W., Young, J. R., Beven, E. G., and DeWolfe, V. G.: Aneurysmectomy in the aged? Surgery 67:34, 1970.
28. Estes, J. E., Jr.: Abdominal aortic aneurysm: a study of one hundred and two cases. Circulation 2:258, 1950.
29. Etheredge, S. N., Yee, J., Smith, J. V., Schonberger, S., and Goldman, M. J.: Successful resection of a large aneurysm of the upper abdominal aorta and replacement with homograft. Surgery 38:1071, 1955.
30. Foster, J. H., Bolasny, B. L., Gobbel, W. G., Jr., and Scott, H. W.: Comparative study of elective resection and expectant treatment of abdominal aortic aneurysm. Surg. Gynec. Obstet. 129:1, 1969.
31. Golden, G. T., Sears, H. F., Wellons, H. A., Jr., and Muller, W. H., Jr.: Paraplegia complicating resection of aneurysms of the infrarenal abdominal aorta. Surgery 73:91, 1973.
32. Gross, R. E.: Treatment of certain aortic coarctations by homologous grafts: Nineteen cases. Ann. Surg. 134:753, 1951.
33. Halsted, W. S.: Cylindrical dilatation of the common carotid artery following partial occlusion of the innominate and ligation of the subclavian. Surg. Gynec. Obstet. 27:547, 1918.
34. Holman, E.: On circumscribed dilatation of an artery immediately distal to a partially occluding band: poststenotic dilatation. Surgery 36:3, 1954.
35. Imparato, A. M., Berman, I. R., Bracco, A., Kim, G. E., and Beaudet, R.: Avoidance of shock and peripheral embolism during surgery of the abdominal aorta. Surgery 73:68, 1973.
36. Johnson, J. M., Gaspar, M. R., Movius, H. J., and Rosental, J. J.: Sudden complete thrombosis of aortic and iliac aneurysms. Arch. Surg. 108:792, 1974.
37. Julian, O.: Personal communication.
38. Kahn, D. R., Vathayanon, S., and Sloan, H.: Resection of descending thoracic aneurysms without left heart bypass. Arch. Surg. 97:336, 1968.
39. Keen, W. S.: *Surgery: Its Principles and Practice.* Philadelphia, W. B. Saunders Co., 1921.
40. LaRoque, G. P.: Ligation of the abdominal aorta for aneurysm of the common iliac artery. J. South. Surg. Assoc. 43:1245, 1931.
41. Leopold, G. R., Goldberger, L. E., and Bernstein, E. F.: Ultrasonic detection and evaluation of abdominal aortic aneurysms. Surgery 72:939, 1972.
42. Linton, R. R.: The arteriosclerotic popliteal aneurysms. A report of 14 patients treated by preliminary lumbar sympathetic ganglionectomy and aneurysmectomy. Surgery 26:41, 1949.
43. McFarland, J., Willerson, J. T., Dinsmore, R., Austen, W. G., Buckley, M., Sanders, C., and DeSanctis, R.: The medical treatment of dissecting aortic aneurysms. N. Eng. J. Med. 286:115, 1972.
44. McKenzie, A. D.: Personal communication.
45. Martin, P., Frawley, J. E., and Sripad, S.: The anatomy and management of aneurysms of the internal iliac artery. Br. J. Surg. 58:111, 1971.
46. Matas, R.: Original memoirs: An operation for the radical cure of aneurysm based upon arteriorrhaphy. Ann. Surg. 37:141, 1903.
47. Matas, R.: Aneurysm of the abdominal aorta at its bifurcation into the common iliac artery. Ann. Surg. 112:909, 1940.
48. May, A. G., DeWeese, J. A., Frank, I., Mahoney, E. B., and Rob, C. G.: Surgical treatment of aortic aneurysms. Surgery 63:711, 1968.
49. Moore, W. S., Cafferata, H. T., Hall, A. D., and Blaisdell, F. W.: In defense of grafts across the inguinal ligament: An evaluation of early and late results of aorto-femoral bypass grafts. Ann. Surg. 168:207, 1968.
50. Mulder, D. G., and Grollman, J. H.: Traumatic disruption of the thoracic aorta. Am. J. Surg. 118:311, 1969.
51. Nobis, P. D.: Aortic occluder: a new instrument. Surgery 68:805, 1970.
52. Palmer, R. F., and Wheat, M. W.: Treatment of dissecting aneurysms of the aorta. Ann. Thorac. Surg. 4:38, 1967.
53. Robicsek, F., Daugherty, H. K., Mullen, D. C., Harbold, N. B., Jr., and Masters, T. N.: Is there a place for wall reinforcement in modern aortic surgery? Arch. Surg. 105:824, 1972.

54. Spencer, F. C., Guerin, P. F., Blaker, H. A., and Bohanson, H. T.: A report of 15 patients with traumatic rupture of the thoracic aorta. J. Thorac. Cardiovasc. Surg. 41:1, 1961.
55. Stahl, W. M., and Stone, A. M.: Prophylactic dieresis with ethacrinic acid for prevention of postoperative renal failure. Ann. Surg. 172:361, 1970.
56. Stokes, J., and Butcher, H. R., Jr.: Abdominal aortic aneurysms. Factors influencing operative mortality and criteria of operability. Arch. Surg. 107:297, 1973.
57. Stoney, R. J., and Wylie, E. J.: Surgical management of arterial lesions of the thoracoabdominal aorta. Am. J. Surg. 126:157, 1973.
58. Szilagyi, D. E., Smith, R. F., DeRusso, F. J., Elliot, J. P., and Sherrin, F. W.: Contribution of abdominal aortic aneurysmectomy to prolongation of life. Ann. Surg. 164:678, 1966.
59. Szilagyi, D. E., Smith, R. F., Elliott, J. P., and Vrandecic, M. P.: Infection in arterial reconstruction with synthetic grafts. Ann. Surg. 176:321, 1972.
60. Thomas, M. L.: Arteriomegaly. Br. J. Surg. 58:690, 1971.
61. Vaughan, G. T.: Ligation of the aorta: Necropsy two years and one month after operation. Ann. Surg. 76:519, 1922.
62. Walker, D. I., Bloor, K., Williams, G., and Gillie, I.: Inflammatory aneurysms of the abdominal aorta. Br. J. Surg. 59:609, 1972.
63. Webb, W. R., Echer, R., Holland, R., and Sugg, W.: Aortic aneurysm with aortic insufficiency. Am. J. Cardiol. 26:416, 1970.
64. Wheat, M. W., Jr., Boruchow, I. B., and Ramsey, H. W.: Surgical treatment of aneurysms of the aortic root. Ann. Thorac. Surg. 12:593, 1971.
65. Wheat, M. W., Palmer, R. F., Bartley, T. D., and Seelman, R. C.: Treatment of dissecting aneurysms of the aorta without surgery. J. Thorac. Cardiovasc. Surg. 59:364, 1965.
66. Whychulis, A. R., Spittell, J. S., Jr., and Wallace, R. B.: Popliteal aneurysms. Surgery 68:942, 1970.
67. Zuber, W. F., Gaspar, M. R., and Rothschild, P. D.: The anterior spinal artery syndrome: A complication of abdominal aortic surgery. Ann. Surg. 172:909, 1970.

Chapter Seventeen

ARTERIAL EMBOLISM IN THE EXTREMITIES

The operation of arterial embolectomy was the first commonly practiced invasion of the arterial tree other than ligation. In its early history the emphasis on urgent operation was based on the propensity of a thrombus to propagate distally to a level from which it could not be recovered and on the belief that reclotting would occur on injured intima after only a few hours. The introduction of heparin to clinical use and the invention of the balloon catheter by Fogarty and associates[7] have greatly altered the approach to arterial embolization.

DIAGNOSIS

The diagnosis of an arterial embolus is based upon the sudden onset of ischemia and the presence of a potential source from which the embolus may have come.

The onset of ischemia is usually dramatic and sudden, and is recognizable because of the onset of pain, followed by hypesthesia, pallor, and coolness. Later, pallor gives way to fixed lividity and a plasticity in the muscles, both of which represent ominous signs.

The level of ischemic change should be followed carefully. The two separate levels of temperature change and sensory adequacy should be recorded frequently, as should motor function. The level of temperature demarcation in the extremity is usually "one segment" below the level of the actual lodgment of the embolus that is, a level just above the ankle usually means distal popliteal occlusion; one at the upper calf suggests an embolus at the adductor hiatus; one at the level of the knee reflects a clot in the common femoral; and one at the high thigh points to an iliac occlusion; bilateral thigh involvement, usually including some change in the buttocks, indicates aortic bifurcation obstruction. Progression of the level upward usually means proximal thrombosis. More frequently, the level drifts downward because of either fragmentation of the clot or an improvement in collateralization.

Clinical diagnosis can be greatly improved by simple biophysical tools. The Doppler sensor used over the artery may be able to directly identify the site of the embolus. Distal pressures measured with the Doppler sensor may identify the adequacy of collateralization. Segmental plethysmography can identify quite exactly the level of the obstruction. Arteriography is the most accurate means of defining the exact level and extent of the obstruction but may usually be deferred until the patient is on the operating table.[17]

The source from which the embolus arose should be identified, and if possible, treated at an appropriate time in order to reduce the risk of recurrent embolism. Emboli from the heart may come from either the mitral or aortic valve and may be either sterile or infected, depending on whether bacterial endocarditis exists. Septic embolization was, in the past, a source of mycotic aneurysms,[1] but the efficacy of antibiotic therapy of endocarditis and success of valve replacement have reduced this complication. Mural thrombi from a recent or even quite old myocardial infarct are also common but may be reduced by the use of anticoagulant therapy after coronary occlusions. Atrial fibrillation on the basis of either cardiac or thyroid disease provides a significant number of emboli. Embolization can also occur at the time of open heart surgery and may not be recognized if the patient does not promptly regain the ability to communicate clearly. Maxwell and associates[13] have described peripheral embolization and mycotic aneurysms derived from candidal endocarditis in the presence of drug usage.

Arterial embolization, even of emboli large enough to occlude the aortic bifurcation, may occur from mural thrombi on ulcerated aortic plaques.

Any proximal aneurysm can spill one or many emboli distally and concomitant thrombosis can propagate proximal to the distal embolization and thrombosis.

The loose compacted fibrin lining of a proximal prosthetic graft can also serve as a source of either single or multiple emboli.

The recovered embolus should always be examined carefully, for a small percentage will be of neoplastic origin from the lungs or from tumor growing in the lumen of the heart, in the aorta, or even in a plastic prosthesis.[9]

DIFFERENTIAL DIAGNOSIS

The differential diagnosis of acute embolization must include acute arterial thrombosis on an atherosclerotic basis, extrinsic compression or trauma, and acute thrombophlebitis.

The distinction between arteriosclerotic thrombosis and embolization may be exceedingly difficult, and, indeed, embolization to an atherosclerotic stenosis may be nearly indistinguishable pathologically. In Table 17–1 are listed some useful criteria, but these only suggest the diagnosis and are not positive means of identification.

Acute thrombosis from extrinsic sources may arise from the entrapment syndromes described in a separate chapter, from extrinsic external pressure (the Saturday night brachial artery palsy from the arm over the back of a chair), or from unrecognized blunt trauma occurring during sleep or other unconsciousness.

Acute thrombophlebitis occasionally has a dramatically sudden onset, with pain, cyanotic pallor and coldness, and loss of palpable distal pulses. The rapid onset of edema, the identification of substantially normal ankle arterial pressures, and the presence of distended superficial veins aid in the distinction. At times, however, acute thrombophlebitis follows a subacute arterial occlusion, and then the true diagnosis can be made only by arteriography. The non-invasive tests such as those reported by Barnes and associates,[2] Cranley,[4] and Gazzaniga and co-workers[8] can help identify the venous component.

MANAGEMENT

The initial use of full heparinization is advocated to reduce the risk of propagation of the clot and concomitant venous thrombosis.

Table 17–1.

	ATHEROSCLEROTIC THROMBOSIS	EMBOLIZATION
Onset	Less dramatic	Sudden: often identifiable to the minute
Level of demarcation	Vague	Sharp but may drift
Prior claudication	Common	Rare
Age of patient	Usually past 40	Any age
Recognizable source for emboli	Possible	Usual
Arteriographic changes	Diffuse atherosclerosis; old collaterals well-developed	Variable atherosclerosis; usually less collateralization

Antispasmodic agents are of little value, for they achieve relief of spasm only in the areas that are not ischemic; the ischemic areas are already maximally vasodilated, and such drugs may only shunt blood away from the critical area. Lumbar paravertebral blocks or stellate ganglion blocks are useful but must be applied with extreme caution in the presence of anticoagulation because of the hazard of retroperitoneal hemorrhage. Continuous epidural blocks may be useful and safer in the lower extremity.

Early decision must be made as to the suitability of the patient for embolectomy, for many patients are in grave condition and should not be operated upon acutely if the limb can be salvaged and blood supply returned toward normal at a later date.

If operative embolectomy is undertaken, the operative procedure can often be accomplished under local anesthesia with an anesthetist standing by to provide good cardiorespiratory support.

SURGICAL TECHNIQUE

Although it has been implied that the use of heparin has allowed embolectomy to be carried out successfully at later times than formerly possible, Thompson and his associates[17] have indicated that delay beyond the 24-hour mark has been associated with a five-fold increase in mortality.[17]

All other things being equal, early operation is mandatory but it is probable that it is in just those very sick patients in whom time is needed to achieve an adequately stable physiologic status that mortality is associated with a delay because of the progression of local ischemia and systemic toxicity. Use of the Fogarty catheter has made it possible to perform almost all peripheral embolectomies through an operative exposure that allows use of local anesthetics.

Preoperative arteriography can be used to delineate the exact status of the embolus, but exact preoperative localization is usually not as important as prompt performance of the operative procedure. If really needed, arteriography can be performed on the operating table. Segmental pressure or plethysmographic curves may establish the upper level of the occlusive process much more quickly and with sufficient accuracy for clinical purposes.

After proximal and distal control of the artery and its necessary collateral branches, a transverse arteriotomy is made. Exploration is ordinarily carried out distally with a Fogarty catheter. Greep and his associates[10] have described the combined technique in which a Dormia ureteral stone-basket has been used to recover significant amounts of embolic material after the Fogarty catheter has seemed to clear the distal tree. This technique may be most pertinent when the embolism lies distal to the arteriotomy and adherent embolus as well as loose clot must be removed.

Use of the Fogarty catheter has been a great advantage, but it is a double-edged sword. There have been documented instances of rupture of the artery or loss of the tip of the catheter.[11] Sawyer and his associates[15] have shown electron microscopic pictures of the ragged intima in a normal artery that is rolled up after several passages of the Foley balloon.

Other measures to retrieve distal emboli include manual manipulation of the extremity, use of an Esmarch bandage to milk the clots out of the arteriotomy, and retrograde flushing techniques such as those described by Olwin and his associates[14] and by Crawford and DeBakey.[5] A distal artery is exposed and cannulated and retrograde irrigation and flushing performed under pressure to dislodge the clots.

When the adequacy of the restoration of arterial patency is uncertain, operative arteriography is of great value. Injection of even relatively innocuous modern contrast material should be followed by generous irrigation of the arterial tree with dilute heparin unless flow is completely restored. If flow is not completely restored, the bolus of contrast material will promptly be emptied into the stagnant venous tree, where it may provoke a venous thrombosis.

Even if total restoration of flow is not possible, delayed embolectomy may allow an improvement in the level of inevitable amputation. For instance, an embolus in the femoral artery may have been associated with both proximal and distal propagation of clot and clearly established gangrene of the foot. If embolectomy can restore flow into the profunda femoris artery and even to some branches of the femoral artery in the thigh, the amputation level may be moved from mid-thigh to below the knee.[12, 17]

It is undoubtedly true that restoration of flow after a protracted period of ischemia may be responsible for sudden cardiovascular collapse. This is in essence a manifestation of declamping shock and is related to the shock that followed crushing wounds in World War II. For a time Stallone and his associates[16] hoped that through-and-through irrigation of the vascular system might reduce this complication, as well as the complication of the pulmonary problems of prolonged ischemia, but this has not been totally successful.[3]

The basic surgical incision will be dictated by the rules of arterial exposure already defined. Certain anatomical localizations demand specific comments.

Saddle Embolus (Aortic Bifurcation)

The introduction of the Fogarty catheter enabled the surgeon to replace the classical transabdominal or retroperitoneal approach to the aortic bifurcation with the bilateral femoral approach. Incisions in the groins allow exposure of the common femoral artery. Once the patency of the distal tree is established, proximal instrumentation allows restoration of flow down the ipsilateral artery. The patient should be fully heparinized so that clotting will not recur in the segment between the aortic bifurcation and the groin. Interrupted sutures are placed and tied only after flushing the aortoiliac system one last time. The other aortofemoral system is cleared in the same way, although passage of the balloon catheter to the aorta must be done with caution so as not to dislodge clot into the first side.

Common Femoral Artery

Clots are cleared from proximal and distal femoral artery and from the profunda branches as well. The presence of adherent clot below the knee may require a separate arteriotomy in popliteal artery or retrograde flushing.

Popliteal Artery

A clot may lodge either at the adductor hiatus or at the distal part of the popliteal artery. An incision over the adductor hiatus will be useful for the former site, but it may be impossible to clear clot from the anterior tibial vessels except by direct approach to the popliteal vessel or by retrograde flushing from the ankle.[14]

Upper Extremity

Clots lodged in the upper extremity can be cleared quite well from the orifice of the subclavian to the brachial artery through brachial incisions over the brachial artery in the upper or lower arm. On some occasions direct exposure of the axillary artery through the clavicular portion of the pectoralis major medial to the humeral attachments of the pectoral muscle itself may allow satisfactory arterial manipulation.

Innominate Artery

Emboli into the innominate artery can be approached through a collar incision removing all the strap muscles from their sternal and clavicular attachments. The most important point here is the protection of the carotid system from distal embolization.

Fasciotomy

The use of fasciotomy, particularly when any significant delay in restoration of flow has occurred, may be limb saving. Although Greep and his associates[10] did not use fasciotomy, most other modern authors advocate its liberal utilization. Fasciotomy should ordinarily be performed in all three compartments of the lower leg, either with a full-length, longitudinal fascial and skin incision[17] or through multiple short, transverse skin incisions through which the fascia may be incised for the full length of the extremity.

RESULTS

Embolectomy rarely is necessary in patients who do not have serious basic disease that constitutes an important threat to life. In the era of the 1940's, embolectomy was likely to be associated with a 35 per cent mortality rate, and most deaths were due to the basic cardiac process. Nearly one-half of the survivors would lose the affected extremity. The mortality reported by Thompson in 1970, however, is only about 15 per cent, and most recent series reported by him lie between 12 and 30 per cent.[17] The commonly reported amputation rates now lie between 5 and 20 per cent if one has used the balloon catheter for more complete embolectomy.[10, 14, 16, 17]

One important implication in the modern era of the management of peripheral arterial embolectomy is the requirement that the surgeon dealing with the embolus identify its source and institute appropriate treatment, whether it be replacement of cardiac valve or removal of a proximal arterial aneurysm.

REFERENCES

1. Barker, W. F.: Mycotic aneurysms. Ann. Surg. *139*:84, 1954.
2. Barnes, R. W., Collicott, P. E., Mozersky, A. J., Summer, D. S., and Strandness, D. E., Jr.: Noninvasive quantitation of maximum venous outflow in acute thrombophlebitis. Surgery *72*:971, 1972.
3. Blaisdell, F. W.: In discussion of Levy and Butcher.[12]
4. Cranley, J. J.: In discussion of Barnes et al.[2]
5. Crawford, E. S., and DeBakey, M. E.: The retrograde flush procedures in embolectomy and thrombectomy. Surgery *40*:737, 1956.
6. Dye, W. S., Olwin, J., Javid, H., and Julian, O. C.: Arterial embolectomy. Arch. Surg. *70*:715, 1955.
7. Fogarty, T. J., Cranley, J. J., Krause, R. J., Strasser, E. S., and Hafner, C. D.: A method of extraction of arterial emboli and thrombi. Surg. Gynec. Obstet. *116*:241, 1963.
8. Gazzaniga, A. B., Pacela, A. F., Bartlett, R. H., and Geraghty, T. R.: Bilateral impedance rheography in the diagnosis of deep venous thrombosis of the legs. Arch. Surg. *104*:515, 1972.

9. Golding, A.: Personal communication; unpublished data.
10. Greep, J. M., Aleman, P. J., Jarret, F., and Bast, T. J.: A combined technique for peripheral arterial embolectomy. Arch. Surg. *105*:869, 1972.
11. Hogg, G. R., and MacDougall, J. T.: An accident of embolectomy associated with the use of the Fogarty catheter. Surgery *61*:717, 1967.
12. Levy, J. F., and Butcher, H. R., Jr.: Arterial emboli: an analysis of 125 patients. Surgery 68:968, 1970.
13. Maxwell, T. M., Olcott, C., and Blaisdell, F. W.: Vascular complications of drug abuse. Arch. Surg. *105*:875, 1972.
14. Olwin, J. H., Dye, W. S., and Julian, O. C.: Late peripheral embolectomy. Arch. Surg. *66*:480, 1953.
15. Sawyer, P. N., Stanczewski, B., Pomerance, A., Lucas, T., Stoner, G., and Srinivasan, S.: Utility of anticoagulant drugs in vascular thrombosis: Electron microscopic and biophysical study. Surgery *74*:263, 1973.
16. Stallone, R. J., Blaisdell, F. W., Cafferata, H. E., and Levin, S. M.: Analysis of morbidity and mortality from arterial embolectomy. Surgery 65:207, 1969.
17. Thompson, J. E., Sigler, L., Raut, P. S., Austin, D. J., and Patman, R. D.: Arterial embolectomy: A 20 year experience with 163 cases. Surgery *67*:212, 1970.

Chapter Eighteen

SURGICAL TECHNIQUES FOR HEMODIALYSIS ACCESS

WILLIAM K. EHRENFELD, M.D.

With the widespread use of hemodialysis, the peripheral vascular surgeon is frequently called upon to provide access to the patient's circulation. This demands a high level of technical skill and ingenuity. The major choices and techniques of operation and the complications encountered in vascular access surgery for acute and chronic hemodialysis will be discussed.

GENERAL CONSIDERATIONS

The shunt or fistula operation for patients in renal failure must be chosen carefully. This is particularly true of the patient in chronic renal failure who will require lifelong dialysis. A properly functioning external shunt or internal fistula is exceedingly important to these patients. The surgeon must consider many factors, including time of initial dialysis, the patient's sex and anatomy, anesthetic management, and operative technique. It is most important to use the least number of peripheral vessels while creating as durable an arteriovenous connection as possible. The individual operative indications and contraindications will be discussed as the techniques are described.

EXTERNAL SHUNTS

Prolonged hemodialysis became feasible after Quinton, Dillard, and Scribner, in 1960, published a report on techniques for cannulation of blood vessels with Teflon and Silastic cannulas.[11] While the need for external shunts has diminished since the introduction of internal fistulas there remain certain indications for their use.

Patients in acute renal failure are best managed with an external Scribner shunt placed on an upper extremity. Dialysis usually lasts for only three to four weeks and the shunt can then be removed. The radial artery and cephalic vein of the upper extremity are used because of ease of cannulation and unrestricted mobility for the patient. If these vessels are compromised, the shunt can be placed at the ankle, utilizing the anterior or posterior tibial artery and adjacent saphenous vein. The second major indication for external shunting exists in conjunction with a planned internal arteriovenous fistula operation in patients with chronic renal failure. Some of these patients need immediate dialysis and are too ill to undergo a more prolonged autogenous fistula operation. In certain other situations a patient with chronic renal failure can tolerate a fistula operation but the fistula cannot be used immediately and a concomitant external shunt must be placed. In both instances the shunt should be placed in the ankle so that the arms can be utilized for internal fistulas. When the arm fistulas are ready for use the ankle shunts can be removed under local anesthesia.

Technique for Scribner External Shunt (Fig. 18–1)

Approximately 8 to 12 ml. of a local anesthetic (1% Xylocaine) is infiltrated about the radial artery and cephalic vein just above the wrist joint. Exposure and cannulation of these vessels are facilitated by perivessel infiltration of a small amount of papaverine to prevent vasospasm. The largest possible Teflon vessel tips that can be comfortably accommodated by the vessels are inserted and fixed into place with 2-0 silk ligatures. The Silastic tubings attached to the vessel tips are brought out of the skin through separate adjacent stab incisions. The proximal loops in the Silastic tubings are positioned in a subcutaneous tunnel to avoid twisting or rotation. The distal loops are attached with a Teflon connecting tip. There should be rapid flow from artery to vein after the clamps are released. The subcutaneous tissue is closed with interrupted 4-0 catgut sutures and the skin is closed with running 5-0 nylon sutures. This same closure is used for all shunt and fistula operations.

Technique for Scribner External Groin Shunt (Fig. 18–2)

An external shunt is often necessary in children because their peripheral vessels are too small for placement of an internal fistula. These vessels are

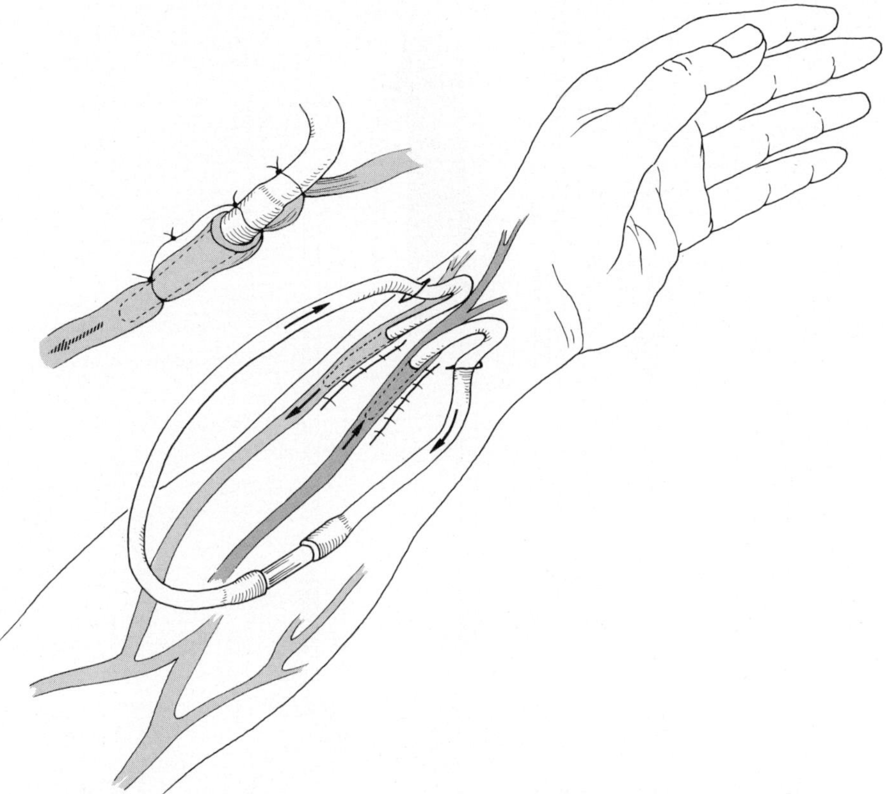

Figure 18–1.   Scribner shunt in place in the forearm. The venous line is in the cephalic vein and the arterial line is in the radial artery. The inset shows the method of securing the Teflon vessel tip and attached Silastic tubing in the vessel.

also frequently too small for cannulation, so that a site allowing cannulation of larger vessels is necessary. Belzer and Kountz have described an external shunt technique utilizing the profunda femoris artery and saphenous vein at the saphenofemoral junction.[2] After a vertical incision is made under local anesthesia the proximal profunda femoris artery and saphenous vein are dissected free. A large proximal profunda arterial branch is mobilized and cannulated with a No. 10 Teflon tip. The arterial tip is initially placed flush with the junction to the main profunda artery and a similar technique is then used for cannulation of the saphenous vein.

There are many advantages to this shunt. The child's hands and arms are free; walking or sitting can be done without difficulty; and high flow rates allow for easy and painless dialysis. This shunt may also be used in adults whose peripheral vessels are unavailable or inadequate for immediate use.

The final external shunt to be described was reported by Thomas in 1970.[14] This shunt is also placed in the groin and utilizes a prosthetic appliqué attached to the arterial and venous Silastic tubings to allow suturing directly to the femoral artery and vein. Be-

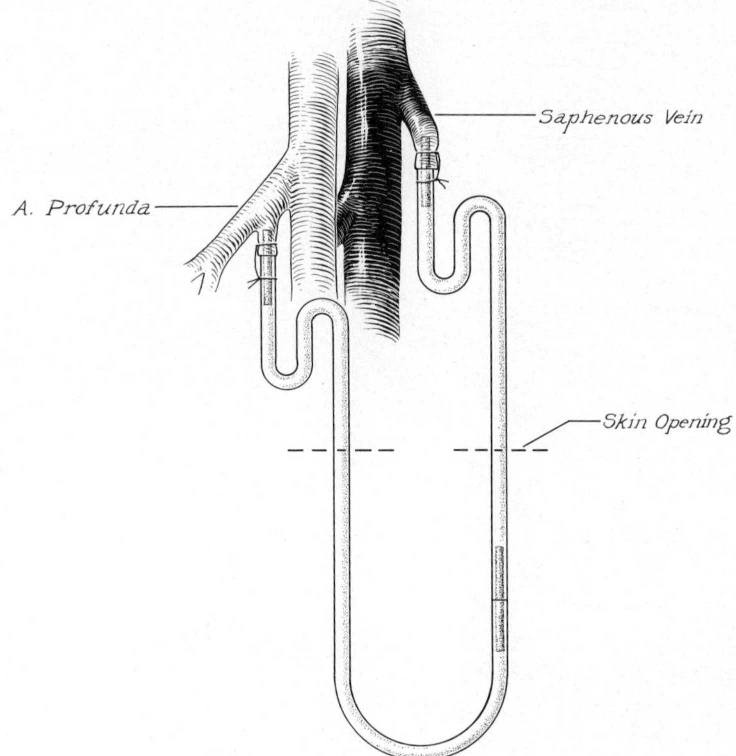

Figure 18–2. Scribner shunt placed in the groin. The venous line is placed in the saphenous vein just proximal to the saphenofemoral junction. The arterial line is placed in a branch of the profunda femoris artery, flush with the main profunda artery.

cause this technique involves permanent or semi-permanent placement the indications are infrequent. However, when indicated it may be very useful in a desperate situation. The shunt can be used immediately, there is high flow, and it should last for a lengthy period of time. This shunt should be placed only after all peripheral access sites for external shunts or internal fistulas are unavailable.

Technique for Thomas External Groin Shunt (Fig. 18–3)

The Thomas shunt is placed after 10 to 20 ml. of a local anesthetic is infiltrated into the groin about the common femoral vein and artery. An oblique skin incision is placed and the vessels are exposed. Longitudinal arteriotomies and venotomies are placed and the Dacron appliqués are fixed into place with running 5-0 prosthetic sutures. The shunt limbs are carefully placed subcutaneously so that the attached Dacron velours are positioned 2 cm. from the skin. The limbs are connected and the incision is closed after wound irrigation with antibiotic solution.

Complications of External Shunts

The major limiting factor of Scribner shunts is their relatively short period of patency. The longest average patency is about six months. For this reason surgical shunt revision and reoperation are frequent, and arteriography through the shunt limbs prior to occlusion is helpful in defining the problem and planning the appropriate revision.[3] The other major problem with external shunts is their propensity to infection because of constant foreign body irritation and exposure to the surrounding skin. Thus, even the most diligent care of the skin and shunt may not preclude infection. When infection occurs in the presence of a Thomas shunt, removal of the shunt is very difficult and may on occasion result in loss of the affected lower limb because of vascular compromise.

INTERNAL SHUNTS (ARTERIOVENOUS FISTULAS)

The most important advances in access surgery for hemodialysis followed the report by Brescia and his associates in 1966.[4] They

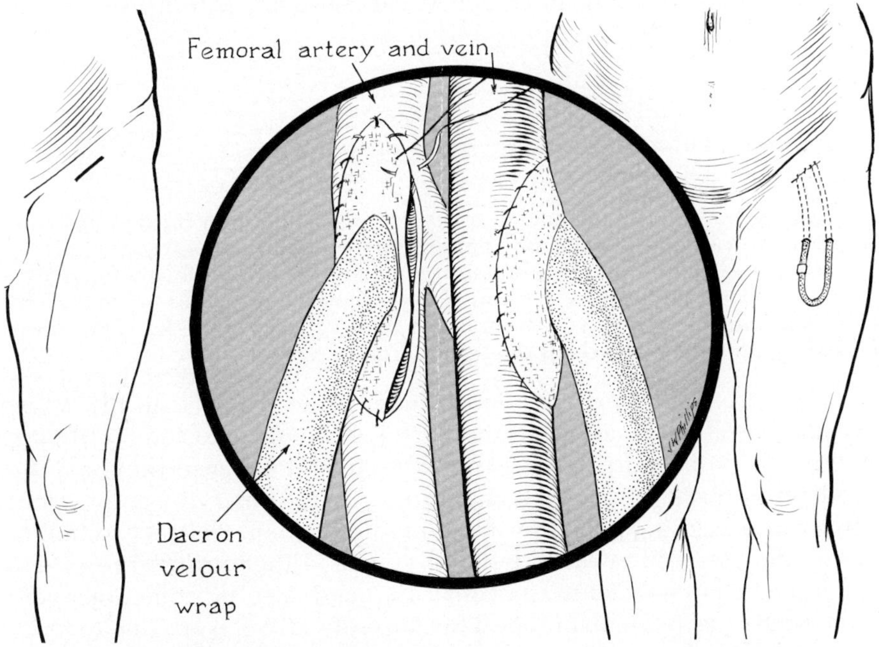

Figure 18–3. Thomas shunt placed in the groin. The prosthetic appliqués attached to the Silastic tubings are sutured to the common femoral artery and vein.

described a surgically created autogenous internal arteriovenous fistula that allows repeated access for hemodialysis and largely removes the clinical and psychological problems associated with external shunts. One of the most satisfying features of this fistula was that it obviated the patient's fear of exsanguination by inadvertent detachment of the Silastic tubings and permitted normal bathing and other activities that are impeded by external shunts. Following this report, numerous modifications and alternative techniques were described and will be discussed.[6, 7, 9, 10, 12]

The most important surgical considerations in patients with chronic renal failure are the location and type of internal arteriovenous fistula to be placed. This planning must take into account the urgency of the hemodialysis and the fact that dialysis will last for the patient's lifetime. When immediate dialysis is necessary it is advisable to place an external shunt in the ankle and to place an autogenous fistula in the non-dominant upper extremity. If dialysis can be deferred for a few weeks, the surgeon has a wide choice of arteriovenous fistula operations. In this instance, the most commonly placed fistula is that described by Brescia and associates and requires a patent radial artery and patent and reasonably sized cephalic vein at the wrist. In women with small cephalic veins, flow through the fistula for three to four weeks is necessary before the efferent veins enlarge sufficiently for easy cannulation. This fistula is best designed for men, in whom it can be used within one to two weeks.

Technique for Radial-Cephalic Arteriovenous Fistula (Fig. 18–4)

The cephalic vein and radial artery are exposed under local anesthesia. Appropriate vascular clamps are applied after the patient is given 2000 IU of heparin intravenously. An end-to-side or side-to-side arteriovenous anastomosis is placed, utilizing a running 7-0 synthetic suture. The length of the fistulous connection may vary from 6 to 8 mm. Patency of the fistula is determined by palpation of a thrill or auscultation of a bruit.

Because some patients have inadequate vessels at the wrist level, several alternate techniques have been advocated utilizing saphenous vein grafts. Graft fistulas are useful because they may be used immediately if necessary, are easier to puncture, and permit earlier and easier conversion from medical center dialysis to home-based dialysis. When a saphenous vein is either unsuitable or unavailable, a bovine heterograft may be used. Use of saphenous vein homografts has been abandoned because of early closure due to stricture and fibrosis.[1]

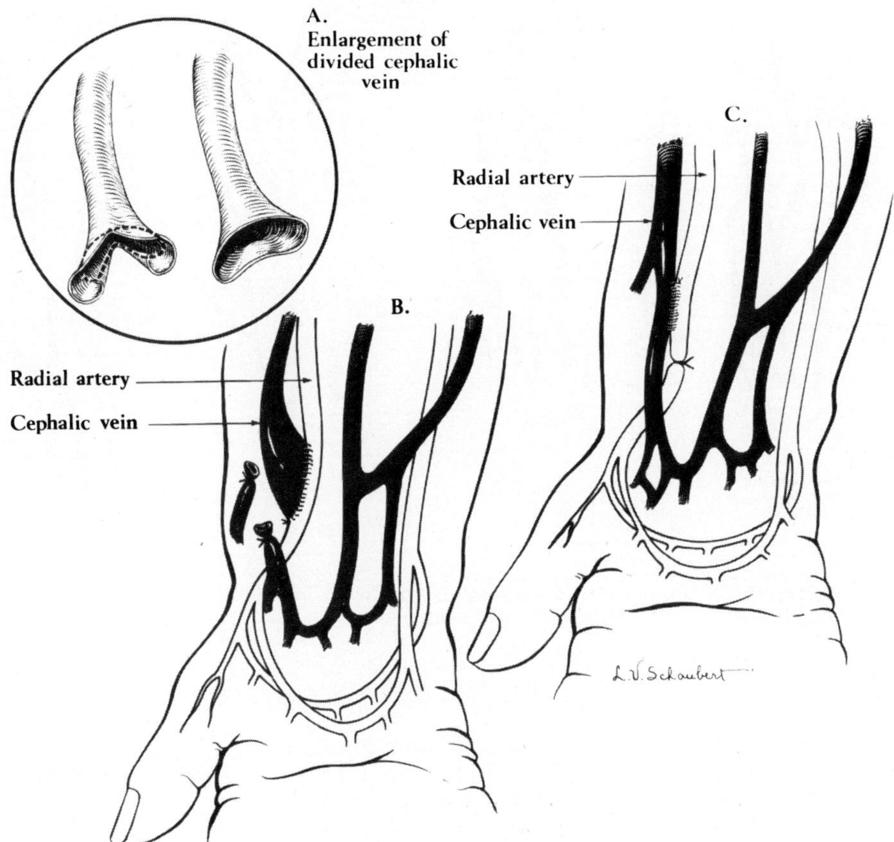

Figure 18–4. Two techniques of radial-cephalic arteriovenous fistulas. (From Ehrenfeld, W. K., Grausz, H., and Wylie, E. J.: Subcutaneous arteriovenous fistulas for hemodialysis. Am. J. Surg. *124*:200, 1972.)

Technique for Graft Arteriovenous Fistulas (Saphenous vein, bovine heterograft) (Fig. 18–5)

General anesthesia is usually employed for these operations. A segment of saphenous vein 20 to 25 cm. long is removed from the thigh. The ulnar or radial artery is exposed at the wrist and the antecubital vein at the upper forearm. A subcutaneous tunnel is made, and after heparin is given end-to-side arteriovenous and venovenous anastomoses are placed, utilizing running 6-0 synthetic sutures. If the arteries at the wrist are inadequate, inflow can be obtained from the brachial artery, with outflow into a cephalic vein at the wrist or into the antecubital vein through a loop graft. If there are no suitable veins in the forearm the axillary vein can be used as an outflow site. *In situ,* saphenous vein fistulas in the thigh are not recommended because of difficulties with needle punction and early closure rate (Fig. 18–6). Adequacy of fistula flow is determined by the force of a palpable thrill or by direct measurement by an electromagnetic flow probe. Satisfactory flow is

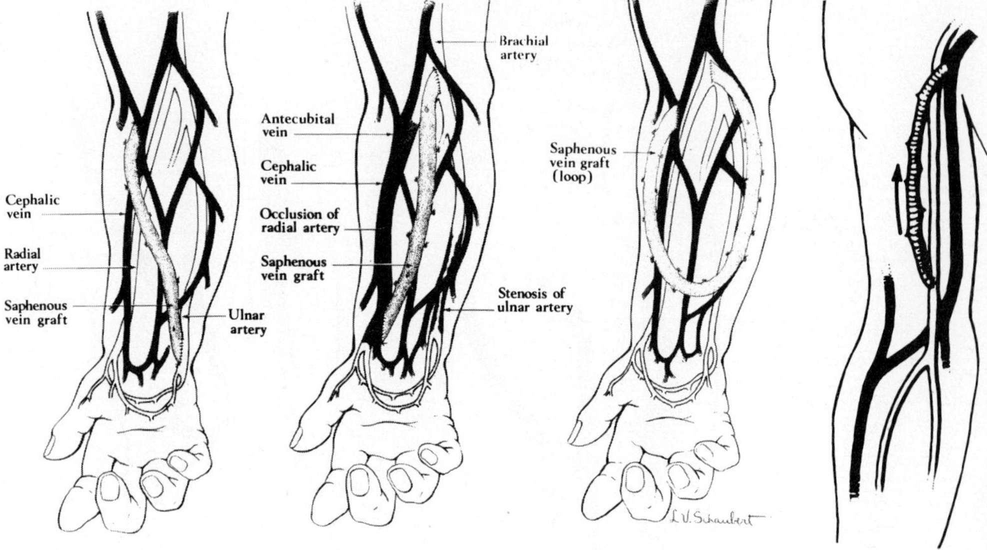

Figure 18–5. Four surgical techniques employed for saphenous vein or bovine heterograft arteriovenous fistulas.

that which exceeds 200 ml. per minute. Forearm graft fistulas have an average flow of 300 to 400 ml. per minute and the upper arm fistulas average 600 to 1000 ml. per minute. If the graft is of sufficient size, dialysis may be performed immediately, although delay will allow better fixation of the graft to the subcutaneous tissue.

Complications of Internal Arteriovenous Fistulas

The complications of arteriovenous fistula operations are both numerous and challenging. The major complications are occlusion, aneurysm formation, infection, "steal" phenomena, and congestive heart failure.

OCCLUSION

Prolonged patency is the objective of all fistula operations, and most should remain patent for several years. The cumulative patency rate is 50 per cent at three and one-half years for the 53 radial-cephalic fistulas in our series. The cumulative patency of the 180 saphenous vein and bovine heterograft fistulas at three and one-half years is 60 per cent. Comparable long term patency rates for these operations have been reported by others.[1, 7, 15]

Acute fistula occlusion indicates improper technique and can be avoided by noting the thrill intensity or flow rate while in the operating room. Operative arteriography may be helpful in delineating the cause of a stenosis or occlusion. Late occlusion is most commonly related to an accelerated intimal fibrosis involving the body of the graft or at one of the anastomoses. Indication of stenosis or impending occlusion is noted by lower flow or increasing outflow resistance during dialysis. Good communication must be maintained between the nephrologist and surgeon so that early attention can be given to a possible impending fistula occlusion. Fistula arteriography through one of the dialysis needles should indicate the area of stenosis (Fig. 18–7). Vascular repair may include resection and reanastomosis or patching of the stenotic zone or relocation of the graft to a more appropriate site. Patching or replacement grafting is applicable to

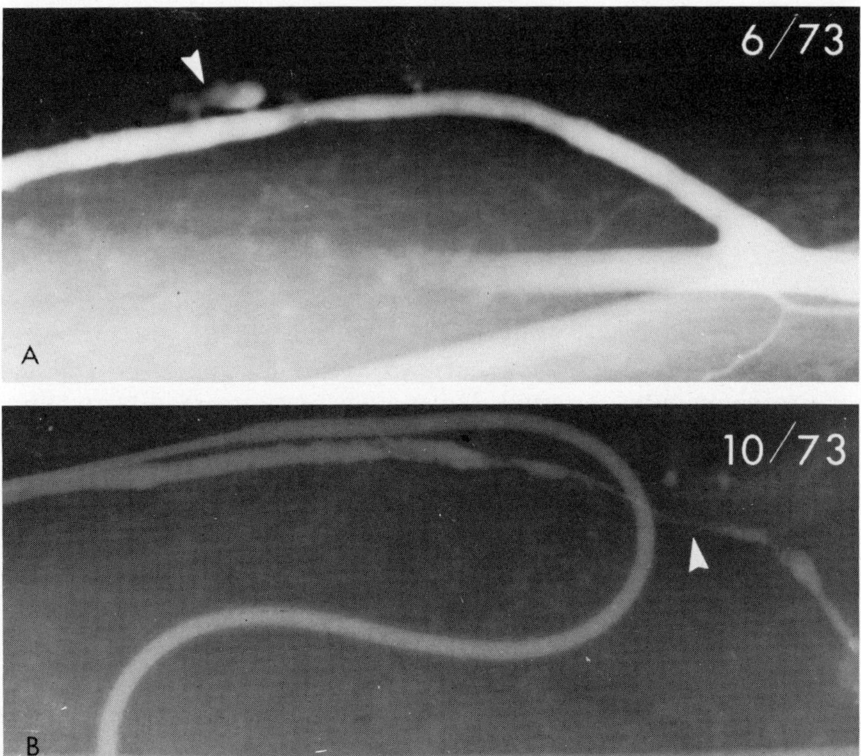

Figure 18–6. *A,* Arteriogram of an *in situ* saphenous vein arteriovenous fistula in the thigh. The graft is widely patent and there are several needle puncture false aneurysms along the course of the vein (arrow). *B,* Arteriogram four months later shows marked narrowing from intimal fibrosis (arrow). This type of arteriovenous fistula is no longer recommended.

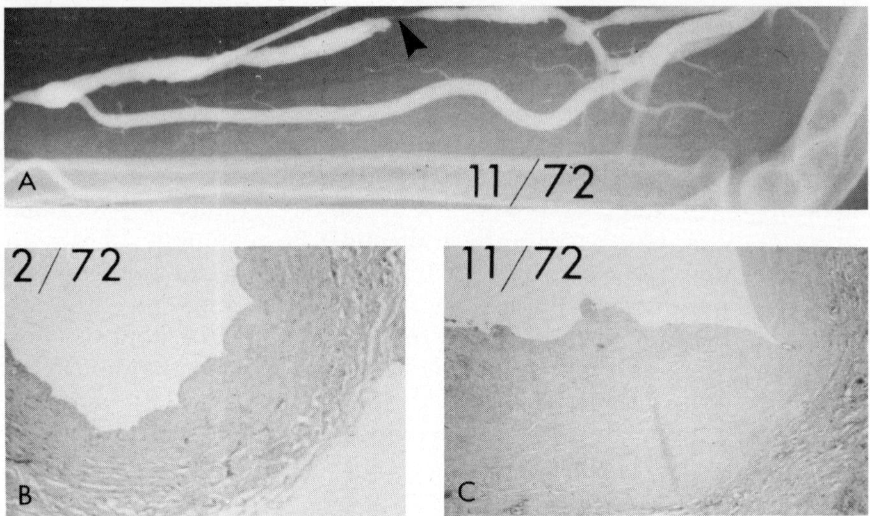

Figure 18–7. *A,* Arteriogram of a saphenous vein arteriovenous fistula in the forearm with an area of marked narrowing (arrow). *B,* Photomicrograph of a section of the vein when first placed. Minimal intimal fibrosis was present at that time. *C,* Photomicrograph of the vein nine months later shows severe narrowing from intimal fibrosis.

bovine heterograft fistulas as well as autogenous graft fistulas. Operative arteriography is indicated if there is any uncertainty about the repair.

ANEURYSM FORMATION

Focal aneurysms, false aneurysms, or diffuse aneurysmal dilatation are commonly observed. False aneurysms are readily repaired by exposure and direct suture of the defect (Fig. 18–8). Focal aneurysms and aneurysmal dilatation are worrisome only if there is significant thinning of the graft and overlying skin (Fig. 18–9). In this instance repair is necessary to avoid disruption and hemorrhage following inadvertent skin abrasion.

INFECTION

Infection of an arteriovenous fistula is a very serious complication. It is gratifying, however, that infection is a relatively rare consequence in view of the thrice weekly insertion of 14 to 16 gauge needles into the fistula for dialysis.

Severe septicemia may occur as a result of systemic bacterial seeding of the circulation directly through the fistula. Bacterial endarteritis and endocarditis are known to result from infected arteriovenous fistulas.[13] The other hazardous sequela of infection is disruption of the fistula with resulting spontaneous hemorrhage. In each instance the fistula must be taken down at the earliest sign of infection to prevent these potentially lethal complications. Further management follows the usual surgical precepts of open drainage and wound care combined with appropriate antibiotic therapy.

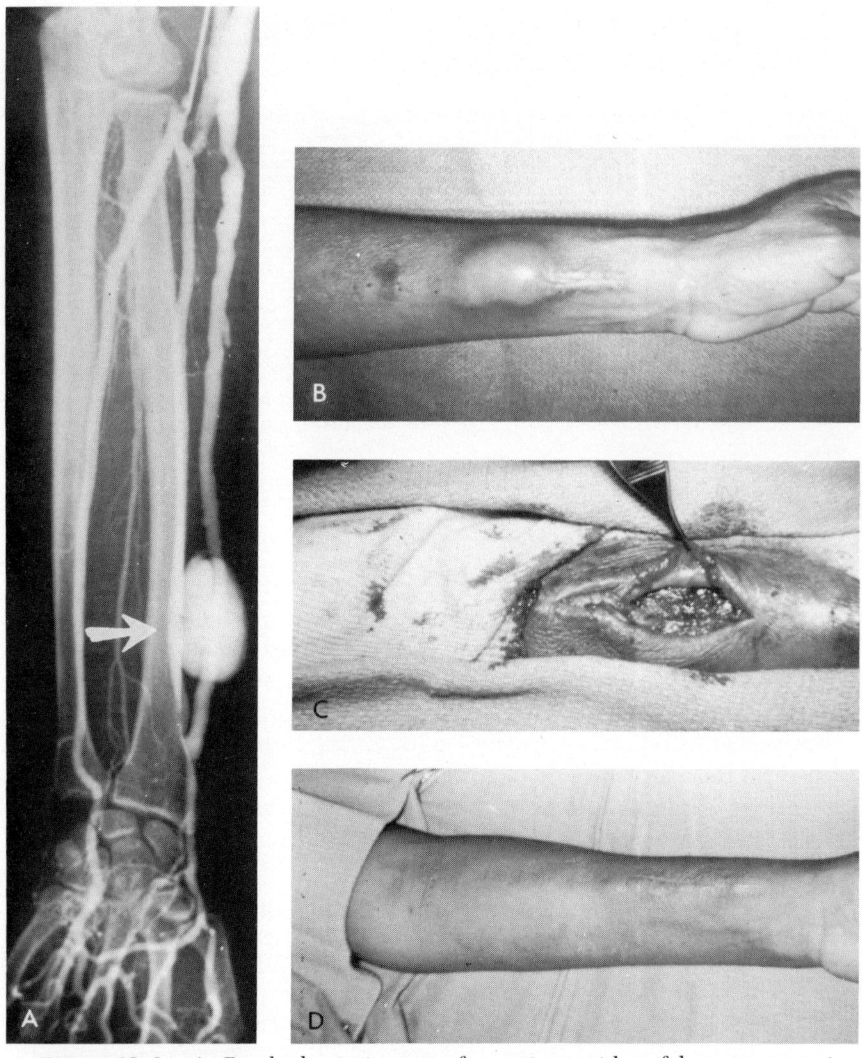

Figure 18–8. *A,* Brachial arteriogram of a patient with a false aneurysm in a saphenous vein arteriovenous fistula (arrow). *B,* Preoperative photograph of the left forearm showing the aneurysm. *C,* Operative photograph showing the false aneurysm sac and the intact adjacent saphenous vein graft. *D,* Photograph of the arm after direct suture repair of the false aneurysm. (From Ehrenfeld, W. K., Grausz, H., and Wylie, E. J.: Subcutaneous arteriovenous fistulas for hemodialysis. Am. J. Surg. *124*:200, 1972.)

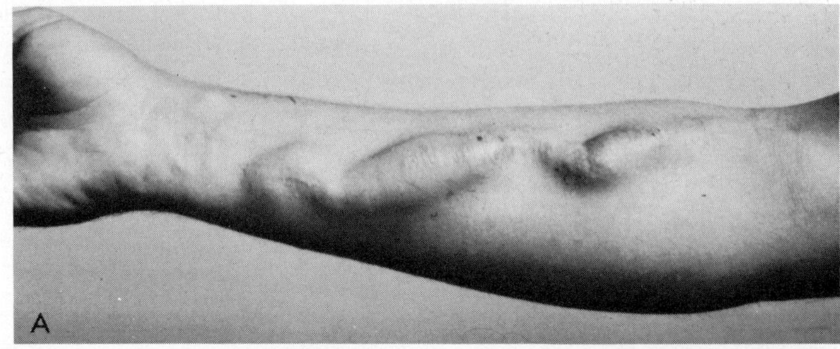

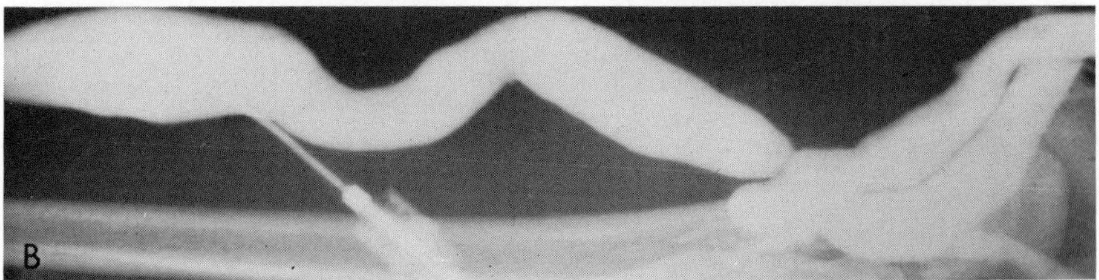

Figure 18–9. *A,* Forearm saphenous vein arteriovenous fistula showing diffuse aneurysmal dilatation. The graft has been patent for three-and-one-half years. *B,* Arteriogram of the fistula shown in *A.* This process is worrisome only if there is thinning of the graft and overlying skin with exposure to abrasion and hemorrhage.

"STEAL" PHENOMENA

The occurrence of vascular "steal" phenomena is also uncommon after creation of an arteriovenous fistula for dialysis, and occurs in less than 2 to 3 per cent of cases. Peripheral vascular impairment usually occurs in the presence of preexisting focal vascular disease (Fig. 18–10), however, ischemia may occur in its absence.[5] Early ischemic symptoms may regress with time, and takedown of a fistula should be delayed until it is apparent that the symptoms are worsening or are permanent. Where there is an obvious threat to viability of the extremity the fistula should be ligated immediately.

CONGESTIVE HEART FAILURE

This complication is rarely caused by a single shunt or fistula in the ankle or forearm.[8] It is more likely to result from a high flow fistula in the upper arm or as a result of the cumulative flows of several shunts and fistulas in one patient. If a flowmeter is available it is desirable to keep flows below 1000 ml. per minute, since renal failure patients in general and elderly renal failure patients in particular are more susceptible to this complication. It is, however, rarely necessary to modify an arteriovenous fistula if the appropriate initial

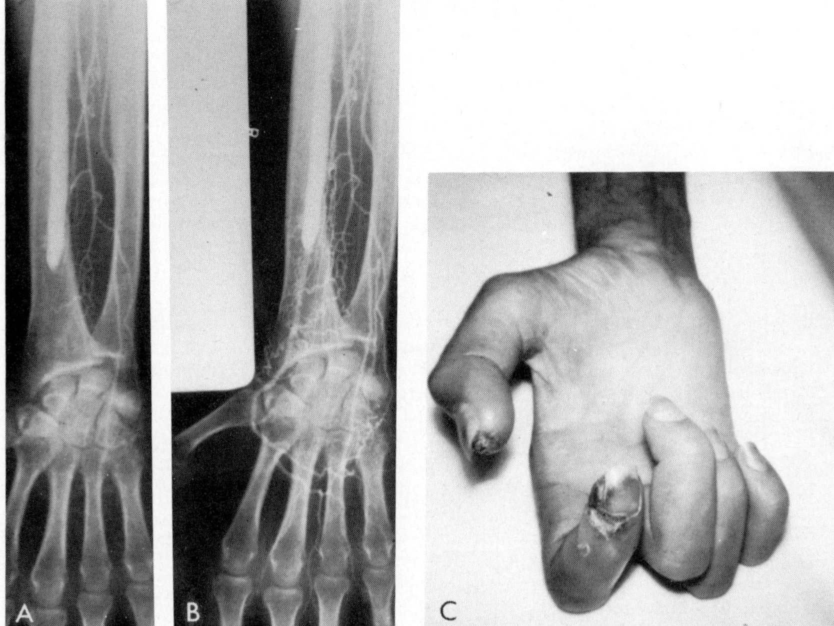

Figure 18–10. *A,* Early phase of a brachial arteriogram showing filling of the saphenous vein graft from the radial artery. There is no antegrade flow in the radial artery distal to the arteriovenous anastomosis. *B,* Later phase arteriogram in the same patient showing retrograde filling of the radial artery and fistula through branches of the ulnar and interosseous arteries. The ulnar artery is diseased and occluded secondary to the underlying renal disease. Digital artery filling of the thumb and index finger is absent. Ischemia of these fingers developed as a result of an apparent "steal" phenomenon. *C,* Photograph of the hand of the patient. Necrosis of the thumb and index fingers healed after cervical sympathectomy. (From Ehrenfeld, W. K., Grausz, H., and Wylie, E. J.: Subcutaneous arteriovenous fistulas for hemodialysis. Am. J. Surg. *124*:200, 1972.)

operation is performed and there is also judicious postoperative medical management.

CONCLUSION

The advent of arteriovenous fistula surgery for hemodialysis in chronic renal failure has dramatically changed the lives of these patients. The problems of repeated vascular access have been lessened. The operations are more durable and the patients are more comfortable. However, a wide range of difficult problems continues to face the vascular surgeon who is responsible for the long term care of these patients. Experience gained from traditional vascular surgery can be successfully applied to this challenging area.

REFERENCES

1. Adar, R., Siegal, A., Bogokowsky, H., and Mozes, M.: The use of arteriovenous autograft and allograft fistulas for chronic hemodialysis. Surg. Gynec. Obst. *136*:941, 1973.
2. Belzer, F. O., and Kountz, S. L.: Arteriovenous Quinton-Scribner shunt with the profunda femoris artery and saphenous vein. Surgery *70*:443, 1971.
3. Berne, T. V., Turner, A. F., and Barbour, B. H.: Angiographic evaluation of Quinton-Scribner shunt malfunction. Surgery *69*:588, 1971.
4. Brescia, M. J., Cimino, J. E., Appel, K., and Hurwich, B. I.: Chronic hemodialysis using venipuncture and surgically created arteriovenous fistula. New. Eng. J. Med. *275*:1089, 1966.
5. Bussell, J. A., Abbott, J. A., and Lim, R. C.: A radial steal syndrome with arteriovenous fistula for hemodialysis. Ann. Intern. Med. *75*:387, 1971.
6. Ehrenfeld, W. K., Grausz, H., and Wylie, E. J.: Subcutaneous arteriovenous fistulas for hemodialysis. Am. J. Surg. *124*:200, 1972.
7. Haimov, M., Burrows, L., Baez, A., Neff, M., and Slifkin, R.: Alternatives for Vascular Access for Hemodialysis: Experience with autogenous saphenous vein autografts and bovine heterografts. Surgery *75*:447, 1974.
8. Johnson, G., Jr., and Blythe, W. B.: Hemodynamic effects of arteriovenous shunts used for hemodialysis. Ann. Surg. *171*:715, 1970.
9. May, J., Tiller, D., Johnson, J., Stewart, J., and Sheil, A. G. R.: Saphenous-vein arteriovenous fistula in regular dialysis treatment. New Eng. J. Med. *280*:770, 1969.
10. Mozes, M., Hurwich, B. J., Adar, R., Eliahou, H. E., and Bogokowsky, H.: Arteriovenous vein graft for chronic hemodialysis: a preliminary report. Surgery *67*:452, 1970.
11. Quinton, W. E., Dillard, D. H., and Scribner, B. H.: Cannulation of blood vessels for prolonged hemodialysis. Trans. Am. Soc. Artif. Intern. Organs *6*:104, 1960.
12. Ries, C. A., Perkins, H. A., and Ehrenfeld, W. K.: Saphenous vein arteriovenous fistulas. J.A.M.A. *226*:665, 1973.
13. Silverman, N. A., Gunnells, J. D., Jr., and Stickle, D. C.: Surgical treatment of staphylococcus aureus endarteritis. Arch. Surg. *108*:730, 1974.
14. Thomas, G. I.: Large-vessel appliqué A-V shunt for hemodialysis. Am. J. Surg. *120*:244, 1970.
15. Zerbino, V. R., Tice, D. A., Katz, L. A., and Nidus, B. D.: A six-year clinical experience with arterio-venous fistulas and bypasses. Surgery *76*:1018, 1974.

Chapter Nineteen

COMPLICATIONS OF VASCULAR SURGERY

Just as postmortem examinations best reveal the true course of disease, so do discussions of complications reveal much about the proper conduct of vascular surgery. Because the nature of severity of systemic diseases varies, different patterns of complications occur, but generally they can be categorized as local and systemic problems (Table 19–1).

The earlier tabulation of complications from the first edition of this book is compared with a later series of 119 consecutive patients reported elsewhere.[2]

One should not try to read specific trends into these figures; in many instances the specific complication was not tabulated for the earlier series.

THROMBOSIS

Thrombosis of the reconstructed segment with associated occulsion within the adjacent arterial tree is critical, since its occurrence negates the operative efforts, and if it progresses there may be further deterioration in the patient's status.

Thrombosis should clearly be understood to indicate reclotting within the reconstructed segment occurring early, rather than as the late recurrence of atherosclerosis and secondary thrombotic disease, either in the reconstructed segment or beyond it.

There are several situations which predispose patients to early thrombosis, and these may be recognizable during the operation.

469

Table 19–1. Summary of Acute Complications

	ORIGINAL SERIES— 1966 183	BARKER, 1971 119
General		
Acute pulmonary insufficiency (? acute MI)	3	4
Asp. pneumonitis	—	3
Tracheostomy	?	4
Superficial wound infection—serious		
hematoma	9	7
Hepatitis	2	5
Intestinal obstruction	—	3
Dehiscence	—	6
Evisceration	—	2
Miscellaneous		
Pancreatitis	not recorded	2
Acute duodenal ulcer	not recorded	1
Delirium tremens	not recorded	1
Related		
Myocardial infarction	4	7
Fatal	1	3
Congestive failure	not recorded	2
Cardiac arrest	not recorded	2
Cerebrovascular accident	—	1
Cerebrovascular arteriosclerosis	—	—
Acute renal failure	1	3
Venous thrombosis	7	9
(Postoperative)	7	6
Pulmonary embolus	7	6
Specific complications		
Acute thrombosis	18	17
Amputation due to thrombosis	7	3
Hemorrhage	8	6
on heparin	not recorded	(3)
Septic reconstruction	4	0
Acute distal edema requiring fasciotomy	—	3
Sympathetic neuralgia, severe	not recorded	1

Most important of these is the lack of an adequate outflow tract, since such a tract is regarded as a *sine qua non* in arterial reconstruction. An outflow tract may be demonstrated by direct visualization or catheterization on preoperative or postoperative arteriography[1, 68] or by flow and pressure measurements.[52]

There are times when nothing can be done to improve the situation. In one such instance endarterectomy had been performed on a popliteal artery of normal caliber, but the branches leading from it were relatively small. The pulse palpable in the reconstructed vessel was of excellent quality—brisk and full, like the distensive pulse characteristic of the prestenotic contour. Pulses were felt in the small distal tree, but on the basis of flow measurements that indicated a flow of less than 50 ml. per minute, early thrombosis and failure were predicted. Despite administration of full doses of heparin, it was not surprising that pedal pulses became undetectable after several days, thus bearing out the flowmeter findings.[10] The distal tree in this circumstance was not amenable to correction, perhaps because of localized hypoplasia, as has been discussed in Chapter Two, and probably contributed to the formation of the original atheroma in the popliteal artery.

Other situations contributing to thrombosis may be correctable; and early in the learning phase most vascular surgeons have met and learned to treat them. One of the most common is the discovery of a plaque causing marked narrowing just beyond the site of anticipated termination of the reconstruction.

Extension of endarterectomy may often be necessary if endarterectomy is the primary form of reconstruction. The combination of endarterectomy and bypass grafting often simply adds the undesirable effects of both operations without combining the good results. A bypass into an area just above a significant obstruction can often be extended to a more distal situation in order to correct the problem. Composite or sequential grafts may be used here.

The presence of debris in a tunnel that was thought to be endarterectomized but which was incompletely freed of all atheromatous and fibrous intimal flaps has been recognized by many as a cause of endarterectomy failure,[3, 10, 11] and this defect must be sought if acute thrombosis supervenes.

When a long tunnel is used it is possible to have the graft twist on itself and become occluded. A line marked on the vein or fabric prosthesis will help avoid this. Furthermore, it is most important to be sure that there is no extrinsic encroachment on the graft. These encroachments may be due to inadequate development of the tunnel, to an acute curve around a muscle group such as around the adductors leading into the popliteal space, or to insufficient dissection under the inguinal ligament. In the postoperative period, the development of a hematoma in a long tunnel may be sufficient to occlude a graft.

Although seventeen acute thromboses were recorded in the second series, only three of these proceeded to amputation, and all of these were in patients whose operation had been performed for attempted limb salvage in the first place.

Recognition of chronic inadequacy of inflow to the segment has long been a factor in selection of patients, and forms the basis for the principle that the more proximal of two discrete lesions must be corrected first.[32]

Thrombosis in the stagnant distal tree should be preventable with careful use of dilute heparin as soon as possible during operation. Spillage of clots which have formed above the proximal clamp

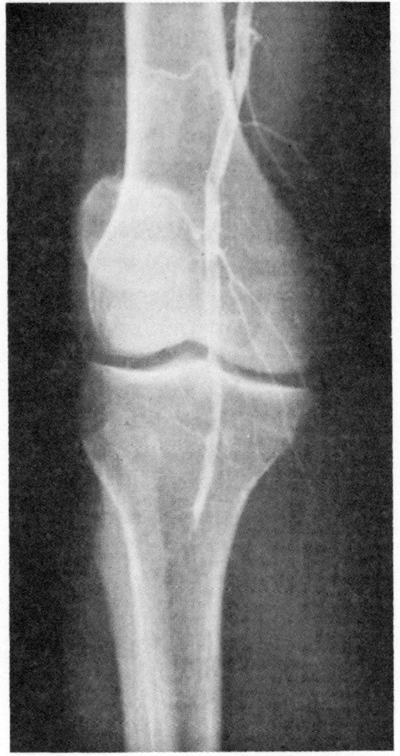

Figure 19–1. Arteriogram of femoral popliteal system showing filling defects caused by thrombi which had migrated into the distal tree during placement of an aortofemoral bypass graft. There is complete occlusion of the distal popliteal trunk. Clots were removed by common femoral arteriotomy, with the aid of a Fogarty catheter.

into the distal tree is another accident which can be prevented by the correct removal of clamps and correct sequence in flushing. In particular might be noted failure to recognize the loose ball of fibrin and atheromatous debris that often lies in the distal aorta above an area of severe aortic or iliac stenosis (Fig. 19–1).

Many surgeons prefer an alternate and appropriate method by giving heparin intravenously to produce total body heparinization, and do not use distal heparinization at all. It should not be necessary to reverse the heparin effect with protamine sulfate unless there is unusual bleeding in the wound at the end of the operation, although most authors recommend such reversal.

Thrombosis is treated by correcting the the anatomical defect, if possible, removing distal clots by means of suction, by retrograde flushing from the posterior tibial artery,[16, 20] and by the use of the Fogarty catheter.[22]

Conservative management of thrombosis with heparinization or thrombolytic enzymes has not proved consistently satisfactory except as it may have prevented further propagation of a thrombus. Nevertheless, these agents should be used as adjuncts to as complete a mechanical correction as possible. The combination of heparin and fibrinolytic agents produces the added hazard of provoking hemorrhage because of the combined effect of heparin on various enzymatic processes in the coagulation cycle and its minor role in preventing platelet aggregation, in addition to the destructive role of fibrinolysins.

Cranley[15] has stressed the importance of avoiding a hematocrit too high to maintain optimal flow. The minor increase of oxygen carrying capacity does not compensate for the increased viscosity and lowered flow rates of a polycythemic bloodstream having a hematocrit level between 40 and 55 per cent.

Intrinsic coagulation defects sometimes produce or contribute to thrombosis. A rare but devastating problem is hypercoagulability associated with cryoglobulinemia. The exact mechanism through which this defect operates to cause occlusion of a reconstructed artery are obscure. In three patients, all women, great quantitative increases in cryoglobulins and increased resistance to heparin were encountered in the face of recurrent intra-arterial thromboses. The following case is representative.

A 41-year-old woman was seen in consultation because of impending gangrene. A year earlier she had suffered an isolated right external iliac occlusion, which took the form of extensive thrombosis superimposed on moderate but well-defined atherosclerosis. An uneventful endarterectomy had been performed by a thoroughly competent surgeon. The patient had been well until 2 weeks prior to admission, when she suddenly manifested signs of serious ischemia due to occlusion of the endarterectomized segment. Repeated attempts at reconstruction failed despite apparent technical perfection. The distal tree, which had been normal, became thrombosed, and gangrene supervened. During this time the patient was demonstrated to have greatly increased (tenfold) cryofibrinogen levels and such resistance to heparin that 400 mg. of sodium heparin every 12 hours produced maximal prolongation of the Lee-White clotting time of only 14 minutes. At amputation thrombosis of all the vessels of the lower leg was apparent.

Heparin alone is known to produce transient pseudocryoglobulinemia,[62] but not of the nature seen in the case presented. Cryofibrinogen levels returned to normal in 6 months in this patient.

Rhodes and his associates have described a syndrome in which a heparin-dependent antibody may be responsible for a thrombocytopenia with both thrombotic and hemorrhagic manifestations. If recognized, cessation of heparin therapy and control of the thrombosis by the use of prothrombin antagonists or by the careful administration of antiaggregating platelet agents such as dipyramidole and aspirin is recommended.[48]

One other mechanism of early failure is the thrombosis that occurs during an episode of postoperative hypotension. Such a case is described.

R.W. was a 59-year-old man who had had two episodes of massive infarction and experienced moderate anginal pain with limited activity. His left foot was markedly ischemic, and arteriography indicated marked stenosis of the left common and external iliac arteries, combined with complete obstruction of the superficial femoral artery. The surgeon underestimated the margin of cardiac reserve and undertook a major reconstructive procedure. This consisted of left lumbar sympathectomy, bypass graft of Dacron from aorta to femoral artery, and reconstruction of the femoral artery that consisted of a combination of endarterectomy of the proximal third and distal third of the femoral artery which was repaired with an autologous saphenous vein patch and joined with a bypass using the same piece of saphenous vein. Excellent pulsations and flow were restored into the distal tree. A few hours postoperatively, however, the patient developed supraventricular tachycardia without evidence of blood loss or clear-cut signs of failure. Administration of 200 ml. of whole blood precipitated an episode of acute congestive failure and hypotension. This was treated successfully with administration of morphine, phlebotomy, and tourniquets to the three uninvolved extremities. During the hour in which circulation was greatly impaired, thrombosis occurred in the femoral reconstructed segment.

Late episodes of thrombosis associated with recurrence of atherosclerosis have already been discussed.

Two factors appear to be responsible for later recurrence of atherosclerosis in a reconstructed segment. First may be the atherogenic propensities of the patient[2, 3, 11, 42, 59] and these should be corrected if possible. The other factor is the mechanical susceptibility of the reconstructed segment itself. Angioplasty can correct any abnormal configuration that increases the vulnerability of the artery, and if necessary, a prosthesis may be used instead of endarterectomy.

Several surgeons have demonstrated the vulnerability of freshly endarterectomized segments of fresh biological grafts in the presence of hyperlipemia.[2, 28, 42, 51]

HEMORRHAGE

Hemorrhage is a hazard with anticoagulant therapy, particularly when this is given immediately after operation, and many surgeons do not give heparin postoperatively. As explained on page 220 there is good reason for using an agent which can control the deposition of whole red clot in the reconstructed segment, and heparin is presently more widely accepted than is the alternative agent, macromolecular dextran.[22, 24] If there is reason to believe that heparin will reduce serum lipids or otherwise stabilize lipid levels during the healing phase, its use might be justified for this reason alone as protection against the deposition of unusual amounts of lipids in the endothelial scar during its early formation.[2]

Heparin used in the dosages we have recommended is not associated with hemorrhage except when hemostasis has been imperfect. In one series, hemorrhage has been reported to occur in 27 per cent of the cases.[49] In the two series presently reported from the University of California at Los Angeles serious hemorrhage has occurred in only 14 of 307 cases, although the definition of "hemorrhage" is an arbitrary one. It is more important to note that of the last 119 cases reported there were six episodes of hemorrhage, and only three of these occurred on heparin, although heparin was used almost routinely in these patients. Some bleeding almost inevitably occurs in all reconstructive surgery. Hemorrhage in separate sympathectomy incisions performed as the first stage of a femoral reconstruction has been an occasional problem.

INFECTION

Not only does hemorrhage have an immediate hemodynamic effect, but it also increases the possibility of infection, and infection, of course, is a predisposing factor in the occurrence of *late* hemorrhage. Infection is therefore one of the dreaded complications of any arterial operation. The combination of extensive wounds, prolonged operating time, general debility of the patient, occasional association of diabetes, and occurrence of many small hematomas even in the absence of heparinization predisposes patients to infection. In our first series there was significant infection in nine of 184 patients and in the second series, in seven of 119 patients. In no second series patient, however, was the infection deep enough to involve the actual reconstruction.

Superficial wound infections may be troublesome but are not necessarily significant unless the infective process reaches the site of arterial reconstruction, as occurred in four instances in the first series (Table 19–2).

The efficacy of giving prophylactic antibiotics has been ques-

Table 19–2.   Postoperative Infection

IDENTIFICATION	SITE	RESTORATION	OUTCOME
M.S.	Iliac artery	Temporary; reinfection	Amputation
F.W.	Iliac artery	Temporary	Fatal hemorrhage
R.M.	Femoral artery	Temporary; prompt failure and reinfection	Fatal bacterial endarteritis
F.R.	Iliac artery	None	Fatal hemorrhage

tioned,[9, 29, 58] although good results have been reported based on the establishment of adequate levels at or prior to operation.[9] Further justification for their use is found in the introduction of synthetic penicillin derivatives. The use of these agents to prevent emergence of a resistant strain of *Staphylococcus,* in combination with cover of a broad spectrum antibiotic, is currently followed. Levels of these agents should be established prior to operation if they are to be used. Protracted therapy with the agents is not necessary and they should usually be stopped within 48 hours of the operation unless there is a continuing specific indication for their therapeutic as opposed to prophylactic use, so as to diminish the risk of superinfection with resistant microbial strains.

The use of fabric prostheses creates a special problem in regard to infection in the prosthesis; i.e., that of an indispensable foreign body that must be removed in order to eradicate the infection. Some favorable results have been achieved with the use of high local concentrations of antibiotics, often with replacement of the prosthesis even in an infected field. Usually, infection in a fabric graft results in ultimate failure of the graft as a conduit, followed by hemorrhage unless the graft is removed. One can sometimes delay extension of sepsis along the fabric to the danger level of the attachment to the host vessel until thrombosis occurs within the prosthesis. Once an infected prosthetic graft becomes occluded, sepsis is apt to spread rapidly along the full length of the graft. An occluded and infected graft, therefore, usually represents a very urgent indication for removal.[8, 50] If the thrombosis does not precipitate a crisis due to ischemia of the limb formerly supplied by the prosthesis, then it may be possible to remove the graft and eradicate the infection without further deterioration of the affected blood supply. If infection reaches the suture line first, the outcome may be fatal.[13, 50, 53, 65]

An example of the successful management of an infected graft is presented.

The patient was a 65-year-old man who had an aortobilateral femoral bypass graft performed for aortoiliac occlusive disease. A small stitch abscess in the left groin complicated the postoperative course. Six weeks later a suture sinus remained, and a piece of silk suture (which had been used in the anastomosis) was extruded. The sinus healed, but in its place appeared a pulsating, hot, red mass, and the patient was transferred to the Medical Center of the University of California at Los Angeles.

Cultures of the closed wound were obtained by fine needle aspirate and revealed staphylococcus aureus (Phage type 80/81); biologically identical staphylococcus aureus was also cultured from the nasopharynx and was found to be susceptible to Staphcillin. Under heavy doses of Staphcillin, the iliac arm of the graft was exposed and found to be free of infection. The graft was divided and a segment resected. The proximal end of the distal portion was ligated and covered with a peritoneal flap. No pulsations could be heard with the Doppler sensor, and the leg appeared cadaveric. It was believed imperative to proceed with immediate revascularization. The distal end of the proximal arm was attached to a new graft, which was led through a new subperitoneal dissection through the obturator canal. An incision medial and distal to the femoral area was carried down to the pectineus, the muscle incised, and the graft led down to the mid-portion of the superficial femoral artery and attached end-to-side, with good restoration of distal flow. Plastic catheters were led down to the new prosthesis and the suprainguinal dissection. These wounds were closed and carefully dressed. The old groin incision was now reopened and after some difficulty with bleeding, the contaminated Dacron, including all of the distal segment, was excised. The common femoral artery was debrided and oversewn with fine polypropylene suture. This area was covered with mobilized sartorius muscle; catheters were also placed here for local irrigation. The patient was kept on heavy antibiotic coverage for a week. The wounds healed unremarkably.

The preferred procedure to be followed in treating an infected graft is as described.

1. The graft is divided through a proximal area which is free of sepsis, and a portion of uninfected graft is removed. All the uninfected graft may be removed, and if feasible, healthy tissue interposed between this area and the distal infected field. Irrigation locally through catheters placed in the wound, using antibiotics and locally effective biological or chemical debriding agents, is advisable especially if any of the proximal graft is left in place. The second stage may be carried out immediately or, if necessary for other reasons, delayed several days.

2. After a delay of no more than five to seven days the distal infected arm of the graft is removed. This will usually include the site of the distal attachment.

3. If the distal point of attachment must be removed the vessel at this site must be repaired with a suture which will not further complicate and support persisting infection. It may be possible to simply ligate the artery, or to oversew it with either fine polypropylene suture or fine wire. If a viable limb can be preserved by removal of the graft and ligation of the vessel, this would probably be the safest thing to do, but viability often cannot be assured. One may assess the viability by means of the Doppler tones. An absent Doppler indicates a very hazardous situation as far as the distal circulation is concerned, and usually demands reconstruction, either immediately or in the very near future.[35] If reconstruction is indicated, a new prosthesis or graft must be brought from clean area. It is preferable to bypass the old reconstruction totally by some form of an extra-anatomic bypass. This may take the form of an axillofemoral bypass, femorofemoral bypass, an iliofemoral bypass through the obturator foramen, or any other route, dependent upon the ingenuity of the surgeon.[5,50,53]

Goldsmith and Beattie have suggested that pedicled omentum may be wrapped around contaminated or exposed arteries (or even vein grafts) to protect against further breakdown and hemorrhage.[27] Porcine grafts have also been suggested as a temporary surface for exposed grafts for a similar purpose,[37] but the surgeon should look on these methods as unusual ways out of a dilemma rather than as the procedure of choice.

According to Wylie,[66, 67] if a graft must be replaced in an infected field, autologous tissue, preferably arterial, should be used, taken from an uninvolved iliac artery, for example. Continuity in the donor site is restored by means of a fabric prosthesis in that area.

Bricker and his associates have, however, called attention to the fact that in experimental grafts in the dog there was a better patency rate in infected veins, but that some Dacron knitted prostheses did heal, and two of the dogs with infected vein grafts did suffer fatal hemorrhages, and they suggest that the vein graft is perhaps not as superior to Dacron as is commonly believed.[8]

GASTROINTESTINAL EFFECTS

Closely related to the problem of infection in fabric prostheses is erosion of a graft into the intestinal tract or development of an aneurysm at the suture line between the aorta and the graft which subsequently ruptures into the duodenum. Humphries[30] and Young[69] in discussing gastrointestinal complications due to major vascular operations within the abdomen, divide them into two main categories.

The first is aortoenteric fistulas, or fistulas associated with erosion of a graft into the intestinal tract. There were two patients in whom the development of an aortoenteric fistula was suspected in our series; however, such a lesion could not be demonstrated at autopsy after death from massive gastrointestinal bleeding. In a third patient there was unequivocal rupture of the aorta in the vicinity of the suture line between the graft and the aortic wall into the duodenum, with massive hemorrhage. This was successfully corrected in another hospital, but the patient died of a pulmonary embolus. A fourth patient developed a fistula from the iliac arm of a Dacron graft into the small bowel. Bowel resection and removal of the graft saved the patient's life, but the leg had to be amputated.

It is most important to cover the graft, especially a bypass graft that lies on top of the aorta and is in an unfavorable position, with as much living tissue as possible so as to diminish the possibility of rupture into the adjacent bowel.[54, 65]

Although end-to-end anastomoses apparently are less at risk than side-to-end, it seems desirable in performing the reconstruction in the treatment of aortic aneurysmal disease to leave enough of the outer wall of the aneurysm that this can be placed over the graft, thus separating the Dacron clearly from its contact with the duodenum at this level. Many surgeons choose to resect the aorta during reconstruction for occlusive disease. Under these circumstances, no aortic shell remains and other tissues such as the omentum may be interposed if desired between the prosthesis and the duodenum and other viscera.

The second major category is of intestinal ischemia. The patient, W.F., reported on page 487, represents our only experience with acute ischemia in the presence of obstructive disease, although several episodes of colonic necrosis in the presence of aneurysm have been encountered.

Perhaps more frequently seen is a form of intestinal angina manifested by abdominal cramps and diarrhea which are stimulated by eating. This is a transient phenomenon, and a similar condition may occur after resection of an aneurysm when internal iliac flow is not restored and division of the inferior mesenteric artery produces functional ischemia but is not severe enough to cause actual necrosis. Similar symptoms due to progression of the basic occlusive disease may occur without operation. Furthermore, episodes of diarrhea and abdominal cramps may follow any operation, due to extreme ileus, minor adhesive band obstruction, or alteration of intestinal flora by antibiotics. Ileus is a commonly recognized complication of any major retroperitoneal dissection, and it not uncommonly follows lumbar sympathectomy. For all these reasons the more subtle forms of functional intestinal ischemia, or intestinal angina, are exceedingly difficult to recognize and prove in the patient operated upon for occlusive disease of the great vessels.

PERIPHERAL NEUROLOGICAL PROBLEMS

Postsympathectomy neuralgia, which is also discussed on page 123, is a distressing but not serious complication of lumbar sympathectomy, whether performed through the flank or through the aortoiliac exposure. It probably occurs to some degree in almost every patient, but in only a small percentage of patients does it demand attention. We have found no means of preventing this complication, or of predicting its occurrence, although it has seemed to be more severe in patients with diabetic neuritis or extensive arteriosclerosis involving both large and small arteries.

Reassurance and mild supportive analgesics are usually all the therapy needed. The use of diphenylhydantoin (Dilantin) and carbamazapine (Tegretol) has been advocated in severe cases.[46] Their effect is probably accomplished by reducing spiking activity in irritated nerve fibers.

One distressing complication in males is the occurrence of sexual impotence after extensive preaortic dissection. Extensive proximal sympathectomy is more likely to cause retrograde ejaculation than impotence. The difficulties in establishing the true etiology of these complications are matched only by the difficulty in treatment, which must lie in the realm of urological prostheses.

Ischemia of the spinal cord due to interference with the origins of the arteria radicularis magna are rare, but may occur unpredictably whenever high aortic dissections are carried out, even when the aorta is not resected.[26, 64, 70] Usubiaga and his associates have described a modification of the syndrome that involves functional transverse section of the cord or damage to the cauda equina.[64] They describe a softening of some of the prevertebral nerve plexuses that may occur as small arterial branches feeding the great nerve plexuses are damaged during prevertebral dissections, especially under regional anesthesia.

Lesser forms of neuritis in the region of the femoral or saphenous nerve may be seen due to operative pressures and trauma, and possibly to inadvertent desiccation.

VENOUS THROMBOSIS

A more hazardous complication of femoral artery surgery is the appearance of deep venous thrombosis. Factors other than those usually operative in the inception of venous thrombosis include local trauma to the femoral vein because of its intimate adherence to the femoral artery, and stagnation of flow in the deep venous system secondary to chronic arterial insufficiency. Acute obstruction of the arterial system during operation is well tolerated, however, especially when intra-arterial heparinization has been used in the distal tree.

Many patients who have extensive and advanced arterial occlusion enter hospital with marked dependent edema; deep venous thrombosis often exists also in these patients. Such patients, however, are not often suitable candidates for arterial reconstruction.

Another source of venous thrombosis is operative angiography; irritating contrast material may be ejected from the artery into the capillary and venous bed and remain there due to stagnant flow for relatively protracted periods. Stagnant flow may be aggravated by spasm in the artery which is induced by the irritating material. This situation may be ameliorated by flushing the system with large quantities of a dilute heparin solution as soon as the films have been taken.

Minor edema of the extremity is a frequent occurrence after successful femoral artery reconstruction. This has been ascribed simply to an increase in perfusion pressure in an endothelial system which has been rendered more permeable to fluids by chronic hypoxia and chronic hypotension. Others have attributed the edema that follows reconstruction to interference with lymphatics, particularly when dissection has been carried out on the course of the saphenous vein at the knee as well as in the groin.[44] It has even been recommended that the opposite saphenous vein be used so as to avoid this extra problem with dissection. Many of these patients show no other stigmata characteristic of venous thrombosis; Homans' sign is equivocal because of dissection in the popliteal space. Lowenberg's sign is applicable only with the cuff well below the area of dissection. Local distention of superficial veins may be a consequence of the effect of sympathectomy. Cyanosis is rarely demonstrable.

Lumbar sympathectomy may, in theory at least, also contribute to the development of deep venous thrombosis. Ablation of sympathetic tone tends to cause shunting of a greater proportion of the arterial input to the superficial vascular bed. It is conceivable that under special circumstances there is actual reduction in the flow through the deep system so that thrombosis is promoted in the susceptible deep veins.

It may not be necessary to use heparin in the presence of vein or Dacron grafts to protect against thrombosis in the reconstruction, but its use postoperatively may be effective in protecting against venous thrombosis.

Major venous thrombosis was encountered in at least 16 patients in the two series. The apparent greater incidence in the second series may be related to the inclusion of patients with more significant distal arterial disease in the occlusive group. This is suggested by the fact that although nine patients in the second series had venous thrombosis, six had had venous thrombosis diagnosed preoperatively, and of the six patients who had pulmonary embolism in the second series, three had had pulmonary embolism before operation.

Two patients in the first series and one in the second succumbed to pulmonary embolism.

The presence of a modest amount of edema is common after arterial reconstructions, especially if there has been interference with lymphatics. This is easily misdiagnosed as venous thrombosis. The use of radioactively tagged fibrinogen uptake studies[43] or phleborheology[4,14] are of help in elucidating the accurate diagnosis. There should be no hesitation in carefully wrapping legs if good peripheral arterial pressures have been restored, or in otherwise pursuing the appropriate therapy of deep venous thrombosis in the postoperative period. Heparin and Coumadin should be used if indicated. Appropriate indications for caval interruption should be chosen, but a prior dissection in the area of the great vessels may be an indication for use of the intracaval umbrella, placed through the jugular vein because of its simplicity.

POSTOPERATIVE ANEURYSM

Aneurysms in segments reconstructed by endarterectomy have occurred very infrequently. The long patch grafts on arterial closures are excluded in our discussion, although with time they may develop into aneurysms. Several patients have developed arterial aneurysms in association with sepsis. Most of these aneurysms ultimately rupture. One patient (in another series) developed an aneurysm in the iliac artery several months after operation; secondary contamination of a hydrarthrosis due to a penicillin reaction was the source of bacteremia which presumably found a nidus in the endarterectomized wall. Aggressive antibiotic therapy controlled the infection; the area remained dilated but stable for more than 6 years. Ultimately, the segment thrombosed and was treated by bypass grafting.

In another series, two patients at the Wadsworth Veterans Hospital in Los Angeles underwent femoral endarterectomy and subsequently manifested significant dilatation without any evidence of infection. One of these patients, who had a short dilated segment that was replaced with saphenous vein, was followed for 11 years; distal pulse is satsifactory and oscillometric readings are normal. During this time, however, he had developed contralateral femoral artery occlusion, cerebral thrombosis, and carcinoma of the tongue. One patient developed multiple aneurysms in a femoral endarterectomy and ultimately had to have all reconstructed segments ligated.

Aneurysms developing at the site of placement of arterial grafts have complicated cases. The following case reports are typical.

M.O., a 44-year-old woman, was subjected to a bypass procedure from the aorta to the common femoral artery; because of occlusion in very small iliac vessels, a Dacron prosthesis was used. The initial result was excellent, but 22 months later she was readmitted with a 5 cm. aneurysm at the site of attachment of the graft in the left femoral triangle. At reoperation, the aneurysm was found to be saccular and to arise from what appeared to be a defect in the wall of the artery just where the toe of the graft had been placed. The remaining wall was of good consistency and the defect was repaired with a patch of Dacron, which extended the toe of the graft. During the following 2 years, the superficial femoral artery has gradually become completely occluded. Serious cardiac disability precludes further operation for this occlusion. The aneurysm has not recurred.

F.W., a 69-year-old male, had had a Dacron graft placed from the left iliac origin to the left common femoral artery because of occlusion of the common iliac artery; grafting rather than endarterectomy was done because of the patient's age and the unusually tenuous arterial wall. The graft was placed using an end-to-end anastomosis proximally and an end-to-side anastomosis in the common femoral artery. There was a prompt restoration of pulses, but 1½ years after operation the superficial femoral artery became stenotic at the same time that an aneurysm developed at the site of anastomosis in the groin. Operation was performed elsewhere to replace the graft at the site of the aneurysm and to restore flow through the femoral artery, but shortly thereafter occlusion recurred and amputation had to be done.

Several factors probably contribute to the formation of aneurysms of the type described in patients M. O. and F. W. The first, infection, has already been discussed.

Second is the peculiar vulnerability of the site of anastomosis into a narrow vessel (Fig. 7–20). Stoney and his associates[57] note that there is a much higher incidence of false aneurysms in oblique graft to host anastomoses than in end-to-end graft to host anastomosis.

Stoney, Albo and Wylie[57] have attributed the formation of aneurysms in this site to the continuing working and tension of the graft at a site of flexion. Darling and Linton[17] have observed a greatly increased late failure rate when fabric grafts must be led from the abdomen as far as the fold of the groin, although Moore and his associates have brought forward strong evidence in favor of carrying the reconstruction across the groin if there is any question as to the adequacy of the anastomosis above the groin.[41] If classic small sutures, as originally advocated by Halsted, are used in the anastomosis, their grasp on the flexible arterial wall may be insufficient to hold the relatively rigid graft, which is placed under tension, and which by reason of its particular mechanical position is subjected to additional tension with flexion and extension. Larger sutures may be less desirable esthetically but will hold the graft more securely. Unfortunately, larger sutures may encroach on the "exit" angle of the anastomosis at its distal limit and produce extreme stenosis. A saphenous vein patch may be used as the means of widening this angle (Fig. 19–2). Lazzarini-Robertson[36] and Taylor[60] suggest use of a square-toed graft placed into a T-shaped incision as a means of preventing this development (Figs. 7–20 and 19–2).

Because they have not had consistently good results following ligation, replacement with additional Dacron, or further grafting, Stoney, Albo and Wylie[57] advocate a different method for treating aneurysms. They use an autologous artery to cross the flexion crease, replacing the donor artery with Dacron at a less vulnerable site. The donor artery is endarterectomized if necessary. Autologous saphenous vein may also be used if the vein is large enough.

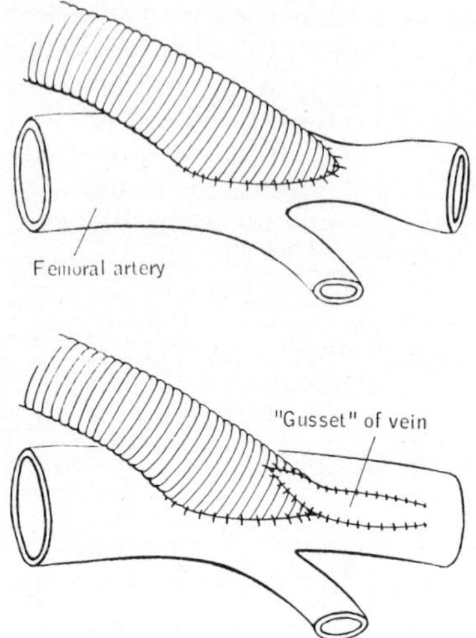

Figure 19–2. Stenosis at site of placement of plastic graft into the junction of the common and superficial femoral arteries. This developed some years after operation and was associated with a local plaque of atheroma. Lower sketch shows a "gusset" of vein placed as a patch to widen the area and continue down the artery as an onlay patch.

Gaspar[25] has suggested that the external iliac artery could be divided and the distal segment withdrawn under the inguinal ligament into the groin. The elastic fabric graft can then be pulled under extreme tension under the ligament also and the anastomosis performed end to end in the groin. On release of tension, the anastomosis will retract above the line of flexion (Fig. 19–3). An end-to-

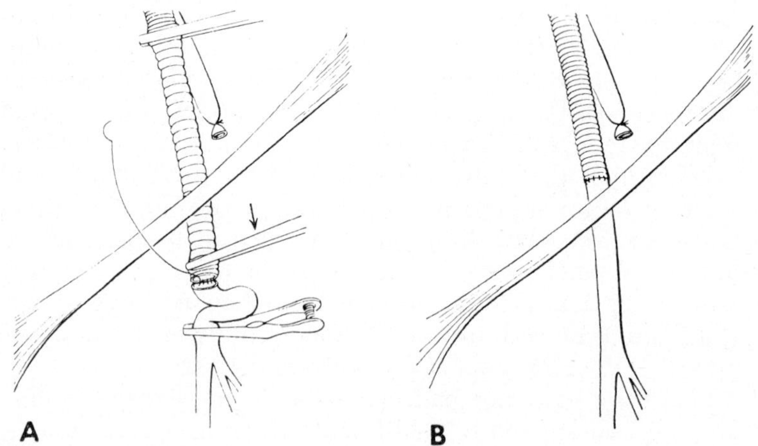

Figure 19–3. A, B, Gaspar's method of avoiding placement of a plastic graft that extends across the fold of the groin. End-to-end anastomosis is made below the ligament, by keeping the elastic graft under maximal tension during the procedure. When the anastomosis is completed and the clamps are removed, the suture line is drawn back up the ligament. The technical advantage is that the anastomosis can be performed in the relatively good exposure of the groin, rather than in the depth of the iliac fossa.

end anastomosis as described, however, does not allow for retrograde flow through the external system into the hypogastric outflow tract.

Another means of avoiding the hazards of avulsion at the toe of the graft is illustrated in Figure 19–4. A strip of Dacron is left at the toe of the graft, but this strip is folded up so as to form the anastomotic line at the toe with a cuff of Dacron. This strip, left untouched in the main suture line, is then tacked down to the adventitia of the femoral artery so as to secure the toe more adequately to the distal vessel.

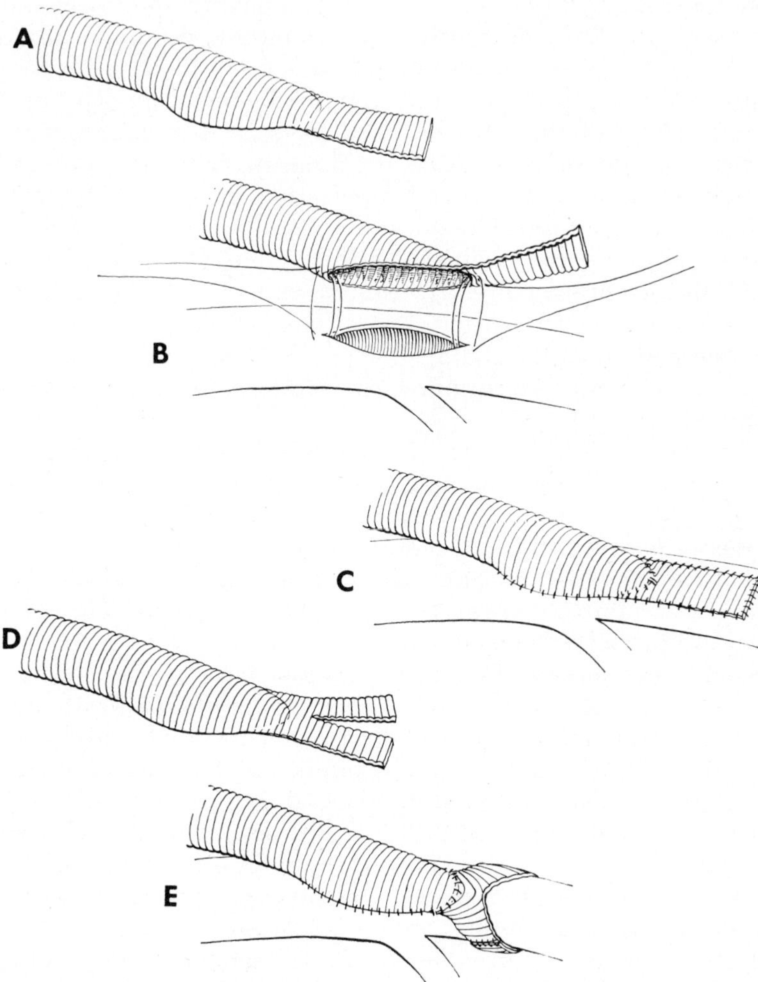

Figure 19–4. A, Plastic graft, in which plastic strip is left at toe. This strip is used to attach tubular graft more securely. B, Arteriotomy is shown as a split, but a T-shaped arteriotomy would be superior. C, Toe of graft as it might be attached to the top of the femoral artery. D, Toe of plastic graft is split so that the two arms can be wrapped around the artery, as in E.

The strip can be split and wrapped around the artery for more secure mechanical attachment, if desired. The sutures placed in the adventitia must be small enough not to encroach on the lumen of the vessel. Interrupted sutures are preferable to continuous sutures, because they eliminate the pursestring effect.

RENAL COMPLICATIONS

Acute renal failure is a grave problem, having both local and systemic origins, following aortic cross-clamping. Kountz[34] reviewed 1659 cases from 10 series, and found an over-all incidence of 3.8 per cent of renal complications with individual series reporting up to 20 per cent. Many of these cases must have been operations for aneurysms. The incidence of acute renal failure following aortic resection for aneurysm, and especially resection for ruptured aneurysm, remains relatively high. On the other hand, acute renal failure following operations for occlusive disease has been less frequent. Three episodes are recorded in the current series; one in a patient who had a bilateral renal artery bypass combined with aortic replacement; one patient suffered diffuse visceral embolizations; one patient died of acute renal failure following hemorrhage (see Table 10–7B, Patients 1, 5 and 6).

The presence of hypertensive vascular disease or renal disease (renovascular *or* parenchymatous), mismatching of transfused blood, episodes of hypotension, and the ill-advised and continuing use of vasopressor amines all seem definitely to contribute to the development of acute renal failure. These factors are applicable to all surgical operations, however, and the specific hazards of lower aortic surgery are probably mechanical.

Kountz has shown[33] that in dogs, cross-clamping the normal aorta below the renal vessels did not cause acute tubular necrosis, and Foster[23] has confirmed this finding in dogs and in monkeys. This procedure did result in a transient and often insignificant decrease in renal blood flow which was ascribed to an increase in sympathetic activity. This observation would agree with that of Powers,[45] who was able to produce a renal lesion by cross-clamping the infrarenal aorta and was able to protect the kidneys from damage by the use of a ganglionic blocking agent, trimethaphan camphor sulfonate (Arfonad).

Further, if there is sufficient renal ischemia, then infrarenal cross-clamping does produce acute tubular necrosis. The investigators found renal hypoxia due to hemorrhage and to renal vein obstruction to be most hazardous. Renal blood flow remained decreased for a prolonged time after blood loss from hemorrhage had been restored, presumably because of arteriolar vasoconstriction. Acute occlusion of the renal artery as a cause of renal ischemia was less serious than chronic renal ischemia of sufficient severity to cause hypertension.

The common practice of the use of either ethacrynic acid or furosemide often in combination with mannitol seems to have protected our series against unusual complications of acute failure.[21, 55, 56]

In humans, atheromatous microemboli have been described[61] and may play a role when cross-clamps are applied near the renal vessels. Probably there is more damage resulting from dislodgment of plaques or thrombotic debris in patients whose occlusion extends to near the renal level. Extraction of such atheromatous debris blindly from the area above the clamp as described on page 146 may be hazardous. Unnecessary manipulation of the upper aorta might fragment or dislodge a large plaque near the orifice of the renal vessels. One of our early reports described such an instance.[3]

W. F., a 45-year-old man, underwent aortoiliac endarterectomy for disease existing primarily at the common iliac level. At the conclusion of the procedure, the small bowel was pale and ischemic, and exploration of the orifice of the superior mesenteric artery showed an obstruction caused by a dislodged plaque. This was removed, and blood was successfully re-established. It was believed that flow into the renal arteries was normal, but 4 days later the patient died from bilateral renal artery occlusion. Both iliac arteries and the superior mesenteric artery were patent, but the renal arteries were occluded by a mixture of fresh clot and old atheromatous debris.

There is no recorded instance of operative injury to the ureter or bladder in the present series.

PULMONARY PROBLEMS

The presence of acute pulmonary insufficiency must have occurred in the earlier group of patients, but may well be hidden in the group described as non-proven myocardial infarcts. Blaisdell has indicated the frequency with which acute postoperative pulmonary insufficiency is incorrectly believed to be due to a myocardial infarction.[6]

The understanding of the management of pulmonary problems has greatly improved in the past ten years.[6, 47] The group of patients operated upon are often elderly and emphysematous; abdominal pain and distention often serve to seriously aggravate any ventilatory deficit.

Preliminary pulmonary preparation of the bad risk patient with postural drainage, expectorants, breathing exercises, and even preliminary antibiotic therapy may be justified. Above all, cessation of smoking is imperative. Planned tracheostomy may even be justified in some patients whose fixed rib cage places an even greater demand on abdominal respiration. This maneuver does indeed reduce upper respiratory dead space, but more than that it allows the use of inhalation therapy without so much likelihood of blowing extra gas by face mask into the gastrointestinal tract. A nasotracheal tube serves a similar purpose but may be very poorly tolerated by some patients. Any protracted endotracheal intubation, especially if a cuff is used to assure an airtight seal, is subject to tracheal erosion and stricture formation. These methods must be used with every precaution to minimize such a complication.

There is an increasing awareness of the frequency with which some degree of tracheal aspiration of gastric juice occurs. Gastric drainage of one form or another is almost mandatory until the patient is fully able to handle his own threatened aspiration—which may be several days. The use of a temporary gastrostomy is a quick, safe and comfortable way to assure prolonged gastric drainage. Either a large Foley or Malecot catheter or a plain (26–30 Fr.) tube can be inserted by the Witzel technique into the mid greater curvature of the stomach and led out through a separate stab wound. The stomach should be sutured to the abdominal wall.

Although these warnings and techniques do not apply so much to the patient who has incisions only in the groin or the legs, aspiration of gastric juice can occur in any patient under any anesthesia; direct nasogastric intubation should be used liberally as a precautionary measure.

Pulmonary embolism, which is of itself a complication of venous thrombosis, is a common and important complication of any surgical procedure. The age of the patients, the frequency of cardiac disorders, the magnitude of the operation, and, above all, the frequency with which peripheral ischemia and venous thrombosis coexist combine to make pulmonary embolism a true hazard. That it has not occurred more frequently in this series is possibly due to the common use of postoperative heparinization, or of one of the dextran solutions. For other reasons, low dose heparin has been in common use much as advocated for prophylaxis against venous thrombosis.[24, 31]

CARDIAC COMPLICATIONS

Myocardial complications are critical; the relative infrequency of their occurrence may be attributed to a conservative attitude in selection of candidates for operation. Myocardial infarction was recognized postoperatively in 11 patients and was fatal in six of these. An increased frequency of myocardial infarction was seen in the second series, again probably related to the inclusion of more poor risk patients for occlusive reconstructions. Late deaths from cardiac disease continue to be common following all forms of vascular reconstructions. This has been most remarkable in our hands in the reconstructions for carotid disease, which is not tabulated in this chapter. DeWeese and Rob have noted a similar high mortality following vein bypass operations for femoral atherosclerosis — a five year mortality rate of 48 per cent.[18]

UNCLASSIFIED COMPLICATIONS

Six patients in the first series have developed severe cerebrovascular arteriosclerosis. By the time the first edition of this book was published, three of these patients had had carotid endarterectomy, one had an endarterectomy of the innominate artery, and two had severe diffuse disease of small intracranial arteries. Two others had suffered cerebrovascular insults, dying of an embolus from mitral stenosis, or a mild stroke secondary to hemorrhage from congenital intracranial aneurysm. Since that time there continues to be an increased occurrence of cerebrovascular occlusive disease, which is being recognized in these patients in years after their reconstruction for peripheral vascular disease.

It had originally been recommended that patients with asymptomatic bruits in the carotid region be studied and be considered for extracranial carotid reconstructions if significant stenotic disease was identified. Treiman and his associates have suggested that cervical bruits are indeed not associated with cerebrovascular accidents in major operations.[63] Nonetheless, careful preoperative evaluation of a patient with carotid bruit is indicated. A bruit which can be proven by ocular plethysmography or by arteriography to be due to turbulence in the external carotid or subclavian system does not need further attention. If the lesion is symptomatic, or if it seems to represent a serious hemodynamic threat to the circulation, then it is likely that extracranial reconstruction should be carried out for a major reconstruction of any other part of the body. The criteria which may serve to identify the proper lesion are suggested below:

1. An insignificant stenosis on one side (greater than five square millimeters on cross section) probably needs no treatment.

2. Bilaterally marginally significant lesions probably do deserve at least one operation — on the carotid serving the dominant side of the brain.

3. A stenosis of critical diameter less than five square millimeters does usually demand endarterectomy.

Seven patients experienced postoperative serum hepatitis: in most the course was benign, but one patient developed acute hepatic necrosis, suffered a myocardial infarction, and died.

There appears to be an increasing incidence of hepatitis related to the use of banked blood. This poses a serious risk for the patient undergoing peripheral vascular reconstruction. One method to reduce this risk is the intraoperative collection and readministration of autologous blood, but Duncan has recently criticized this because of the occurrence of clotting defects in such patients.[19] A second method, which may be of more general utility, is the preoperative collection of one or more units of blood and the subsequent administration of this autologous blood during the performance of elective operation.[39]

Severe gastrointestinal hemorrhage occurred in four patients. In one case, it was due to a proved aortoduodenal fistula from a defect at the level of take-off of an aortofemoral bypass prosthesis that occurred 3½ years after the original operation. The defect was successfully repaired elsewhere. Another patient developed bleeding from a Dacron graft that eroded into a loop of small intestine. A third patient died of gastrointestinal hemorrhage 16 months after operation. Autopsy was not done, and the site of bleeding remains in doubt. A fourth patient hemorrhaged fatally 3 weeks after operation. At autopsy no lesion or site could be identified as the source of bleeding.

The occurrence of a classical acute duodenal ulcer should be distinguished from superficial stress ulcerations. Bouhoutsos, Barabas and Martin have indicated the frequent concomitant ulcer and aneurysmal disease.[7]

Pancreatitis as a nonspecific complication is a difficult diagnosis in the presence of anticipated abdominal pain and protracted ileus. In one instance, acute pancreatitis was associated with such dramatic fibrinolysis that active bleeding through a knitted prosthesis occurred a week after operation.

Dehiscence and evisceration represent complications that should ordinarily be considered preventable. The combination of pulmonary problems, protracted ileus, long vertical wounds, and occasional wound hematomas make dehiscence a special hazard and for that reason sutures are advocated as part of the routine closure.

Postoperative intestinal obstruction due to adhesions is a hazard of any intraabdominal operation, but prolonged evisceration and congestion seem unusually likely to produce such adhesions. The prolonged ileus that at times follows major abdominal arterial operations may merge with obstruction with fibrinous bands but usually deserves conservative management.

It has appeared to us that the patients operated upon for aneurysm have had more severe cardiovascular and cerebrovascular disease, but this may be a peculiarity of selection. We have rejected few patients with aneurysm, but many patients have been denied operation for occlusive disease on the basis of associated cardiovascular or cerebrovascular disease.

Complications of arterial surgery do remain a serious problem but improvements in patient selection and in surgical technique are helping to reduce the number of complications. In this respect, Dr. Jack Cannon's comment[11] justifies repetition:

"It is now quite apparent that when patients are carefully selected for operation, and when the procedure is gently, carefully and meticulously performed, excellent results can be anticipated. It must be remembered, however, that there is little leeway for error since disaster is near at hand until the wounds are well healed."

REFERENCES

1. Barker, W. F.: Distal operative angiography as an aid in endarterectomy. Surgery 36:233, 1954.
2. Barker, W. F.: Management of complications of vascular repair. *In* Dale, W. A.: Management of Arterial Occlusive Disease. Chicago, Year Book Medical Publishers, Inc., 1971.
3. Barker, W. F., and Cannon, J. A.: An evaluation of endarterectomy. Arch. Surg. 66:488, 1953.
4. Barnes, R. W., Collicott, P. E., Mozersky, D. J., Summer, D. S., and Strandness, D. E. Jr.: Noninvasive quantitation of maximum venous outflow in acute thrombophlebitis. Surgery 72:971, 1972.
5. Blaisdell, F. W., and Hall, A. D.: Axillary-femoral artery bypass for lower extremity ischemia. Surgery 54:563, 1963.
6. Blaisdell, F. W., and Schlobohm, R. M.: The respiratory distress syndrome: a review. Surgery 74:251, 1973.
7. Bouhoutsos, J., Barabas, A., and Martin, P.: The association of peptic ulcer and abdominal aortic aneurysm and its significance. Brit. J. Surg. 60:302, 1973.
8. Bricker, D. L., Beall, A. C., Jr., and DeBakey, M. E.: The differential response to infection of autogenous vein versus Dacron arterial prostheses. Chest 58:566, 1970.
9. Burke, J. F.: The effective period of preventive antibiotic action in experimental incisions and dermal lesions. Surgery 50:161, 1961.
10. Cannon, J. A.: Personal communication.
11. Cannon, J. A., Kawakami, I. G., and Barker, W. F.: The present status of aortoiliac endarterectomy for obliterative atherosclerosis. Arch. Surg. 82:813, 1961.
12. Cannon, J. A., Van de Water, J., and Barker, W. F.: Experience with the surgical management of 100 consecutive cases of abdominal aortic aneurysm. Am. J. Surg. 106:128, 1963.
13. Carter, S. C., Cohen, A., and Whelan, T. J.: Clinical experience with management of the infected dacron graft. Ann. Surg. 158:249, 1963.
14. Cranley, J. J., in discussion of Barnes, R. W., Collicott, P. E., Mozersky, D. J., Summer, D. S., and Strandness, D. E. Jr.: Noninvasive quantitation of maximum venous outflow in acute thrombophlebitis. Surgery 72:971, 1972.
15. Cranley, J. J., Fogarty, T. J., Krause, R. J., Strasser, E. S., and Hafner, C. D.: Phlebotomy for moderate erythrocytemia. J.A.M.A. 186:206, 1963.

16. Crawford, E. S., and DeBakey, M. E.: The retrograde flush procedure in embolectomy and thrombectomy. Surgery *40*:737, 1956.
17. Darling, R. C., and Linton, R. R.: Management of the late failure of arterial reconstruction of the lower extremities. New Eng. J. Med. *270*:609, 1964.
18. DeWeese, J. A., and Rob, C. G.: Autogenous venous bypass grafts five years later. Ann. Surg. *174*:346, 1971.
19. Duncan, S. E., Edwards, W. H., and Dale, W. A.: Caution regarding autotransfusion. Surg. Vol. 76, Dec. 1974.
20. Dye, W. S., Olwin, J., Javid, H., and Julian, O. C.: Arterial embolectomy. Arch. Surg. *70*:720, 1955.
21. Eng, K., and Stahl, W. M.: Correction of the renal hemodynamic changes produced by surgical trauma. Ann. Surg. *174*:19, 1971.
22. Fogarty, T. J., Cranley, J. J., Krause, R. J., Strasser, F. S., and Hafner, C. D.: A method for extraction of arterial emboli and thrombi. Surg. Gynec. Obstet. *116*:241, 1963.
23. Foster, J. H., Adkins, R. B., Chamberlain, N. O., Symbas, P. N., and Harris, A. P.: The renal effects of lower abdominal aortic cross-clamping, Report of negative results in dogs and monkeys. J.A.M.A. *183*:451, 1963.
24. Gallus, A. S., Hirsh, J., Tuttle, R. J., Trebilcock, R., O'Brien, S. E., Carroll, J. J., Minden, J. H., and Hudecki, S. M.: Small subcutaneous doses of heparin in prevention of venous thrombosis. N. Eng. J. Med. *288*:545, 1973.
25. Gaspar, M.: Discussion of paper by Stoney, R. J., Albo, R. J., and Wylie, E. J.: False aneurysms after arterial grafting. Am. J. Surg. *110*:153, 1965.
26. Golden, G. T., Sears, H. F., Wellons, H. A., and Muller, W. H., Jr.: Paraplegia complicating resection of aneurysms of the infrarenal abdominal aorta. Surgery *73*:91, 1973.
27. Goldsmith, S., and Beattie, E. J., Jr.: Carotid artery protection by pedicled omental wrapping. Surg. Gynec. Obstet. *130*:57, 1970.
28. Gryska, P. F.: The development of atheroma in arteries subjected to experimental thromboendarterectomy. Surgery *45*:655, 1959.
29. Howard, J. M., et al.: Postoperative wound infections. The influence of ultraviolet irradiation of the operating room and of the various other factors. Ann. Surg. (Supplement) *160*:1, 1964.
30. Humphries, A. W., Young, J. R., DeWolfe, V. G., and LeFevre, R. A.: Complications of abdominal aortic surgery. I. Aortoenteric fistula. Arch. Surg. 86:43, 1963.
31. Kakkar, V. V., Corrigan, T., Spindler, J., Fossard, D. P., Flute, P. T., Crellin, R. Q., Wessler, S., and Yin, E. T.: Efficacy of low doses of heparin in prevention of deep vein thrombosis after major surgery: a double blind, randomised trial. Lancet 2:101, 1972.
32. Kirkpatrick, J. R., and Miller, D. R.: Effects of decreased arterial inflow and runoff on vein graft patency. Surgery 69:870, 1971
33. Kountz, S. L., and Cohn, R.: Aortic blood flow following lower aortic resection and sympathectomy. Surgery 53:173, 1963.
34. Kountz, S. L., Tuttle, K. L., Cohn, L. H., Eschelman, L. T., and Cohn, R.: Factors responsible for acute tubular necrosis following lower aortic surgery. J.A.M.A. *183*:447, 1963.
35. Lavenson, G. S., Rich, N. C., and Strandness, D. E.: Ultrasonic flow detector value in combat vascular injuries. Arch. Surg. *103*:644, 1971.
36. Lazzarini-Robertson, A. A., Jr.: Hemodynamic principles and end-to-side vascular anastomoses. Arch. Surg. 82:384, 1961.
37. Ledgerwood, A. M., and Lucas, C. E.: Massive thigh injuries with vascular disruption. Role of porcine skin grafting of exposed arterial vein grafts. Arch. Surg. *107*:201, 1973.
38. Louw, J. H.: The treatment of combined aortoiliac and femoropopliteal occlusive disease by splenofemoral and axillofemoral bypass grafts. Surgery 55:387, 1964.
39. McKittrick, J. E.: Banked autologous blood in elective surgery. Amer. J. Surg. *128*:137, 1974.

40. Moncrief, J. A., Darin, J. C., Canizaro, P. C., and Sawyer, R. B.: Use of dextran to prevent arterial and venous thrombosis. Ann. Surg. *158*:553, 1963.
41. Moore, W. S., Cafferata, H. T., Hall, A. D., and Blaisdell, F. W.: In defense of grafts across the inguinal ligament: an evaluation of early and late results of aorto-femoral bypass grafts. Ann. Surg. *168*:207, 1968.
42. Pilcher, D. B., and Barker, W. F.: Retardation of experimental atherosclerosis in endarterectomized arteries by the administration of heparin and dextran. Amer. J. Surg. *120*:270–274, 1970.
43. Pollak, E. W., Webber, M. M., Barker, W. F., Victery, W., Cragin, M., and Witt, W.: Autologous ^{125}I labeled fibrinogen uptake test in the management of venous thrombosis. A prospective study. Arch. Surg. *109*:48, 1974.
44. Porter, J. M., Lindell, T. D., and Lakin, P. C.: Leg edema following femoral popliteal autogenous vein bypass. Arch. Surg. *105*:883, 1972.
45. Powers, S. R., Jr., Boba, A., and Stein, A.: The mechanism and prevention of distal tubular necrosis following aneurysmectomy. Surgery *42*:156, 1957.
46. Raskin, N. H., Levinson, S. A., Hoffman, P. M., Pickett, J. B. E., III, Fields, H. L.: Postsympathectomy neuralgia. Amelioration with diphenylhydantoin and carbamazepine. Amer. Jr. Surg. *128*:75, 1974.
47. Reul, G. J., Jr., Greenberg, D. S., Lefrak, E. A., McCollum, W. B., Beall, A. C. Jr., and Jordan, G. L. Jr., Prevention of post-traumatic pulmonary insufficiency: fine screen filtration of blood. Arch Surg. *106*:386, 1973.
48. Rhodes, G. R., Dixon, R. H., and Silver, D.: Heparin induced thrombocytopenia with thrombotic and hemorrhagic manifestations. Surg. Gynec. Obstet. *136*:409, 1973.
49. Salzman, E. W.: The limitations of heparin therapy after arterial reconstruction. Surgery 57:131, 1965.
50. Scott, H. W., Barker, W. F., Cannon, J. A., Rob, C. G., and Whelan, T. G.: Management of infected wounds and grafts. *In* Dale, W. A. (Ed.): Management of Arterial Occlusive Disease. Chicago, Ill. Year Book Medical Publishers, Inc., 1971.
51. Scott, H. W., Morgan, C. V., Bolasny, B. L., Lanier, V. C., Younger, K., and Butts, W.: Experimental atherosclerosis in autogenous venous grafts. Arch. Surg. *101*:677, 1970.
52. Sharf, A. G., and Acker, E. D.: The outflow tract of the lower extremity. Western J. Surg. *68*:312, 1960.
53. Shaw, R. S., and Baue, A. E.: Management of sepsis complicating arterial reconstructive surgery. Surgery *53*:75, 1963.
54. Sproul, G.: Rupture of an infected aortic graft into jejunum: resection and survival. J.A.M.A. *182*:1118, 1962.
55. Stahl, W. M., and Stone, A. M.: Prophylactic diuresis with ethacrynic acid for prevention of postoperative renal failure. Ann. Surg. *172*:361, 1970.
56. Stone, A. M., and Stahl, W. M.: Effect of ethacrynic acid and furosemide on renal function in hypovolemia. Ann. Surg. *174*:1, 1971.
57. Stoney, R. J., Albo, R. J., and Wylie, E. J.: False aneurysm after arterial grafting. Am. J. Surg. *110*:153, 1965.
58. Szilagyi, D. E., Smith, R. F., Elliott, J. P., and Vrandecic, M. T.: Infection in arterial reconstruction with synthetic grafts. Ann. Surg. *176*:321, 1972.
59. Tarizzo, R. A., Alexander, R. W., Beattie, E. J. Jr., and Economou, S. G.: Atherosclerosis in synthetic vascular grafts. Arch. Surg. *82*:826, 1961.
60. Taylor, G. W.: Personal communication.
61. Thurlbeck, W. M., and Castleman, B.: Atheromatous emboli to the kidneys after aortic surgery. New Eng. J. Med. *257*:442, 1958.
62. Tishcoff, G. H.: Personal communication.
63. Treiman, R. L., Foran, R. F., Shore, E. H., and Levin, P.: Carotid bruit. Significance in patients undergoing an abdominal aortic operation. Arch. Surg. *106*:803, 1973.
64. Usubiaga, J. E., Kolodny, J., and Usubiaga, L. E.: Neurological complications of prevertebral surgery under regional anesthesia. Surgery 68:304, 1970.
65. Van de Water, J. M., and Gaal, P. G.: Management of patients with infected vascular prostheses. Amer. Surg. *31*:651, 1965.

66. Wylie, E. J.: Discussion of paper by Krippaehne, W. W., Hunt, T. K., Jackson, D. S., and Dunphy, J. E.: Studies on the effect of stress on transplants of autologous and homologous connective tissue. Am. J. Surg. *104*:267, 1962.
67. Wylie, E. J.: Vascular replacement with arterial autografts. Surgery *57*:14, 1965.
68. Wylie, E. J., and Goldman, L.: The role of aortography in the determination of operability in arteriosclerosis of the lower extremities. Ann. Surg. *148*:325, 1958.
69. Young, J. R., Humphries, A. W., DeWolfe, V. G., and LeFevre, F. A.: Complications of abdominal aortic surgery. II. Intestinal ischemia. Arch. Surg. *86*:51, 1963.
70. Zuber, W. F., Gaspar, M. R., Rothschild, P. D.: The anterior spinal artery syndrome—a complication of abdominal aortic surgery. Ann. Surg. *72*:909, 1970.